Study Guide for Medical-Surgical Nursing
Concepts for Interprofessional Collaborative Care

Tenth Edition

Donna D. Ignatavicius,
MS, RN, CNE, CNEcl, ANEF
Speaker and Nursing Education
Consultant;
Founder, Boot Camp for Nurse
Educators;
President, DI Associates, Inc.
Littleton, Colorado

Cherie R. Rebar,
PhD, MBA, RN, COI
Subject Matter Expert and Nursing
Education Consultant
Beavercreek, Ohio;
Professor of Nursing
Wittenberg University
Springfield, Ohio

M. Linda Workman, PhD, RN, FAAN
Visiting Professor, Frances Payne
Bolton
 School of Nursing, Case Western
 Reserve University, Cleveland, Ohio
Author and Consultant
 Cincinnati, Ohio

Nicole M. Heimgartner,
DNP, RN, COI
Subject Matter Expert and Nursing
Education Consultant
Louisville, Kentucky;
Adjunct Faculty
American Sentinel University
Aurora, Colorado

Guide prepared by

Linda A. LaCharity, PhD, RN
Retired Accelerated Program Director
and Assistant Professor
College of Nursing
University of Cincinnati
Cincinnati, Ohio

M. Linda Workman, PhD, RN, FAAN
Visiting Professor, Frances Payne Bolton
 School of Nursing, Case Western
 Reserve University, Cleveland, Ohio
Author and Consultant
 Cincinnati, Ohio

Contributors

Donna D. Ignatavicius, MS, RN, CNE,
CNEcl, ANEF
Speaker and Nursing Education
Consultant;
Founder, Boot Camp for Nurse
Educators;
President, DI Associates, Inc.
Littleton, Colorado

Linda Anne Silvestri, PhD, RN, FAAN
Nursing Instructor, University of
Nevada, Las Vegas
Las Vegas, Nevada
President, Nursing Reviews, Inc. and
Professional Nursing Seminars, Inc.,
Henderson, Nevada
Next Generation NCLEX® (NGN)
Thought Leader,
Elsevier, Inc.

Elsevier
3251 Riverport Lane
St. Louis, Missouri 63043

STUDY GUIDE FOR MEDICAL-SURGICAL NURSING, TENTH EDITION   ISBN: 978-0-323-68147-6

Previous editions copyrighted 2018, 2016, 2013, 2010, 2006, 1999, 1995, and 1991

Library of Congress Control Number: 2020940755

Executive Content Strategist: Lee Henderson
Content Development Specialist: Laura Goodrich
Publishing Services Manager: Deepthi Unni
Project Manager: Radjan Lourde Selvanadin

Printed in the United States of America

Last digit is the print number: 9 8 7 6 5 4 3 2

Working together
to grow libraries in
developing countries

ELSEVIER   Book Aid International

www.elsevier.com • www.bookaid.org

Preface

The *Study Guide for Medical-Surgical Nursing: Concepts for Interprofessional Collaborative Care,* 10th Edition, is a companion publication for Ignatavicius, Workman, Rebar, and Heimgartner's *Medical-Surgical Nursing: Patient-Centered Collaborative Care,* 10th Edition. This Study Guide, written by experts in the fields of adult medical-surgical nursing and nursing education, will help to ensure mastery of the textbook content and help you learn about collaborative practice in the care of the adult medical-surgical patient.

The 10th Edition has been carefully revised and updated for an increased emphasis on utilization of clinical judgment skills.

The overall organization of the *Study Guide for Medical-Surgical Nursing: Concepts for Interprofessional Collaborative Care* directly corresponds to the unit/chapter name and number in the textbook so that you or your instructor can readily select the corresponding learning exercises in the Study Guide. Chapters are focused on

- **Study/Review Questions** that are designed to encourage prioritizing, use clinical judgment, participate in interprofessional collaboration, and apply of the steps of the nursing process. Questions have been updated to focus on the question formats of the NCLEX examination including next generation testing, and emphasize the NCLEX priorities of safety, patient-centered care, and evidence-based practice.

Answers and rationales to the Study/Review Questions are provided at the ends of each chapter of the Study Guide.

The *Study Guide for Medical-Surgical Nursing: Concepts for Interprofessional Collaborative Care* is a practical tool to help you prepare for classroom examinations and standardized tests as well serve as a review for clinical practice. This improved format will help you review and apply medical-surgical content and help you prepare for the NCLEX Examination.

In addition to answering NCLEX®-style test items to prepare for the nursing licensure examination, students have the opportunity to practice answering new item types that will be part of the Next-Generation NCLEX® (NGN). These new items are integrated into 10 unfolding case studies to help students develop the six cognitive skills of the National Council of State Boards of Nursing Clinical Judgment Measurement Model (NCJMM). Beginning as early as 2023, the new NGN item types will be part of the nursing licensure examination.

Contents

Unit XIII: Interprofessional Collaboration for Patients with Problems of the Endocrine System

Unit XIV: Interprofessional Collaboration for Patients with Problems of the Renal/Urinary System

Unit XV: Interprofessional Collaboration for Patients with Problems of the Reproductive System

1 CHAPTER

Overview of Professional Nursing Concepts for Medical-Surgical Nursing

1. Which nursing actions performed for a client are most consistent with the attributes of patient-centered care? **Select all that apply.**
   A. Asking the client's visitor to explain his or her relationship to the client
   B. Ensuring the client's side rails are in the up position whenever the client is in bed
   C. Asking the health care provider to prescribe the daily vitamin C the client takes at home
   D. Coaxing the client to take a prescribed medication that the client says makes him or her vomit
   E. Assigning a nursing assistant rather than a licensed practical nurse or vocational nurse LPN/LVN to give the client a back rub
   F. Ensuring the presence of a professional interpreter when providing discharge instructions to the client and family whose English is poor

2. Which nursing action is the best example of patient-centered care?
   A. Determining the family's thoughts and fears when asking them to consider a do-not-resuscitate option
   B. Using two separate identifiers when administering medication to prevent a "wrong-patient" error
   C. Ensuring medications are administered within 15 minutes of their prescribed schedule
   D. Using sterile technique when inserting a urinary catheter

3. Which nursing action supports patient-centered care for a fearful client about to have a colonoscopy who refuses to be sedated until the family pastor can pray with him before the procedure?
   A. Offering to pray with the client
   B. Calling the hospital-based chaplain to intervene
   C. Moving the client's procedure time until after his pastor arrives
   D. Explaining that delaying the procedure will disrupt agency efficiency

4. Which response by a nurse to a client's fear that his wide bed with traction equipment might prevent him from being moved to safety if a fire occurred on the unit demonstrates the most respect for the client's concerns?
   A. This room is equipped with an automatic sprinkler system that will quickly put out a fire.
   B. We would disconnect your traction, lift you to the floor with a sheet, and pull you to a safe area.
   C. Your fears are groundless because this is a brand new building made of fire-resistant materials.
   D. The fire department is less than 1 mile away and has a practiced response time to this facility of under 2 minutes.

5. Which professional nursing concepts are exemplified in an interaction in which a nurse at a rehabilitation center is working with a client who is Muslim and a registered dietitian nutritionist to honor the client's request for a Halal-restricted diet? **Select all that apply.**
   A. Autonomy
   B. Evidence-based practice
   C. Clinical judgement
   D. Patient-centered care
   E. Quality improvement
   F. Systems thinking
   G. Teamwork and collaboration
   H. Safety

6. The Emergency Department nurse is admitting a 58-year-old client with atypical chest pain. Which actions would the nurse delegate to the experienced AP? **Select all that apply.**
   A. Label and place the client's belongings in a plastic bag
   B. Insert a saline lock and draw blood samples for lab
   C. Check admission vital signs and record
   D. Complete a 12-lead ECG for the client
   E. Assess the client's level of chest pain
   F. Place the client on a continuous cardiac monitor
   G. Assist the client to use the bathroom
   H. Use pulse oximetry to check the client's oxygen saturation

7. The nurse is administering the client's 9 a.m. medications when the client, who was admitted at 4 a.m. and has asthma, asks why he is not receiving his inhaled corticosteroid. Which process would the nurse use to assure that the client receives the medications he was taking at home while he is hospitalized?
   A. Systems thinking
   B. Clinical judgment
   C. Medication reconciliation
   D. Teamwork collaboration

8. Which of the following are cognitive skills of Clinical Judgment that are recognized by the National Council of State Boards of Nursing (NCSBN)? **Select all that apply.**
   A. Recognizes cues
   B. Assesses clients
   C. Analyzes cues
   D. Prioritizes hypotheses
   E. Plans and implements actions
   F. Generate solutions
   G. Take action
   H. Evaluate outcomes

9. Which principle of ethics is violated most when a nurse fails to readminister pain medication to a client with advanced cancer within the next hour as was promised?
   A. Autonomy
   B. Beneficence
   C. Fidelity
   D. Veracity

10. When using the Situation, Background, Assessment, Recommendation (SBAR) method of communicating a client's condition, the nurse would include which information in the background section?
   A. Request fingerstick glucose monitoring.
   B. Patient states that he feels dizzy and lightheaded.
   C. Admission diagnosis is new-onset type 2 diabetes.
   D. Blood pressure is 130/90 mm Hg; heart rate is 89 beats per minute.

11. Which information communicated by a nurse handing-off a client from the intensive care unit (ICU) to a receiving nurse in the step-down unit is **most relevant** to continuity of care in this transition?
   A. Informing the receiving nurse that the client's family has not yet visited today
   B. Reporting that the client's blood pressure usually rises when coffee is ingested
   C. Describing the client's successful progression from NPO status to that of a regular diet
   D. Explaining that the client's right ear is deaf and she hears only when the speaker is on the left.

12. The nurse is providing care for four clients. Which best provides an example of the clinical judgment term failure to rescue (FTR)?
    A. The client with a respiratory problem expresses interest in smoking cessation but the nurse waits to put in a consult until the next day.
    B. The client with pneumonia develops a fever of 101.9°F (38.8°C) and the nurse does not notify the health care provider.
    C. The client with chest pain develops pain while ambulating in the hall; the nurse immediately has the client sit down, checks HR and blood pressure, then notifies the health care provider.
    D. The client with altered level of consciousness experiences a fall when trying to go to the bathroom alone and the nurse first assesses the patient, then reports the incident.

13. Which nursing activity most closely demonstrates the concept of telenursing?
    A. Completing an online distance learning course toward earning a bachelor of science in nursing (BSN) degree
    B. Directing clients to proven factual internet sites for a variety of resources to learn more about their newly diagnosed diabetes
    C. Using a cell phone camera to directly observe a client while he or she is actually taking prescribed medication for tuberculosis therapy
    D. Teaching a client who cannot speak because of the presence of an endotracheal tube how to communicate pain level using a computer picture board

Chapter 1 Answer Key

1. **C, F**
   Options B and E are standard nursing care actions and do not take into consideration the client's preferences, values, and needs. Option A is a violation of the client's privacy. Option D is a violation of the client's autonomy. Only options C and F are client-specific and take into consideration his or her preferences (C), values, and needs (F).

2. **A**
   Although safety is always a priority when providing care, patient-centered care specifically takes into consideration and respects the patient and family's preferences, values, and needs.

3. **C**
   The concern about agency efficiency is agency-centered, not patient-centered. Offering to pray with the client and/or having the agency's chaplain is a reasonable suggestion if the client's own pastor cannot be there; however, the most patient-centered option is changing the client's procedure time to allow him to pray with his own pastor.

4. **B**
   Although the sprinkler system, fire department response time, and fire-resistant building materials may provide some reassurance of security, only response B, which explains exactly how moving him to safety would be accomplished, shows respect for his concerns. Telling him his personal fears are groundless should never occur.

5. **A, D, G**
   By working with both the client and a registered dietitian nutritionist, the nurse is using teamwork and collaboration. The honoring of the client's request not only demonstrates patient-centered care but also allows the client to help self-manage his or her diet. This interaction does not demonstrate evidence-based practice, quality improvement, systems thinking, clinical judgment, or physical safety.

6. **A, C, D, F, G, H**
   Invasive procedures (e.g. saline locks, venipuncture) require additional training and are beyond the scope of practice for a AP. Assessment also

requires additional skill and education at the professional nurse level. An AP's scope of practice includes assistance with activities of daily living (ADL), checking and recording vital signs, ambulation, and feeding. An experienced AP could receive extra training for skills specific to the ED (e.g. ECG, placement of monitor leads) and then be delegated those actions. However, the RN would be responsible for supervising and assuring that the AP possesses these skills before delegating these actions.

7. C

Medication reconciliation is a formal process in which a client's actual current medications are compared to his or her medications during a care transition such as facility admission, transfer, or discharge.

8. A, C, D, F, G, H

The NCSBN recognizes six cognitive skills of clinical judgment that can be measured and serve as a basis for the new types of test items on the NCLEX national nursing licensure examination. The skills include recognizes cues, analyzes cues, prioritizes hypotheses, generates solutions, takes action, and evaluates outcomes. Responses B and E are from Tanner's model of clinical judgment.

9. C

Nearly all the ethical principles listed are violated to some degree when the nurse fails to follow-through with an action that was promised; however, fidelity is most violated in this situation. Fidelity is the ethical principle in which the nurse always follows through with their obligations to clients or their promises in order to ensure quality care that is patient-centered. It is related to veracity, which is the obligation to be truthful.

10. C

The only background information presented is the admission diagnosis. Option B is the current situation, option D is assessment findings, and option A is a recommendation.

11. D.

Any client problem that interferes with his or her ability to comprehend or communicate successfully has the potential to affect safety. Clearly communicating this client's hearing problem will contribute more to the continuity of care in the transition to a new unit more than knowing that the client's family has not yet been in today or that the client is now eating a regular diet. Knowing that coffee raises the client's blood pressure (and we don't know by how much) is less relevant to continuity of care than is the hearing problem.

12. B.

FTR is the inability of a nurse or other health care team member to save a client's life in a timely manner when a health care issue or medical complication occurs. Clients often have changes in signs and symptoms that are subtle. Failure to recognize those changes or to accurately interpret them leads to actions which may improve the client's condition not being implemented (FTR).

13. C

Telenursing, similar to telehealth, uses technology in the care of clients at a distance in order to monitor changes in condition or ensure the correct performance of specific therapies. Completing a BSN online does not involve a client. Directing clients to factual and legitimate internet information sites may or may not result in the client actually using the sites and is not limited to clients at a distance. Teaching a client how to use a computer to communicate with a picture board is again, not providing care at a distance.

2
CHAPTER

Clinical Judgment and Systems Thinking

1. Which type of health factor is best described when a client tells the nurse that she believes health is important and that people should be willing to take steps to maintain their health such as getting annual flu shots?
   A. Evidence-based methods to reduce health inequities
   B. Policy and health care reform
   C. Emerging new technologies
   D. Behavioral social determinants of health

2. Which QSEN competency is best demonstrated when the nurse places a bed alarm on the bed of a client with mental status changes?
   A. Patient-centered care
   B. Safety
   C. Evidence-based practice
   D. Teamwork and collaboration

3. Which process best describes the nurse's actions when his or her assessment reveals an oral temperature of 102.2°F (39°C) and new crackles in all lobes of the lungs, and then notifies the health care provider of these findings?
   A. Clinical reasoning
   B. Clinical judgment
   C. Critical thinking
   D. Patient-centered care

4. The nurse admits a client with COPD to the medical care unit and during initial assessment discovers these findings. Which data are relevant and directly related to client outcomes or priority of care for this client? **Select all that apply.**
   A. Client describes shortness of breath when climbing stairs
   B. Client tells the nurse that he had his gall bladder removed a year ago
   C. Client's medications include an albuterol inhaler which he uses as needed
   D. Client states that his health care provider (HCP) may prescribe home oxygen
   E. Client's daughter is pregnant with her fourth child
   F. Client's wife still smokes a pack of cigarettes every day
   G. Client's pulse oximetry reading is 89%
   H. Client has crackles and wheezes bilaterally in lungs

5. Using clinical judgment, which actions will the nurse take for a client with COPD admitted to the medical care unit? **Select all that apply.**
   A. Preparing the client for the possibility of a tracheostomy
   B. Monitoring for changes in respiratory status
   C. Applying oxygen as prescribed by the health care provider
   D. Elevating the head of the client's bed to a position of comfort
   E. Teaching the client to perform effective coughing to eliminate excess mucus
   F. Administering acetaminophen 650 mg every 8 hours to prevent fever
   G. Instructing the client how to use metered-dose inhalers
   H. Performing airway suctioning every 3 to 4 hours on a regular schedule

6. At an office visit for an annual check-up, the client tells the nurse and HCP about increased shortness of breath and occasional chest discomfort when performing yard work; the HCP makes a referral to a cardiologist. Which term best describes this situation?
    A.   Primary health care
    B.   Inpatient care
    C.   Community health care
    D.   Managed health care

7. Which of these are examples of types of long-term care services? **Select all that apply.**
    A.   Nursing care
    B.   Rehabilitation care
    C.   Mental health
    D.   Hospice services
    E.   Dementia care
    F.   Respite care
    G.   Home health care
    H.   End-of-life care

8. Which statement is **specific** to the role of nurse practitioners?
    A.   Focus on identification of the cause of health problems
    B.   Educated and practice according to a medical model
    C.   Involved in direct care of clients throughout the health care system
    D.   Emphasizes patient-centered care that involves promotion of health and wellness

9. The critical care nurse is providing care for a client who is intubated, and wants to prevent ventilator-associated pneumonia (VAP). What actions will the nurse take to facilitate the progression from clinical judgment (frequent oral care) to systematic change in this critical care unit? **Select all that apply.**
    A.   Place a sign over the client's bed reminding other nurses about oral care.
    B.   Provide a unit educational unit covering the research and the results.
    C.   Make copies of the research and results available to the nurses on the unit.
    D.   Instruct all nurses providing care for this client to provide suction every 2 hours.
    E.   Remind the nurses taking responsibility of the client's care about oral care.
    F.   Teach all nurses to lower the head of the bed and provide oral suction before each position change.

10. What is the goal of systems thinking for nursing when moving from clinical judgment to systems thinking?
    A.   To recognize cues, generate hypotheses, take actions, and evaluate outcomes
    B.   To use logic and reasoning to identify the strengths and weaknesses of alternative health care solutions, conclusions, or approaches to clinical problems
    C.   To encourage the nurse to develop awareness of the interrelationships that exist between individual care and the context of health care safety and quality
    D.   To collect cues, process the information, come to an understanding of a patient problem, plan and implement interventions, evaluate outcomes, and reflect on or learn from the process

11. Which nursing action reflects the use of clinical judgment to adapt client care based on a change in care environment?
    A. Asking a family to bring in the client's favorite food from home to help meet his or her nutritional needs
    B. Teaching family members to use clean supplies instead of sterile supplies when changing a wound dressing at home
    C. Convening an interprofessional team conference to determine the readiness of the family and client with complex care needs for discharge
    D. Assigning a licensed practical nurse/licensed vocational nurse (LPN/LVN) instead of a nursing assistant to provide morning care to a client whose condition has become less stable

12. Which actions by a nurse best exemplifies the use of systems thinking to prevent pressure injury on a medical-surgical nursing unit? **Select all that apply.**
    A. Attending a workshop to learn about different types of pressure injury dressings
    B. Performing an electronic literature search to explore techniques for pressure injury prevention
    C. Reviewing client records for the past 12 months to determine the rate of pressure injury development
    D. Examining the skin of a 93-year-old client at least daily for the presence of pressure injury indicators
    E. Using an evidence-based practice assessment tool to identify all admitted clients at increased potential risk for pressure injury
    F. Collaborating with unit registered nurses to develop a "turning team" to ensure regular repositioning of all clients at risk for pressure injury

Chapter 2 Answer Key

1. D
   Behavioral and social determinants of health include what "health" means to the client within the context of his or her culture and what actions he or she is willing to take to achieve or maintain health. This client is taking responsibility for her health.

2. B
   Within the QSEN competencies, safety includes designing all nursing care with the focus on safety at the forefront of planning and execution of care at the individual and systems level. The most important concern for this client is safety.

3. A
   Clinical reasoning is the process by which nurses collect cues, process the information, come to an understanding of a patient problem or situation, plan and implement interventions, evaluate outcomes, and reflect on and learn from the process. This nurse recognized the cues that the client's situation was getting worse and notified the HCP so that the plan of care could be modified to improve his or her condition.

4. A, C, D, F, G, H
   When a nurse assesses a patient using clinical judgment, the first step of a six-step process is to recognize cues and determine which cues are relevant (directly related to the client outcomes or the priority of care) versus those which are irrelevant (unrelated to the client outcomes or priority of care). Removal of his gall bladder a year ago and his daughter's fourth pregnancy are not relevant at this time. The remaining responses are relevant.

5. B, C, D, E, G
   The actions that the nurse takes are performed to address the highest priorities of care. Most patients do not need to have a tracheostomy. Around-the-clock acetaminophen is not usually prescribed. Suctioning is only performed as needed, not on a routine schedule. The other responses are appropriate actions for a client with COPD.

6. A
   Primary health care is generally provided by a primary care provider. That person becomes a

"gatekeeper" for the client's care. Primary care ranges from prevention to management of chronic health conditions.

7. A, B, C, E, F, H

Long-term care is a complex system within a larger system of the U.S. health care delivery system. Care is highly individualized and well coordinated to help provide partial or total care, sometimes indefinitely. Hospice care and home health care are types of community-based care. The rest of the responses are types of long-term care.

8. D

While A is true of nurse practitioners, it is also true of physicians and physician assistants and therefore not specific to nurse practitioners. Nurse practitioners are educated and practice according to a nursing model which emphasizes client-centered care including promotion of health and wellness, and quality of life across the lifespan.

9. A, B, C, E

To move from clinical judgment to systems thinking, nurses must move from focus on individual nursing actions to focus on nursing actions and relationships within a nursing unit or organization. The goal is to add enhanced methods to promote safety and increase quality of care. Suctioning does not help to prevent VAP but all strategies that encourage frequent oral care have the potential to decrease the incidence of VAP.

10. C

The goal of systems thinking is to encourage the nurse to develop awareness of the interrelationships that exist between individual care and the overall context of health care safety and quality. Nurses need to address quality and safety concerns.

11. B

Care of a wound in the home does not require sterile supplies or technique because the home environment has fewer environmental pathogens than does an acute care setting or other health care setting. All the other actions focus on changing client conditions rather than changing environmental conditions.

12. B, C, E, F

Systems thinking reflects the general care and well-being of all clients. The process begins with knowledge of problem prevention (option B), identifying whether a problem exists as a systemic issue beyond the care of one client (option C), using the evidence for best practice (option E), and formulating a potential action plan (option F). Option A is describing an action for management of pressure injury, not prevention. Option D is focused on one client, not on a possible system problem. Also, it is focused on early detection rather than on primary prevention.

3

CHAPTER

Overview of Health Concepts for Medical-Surgical Nursing

1. Which medical-surgical nursing concept does the nurse expect to be **most affected** by a client's recent episodes of nausea and vomiting?
   A. Acid-base imbalance
   B. Cellular regulation
   C. Gas exchange
   D. Immunity

2. Which action for correction does the nurse expect to occur in the client who has a pH of 7.49?
   A. Kidneys reabsorb bicarbonate
   B. Respiratory rate increases
   C. Kidneys excrete H+ ions
   D. Lungs decrease CO_2 excretion

3. Which client action is **most likely** to promote acid-base balance?
   A. Client with immunodeficiency avoids eating undercooked meat
   B. Client with COPD quits smoking
   C. Client with alkalosis uses daily antacids
   D. Client with heart disease reduces fat intake

4. Which medical-surgical concept does the nurse view as altered in a client who has a thick, ridge-like, large scar over the site of surgery to repair a fractured femur performed 3 years ago?
   A. Mobility
   B. Infection
   C. Cellular regulation
   D. Sensory perception

5. Which topics are **most relevant** for the nurse to include when teaching a client about cancer prevention from impaired cellular regulation? **Select all that apply**.
   A. Protect exposed skin with sunscreen of at least 30 SPF.
   B. Consume a diet low in fiber and high in saturated fats.
   C. Greatly reduce or stop using tobacco in any form.
   D. Get regular exercise.
   E. Determine who in your family has ever been diagnosed with heart disease.
   F. Avoid exposure to environmental chemicals and particulate matter.
   G. Avoid eye strain by wearing prescribed corrective lenses.
   H. Drink at least 3 liters of water daily unless another health problem requires fluid restriction.

6. When caring for a client who is a smoker with a history of polycythemia and immobility issues, which medical/surgical concepts are the nurse's **highest priority**? **Select all that apply**.
   A. Infection
   B. Clotting
   C. Fluid and electrolyte imbalance
   D. Pain
   E. Gas exchange
   F. Sexuality

7. With which client health problem does the nurse try to **prevent harm** by remaining alert for the potential of reduced clotting?
   A. Atrial fibrillation
   B. Bone fracture
   C. Cirrhosis of the liver
   D. Chronically elevated blood glucose levels

8. Assessment for which physiological consequence of impaired clotting does the nurse perform regularly to **prevent harm** for the client with a deep vein thrombosis of the calf?
   A. Pulmonary embolus
   B. Superficial phlebitis
   C. Hemorrhagic stroke
   D. Myocardial infarction

9. Which signs and symptoms are indicators of inadequate clotting? **Select all that apply**.
   A. Purpural lesions
   B. Localized itching
   C. Ecchymosis
   D. Prolonged bleeding
   E. Skin dryness and poor turgor
   F. Hematuria

10. Which statement by a client indicates to the nurse that additional teaching is needed to **prevent harm** from the risk for increased clotting?
    A. "I will cross my legs only when sitting down."
    B. "I will drink plenty of fluids so that I will not become dehydrated."
    C. "I will get up and move for 10 minutes every hour while working at the computer."
    D. "I will notify my health care provider if I see redness or swelling in my leg."

11. How will the nurse document the client's cognitive status when he or she experiences recent confusion with a rapid onset?
    A. Delirium
    B. Amnesia
    C. Dementia
    D. Intermittent confusion

12. Which nursing actions are appropriate when caring for a client with dementia? **Select all that apply.**
    A. Reorienting the client to the date and place every shift
    B. Providing a safe environment
    C. Correcting the client when he or she tells the nurse that the baby is crying
    D. Observing for delusions or hallucinations
    E. Teaching the family how to make the home environment safer
    F. Having the client sign his or her own informed consent statement

13. Which action may the nurse safely delegate to a assistive personnel (AP) when caring for a client who has urinary incontinence?
    A. Instructing the client about the causes of incontinence
    B. Assessing the client's skin for redness or breakdown
    C. Monitoring the client for symptoms of electrolyte imbalance
    D. Assisting the client to the bathroom every 2 hours.

14. Which nursing assessment finding for a client with fluid volume excess supports the continued presence of this condition?
    A. Weak thready pulses
    B. Increased blood pressure
    C. Decreased heart rate
    D. Poor skin turgor

15. Which health promotion strategies and actions are **most appropriate** for the nurse to perform when caring for a client who has a chronic health problem that interferes with gas exchange? **Select all that apply**.
    A. Instructing the client to obtain influenza and pneumonia immunizations
    B. Encouraging the client to sleep flat in a side-lying position on his or her left side
    C. Reminding the client to wash hands thoroughly after using the commode
    D. Administering bronchodilators as ordered by the health care provider
    E. Reminding the client to use incentive spirometry every hour while awake
    F. Instructing the client to increase the oxygen flow rate gradually throughout the day

16. With which clients is the nurse especially vigilant in actions to prevent infection? **Select all that apply**.
    A. 24-year-old who fractured a leg while hiking
    B. 28-year-old undergoing cancer chemotherapy
    C. 30-year-old who has never received an influenza vaccination
    D. 40-year-old who has severe allergies
    E. 55-year-old who takes oral prednisone daily for rheumatoid arthritis
    F. 80-year-old with chronic obstructive pulmonary disease (COPD)

17. Which signs and symptoms in a client with a wound infection indicate to the nurse that the infection may have progressed from localized to systemic? **Select all that apply**.
    A. Temperature is 102.2°F (39°C).
    B. Wound edges are red.
    C. Total leukocyte count is 14,000 cells/mm³ (14 × 10⁹/L).
    D. Client reports the wound is more painful than the surrounding tissue.
    E. Purulent exudate is present.
    F. The infection has been present for 5 days.

18. Which conditions or health problems demonstrate the presence of inflammation without infection? **Select all that apply**.
    A. Allergic rhinitis
    B. Viral hepatitis
    C. Rheumatoid arthritis
    D. Cellulitis
    E. Appendicitis
    F. Simple cholecystitis
    G. Tuberculosis

19. Why is chronic inflammation treated?
    A. Chronic inflammation usually becomes an infectious process over time.
    B. Treatment is required to prevent the client from becoming immunosuppressed.
    C. The cell actions associated with chronic inflammation often lead to tissue damage.
    D. The presence of chronic inflammation increases the risk for development of autoimmune disorders.

20. Which client does the nurse recognize to be at highest risk for impaired mobility?
    A. Client with unrepaired hip fracture
    B. Client with mild seasonal asthma
    C. Post–cardiac-catheterization client on bedrest for 12 hours.
    D. Client with fractured right radius

21. For which common physiologic complications will the nurse observe in a client with impaired mobility? **Select all that apply**.
    A. Pressure injuries
    B. Bloody diarrhea
    C. Changes in sleep-wake cycle
    D. Sensory deprivation
    E. Muscle atrophy
    F. Kidney stones
    G. Depression

22. Which nursing actions are **most appropriate** for the nurse caring for a client with poor nutrition from bulimia nervosa to implement? **Select all that apply**.
    A. Administering high-protein nutritional supplements
    B. Assessing for dry skin and dry or brittle hair
    C. Encouraging regular, strenuous exercise at least twice a day
    D. Stressing the need for intake of high-fat foods for weight gain
    E. Monitoring serum albumin and pre-albumin levels
    F. Teaching about bariatric surgery

23. Which assessment findings support the nurse's suspicion that a client has impaired central perfusion? **Select all that apply**.
    A. Dizziness
    B. Decreased hair distribution
    C. Pallor of extremities
    D. Difficulty breathing
    E. Chest pain
    F. Cyanosis of extremities

24. Which client report of pain would indicate to the nurse the possibility of persistent pain rather than acute pain?
    A. The exact location is hard to determine.
    B. It first started immediately after a sports injury.
    C. Its presence reminds the client to protect the area.
    D. The level has improved every day since the injury occurred.

25. Which question would the nurse be sure to ask a client who has impaired sensory perception related to smell and taste?
    A. "Have you ever been told that your blood sugar is high?"
    B. "Do you usually eat a lot of physically hot or spicy foods?"
    C. "Do you have any dry mouth side effects with your prescribed drugs?"
    D. "Have you experienced any other problems with your senses for vision or touch?

Chapter 3 Answer Key

1. **A.**
   Excessive emesis is one of the most common risk factors for acid-base imbalance.

2. **D.**
   When the body has an impaired acid-base balance, several mechanisms are activated in an attempt to correct the imbalance, a process referred to as compensation. If the client's pH is alkalotic (greater than 7.45), the lungs try to release carbon dioxide (directly related to hydrogen ions) through decreased and shallower respirations and bring the pH back to the normal range.

3. **B.**
   The best way for an individual to maintain acid-base balance is to practice health promotion measures, including living a healthy lifestyle. For example, most cases of COPD can be prevented by avoiding or quitting smoking.

4. **C.**
   Reduced control over cellular regulation can lead to excessive growth of normal cells, such as those involved in scar tissue formation, and in this case results in benign excessive growth of a skin keloid. Inflammation is no longer present 3 years later. A keloid in this location does not interfere with mobility or sensory perception.

5. **A, C, D, F**
   Primary health promotion strategies to prevent impaired cellular regulation include teaching clients to:
   - Protect exposed skin with sunscreen of at least 30 SPF.
   - Minimize exposure to sunlight or other source of ultraviolet light such as tanning beds (to prevent skin cancers).
   - Stop smoking or other tobacco use if applicable (to prevent many cancer types, including lung, oral, and bladder cancers).
   - Consume a diet low in saturated fat and high in fiber (to prevent breast and colon cancer).
   - Increase physical activity and regular exercise (to prevent all cancer types).
   - Avoid exposure to environmental hazards (to prevent all cancer types).

6. **B, E**
   Common risk factors for increased clotting include immobility or decreased mobility, health problems such as polycythemia, and smoking. Immobility slows venous blood flow to the heart and can result in venous stasis and venous thromboembolism (VTE). Polycythemia causes an excessive production of red blood cells, which can lead to multiple clots. When clots are present in circulation, perfusion to the tissues is reduced resulting in impaired gas exchange. A smoking history also increases the risk for many types of problems that can result in poor gas exchange.

CHAPTER 5

Assessment and Concepts of Care for Patients with Pain

1. Which common causes of persistent (chronic) pain are most associated with long-term disability? **Select all that apply**.
   A. Compound femur fracture
   B. Diabetic neuropathy
   C. Osteoarthritis
   D. Rheumatoid arthritis
   E. Scald burn to the arm
   F. Surgical repair of a torn ligament

2. Why are older residents in nursing homes at high risk for inadequate pain management?
   A. Many nursing home residents lack the verbal ability to describe or report pain.
   B. Nursing home clients are often too confused or have dementia and do not recognize pain.
   C. Many nurses worry about overdosing older clients, who are more sensitive to the effects of pain medications.
   D. Clients in nursing homes are more likely to have persistent (chronic) pain rather than the more easily identified acute types of pain.

3. Which observation after administering prescribed pain medication to a client who reported persistent (chronic) leg pain level of a 7 on a 0 to 10 scale indicates to the nurse that the functional goal of therapy is being met?
   A. Client is engaging in conversation with visitors.
   B. Pulse, blood pressure, and respirations are within the client's usual range.
   C. Client is able to ambulate independently to the bathroom without distress.
   D. Client uses his or her arms to lift the leg when changing positions while in bed.

4. Which question is **most** appropriate for a nurse to ask to assess pain in a client who was just transferred to the unit from the postanesthesia recovery area after abdominal surgery?
   A. "How bad is your pain? Is it better than before?"
   B. "The pain is probably pretty bad at the incision site. Right?"
   C. "Can you tell me about any pain or discomfort you are having?"
   D. "Which problem is bothering you more, your pain or your nausea?"

5. Which behavior(s) by a client with cognitive impairment indicate(s) to the nurse the possibility that the client is experiencing pain? **Select all that apply**.
   A. Has no interest in attending a musical entertainment that he or she always enjoyed in the past
   B. Attempting to slap assistive personnel who are providing care
   C. Restlessness and pulling at the bed clothes
   D. Grimacing when being turned
   E. Refusal to eat or drink
   F. Inability to sleep

6. The nurse considers the pain reported by a client with which health problem **more** likely to likely reflect acute pain rather than persistent (chronic) pain?
   A. Peripheral vascular disease with a foot that is suddenly cold and blue
   B. Diabetic neuropathy with tingling and burning sensation in lower leg
   C. Development of osteoarthritis in an old sports injury of a fractured ankle
   D. Spinal stenosis with intermittent pain down the right leg for past 6 months

7. Which action does the nurse take or perform **first** when caring for a client on the first post-operative day after major abdominal surgery who states he or she has no pain, but blood pressure and pulse are elevated and the client is diaphoretic and appears anxious?
    A. Believe and document the client's self-report of "I have no pain."
    B. Call the health care provider and report the vital signs, diaphoresis, and anxiety.
    C. Assess the client for postoperative complications or barriers to reporting pain.
    D. Ask the client whether he or she has ever had a pain experience.

8. An older client tells the home health nurse that he took two tablets of arthritis-strength extended-release acetaminophen at 6:00 a.m. and two tablets of hydrocodone at 2:00 p.m. and that he plans to take one dose of an over-the-counter product that contains acetaminophen, doxylamine succinate, and dextromethorphan to sleep tonight. Which action would the nurse take **first to prevent harm**?
    A. Call poison control because the client has exceeded the recommended dose of acetaminophen.
    B. Tell the client to call the health care provider and report all medications that he takes.
    C. Educate the client about the acetaminophen in each product and the maximum dosage/day.
    D. Record the medications, frequency, and dosage in the medication reconciliation record.

9. Which statement made by a nurse regarding a client's report of pain reflects personal bias?
    A. "This client wants more pain medication 2 hours before it is scheduled, so I need to inform the health care provider that the dosage or schedule may need adjustment."
    B. "I was not going to give the client the scheduled pain medication because he was sleeping; however, I don't want to skip dose and have the pain level escalate."
    C. "The client says the pain is worse now than it was on the day after surgery. I wonder if something else is causing the pain."
    D. "With all of her laughing and talking with friends, her pain cannot possibly be as bad as she reports it to be."

10. Which observation indicates to the nurse that a client with rheumatoid arthritis who has had persistent (chronic) pain for years and now has an exacerbation that started this morning has a physiologic adaptation to pain?
    A. Pupils are dilated.
    B. Breathing is shallow.
    C. Pulse rate is 70 beats/min.
    D. Temperature is 98.6°F (37°C).

11. With which client does the nurse expect to administer gabapentin?
    A. A client who has persistent burning and tingling sensation in the lower extremities
    B. A client who reports a gnawing and burning discomfort in the epigastric area between meals
    C. A client who expresses fear, anxiety, and uncertainty related to episodes of angina
    D. A client who is 1 day postoperative from cardiac bypass graft surgery

12. Which behavior exemplifies the nurse's primary role in assessing and managing the client's pain?
    A. Administers pain medication as ordered if pain is sufficient to warrant therapy
    B. Listens to the client's self-report and forms an opinion about the veracity of the description
    C. Observes for concurrent verbal reports and nonverbal signs to substantiate presence of pain
    D. Listens to and accepts the self-report of pain and assesses client's preferences and values

13. Which physiologic responses indicate to the nurse that the client is experiencing acute pain? **Select all that apply**.
    A. Diaphoresis
    B. Somnolence
    C. Bradypnea
    D. Hypotension
    E. Tachycardia
    F. Dilated pupils

14. Which side effect does the nurse assess for in a client who has been using an opioid analgesic for the past 5 days?
    A. Addiction
    B. Hallucinations
    C. Constipation
    D. Excessive thirst

15. Which pain scale will the nurse use to most accurately assess the pain level of an adult client who has either a language barrier or reading problems?
    A. 0 to 10 numeric rating scale
    B. FACES (smile to frown)
    C. Vertical presentation scale
    D. Pasero Opioid-Induced Sedation Scale

16. Which outcome indicates to the nurse assessing that a client's pain control medication is effective 45 minutes after receiving pain medication for pain intensity rated as the "worst possible?"
    A. Client reports that the pain level is 4/10.
    B. Client is drowsy and has trouble staying awake.
    C. Client tolerates the dressing change without grimacing.
    D. Client is also receiving a medication to reduce anxiety.

17. Which strategy will the nurse use to help an older adult client who reports having "pain all over" to accurately identify which areas of the body are painful?
    A. Start with gentle palpation on the abdomen and chest.
    B. Focus on the hand and fingers of one extremity.
    C. Direct the client to find one area that does not hurt.
    D. Provide examples and comparisons of severe pain.

18. Which assessment question does the home health nurse ask an older adult client who is taking naproxen twice daily for pain to assess for adverse effects?
    A. "Have you noticed unusual fatigue, restlessness, or feelings of depression?"
    B. "Do you notice dry mouth, dizziness, mental clouding, or weight gain?"
    C. "Are you experiencing constipation, itching, or excessive sleepiness?"
    D. "Have you had any gastric discomfort, vomiting, bleeding, or bruising?"

19. Which statement is the best response for a nurse to use when interviewing a client who frequently comes to the clinic to obtain medication for chronic back pain says, "I know you guys think I am faking, but I hurt and I am really sick of your attitude"?
    A. "Tell me about your pain and how it is affecting your life."
    B. "Would you prefer to speak with a nurse who is a pain specialist?"
    C. "I know you are frustrated, but you are unfairly judging me."
    D. "We are trying our best but sometimes you just have to learn to live with the pain."

20. Which is the **priority** action for the nurse to take after assessing a client with severe dementia at a score of 9 using the Pain Assessment in Advanced Dementia (PAINAD) Scale?
    A. Speak calmly to the client and explain that repositioning will make him more comfortable.
    B. Contact the family and ask how the client would typically respond to discomfort.
    C. Gently reassure the client and continue routine observation for discomfort or pain.
    D. Assess the client for the source of the pain and immediately inform the primary health care provider.

21. How many mL of morphine will the nurse administer by IV push to a client who is prescribed to receive 3 mg when the drug is available in a solution of 5 mg/mL?
    A. 0.2 mL
    B. 0.4 mL
    C. 0.6 mL
    D. 0.8 mL

22. On reassessing a client for pain relief 1 hour after administering 15 mg of morphine intramuscularly, the nurse finds the client sleeping and has a respiratory rate of 10 breaths/min. What is the nurse's best **first** action to prevent harm?
    A. Attempt to arouse the patient by calling his or her name and lightly shaking the arm.
    B. Administer oxygen by mask or nasal cannula and notify the prescriber.
    C. Check the patient's oxygen saturation and raise the head of the bed.
    D. Document the finding as the only action.

23. What is the nurse's best response to the spouse of a client receiving an extended-release form of oral morphine for severe cancer pain who explains that the client has difficulty swallowing and asks if the tablets can be crushed and given with applesauce or pudding?
    A. "That is an excellent solution and will make swallowing pain medication much easier."
    B. "We can ask the oncology health care provider to place a feeding tube for medication administration."
    C. "You can dissolve the tablets in water and mix it with juice before administering it."
    D. "I will contact the health care provider to change the prescription for a different form of morphine."

24. With which client is the nurse **most** likely to question a prescription for patient-controlled analgesia?
    A. 32-year-old with severe burns and a history of opioid use disorder
    B. 76-year-old with multiple injuries sustained during an accident
    C. 34-year-old with functional blindness who had abdominal surgery
    D. 25-year-old with intermittent lucidity after a severe head injury

25. By which route does the nurse anticipate administering pain medication to a client who has a severe burn on the hand and forearm and reports pain that is severe and escalating?
    A. Oral
    B. Intravenous
    C. Intranasal
    D. Subcutaneous

26. What is the appropriate action for the nurse to take when a client is prescribed both an around-the-clock opioid and a daily NSAID dose after orthopedic surgery?
    A. Ensure to separate administering the two drugs by at least 4 hours.
    B. Administer both drugs as prescribed and assess the client's level of pain relief.
    C. Notify the surgeon that two different classes of pain medication were prescribed.
    D. Use clinical judgment to determine which of the two drugs to administer based on assessment of the client's pain level.

27. Which term will the nurse use to describe a client's response of increasing morphine dosage needs over time to manage severe cancer pain?
    A. Addiction
    B. Pseudoaddiction
    C. Tolerance
    D. Dependence

28. Which drug prescription for an older adult client in acute pain does the nurse question because of the possibility of severe adverse effects?
    A. Ibuprofen
    B. Morphine
    C. Meperidine
    D. Acetaminophen with hydrocodone

29. What is the nurse's best response to a daughter caring for her 79-year-old father, who has been prescribed multimodal analgesia, when the daughter asks if just using one drug would be easier and less expensive?
    A. "The doctor always prescribes this combination of medications as the best therapy."
    B. "Older adults often do better with fewer medications; let me call the doctor."
    C. "Just see how it goes for your dad. You may be able to gradually reduce the number of drugs."
    D. "Combining different types of pain medication gives greater relief with lower doses and fewer side effects."

30. The family of a client who is 3 hours postoperative and receiving IV morphine for pain management asks the nurse when the client could take oral pain medication because he is scheduled to be discharged tomorrow. What will the nurse tell the family?
    A. We will teach you how to give IV drugs before he is discharged.
    B. When the surgeon determines he is ready
    C. When he is able to tolerate oral intake
    D. When we discontinue the IV line

31. What is the best way for a nurse to determine when to administer a prn analgesic with a prescription of "every 4–6 hours as needed" for a client who is also receiving around-the-clock analgesic medication?
    A. Automatically administer a dose every 6 hours to ensure adequate relief.
    B. Contact the health care provider and ask for specific parameters for prn dosing.
    C. Review the medication administration record to see how often the client received it on the previous shift.
    D. Assess the client for breakthrough pain and also administer it in advance of painful procedures.

32. What is the **priority** issue for a nurse to consider before administering a dose of morphine to a younger client in severe pain who is opioid naïve?
    A. Decreased analgesia may occur because the client is opioid naïve.
    B. The client is more likely to develop drug tolerance than someone who has received it before.
    C. Excessive sedation can progress to clinically significant respiratory depression.
    D. An order for a prn one-time dose of naloxone is needed for possible adverse effects.

33. What action does the nurse perform **first** on finding a client who is receiving opioid medication via a patient-controlled analgesia device very drowsy and difficult to arouse?
    A. Wake the client and tell the client to stop pushing the button so frequently.
    B. Stay with the client and discontinue the basal rate.
    C. Take no immediate action and increase the frequency of assessment.
    D. Ask the primary health care provider to change the pain medication to a nonopioid drug.

34. The nurse expects which physiologic responses with a client who is taking a mu opioid agonist intravenously? **Select all that apply.**
    A. An increase in dosage yields an increase in pain relief.
    B. A dose ceiling effect occurs and intensifies pain perception.
    C. Analgesia is reversed at the peak effect.
    D. Peak comfort occurs within 20 to 30 minutes.
    E. Pupils become widely dilated.
    F. Gastrointestinal peristalsis slows.

35. Which information will the nurse need to understand when caring for a hospitalized client who has an intrathecal implanted pump for pain management? **Select all that apply**.
    A. Assess for cerebral spinal fluid leak if the client reports a headache.
    B. Morphine is the drug most often used.
    C. Higher doses of analgesic are needed compared with patient-controlled analgesia delivered intravenously.
    D. These devices are used exclusively to deliver single bolus doses during surgical procedures.
    E. This form of analgesia avoids the risk for respiratory depression.
    F. An abdominal binder may be prescribed to keep the pump in the proper position.

36. Which analgesic type does the nurse expect to be prescribed to reduce the pain and discomfort from inflammation for a client who has a history of rheumatoid arthritis and is also being treated for acute pain from a wrist sprain?
    A. Acetaminophen
    B. Local anesthetic
    C. NSAID
    D. Opioid agonist/antagonist

37. What action will the nurse take when seeing that a client is prescribed to receive acetaminophen and celecoxib at the same time?
    A. Request that the health care provider change the prescription so that administration of these two drugs is staggered.
    B. Ask the client which one he or she prefers to take; administer the preferred drug and assess for relief.
    C. Administer the acetaminophen because it is less likely to cause gastric irritation and bleeding.
    D. Administer the medications as prescribed and document the client's response.

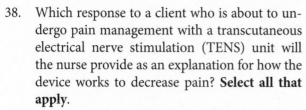

38. Which response to a client who is about to undergo pain management with a transcutaneous electrical nerve stimulation (TENS) unit will the nurse provide as an explanation for how the device works to decrease pain? **Select all that apply**.
   A. Increases comfort by promoting better blood flow to the area
   B. Changes your sensation of pain at the site to feelings of "pins and needles"
   C. Increases secretion of brain hormones similar to morphine to reduce pain
   D. Distracts your mind from the presence of pain

39. Which client actions during the use of fentanyl patches for pain control will the nurse correct to **prevent harm**, especially respiratory depression? **Select all that apply**.
   A. Folding the patch in half
   B. Returning the used patches to the clinic for disposal
   C. Placing a heating pad over the patch
   D. Placing a new patch and retaining the old ones in their current positions
   E. Washing the area before applying a new patch
   F. Using adhesive tape over the patch to keep it in place

40. How much time does the nurse expect to pass between the first dosage level and a change of dosage level with transdermal fentanyl administration when starting the titration of this medication until the client experiences adequate pain control?
   A. At least 24 hours
   B. Between 5 and 15 minutes if the pain is severe
   C. About 2 to 3 days
   D. Varies by the prescribed frequency of patch changes

41. Which common side effects will the nurse assess for in a client receiving (NSAIDs) therapy for pain management? **Select all that apply**.
   A. Bleeding
   B. Constipation
   C. Drowsiness
   D. Dry mouth
   E. Gastrointestinal ulcers
   F. Hypertension
   G. Memory loss (temporary)

42. Which side effects does the nurse assess for in a client who is using cannabis (medical marijuana) to help manage persistent pain? **Select all that apply**.
   A. Increased heart rate
   B. Impaired attention
   C. Increased appetite
   D. Diaphoresis
   E. Dry mouth
   F. Tremors

43. Which actions will the nurse in the emergency department take to **prevent harm** after a possible fentanyl/carfentanyl exposure while caring for a client admitted with indications of an opioid overdose? **Select all that apply**.
   A. Immediately alert his or her co-workers if drowsiness, difficulty breathing, or clammy skin are experienced.
   B. Shake bed linen thoroughly after client use to prevent transferring contaminants to laundry workers.
   C. Wear personal protective equipment while cleaning all surfaces contacted by the client.
   D. First clean hands using an alcohol-based hand rub.
   E. Avoid touching his or her mouth, nose, or eyes.
   F. Report any new onset of diarrhea.

44. A nurse observes a colleague preparing to administer an injection of normal saline as a placebo to a client who states that their pain was not relieved by opioid injected 2 hours ago. What is the nurse's **best first** action?
    A. Reinforce to the client that this injection is highly likely to relieve his current pain.
    B. Ignore the incident and allow the colleague to use his or her own clinical judgment.
    C. Take the syringe from the colleague and write up an incident report.
    D. Remind the colleague that using a placebo is deceitful and unethical.

Chapter 5 Answer Key

1. B, C, D
   The pain associated with diabetic neuropathy, osteoarthritis, and rheumatoid arthritis is not only persistent, it is usually also progressive. The nature of both the pain and the disease generally decreases the client's activity level, leading to a decline in function and quality of life. The other listed causes of pain produce acute pain that improves over time.

2. A.
   Although some clients have dementia or another type of cognitive decline, they can feel both acute and persistent pain. Confused clients and those with reduced verbal skills are often unable to report pain or adequately describe its quality.

3. C
   Pain in an extremity is reflected as reduced function and use of the extremity. The client may limit its movement and guard it to prevent more pain. Actually, using the extremity in a normal way indicates that the pain is reduced enough to permit function.

4. C
   Pain is a personal experience and only the client can adequately describe his or her pain experience. The nurse asks the client to describe the presence and intensity of his or her pain and neither presumes its presence or intensity nor tell the client what his or her pain level should be.

5. A, B, C, D, E, F
   A client in pain experiences both physiologic and behavioral responses. Behavioral changes are often observed as restlessness, an inability to concentrate, loss of interest in activities that used to bring pleasure, and disturbances in eating or sleeping.

6. A
   The only health problem listed with a sudden change that could produce pain is option A. Everything else is a chronic problem with a gradual pain onset.

7. C
   Although "pain is whatever the client says it is occurring when the client says it does," the client is exhibiting many of the indicators of acute pain. Some clients have misconceptions about the meaning of pain or about the consequences of taking pain medication and underreport their pain. The nurse must use clinical judgment and explore possible reasons the client would insist that pain is not present.

8. C
   Acetaminophen when taken in high doses and/or daily can be toxic to the liver. For this reason, there is a maximum daily dose for adults. Clients often are unaware of this maximum or of the presence of acetaminophen in other over-the-counter or combination drugs.

9. D

This nurse is projecting what he or she believes that a person in pain would or would not be able to do. Even a person in extreme pain may be able to hide that pain from friends or relatives for short periods of time. Pain is whatever the client says it is occurring whenever he or she says it does.

10. C

Clients who have had persistent pain for a long time often have adapted to the pain experience and no longer respond to either the presence of persistent pain or new-onset acute pain with the expected sympathetic nervous system responses of diaphoresis, increased heart rate and blood pressure, and increased respiratory rate.

11. A

Gabapentin is an antiepileptic drug that works on nerves and neurotransmitters to reduce seizure activity. It also reduces neuropathic pain, which is characterized by burning and tingling sensations in the affected areas.

12. D

The pain experience is highly personal and the client is the only person who can adequately determine the presence and intensity of the pain experience. The nurse accepts the client's report of pain and takes into consideration his or her values and preferences.

13. A, E, F

Acute pain is a stressor that causes a client to have a sympathetic nervous system reaction similar to the "fight or flight" responses. These responses include diaphoresis, increased heart rate and blood pressure, and increased respiratory rate.

14. C

The most common side effect of opioids is constipation because these drugs slow intestinal movement. Most clients who are on opioids for 2 or more days experience constipation. Assess clients who are prescribed opioids for constipation and the need for stool softeners or laxatives.

15. B

The FACES pain-rating scale does not rely on reading skills and requires less language comprehension for a client to indicate pain level than any of the other listed scales.

16. A

The most reliable indicator of pain relief is the client's self-report of reduced pain. Being drowsy or actually sleeping does not mean that pain is absent. Tolerating a dressing change without grimacing may only indicate that the dressing change manipulation is not the source of the pain. Although anxiety may increase pain perception, receiving an antianxiety medication does not indicate pain reduction.

17. B

By focusing on specific body areas one at a time, clients are better able to separate areas that really aren't painful from those that are. This strategy helps clients understand the origin of the pain better.

18. D

Naproxen is a fairly powerful NSAID. All NSAIDs increase the risk for gastric upset, gastrointestinal ulcers, and also reduce platelet action, which increases the risk for bleeding.

19. A

All clients must be treated with respect and have their pain issues relieved. Determining how much the pain interferes with the client's lifestyle and quality of life not only demonstrates interest in that client as an individual, but can also help in assessing pain severity. Nurses should not take comments personally. Although offering a referral to a pain specialist may be done eventually, a thorough pain assessment is performed first. Learning to "live with the pain" takes away all hope for effective pain management and should not be said to the client.

20. D

A score of 9 (out of a possible 10) on the PAINAD scale indicates severe pain. The nurse must assess further to determine the pain source. Even if the source is not determined, this client's condition needs to be reported to the primary health care provider immediately for appropriate intervention.

21. C

Have 5 mg in 1 mL. *Want* 3 mg in X mL. 1 × 3 divided by 5 = 0.6 mL

22. A

Many clients experience some degree of respiratory depression with opioid analgesics. If the client can be aroused with minimally-intrusive techniques and the respiratory rate increases spontaneously, no further intervention is required.

23. D

Extended-release tablets must not be chewed, crushed, or dissolved before administering it because these actions can cause a drug overdose from releasing too much drug at a time. The best action is to contact the oncology health care provider with the information about the client's difficulty swallowing because a different form of morphine or a different drug may be needed to control the pain.

24. D

In order for a client to use patient-controlled analgesia effectively, he or she must have both adequate cognition and the physical ability to use the pump. Intermittent lucidity interferes with the client's understanding of the pump's purpose and controls. Blindness is not a hindrance and neither is age. Clients who have a history of opioid use disorder still require pain medications when conditions cause severe pain, as with a burn injury.

25. B

The client has severe acute pain that is escalating and needs to have pain medication delivered as quickly as possible by the most effective route, which is intravenous.

26. B

Often, the best pain relief is achieved when multimodal drugs are prescribed. The NSAID may reduce the pain caused at the site of the surgery and the opioid medication can alter the client's

perception of pain. Neither drug interferes with the action of the other and both should be administered as prescribed.

27. C

With long-term opioid use, clients can develop tolerance in which side effects are less severe and the main effect of pain relief requires higher dosages of the drug. This is a physiologic response in which the body adapts to morphine presence in several ways, one of which is by increasing its rate of degradation and elimination. It is purely a physical response and does not have a behavioral component in the way that pseudoaddiction, addiction, or dependence do.

28. C

Meperidine, an older type of synthetic opioid that is no longer recommended for pain management in anyone, converts into a metabolite that can be toxic, especially to older adults who may have reduced excretion of the metabolite. The metabolite can cause delirium, tremors, irritability, myoclonus, and seizures. Although every drug can have adverse effects, the other drugs in this list usually have less problems in older adults.

29. D

Multimodal drug therapy using different types of drugs may help reduce the problems at the source of the pain in addition to altering the client's perception of pain, thus providing better pain management. Also, the amounts of the different drugs may be reduced, thus reducing the incidence and intensity of possible side effects.

30. C

The vast majority of clients are able to take an oral analgesic as soon as they can tolerate food and liquids after surgery, regardless of when the IV access is discontinued. Very few clients require IV medication at home after surgery.

31. D

Clients on around-the-clock pain medication may have periods in which the medication does not fully cover the pain and will experience acute pain during painful procedures. PRN drugs are not administered automatically, only when the client requires it. In this case, the client can receive the medication every 4 to 6 hours, which is the specific parameter prescribed. When a painful procedure is scheduled and the client has not received the PRN drug within the past 4 hours, the nurse would administer it before the procedure. Although reviewing when the client requested and received the PRN drug earlier can provide information about overall pain management, it does not dictate his or her individual need in the moment.

32. C
The analgesic effects and side effects, including respiratory depression, are more likely to occur at lower doses in a client who is opioid naïve than in one who has received the drug in the recent past. An order for naloxone is not needed because its use is permitted whenever indications of severe respiratory depression or overdose are present.

33. B
The basal dose of the drug may be set at too high a rate and should be discontinued until a reevaluation can be performed. The client is at risk for respiratory depression and requires continuous monitoring until the level of consciousness reliably increases.

34. A, F
Mu receptors are located in the brain and elsewhere in the body, causing opioid agonist effects. When administered intravenously, pain relief increases with the dosage and occurs within 1 or 2 minutes. A ceiling effect does not occur and an agonist does not reverse the analgesic effect. Pupils are constricted and GI peristalsis slows.

35. A, B, F
An intrathecal pump is a form of intraspinal analgesia and can be used as a single bolus for acute pain or as a continuous infusion for management of persistent pain. Morphine is the drug most commonly placed in the cerebral spinal fluid in the subarachnoid space and its dosage is considerably lower than when administered any other way. The location of drug placement does increase the risk for respiratory depression, and one complication is a cerebrospinal fluid leak,

which often manifests as a headache. For the pump to work properly, it must remain flat and an abdominal binder may be used to maintain its proper position.

36. C
NSAIDs can greatly reduce pain caused by inflammation and swelling. Acetaminophen has few, if any, anti-inflammatory properties and a local anesthetic has none. Although opioid agonists can help relieve acute pain, an agonist/antagonist has many side effects and does not affect inflammation.

37. D
These two drugs are from different categories and help relieve pain in different ways. They do not interfere with each other and can be given together without ill effects.

38. B
A TENS unit uses electrical stimulation to increase the sensation of "tingling" or "pins and needles" and reduce the sensation of pain transmitted along sensory nerve tracts. It does not alter blood flow, increase brain secretion of hormones, or truly distract the client.

39. A, C, D
Using a heating pad at the patch site increases its movement across the skin and increases blood flow to the area. Both actions allow the drug to be absorbed more rapidly and increase the risk for complications, especially respiratory depression. Although not a lot of drug remains in the old patches, enough drug could be present to increase the blood level of the drug and increase the risk for side effects. Folding the patch in half would reduce drug absorption. Returning used patches to the clinic for disposal does not increase the client's risk for overdose. Washing the area (and drying it) increases the adhesive properties of the patch and not its absorption properties. The same is true for applying tape over the patch.

40. A
Although the frequency of dosage increases may be as often as 10 to 15 minutes for IV opioids, at least 24 hours is used as the titration time

average before increasing the dose of transdermal fentanyl. This medication patch is formulated as continuous release to help maintain a constant effective blood level of the drug. The client is reassessed after at least 24 hours of transdermal fentanyl therapy to determine effectiveness and the need to manage breakthrough pain before increasing the fentanyl dose.

41. A, E, F

NSAIDs disrupt platelet action and reduce clotting, which increases the risk for bleeding in response to minor trauma. NSAIDs also reduce the thick, gel-like coating of the stomach, allowing normal stomach acids to irritate the stomach lining and form ulcers. Finally, NSAIDs cause the kidneys to retain more sodium and water. These enter the bloodstream and raise blood pressure.

42. A, B, C, E

Medical marijuana has common side effects of increased heart rate, impaired attention, increased appetite, and dry mouth. This preparation does not contain THC, a major component of nonmedical marijuana, which is psychoactive and responsible for side effects that are not associated with cannabis.

43. A, C, E

Fentanyl/carfentanyl can be absorbed through the skin, especially mucous membranes, and cause overdose symptoms (drowsiness, difficulty breathing, change in cognition or level of consciousness, cold clammy skin, etc.) in any person who comes into contact with the drug.

Shaking linens used by a client could aerosolize the drug (powder form) and increase the spread of this contaminant in the immediate environment and must be avoided. Soap and water are used to clean the hands because using alcohol-based hand rubs can enhance skin absorption of the drug.

44. D

This action is both deceitful and unethical. It negates the client's concerns and prevents proper pain management. Reminding the colleague allows him or her to reflect on the proposed behavior and think about other options. Being confrontational is not the best first step. Nurses have an obligation to do what is right. Supporting or ignoring deceitful behavior is not appropriate professional behavior.

6 CHAPTER

Concepts of Genetics and Genomics

1. What is the current greatest benefit of genomic health care for adult clients?
   A. Allows the use of genetic engineering to alter or "edit" mutated genes to reduce the risk for future development of a specific disorder
   B. Establishes the level of personal risk for the development of a specific disorder and directs possible prevention strategies
   C. Pin-points the specific ancestor within an extended family responsible for transmitting an inherited disorder
   D. Identifying the actual presence of a specific disorder before symptoms develop

2. What is the major reason medical-surgical nurses need to understand the genetic basis for diseases?
   A. Nurses must be prepared to offer genetic counseling at the bedside.
   B. Clients read about genetics and ask questions about this topic.
   C. Many serious adult-onset diseases have a genetic component.
   D. Most adult-onset diseases can cause genetic anomalies.

3. A client asks the nurse to explain the term "microbiome." Which explanation is most accurate?
   A. Microbiome is a new genetics concern because it refers to microorganisms that are pathogenic.
   B. Microbiome is all the microorganisms that move from place to place within the human body.
   C. Microbiome is the bacteria or viruses that allow disease-causing genetic mutations to occur.
   D. Microbiome is the genomes of all the microorganisms that coexist in and on a person.

4. What concept is exemplified by the fact that estrogen is secreted only by the ovaries and adrenal glands even though the estrogen gene is present in every cell type?
   A. Selective gene expression
   B. Beneficial gene mutation
   C. Reduced penetrance
   D. Genomic instability

5. When taking a client's history, which information suggests to the nurse that the client may have an increased genetic risk for a disease or disorder? **Select all that apply.**
   A. First-degree relative has type 2 diabetes mellitus.
   B. Client was exposed to the agent orange carcinogen during a war.
   C. Client has been diagnosed with two different types of cancer.
   D. Sister was diagnosed with breast cancer at 24 years of age.
   E. Father had rheumatic fever at 10 years of age.
   F. Client reports never engaging in regular exercise.

6. Which situation is most likely to be caused by a genetic polymorphism?
   A. A client reports pain relief from morphine but not from an equigesic dose of codeine.
   B. The intestinal microbiome of a client is changed by 3 weeks of antibiotic therapy.
   C. The son of an adult male with hemophilia is neither a hemophiliac nor a carrier of the trait.
   D. Blood type can be determined by a simple laboratory test rather than by analysis of DNA sequencing.

7. The nurse is aware that which type of genetic testing examines a client's chromosomes for variations in number or structure.
   A. Cytogenetic testing
   B. Presymptomatic testing
   C. Predictive testing
   D. Direct DNA sequencing of a specific gene

8. A client's genetic sequence for a specific protein has a mutation. Which outcomes does the nurse expect to result from this mutation? **Select all that apply**.
   A. Function of the protein may be reduced.
   B. Function of the protein may be the same.
   C. Function of the protein may be eliminated.
   D. Function of the protein may result in a totally different protein.
   E. Function of the protein may be normal or expected.
   F. Function of the protein may be enhanced.

9. Which statement regarding the influence of epigenetic changes on gene expression is **always** true?
   A. The change must be inherited from the parent of the same gender as the child for expression to be affected.
   B. Although gene expression is changed by inheriting these changes, the gene's DNA sequence remains unaffected.
   C. Epigenetic changes must first occur in the parental somatic cells in order to be inherited.
   D. These changes occur throughout the genome rather than in the area of any single specific gene.

10. When constructing a pedigree around a client's specific health problem, what is the minimal number of generations the nurse needs to obtain information about to accurately assess the presence or absence of a genetic factor in disease development?
    A. 1
    B. 2
    C. 3
    D. 4

11. How does the nurse expect warfarin therapy to be specifically modified for a Caucasian client with a CYP variation that slows the metabolism of warfarin?
    A. The drug will need to be administered by the intravenous route only.
    B. The drug will need to be administered by transdermal patch only.
    C. Higher drug doses are needed to reach the target anticoagulation level.
    D. Lower drug doses are needed to reach the target anticoagulation level.

12. Which criteria does the nurse use to determine if the inheritance of a specific health problem, such as type 2 diabetes mellitus, is autosomal dominant (AD)? **Select all that apply.**
    A. The trait/disorder appears in every other generation.
    B. The risk for the affected person to pass the trait/disorder to a child is 50% with each pregnancy.
    C. Unaffected people do not have affected children.
    D. The trait/disorder is found equally in males and females.
    E. For the trait/disorder to be expressed, both alleles must be dominant.
    F. The trait/disorder will appear in less than 25% of the entire family (kindred).

13. Which statement by a client who has just been diagnosed with a genetic health problem that has an autosomal recessive pattern of inheritance indicates to the nurse that the client has correct understanding regarding the diagnosis?
    A. If my wife doesn't have the problem and is not a carrier, my children will not have this problem.
    B. We should make certain to abort any pregnancy with a boy to prevent transmitting this gene on to our children.
    C. I wish only one of my genes (alleles) was affected so I could remain healthy by replacing it with a normal gene.
    D. Luckily, since I do have the problem and the risk is only 25% because my parents are both carriers, neither of my two brothers will get this disease.

14. Why are the male offspring of men with an X-linked recessive disorder not affected with the disorder if their mothers are not carriers?
    A. Males have only one X chromosome.
    B. Sons do not inherit an X chromosome from their fathers.
    C. X-linked recessive disorders usually skip a generation.
    D. X-linked recessive disorders have dominant expression in males.

15. The nurse is expected to use which "key" action when providing any level of genetic counseling to a client?
    A. Being nondirective
    B. Providing both information and advice to the client
    C. Ensuring that the client actually follows through with prescribed genetic testing
    D. Collaborating with the primary health-care provider to notify all family members of a client's genetic risk

16. A client whose mother has Huntington disease (HD) is told by a primary health care provider that the client must have genetic testing for this disorder. The nurse who witnesses this interaction knows which of the following principles of professional and ethical behavior is/are being violated in this situation? **Select all that apply.**
    A. Right to know versus the right not to know
    B. Confidentiality
    C. Nondirective
    D. Beneficence
    E. Autonomy
    F. Coercion

17. Which actions are consistent with the expected role of the medical-surgical nurse in genetic testing? **Select all that apply.**
    A. Ensuring that the client's rights are respected.
    B. Providing complete information on the results of the testing.
    C. Referring the client to a genetic counselor.
    D. Always being present when the client receives genetic counseling.
    E. Teaching clients about the nature of genetic testing.
    F. Establishing whether or not the client understands the information provided.

18. Which statements about gene mutations or variations are accurate? **Select all that apply.**
    A. All gene mutations are serious and potentially deadly.
    B. Gene variations that increase the risk for a disorder are *susceptibility* genes.
    C. Mutations that occur in the body cells (somatic) can be passed from parents to children.
    D. Germline mutations (sex cells) cannot be passed from parents to children.
    E. Gene variations that decrease the risk for a disorder are *protective* or *resistance* genes.
    F. Somatic cell gene mutations may cause increased risk for cancer in cells.

19. For which disorders is predisposition genetic testing performed? **Select all that apply.**
    A. Sickle cell disease
    B. *BRCA1* mutation breast cancer
    C. Huntington disease
    D. Type 1 diabetes mellitus
    E. Lung cancer
    F. Hereditary colorectal cancers

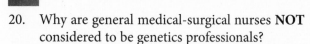

20. Why are general medical-surgical nurses **NOT** considered to be genetics professionals?
    A. The typical clients seen by these health professionals have acute conditions rather than chronic conditions, and thus genetic influence is irrelevant.
    B. Most of today's nurses were educated before completion of the human genome research project.
    C. These professionals have minimal experience with genetics laboratory techniques.
    D. The focus of basic nursing education is the study of nursing rather than genetics.

Chapter 6 Answer Key

1. B
   By identifying personal risk for developing a specific disorder, clients would be available to either take advantage of primary prevention strategies to prevent development of the disorder or participate in monitoring strategies for secondary prevention that would help identify the problem early when therapy may modify or delay the serious consequences of the disorder. At the present time, mutated genes cannot be modified or edited. Identifying the original ancestor who first transmitted the gene to his or her children and further generations does nothing to benefit the client. Although some types of genetic testing can identify the presence of a disorder before symptoms develop, this action does not usually alter the course of the disorder.

2. C
   At one time, only childhood problems and birth defects were thought to have a genetic basis. Current state of the science indicates that many common adult-onset disorders, such as heart disease, hypertension, diabetes, adult-onset hearing loss, COPD, cancer, and many others, have one or more genetic components. Some of these can be modified.

3. D
   Many "normal flora" microorganisms exist on and in the human body that play a role in maintaining health and are not pathogens. These organisms differ from person to person depending on environmental conditions. Alterations in a person's microbiome can increase the risk for many diseases.

4. A
   Part of cellular regulation is the selective expression or "turning on" of specific genes in cells to allow them to perform their normal physiologic functions to make the whole body work well. Expression of normal genes in their proper cells only is not a mutation of any kind. Penetrance is related to whether a gene is expressed at all anywhere when it is present. Genomic instability is a condition in which gene changes constantly occur, reducing function and increasing the risk for cancer development if cellular regulation is lost.

5. A, C, D
   The client's history reveals several red flags associated with an increased risk for any genetic problem, including having a first-degree relative with an identified genetic problem, having more than one type of cancer, and having a first-degree relative with a cancer diagnosis at an early age. Exposure to a carcinogen is an environmental factor, not a genetic one, as is never exercising. An infection in a parent long ago does not constitute an increased genetic risk.

6. A

A polymorphism is a variation in a gene that somewhat alters the function of the protein coded by it. A common polymorphism is one that occurs in a specific enzyme that prevents the conversion of codeine at the tissue level into morphine. Thus clients with this polymorphism do obtain pain relief when given morphine but not when given codeine.

7. A

The type of test that examines chromosomes is cytogenetic testing. Presymptomatic testing determines whether one specific gene mutation is present, so that clients can prepare for a problem before symptoms appear. Predictive testing tests an asymptomatic person to determine future genetic risk. Direct DNA sequencing is performed at the gene level, not the chromosomal level.

8. A, C

A mutation in a gene coding for a protein either reduces or eliminates the function of that protein. A variation or polymorphism can result in the function remaining the same (normal), or even be enhanced. Gene mutations do not change one protein into another protein.

9. B

Epigenetic events affect gene expression but do not change DNA sequences. These influences are not related to the gender of the parent transmitting them. Most likely, changes occurring in the gametes (ova and sperm) or in all body cells are the events that can be transmitted to the next generation. Thus, the changes can occur throughout the genome or in areas of single genes.

10. C

Unless a pedigree shows at least three generations, no supportable conclusions regarding transmission patterns can be made.

11. D

Slower metabolism of the drug allows it to remain as an active drug in the client's system longer and continue to reduce blood clotting to a greater degree. Thus this client's dose must be lower than average to achieve the same level of effect without greatly increasing the client's risk for bleeding. Warfarin is only an oral drug.

12. B, C, D

For a genetic trait or disorder to be transmitted following an autosomal dominant pattern of inheritance, the problem or trait appears in every generation and only one allele needs to be dominant for it to be expressed. With two possible alleles (one dominant and one recessive or not mutated), the risk for an affected person expressing the trait/disorder to transmit it to his or her children is 50% with each pregnancy. With the gene being on an autosome and not a sex chromosome, the trait/disorder would be about equally expressed in males and females. A person who does not express the trait/disorder, and thus does not have the allele for it, cannot pass the trait/disorder to his or her children. With the allele for the disorder having a 50% risk for transmission, the expected rate of its appearance within the family is at least 50%.

13. A

Because this client can only contribute one of his two affected alleles to any child and his wife is not a carrier, none of their children will be affected but all of them will be carriers. With the disorder being autosomal, males and females would be affected equally. At this time, gene replacement is not a therapeutic option. The risk is 25% with each pregnancy, not for these specific siblings. Thus, each of three brothers have an equal 25% risk for developing the disorder.

14. B

If at conception a zygote inherited an X chromosome from its father, the resulting child would be a girl. Sons do not inherit an X chromosome from their fathers and do not inherit a Y chromosome from their mothers.

15. A

Regardless of the genetics preparation of a health care professional who is providing any level of genetic counseling, a "key" feature is to be nondirective. The client alone is the only person who must make the decision to have or not have genetic testing and is not required to share the results with anyone. Also, no matter how intense or great the risk is for the client to develop the genetic disorder, he or she has the right to refuse to participate in testing at any level.

16. A, C, E, F
All professionals involved in genetic testing or counseling must respect the client's autonomy and self determination in making a decision and not coerce him or her into an action. In this situation, confidentiality has not been violated. At this point, beneficence has not been violated and the health care professional does have good intentions. However, if the client is actually coerced into having the test and it is positive, his or her psychosocial health may be detrimentally affected.

17. A, C, E, F
Although medical-surgical nurses are not considered genetic professionals, they are client and family advocates. The advocacy role includes ensuring that whomever is providing genetic counseling or test respects the client's rights, obtains informed consent, and respects the client's decisions. Advocacy also includes determining whether the client understands what he or she is told about genetic testing. Another role is assisting the client and family to find the right level of genetic counseling before genetic testing occurs. The nurse also can help the client understand just what genetic testing is and how it is different from other tests. The nurse may be present when genetic counseling occurs only if the client requests this.

18. B, E, F
Not all gene mutations are deadly or serious, depending on the nature of the gene involved. Susceptibility gene variations increase the risk for developing a specific disorder, whereas protective or resistance gene variations reduce the risk for developing a specific disorder. Germline mutations occur before conception and can be passed from parent to child; however, somatic mutations occur after conception and cannot be passed from parent to child but do increase the risk for cancer development in the cells that have a somatic mutation.

19. B, F
An increased risk for development of both *BRCA1* mutation breast cancer and hereditary colorectal cancer can be assessed with predisposition genetic testing although an individual with a positive test still has a chance for not developing either disease. Sickle cell disease testing would be for carrier status or actual diagnosis of the disorder. Huntington disease testing is done as presymptomatic genetic testing because if the mutation is present, the client will develop Huntington disease. There is no predisposition genetic testing available for any type of diabetes mellitus. Lung cancer is an environmental exposure cancer development with no genetic predisposition testing available.

20. D
The title of genetics professional implies that the individual has extensive education and often, special credentialing in some aspect of the broad genetics field. By these criteria, a person with an entry-level degree in a health care profession, such as registered nurse, registered dietitian nutritionist, physical therapist, pharmacist, or physician/surgeon, is not a genetics professional because genetics was not the focus of their professional education. Although knowledge of genetics laboratory techniques is helpful to genetics professionals, clinical geneticists are not expert technicians. Acute health problems often have a genetic input to the disorder, as does the client's response to therapy.

7
CHAPTER

Concepts of Rehabilitation for Chronic and Disabling Health Problems

1. In which settings would the older adult client receive post-acute care after being discharged from an acute care facility? **Select all that apply.**
    A. Inpatient rehabilitation facility
    B. Skilled nursing facility
    C. Physical therapy clinic
    D. Long-term care hospital
    E. Home health agency
    F. Community acute care facility

2. After a car crash, an older adult is unable to perform activities of daily living, such as bathing, without assistance. Which term does this exemplify?
    A. Rehabilitation
    B. Paresis
    C. Aphasia
    D. Disability

3. The client wears street clothes and makes decisions about how their day will be planned. In which type of rehabilitation setting does the nurse find the client? **Select all that apply.**
    A. Skilled nursing facility
    B. Short-term rehabilitation facility
    C. Acute care facility
    D. Custodial nursing home
    E. Assisted-living facility
    F. Long-term care nursing home

4. When caring for a client, which responsibilities are part of the nurse's role as a member of the rehabilitation team? **Select all that apply.**
    A. Directs all members of the rehabilitation team
    B. Coordinates rehabilitation team activities
    C. Plans for continuity of care when the client is discharged
    D. Delegates or assigns client care only to the assistive personnel (AP)
    E. Creates a therapeutic rehabilitation milieu
    F. Advocates for the client and family

5. Which member of the rehabilitation team would **best** help a client with self-feeding, bathing, and dressing?
    A. Rehabilitation nurse
    B. Occupational therapist
    C. Physical therapist
    D. Recreational therapist

6. Which statement **best** describes the desired outcome of rehabilitation?
    A. To restore and maintain the client's capacities to the best extent possible
    B. To rely on a specific plan of care standardized based on the medical diagnosis
    C. To identify one conceptual framework to serve as the sole model for the practice of rehabilitation nursing
    D. To enable clients and families to identify strategies to successfully meet short-term goals

7. Which are the features of the rehabilitation milieu that the nurse would create for rehabilitation clients? **Select all that apply.**
   A. Making the unit more regimented and schedule oriented
   B. Allowing clients to practice self-management skills
   C. Delegating most client bathing tasks to the AP
   D. Encouraging clients and providing emotional support
   E. Promoting self-esteem
   F. Keeping family and friend visits to a minimum for the first 2 weeks

8. Which factors will the nurse assess when implementing a position change schedule for an older adult rehabilitation client? **Select all that apply.**
   A. Ability of the client to change positions independently
   B. Type or injury the client sustained
   C. Presence of abnormal breath sounds
   D. Condition of client's skin with each position change
   E. Age of the client
   F. Frailty of the client

9. When an assistive personnel (AP) is turning and repositioning an older adult rehabilitation client, for which action must the nurse intervene?
   A. AP carefully cleans and dries the skin after an incontinence episode
   B. AP assists the client to turn and reposition in bed every 2 hours
   C. AP uses pillows to support the client while turned on their side
   D. AP rubs and massages a reddened area on the client's hip

10. The client's dietary history reveals low fluid intake as well as little fiber intake. For which **priority** gastrointestinal problem will the RN create a plan to avoid?
    A. Diarrhea
    B. Electrolyte imbalance
    C. Constipation
    D. Emaciation

11. Which assessment findings would the nurse expect to find when admitting a client with a history of decreased cardiac output to the rehabilitation program?
    A. Ability to ambulate without chest pains
    B. Feeling rested upon awakening from sleep
    C. Ability to move from sitting to standing position easily
    D. Fatigue, chest pain, and the need for rest periods

12. The occupational therapist is teaching a client about activities of daily living (ADLs) and independent activities of daily living (IADLs). Which activities are IADLs? **Select all that apply.**
    A. Cooking a meal
    B. Ambulating to the bathroom
    C. Shopping for groceries
    D. Getting out of bed into a chair
    E. Using a telephone
    F. Bathing

13. Which statements correctly describe the Functional Independence Measure (FIM)? **Select all that apply.**
    A. It tries to measure what a person should do, whatever the diagnosis or impairment.
    B. It tries to measure what a person actually does, whatever the diagnosis or impairment.
    C. It is a basic indicator of the severity of a disability.
    D. Evaluation may be done at specified times during therapy to determine client progress.
    E. The assessment may be performed by various health care disciplines.
    F. Categories for assessment are self-care, sphincter control, mobility and locomotion, communication, and cognition.

14. Which option **best** describes the purpose of a vocational assessment that a nurse will do for a client in rehabilitation?
    A. Demonstrates improvements in physical, social, cognitive, and emotional functions
    B. Assists the client to find meaningful training, education, or employment after discharge from a rehabilitation setting
    C. Evaluates and retrains clients with deficits that distort consonant and vowel production
    D. Identifies resources to assist with client injuries that cause deficits in cognition

15. Which abilities does manual muscle testing performed by physical therapy (PT) for a rehabilitation client determine?
    A. Range of motion and resistance to gravity
    B. Body flexibility and muscle strength
    C. Voluntary versus involuntary movement
    D. Muscle strength and pain on movement

16. During a psychosocial assessment of a rehabilitation client, the nurse discovers that the client's only support system is a married son who lives 2,500 miles away. For which **priority** complication must the nurse plan to monitor?
    A. Panic
    B. Depression
    C. Fear
    D. Anxiety

17. While assisting a client with hemiplegia to dress, what instructions from the occupational therapist (OT) would the nurse be sure to reinforce?
    A. Use the strong arm to lift the shirt over both arms and then pull the shirt over the head.
    B. Button all the buttons, then slide the shirt over the head and put both arms in the sleeves.
    C. Put on the shirt by first placing the unaffected arm into the sleeve, followed by the affected arm.
    D. Put the shirt on by first placing the affected arm into the sleeve, followed by the unaffected arm.

18. Which findings would be **relevant data** when the nurse assesses the musculoskeletal system of an older adult rehabilitation client? **Select all that apply.**
    A. Range of motion
    B. Fluid intake
    C. Functional ability
    D. Weight loss or gain
    E. Endurance
    F. Muscle strength
    G. Sensation

19. Which assistive device would the nurse recommend for a client who can no longer tie their shoes?
    A. Long-handled reacher
    B. Velcro shoe closer
    C. Extended shoehorn
    D. Hook and loop fastener

20. Which practices should be taught by the RN to staff and followed by the staff for safe handling and mobility of clients?
    A. Keep the client about 2 to 3 feet from your body to prevent reaching.
    B. Maintain a narrow but stable base with your feet.
    C. Keep the client or work directly in front of you to prevent your spine from rotating.
    D. Position the bed at hip level while providing direct care and at waist level when moving clients.

21. Which methods of transfer would a nurse use for a rehabilitation client at a facility that follows a no-lift or limited-lift policy? **Select all that apply.**
    A. An electric-powered, portable sit-to-stand device
    B. No transfers for clients who are unable to move independently
    C. Independent movement of a client when they are able
    D. Multiple staff assistance when physically lifting a patient
    E. Mechanical full-body lift that is ceiling or wall mounted, or is portable
    F. Following all facility guidelines for safe patient transfer

22. Which actions would the nurse teach clients and families to **best** prevent pressure injury from immobility in an older adult rehabilitation client? **Select all that apply.**
    A. Provide foods high in protein, carbohydrates, and vitamins for sufficient nutrition.
    B. Use pressure-relieving devices when turning and repositioning is difficult.
    C. Maintain good skin care by keeping the skin clean and dry, and applying a moisturizer.
    D. Inspect the skin after each repositioning for reddened areas.
    E. Report reddened areas that do not fade within 30 minutes after pressure relief to the HCP.
    F. Massage reddened areas to facilitate blood flow with oxygen and nutrient delivery.
    G. Change positions often to relieve pressure on all bony prominences.

23. Which instructions would the nurse give the AP when caring for an older adult rehabilitation client who sits in a wheelchair most of the day, to **prevent harm**? **Select all that apply.**
    A. "Be sure to place the special gel pad on the wheelchair seat before getting the client up."
    B. "Make sure that the client gets back in the bed for all meals."
    C. "The client will need to be repositioned every 1 to 2 hours."
    D. "If the client is sleeping in the wheelchair, do not wake him or her for repositioning."
    E. "Remind the client to perform pressure relief by using arms to lift buttocks off the seat for 20 seconds every hour."
    F. "Teach the client to do arm exercises to strengthen their arms to perform pressure relief, sometimes called wheelchair push-ups."

24. How will the nurse recognize that a client with a lower motor neuron injury below T12 has a flaccid bladder?
    A. The client has incontinence due to loss of sensation.
    B. The client has incontinence and inability to empty the bladder completely.
    C. The client has urinary retention with dribbling due to overflow of urine.
    D. The client has incontinence caused by inability to wait for a commode or bedpan.

25. Which teaching points would the nurse include when teaching a client with a flaccid bladder about intermittent catheterization? **Select all that apply.**
    A. The procedure is completed as a sterile procedure at all times.
    B. A catheter is inserted every few hours to drain the urine after the client attempts to void.
    C. The Crede and Valsalva maneuvers are tried for voiding before the catheter is inserted.
    D. A residual of less than 100 to 150 mL leads to increasing the time between catheter insertions.
    E. The maximum time between catheter insertions to drain urine is 4 hours.
    F. A specialized appliance to help perform the catheter insertion can be used at home when problems with dexterity occur.

26. For which older adult rehabilitation client with constipation must the nurse **avoid** performing digital stimulation to induce evacuation of stool to **prevent harm**?
    A. Client with spinal cord injury resulting from a diving accident
    B. Client with myocardial infarction who is beginning cardiac rehabilitation
    C. Client with multiple sclerosis
    D. Client with bowel incontinence caused by cognitive deficit

27. Which prescribed action does the nurse expect from the HCP for a client who does regular intermittent urinary catheterization?
   A. Immediate antibiotic treatment for the chronic bacteriuria found on urinalysis
   B. Insertion of an indwelling urinary catheter for accurate measurement of output
   C. No treatment of the bacteriuria if the client has no symptoms of urinary tract infection
   D. Testing of all care providers to determine if they are positive for bacteriuria

28. Which action would the nurse assign to the assistive personnel (AP) when caring for a client with overactive bladder?
   A. Assess the client's bladder for fullness after each voiding.
   B. Perform a bladder scan at the bedside after each intermittent catheter insertion.
   C. Toilet the client every 2 hours during the day and every 3 to 4 hours at night.
   D. Insert an intermittent urinary catheter sterilely every 4 hours.

29. Which finding in an older adult client with mild overactive bladder who is receiving oxybutynin will the nurse report to the HCP?
   A. Burning on voiding
   B. Dribbling at night
   C. Sudden voiding
   D. Hallucinations

30. The older adult rehabilitation client with hypertension is taking antihypertensive drugs. Before assigning the AP to assist the client to rise from the bed, what is the nurse's **priority** assessment?
   A. Check blood pressure in both arms.
   B. Perform a gait assessment.
   C. Ask the client about chest pain with activity.
   D. Complete a set of orthostatic vital signs.

31. For a client in a long-term setting, which are foci for the coordinated efforts of restorative nursing programs? **Select all that apply.**
   A. Bed mobility
   B. Nutrition
   C. Communication
   D. Walking
   E. Passive range of motion
   F. Dressing

32. A rehabilitation client becomes easily fatigued when walking. Which assistive device would be **best** for the nurse to recommend for this client?
   A. Wheelchair
   B. Cane with a wide base
   C. Walker with a seat
   D. Electric scooter

33. What is the **first** step for patient safety that the nurse takes when providing gait training with assistive devices such as walkers or canes?
   A. Apply a transfer belt around the client's waist.
   B. Instruct the client to take small steps.
   C. Ensure that the client's body is well balanced.
   D. Guide the client into a standing position.

34. Which action does the nurse use with a client when describing the cane-centered procedure for gait training?
   A. Remind the client to place the weak hand on the cane.
   B. The client should move the cane and stronger leg forward at the same time.
   C. The height of the cane should be even with the client's wrist when the arm is at their side.
   D. Instruct the client to take small steps.

35. Which actions will a nurse consider when administering a bisacodyl suppository to a rehabilitation client with flaccid bowel and constipation? **Select all that apply.**
    A. Gather the suppository, a lubricant, and a glove for insertion.
    B. Administer the suppository when the client expects to have a bowel movement (e.g., after a meal).
    C. Place the suppository against the bowel wall to stimulate the sacral reflex arc and promote rectal emptying.
    D. Expect results to occur within 30 minutes to an hour.
    E. Using a suppository every second or third day is usually effective in re-establishing a defecation pattern.
    F. If this is not successful, it may be necessary to use digital stimulation.

36. Which action does the nurse implement when caring for a rehabilitation client who shows fatigue?
    A. Get everything done in the morning so that the client can rest throughout the afternoon.
    B. Schedule frequent rest periods throughout the day, especially before activities.
    C. Instruct the client to perform major tasks in the afternoon when they have more energy.
    D. Encourage the client to complete all morning care before breakfast.

Chapter 7 Answer Key

1. A, B, D, E
   Option C is a clinic focused primarily on physical aspects of rehabilitation. Option F is an acute care facility which is not focused on the long-term needs of an older adult client. The remaining options are appropriate for longer-term needs which will vary in terms of the amount and type of rehabilitation, nursing care, health care provider, and other services offered. The goal of these facilities is to minimize activity limitation and to maximize participation in meaningful activities.

2. D
   Disability is a physical or mental condition that limits a person's movements, senses, or activities. Aphasia is inability to use or comprehend spoken or written language due to brain injury or disease. Paresis is weakness. Rehabilitation is the philosophy of practice and an attitude toward caring for clients with disabilities and chronic health conditions.

3. A, D, E
   Clients in skilled nursing facilities, custodial nursing homes, and assisted-living facilities are called residents. They live at the facility and have all the rights of anyone living in their home. They wear street clothes and have choices in what they eat and how they plan each day.

4. B, C, E, F
   The nurse's role in the rehabilitation setting is complex, including advocating for the client and family, creating a therapeutic milieu, providing and coordinating whole-person care, coordinating rehabilitation team activities, acting as a resource for the rehabilitation team, communicating with all members of the rehabilitation team, planning for continuity of care when a client is discharged, and evaluating the effectiveness or the plan of care for the client and family. The nurse would delegate or assign client care to other members of the team besides APs, and would not direct all members of the team.

5. B
   An occupational therapist works with a client to develop fine motor skills used in ADLs such as eating, bathing, grooming and dressing. PT focuses on helping a client by concentrating on gross mobility such as walking with assistive devices, or transferring (e.g., moving into and out of bed). A rehabilitation nurse's role is complex (see Table 7.1 in your textbook). Recreational

therapists help clients to continue or develop recreation or leisure interests.

6.   A

The desired outcome of rehabilitation is that the client will return to the best possible physical, mental, social, vocational, and economic capacity and participate in society. It is not limited to return of function, but includes education and therapy.

7.   B, D, E

The rehabilitation milieu should include allowing clients to practice self-management skills, encouraging clients and providing emotional support, promoting self-esteem, and making the unit more homelike. Clients are encouraged to do most if not all of their self-care, with APs only helping as needed. Families and friends are encouraged to visit.

8.   A, B, D, E, F

The best intervention to prevent pressure injury and maintain tissue integrity is frequent position changes in combination with adequate skin care and sufficient nutritional intake. Clients should be repositioned at the minimum every 2 hours. If a client can reposition independently, nursing staff need to remind them to do this; however, if they are unable to reposition themselves, then staff must assist (e.g., can be delegated to APs). An older adult who is frail or has thin skin may need turning more often. Clients need skin assessment with each turn (e.g., if redness does not fade in 30 minutes, the client may have stage I pressure area). Also be aware that clients who sit in wheelchairs for long periods need to be repositioned every 1 to 2 hours.

9.   D

The nurse must teach the AP to *avoid* rubbing reddened areas to prevent damage to the client's fragile capillary system. The other options are appropriate for the AP when assisting a client to turn and reposition in bed. The AP would also apply a moisturizer after cleaning and carefully drying soiled area, and if prescribed could use a topical barrier cream for a client who is incontinent.

10.   C

Most rehabilitation clients are at risk for constipation (especially older adults). Nurses must teach clients and families the importance of adequate fluid intake (at least 8 glasses a day) and fiber in the diet (20 to 35 g a day). Encourage whole grains, legumes and bran cereals, as well as five servings of fruit and vegetables. Another important point is to have the client sit upright on a bedside commode or toilet to facilitate defecation.

11.   D

Altered cardiac status can affect a client's cardiac output (e.g., decrease) and lead to activity intolerance. Signs and symptoms of decreased cardiac output include fatigue and chest pain. The nurse must assess the client for what causes and what relieves these symptoms. They may need drug therapy for the chest pain and often need rest periods for symptom relief. Activity levels may need to be modified for these clients.

12.   A, C, E

IADLs are independent living skills often requiring fine motor skills and taught by occupational therapists. These include cooking, shopping, and using a telephone. Ambulating to the bathroom, getting up into a chair, and bathing fall into the category of ADLs that focus on more gross motor skills.

13.   B, C, D, E, F

The FIM is a commonly used assessment tool intended to measure the burden of care for a client. Categories of assessment are self-care, sphincter control, mobility and locomotion, communication, and cognition. It does not try to measure what a client should do or how the client would perform under different circumstances.

14.   B

A vocational rehabilitation assessment is the process of identifying and appraising an individual's level of functioning in relation to **vocational** preparation, employment selection, and career decision making. The rehabilitation team assesses the cognitive and physical demands of the client's job to determine whether they can return to a position or if retraining in another field is necessary.

15. A

The PT is responsible for manual muscle testing. The test identifies a client's range of motion (ROM) and resistance against gravity. During the procedure, the PT determines the degree of strength present in each body segment.

16. B.

For a rehabilitation client, the nurse must assess the availability of support systems (e.g., family, friends). Clients who do not have support systems are more likely to develop depression. The nurse should ask a client what is important to them and what gives their life meaning (e.g., cultural, spiritual, religious). This may give clues to possible support systems.

17. D

The nurse must reinforce the OT's teaching about putting on a shirt. The client should first place the affected arm into a sleeve, followed by placing the unaffected arm into the other sleeve. This allows the client to use the strong (unaffected) arm to move the weak (affected) arm.

18. A, C, E, F

Relevant data for assessment of the musculoskeletal system is listed in Table 7.3 of your textbook. These data include functional ability, range of motion, endurance, and muscle strength. Weight gain or loss is relevant to assessment of the GI system, sensation to the neurologic system, and fluid intake to the renal-urinary system.

19. B

Velcro shoe closure or elastic shoelaces would be the best choices because they eliminate the need for tying shoes.

20. C

Safe client handling and mobility recommends teaching staff about and using these general practices: Maintain a wide, stable base with your feet; Place the bed at waist level while providing care and at hip level when moving clients; Keep the client or work directly in front of you to prevent your spine from rotating; Keep the client as close to your body as possible to prevent reaching; and Use appropriate safe client handling equipment (e.g., mechanical lifts).

21. A, C, E, F

When a facility has a no-lift or limited-lift policy, this means that the nursing staff and therapists either rely on the patient independently to move and transfer, or use a powered mechanical full-body lift that is mounted (ceiling, wall) or portable. Most lifts use slings that are comfortable, safe, and easily applied. Electric-powered sit-to-stand devices may also be used.

22. A, C, D, E, G

Pressure-relieving devices do not eliminate the need for repositioning. Rubbing or massaging reddened areas that to not fade should be avoided as these findings may indicate pre-pressure injury or stage I pressure areas. The remaining options are all appropriate to use to prevent pressure injuries and must be taught to clients and families. The nurse would also teach about the use of topical barrier creams or ointments to protect skin from moisture especially when a client is incontinent.

23. A, C, E

Clients in a wheelchair are evaluated for the best seating pad that is both comfortable and reduces pressure over bony prominences; they still need to be repositioned every 1 to 2 hours. They are taught arm strengthening exercises to facilitate performing pressure relieving (lifting buttocks from seat for 20 seconds or more every hour). Clients may sit up in the wheelchair to consume meals. If a client is not repositioned every 1 to 2 hours, the risk for pressure injury increases. The PT or OT would be responsible for teaching the client arm strengthening exercises.

24. C

An underactive flaccid (areflexive) bladder results in urinary retention and overflow which manifests as dribbling. There is often interference with the reflex arc that can cause inaccurate interpretation of impulses to the brain so that the bladder fills and there is a failure to respond with a message for the bladder to contract.

25. B, C, D, F

At home, the client (or a family member or friend) will use clean technique for catheter insertion. The client should not go beyond 8 hours between catheter insertions. The remaining options are appropriate for a client needing intermittent urinary catheter insertion and should be taught by the nurse. The nurse should also teach the client and family how to perform the Crede and Valsalva maneuvers.

26. B

Digital stimulation is an example of a triggering technique that can cause a client to evacuate stool. However, it should **not** be used with clients who have cardiac disease because of the risk for inducing a vagal response that leads to a rapid decrease in heart rate (bradycardia).

27. C

Most clients who require intermittent catheterization have chronic bacteriuria (bacteria in the urine). Unless a client develops symptoms of urinary tract infection (e.g., fever, burning when voiding), the infection is not treated.

28. C

Toileting is within the scope of practice for an AP. The nurse would provide the AP with specific instructions as to the timing of the toileting and tell the AP to report the results of each toileting attempt. Assessing, inserting urinary catheters, and completing bedside bladder scans require additional training and skill and should be completed by licensed nurses.

29. D

Oxybutynin is a urinary antispasmodic drug. When these drugs are used in older adults, nurses must observe for, document, and report hallucinations, delirium, or other acute cognitive changes caused by anticholinergic effects of these drugs. Burning is associated with urinary tract infection and dribbling with flaccid bladder. Sudden voiding is associated with overactive bladder, but is not a side effect of these drugs.

30. D

A client receiving antihypertensive drugs should always be assessed for orthostatic hypotension, which is a common problem in older adults and often the cause of falls. The other assessments are important, but not as urgent a priority as assessing orthostatic vital signs. Orthostatic hypotension is indicated by a drop of more than 20 mm Hg in systolic pressure and 10 mm Hg in diastolic pressure when a client moves from lying to sitting or sitting to standing positions.

31. A, C, D, F

Restorative nursing programs are often in skilled nursing facilities (SNF). Federal regulations require a plan to prevent residents from losing their functional skills while in the facility. The foci of these coordinated efforts include bed mobility, walking, transfers, dressing, grooming, active range of motion, and communication.

32. C

A walker with a seat would give the client the option to sit down and rest when fatigued, but would still preserve the ability to walk. The wheelchair and scooter may risk the client's loss of walking stamina and increase risk for immobility. The care cane does not provide a place for the client to sit and rest.

33. A

For best practices with gait training with ambulatory aids, the first step is to apply a transfer belt around the client's waist. Second would be to guide the client to a standing position. The client must be reminded to place both hands on the walker and then the client's body must be well-balanced. (See the QSEN Best Practice for Patient Safety and Quality Care - Gait Training with Selected Aids box in your text)

34. C

The height of the cane should be even with the client's wrist when the arm is placed at his or her side. The client should place the strong hand on the cane. The sequence to perform when using the cane is: move the cane and weaker leg forward at the same time, move the stronger leg one step forward, then check balance and repeat the sequence.

35. A, B, C, E
With a bisacodyl suppository, results are expected within 15 to 30 minutes. Drug therapy is not the first choice for treating constipation. When other strategies such as consistent toileting, dietary modifications, or digital stimulation are not successful, drug therapies are tried. The remaining options are accurate and should be considered before administering this type of suppository.

36. B
For this client, the nurse must plan methods for using limited energy resources. Scheduling frequent rest periods through the day, especially before activities, is a good strategy. Major tasks should be scheduled in the morning when most clients have more energy, but trying to do everything in the morning can lead to more fatigue. It is unrealistic to expect a client with fatigue to complete all morning care before breakfast.

8
CHAPTER

Concepts of Care for Patients at End-of-Life

1. Which statements are true about the nature of death in the United States? **Select all that apply.**
   A. Most deaths occur suddenly and unexpectedly.
   B. Most people die after a long period of chronic illness.
   C. Most people die after the age of 75.
   D. The most common cause of death is heart disease.
   E. Medicare covers the cost of death for most people.
   F. Most people die at home just as they wish.

2. Which are the manifestations of death? **Select all that apply**
   A. Loss of heartbeat
   B. Unresponsiveness to physical or verbal stimuli
   C. Absence of spontaneous respirations
   D. Lack of deep tendon reflexes
   E. Irreversible brain dysfunction
   F. Oliguria or no urine output

3. Which client and family have the **most** accurate understanding of hospice care?
   A. Family expects that client will resist hospice and therefore, an involuntary order is needed.
   B. Dying client and family believe it is important to focus on facilitating quality of life.
   C. Family believes that dying client receives home care when no funds are available for care in a facility.
   D. Client and family expect round-the-clock nursing care from hospice staff.

4. Which action will the nurse perform when the assistive personnel (AP) reports that the client now has a "death rattle?"
   A. Perform oropharyngeal suctioning to remove the secretions.
   B. Call the health care provider and family to notify them that the client has died.
   C. Instruct the AP to bring a postmortem pack to the client's bedside.
   D. Have the AP assist the nurse in turning the client on the side to reduce gurgling.

5. Which **priority** HCP-prescribed action would the nurse expect for a dying client with dyspnea, crackles on auscultation, peripheral edema, and other signs of heart failure?
   A. Antibiotics to prevent a possible respiratory infection
   B. Insertion of a urinary catheter for accurate measurement of output
   C. Administration of the diuretic furosemide
   D. Offer an electric fan as a comfort measure

6. The client has a durable power of attorney for health care (DPOAHC), also called a health care proxy. When would the nurse contact the designated person?
   A. The client is discovered at 3:00 a.m. in a comatose state.
   B. The client refuses to eat unless given a beer with dinner.
   C. The client is difficult to arouse for midnight vital signs.
   D. The client has an unexpected episode of dizziness.

7. What is the nurse's **best** action when a client, with a living will and do-not-resuscitate order, is dying and the daughter tells the nurse that she wants everything done to save her parent's life?
   A. Call and notify the HCP about the daughter's wishes and change the plan of care.
   B. Initiate a CODE and bring the crash cart to the client's bedside.
   C. Inform the daughter that further actions are not warranted.
   D. Respect the client's wishes and ask the chaplain to stay with the daughter.

8. Which actions are examples of passive euthanasia? **Select all that apply.**
   A. Terminating IV fluids
   B. Giving a large dose of intravenous morphine
   C. Suspending telemetry heart monitoring
   D. Administering a drug that will stop the heart
   E. Discontinuing a mechanical ventilator
   F. Turning off a temporary pacemaker

9. Which action would the nurse take when assessing a dying client with findings including coldness of extremities that are also mottled and cyanotic?
   A. Gently rub the extremities to stimulate circulation.
   B. Administer warmed oral and intravenous fluids.
   C. Reposition the client with the lower extremities dependent.
   D. Cover the client with a warm blanket.

10. Which client statement represents the symptoms **most** feared and perceived as distressing by dying clients?
    A. "I'm hoping that my health care provider prescribes a lot of pain medication."
    B. "I fear my family will be upset when I can no longer recognize them."
    C. "If I become nauseated, my wife will be distressed that I can't eat or drink."
    D. "Being short of breath frightens me and will scare my family members."

11. The use of cannabinoid-based medicines (CBM, medical marijuana) is increasing in palliative and end-of-life care. For which symptoms would the nurse expect to see these drugs prescribed for a dying client? **Select all that apply.**
    A. Pain
    B. Fatigue
    C. Difficulty with breathing
    D. Loss of appetite
    E. Anxiety
    F. Difficulty sleeping
    G. Decrease in urine output

12. What is the nurse's **best** response when the spouse of a dying client expresses concern that the client has no appetite and eats very little?
    A. Keep fluids and finger foods at the bedside for easy access when a dying client is hungry or thirsty.
    B. Explain to the spouse that loss of appetite is normal when a client nears death and teach about the risk for aspiration.
    C. Encourage the spouse to feed the client as much as he will take to maintain adequate nutrition.
    D. Request that the health care provider prescribe a dietary nutrition consult to include foods that the client prefers.

13. A client in hospice is deteriorating and the family is concerned about restlessness. Which are the **best** actions for the nurse to perform?
    A. Assess for pain, provide analgesics, and make the client as comfortable as possible.
    B. Initiate intravenous hydration to provide the client with necessary fluids.
    C. Notify the health care provider and request an order for transfer to the hospital.
    D. Encourage family members to assist the client to eat in order to gain energy.

14. Which action is **most** likely to be implemented **first** when a client near dying tells the nurse about an uncomfortable feeling of breathlessness?
    A. 10 mg furosemide IV
    B. 2 L oxygen by nasal cannula
    C. Albuterol puff by metered-dose inhaler
    D. 5 mg morphine sulfate IV

15. When caring for a client of the Jewish faith who is dying, which cultural concept must the nurse keep in mind?
    A. A client who is extremely ill and dying should not be left alone.
    B. Upon death, a priest may say a prayer and light a candle.
    C. Death is viewed a dying person may wish to die facing Mecca.
    D. On death, the eyelids should be left open but the body should be covered.

16. A dying client receiving morphine sulfate for pain is at increased risk for acute renal failure. Which assessment finding will the nurse observe that indicates worsening of renal failure and failure to excrete the morphine?
    A. Adequate pain relief
    B. Crackles and wheezes in the lungs
    C. Color, clarity, and amount of urine
    D. Signs of confusion or delirium

17. Which actions would the nurse assign to the assistive personnel (AP) for postmortem care of a client? **Select all that apply.**
    A. Ask family if they wish to help wash the client's body.
    B. Straighten the client and lower the bed to a flat position.
    C. Remove dentures, then clean and carefully store them.
    D. Wash the client and comb the hair.
    E. Place pads under the hips and around the perineum.
    F. Place a pillow under the client's head.
    G. Clean and straighten up the client's room or unit.

Chapter 8 Answer Key

1. B, D, E,
   In the United States, most deaths occur after a long chronic illness (few die suddenly or unexpectedly). Most people die after the age of 65 and are eligible for Medicare. The most common cause of death is heart disease (see Table 8.1 for other common causes). While most people wish for a peaceful death at home, most die in acute, long-term, and hospice facilities.

2. A, C, E
   The definition of death is the cessation of tissue and organ function, manifested by no heartbeat, absence of spontaneous respirations, and irreversible brain dysfunction. A client may or may not experience unresponsiveness to stimuli, oliguria, and loss of DTRs before death occurs.

3. B
   Hospice does provide care for dying clients, but the focus of hospice care is quality of life. Actions are planned to meet the clients' needs (physical, social, psychological, or spiritual). A coordinated interdisciplinary team works together to meet these needs and provide the best quality of care for the time the client has left.

4. D.
   A death rattle is heard with loud, wet respirations and this is upsetting to family, friends, and care providers. Repositioning the client to one side reduces the gurgling. The nurse should also place a small towel under the client's mouth to collect the secretions. One other action that may help is to administer an anticholinergic (e.g., 1% atropine ophthalmic) to help dry the secretions. Suctioning is not recommended because it is not effective and is often upsetting to the client.

5. C
   When a dying client shows symptoms of heart failure, the HCP may prescribe a diuretic such as furosemide to decrease blood volume, reduce vascular congestion, and decrease the workload on the heart. It can be given orally, intravenously, or subcutaneously. IV is the preferred route because it works very quickly (within minutes) and can help the client feel more comfortable. Other nonpharmacological measures could include limiting exertion, inserting a urinary catheter, elevating the client's head of bed or placing the client in a reclining chair, applying cool cloths to

the face, and encouraging therapies such as imagery and deep breathing.

6. A

The designated DPOAHC does not make decisions for the client until the HCP states that the client lacks capacity to make his or her own decisions. Usually this is because of cognitive impairment (e.g., coma). To have decision-making ability, the client must be able to receive information; evaluate, deliberate, and mentally manipulate information; and communicate a treatment preference. When the client can no longer make decisions, the DPOAHC steps in to make the decisions.

7. D

A living will identifies what a client wants and does not want when near death. A DNR order, signed by a physician or the primary HCP instructs that CPR is not to be attempted. These are meant for clients with life-limiting conditions where resuscitation is not wise. The nurse should notify the HCP but the plan of care should not be changed. Asking the chaplain or someone else to sit with the daughter is a good move. A CODE should not be initiated. CPR can be violent and uncomfortable, as well as prevent a peaceful death.

8. A, C, E, F

Withholding or withdrawing life-sustaining therapy (passive euthanasia) involves discontinuing one or more therapies that might prolong the life of a client who cannot be cured by the therapy. Withdrawing the interventions does not directly cause death. The cause of death is the progression of the client's disease and poor status. Examples include discontinuing heart monitoring, IV fluids, and mechanical ventilation or turning off a temporary pacemaker. Active euthanasia involves the HCP taking action that purposefully and directly causes death. Examples include giving drugs that can stop the heart or large doses of morphine sulfate.

9. D

When death is approaching, a comfort measure for coolness of extremities that may become discolored or mottled is to cover the client with a warm blanket. Avoid the use of electric blankets, hot water bottles, or electric heating pads to warm the extremities.

10. A

Pain is the symptom that dying clients fear the most. Opioid and nonopioid drugs are important in managing pain near the end of life. Shortness of breath, nausea, and in some cases, clients not recognizing family or friends are also fearful symptoms and must be treated, but pain is the most feared and distressful symptom for dying clients.

11. A, B, D, E, F

Most clients have CBM prescribed for pain. Other symptoms for which these drugs have been positively effective include fatigue, anorexia, sleep problems, anxiety, and nausea and vomiting. Lots of research is continuing with regard to the effectiveness of CBM in palliative and end-of-life care.

12. B

As death approaches, anorexia is one of the symptoms that normally occurs. Combined with dysphagia (difficulty swallowing), the risk for aspiration increases. While giving the client something to eat when hunger occurs, avoid forcing the client to eat too much.

13. A

When dying clients become restless or agitated, the cause is often pain. The nurse should assess for pain, provide prescribed pain medication (remember this is the greatest fear of dying clients), and perform actions to make the client as comfortable as possible (e.g., reposition, playing soothing music, speaking quietly, and keeping the room dim and noise to a minimum). The other three options do not attempt to solve the problem.

14. D

Opioids like morphine sulfate are the standard treatment for dyspnea near death. Morphine works by altering the sense of air hunger, reducing anxiety and associated oxygen consumption, and reducing pulmonary congestion.

Furosemide is a diuretic and albuterol is a bronchodilator. Oxygen therapy for dyspnea near death is not a standard of care for all dying clients, however, if a client does not respond to morphine therapy, he or she may be placed on oxygen (2 to 6 L nasal cannula).

15. A

Individuals of Jewish faith believe a person should not be left alone at the end of life. A Greek Orthodox practice surrounding death is to have a priest say a prayer and light a candle after the death. Individuals of the Muslim faith may wish to face Mecca during the end of life. The eyelids should always be closed, not left open.

16. D

When a client develops kidney failure, the failing kidney is unable to excrete the metabolites of morphine; therefore, the level of the drug increases and this leads to delirium and confusion. When this happens, the HCP considers changing pain drug from morphine to fentanyl which does not have active metabolites and can be administered transdermally.

17. B, D, E, F, G

The AP's scope of practice would include manipulating client beds, washing the client (if the family does not wish to participate), placing a pillow under the head, straightening the room, and placing pads under the client's hips and perineum. The nurse should ask the family if they would like to assist in washing the body. Dentures should be inserted if the client wore them. See the box in your text titled Best Practice for Patient Safety & Quality Care QSEN Postmortem Care for more information.

CHAPTER 9

Concepts of Care for Perioperative Patients

1. Which statements **best** describe the preoperative period when a client is being prepared for surgery? **Select all that apply.**
   A. It begins when the client makes an appointment with a surgeon to discuss the need for surgery.
   B. It ends when the client is transferred to the surgical suite.
   C. It is a time during which a client's need for surgery is established.
   D. During this time, the client receives testing and education related to the impending surgery.
   E. It begins when the client is scheduled for surgery.
   F. It is a time when clients and families receive instruction for after discharge.

2. Which is the **most** important priority for nurses when caring for a client preoperatively?
   A. Client safety
   B. Client diagnostic testing
   C. Client care documentation
   D. Client teaching

3. What are the advantages for clients whose surgery is accomplished in a same-day surgery center (outpatient surgery center)? **Select all that apply.**
   A. Cost-effective care
   B. Increased postsurgery responsibility for client
   C. Decreased need for anesthesia
   D. High degree of client satisfaction
   E. Service-oriented processes
   F. Case manager to coordinate postdischarge care

4. What is the **most** appropriate category of surgery for a client who can barely ambulate with a walker at home, who is having a left total knee replacement?
   A. Urgent
   B. Palliative
   C. Reconstructive
   D. Simple

5. What is the **best** classification for the surgery when a female client has a biopsy of a nodule found in the right breast?
   A. Cosmetic
   B. Diagnostic
   C. Minor
   D. Palliative

6. What is the **best** classification for surgery when a client with Crohn's disease has a colostomy?
   A. Preventative
   B. Reconstructive
   C. Curative
   D. Palliative

7. A client with appendicitis is to have an uncomplicated appendectomy performed. What is the **best** classification for this surgery?
   A. Elective
   B. Curative
   C. Diagnostic
   D. Minor

8. An older client is having a cataract removal surgery. What is the **best** category for this surgery?
    A. Urgent
    B. Emergent
    C. Elective
    D. Cosmetic

9. A hypertensive client with a large abdominal aortic aneurysm is having a surgical repair. What is the **best** category for this surgery?
    A. Urgent
    B. Emergent
    C. Radical
    D. Curative

10. Which surgical approach does the nurse expect will be used for a client having an uncomplicated cholecystectomy at the same-day surgery clinic?
    A. Simple
    B. Open
    C. Minimally invasive
    D. Radical

11. What is the nurse's **priority** action when interviewing a preoperative client who had a right hip replacement?
    A. Document this in the client's preoperative chart.
    B. Mark the right hip with an indelible pen.
    C. Use caution when positioning the client.
    D. Communicate this to the operative personnel.

12. Which manifestations would the nurse expect for a client with a history of malignant hyperthermia (MH)? **Select all that apply.**
    A. High body temperature
    B. Decreased serum calcium level
    C. Tachypnea
    D. Skin mottling
    E. Muscle rigidity of jaw and upper chest
    F. Increased serum potassium level

13. Which are the **most** sensitive indicators of malignant hyperthermia that the nurse would monitor for in a client? **Select all that apply.**
    A. Rise in the end-tidal carbon dioxide level with a decrease in oxygen saturation
    B. Extremely high temperature
    C. Increased metabolic rate
    D. Hypotension
    E. Tachycardia
    F. Cyanosis

14. When the nurse is screening a preoperative client, which factors increase the risk for complications during the perioperative period? **Select all that apply.**
    A. Age 72
    B. 35 pounds overweight
    C. Walks half a mile every day
    D. History of hernia repair surgery
    E. Smokes half a pack of cigarettes per day
    F. Type 2 diabetes

15. Which classification will a client having surgery, who also had a myocardial infarction (MI) 6 weeks ago, fit **best** based on the American Society of Anesthesiologists (ASA) system?
    A. ASA class I
    B. ASA class II
    C. ASA class III
    D. ASA class IV

16. What is the nurse's best response when a preoperative client speaks about fear of a reaction if blood is given during his or her surgery?
    A. "The likelihood that you will need a blood transfusion during your surgery is minimal, so do not worry about it."
    B. "You could donate some of your own blood, which is an autologous donation, a few weeks before your surgery."
    C. "With today's technology and procedures, it is very unlikely that you would have a reaction to donated blood."
    D. "The nursing staff follows very strict rules and procedures to prevent such an event from ever happening."

17. Which common laboratory tests does the nurse expect will be completed on a client prior to surgery? **Select all that apply.**
    A. Lipid profile
    B. Urinalysis
    C. Metabolic panel
    D. Clotting studies
    E. Complete blood count
    F. Fasting blood glucose

18. Informed consent implies to the nurse that a client understands which of the following? **Select all that apply.**
    A. The nature and reason for the surgery
    B. The length of stay in the hospital
    C. Who will be performing the surgery
    D. Information about the surgeon's experience
    E. The risks associated with the surgical procedure and its potential outcomes
    F. The risks associated with the use of anesthesia

19. Which statement **best** describes the interprofessional collaborative roles of the nurse and surgeon when obtaining informed consent?
    A. The nurse is responsible for having the informed consent form on the chart for the surgeon to witness.
    B. The nurse may serve as a witness that the client has been informed by the surgeon before surgery is performed.
    C. The nurse may serve as witness to the client's signature after the surgeon has the consent form signed, but before preoperative sedation is given and surgery is performed.
    D. The nurse has no duties regarding the consent form if the client has signed the informed consent form for the surgeon, even if the client then asks additional questions about the surgery.

20. After a client is prepared for surgery and before preoperative drugs are given and the client is transferred to surgery, which intervention can the nurse delegate to the assistive personnel (AP)?
    A. Assist the client to the bathroom to empty his or her bladder.
    B. Help the client to remove the hospital gown.
    C. Recheck the client's identity with another AP.
    D. Teach the client to use incentive spirometry.

21. Which postoperative interventions would the preoperative nurse typically teach a client to prevent complications following surgery? **Select all that apply.**
    A. Range-of-motion exercises
    B. Massaging of lower extremities
    C. Incision splinting
    D. Deep breathing exercises
    E. Use of incentive spirometry
    F. Taking pain drugs when experiencing severe pain

22. A blind client is to have a surgical procedure. What is the nurse's **best** response when the client asks if he or she will be permitted to sign the consent form?
    A. "Yes, but you will need to make an X instead of signing your name."
    B. "No, but you can give instructions for a responsible adult to sign for you."
    C. "Yes, but your signature will need to be witnessed by two people."
    D. "No, but your next of kin can sign the informed consent for you."

23. Which drugs usually taken daily by a client would the surgeon instruct the nurse to be sure to administer prior to surgery? **Select all that apply.**
    A. Daily multivitamin
    B. Anticonvulsant
    C. Stool softener
    D. Beta blocker
    E. Daily chewable aspirin
    F. Anticoagulant

24. What would the nurse suspect when assessing an older preoperative client and finding brittle nails; dry, flaky skin; muscle wasting; and dry, sparse hair?
    A. Poor fluid and nutrition status
    B. Improper client care by the home care giver
    C. Expected physiological changes that occur with aging
    D. Depression of the client related to the aging process

25. A preoperative client's vital signs before transport to the surgery holding area are: (BP 90/60 mm Hg, HR 110/minute, RR 24/minute, T 100.9°F [38.3°C]). What is the nurse's **priority** action?
    A. Administer acetaminophen with just a sip of water.
    B. Recheck the vital signs in 15 minutes.
    C. Call and notify the surgeon immediately.
    D. Instruct the client to cough and take deep breaths.

26. Which phase of client care in a postanesthesia care unit (PACU) requires the nurse to perform the most intensive observations and assessments?
    A. Phase I
    B. Phase II
    C. Phase III
    D. Phase IV

27. Which action does the nurse perform **first** for a postoperative client arriving on the medical-surgical unit after discharge from the postanesthesia care unit (PACU)?
    A. Calculate the client-controlled analgesia (PCA) pump maximum dose per hour to avoid an overdose.
    B. Compare the client's core body temperature with bilateral peripheral temperatures.
    C. Determine the client's level of consciousness and cognition.
    D. Assess respiratory status for adequate gas exchange.

28. Which client signs and symptoms does the nurse consider postoperative complications rather than expected responses to the experience? **Select all that apply**.
    A. Core body temperature of 95.2°F (35.1°C)
    B. Pain at the surgical site
    C. Pulmonary embolism
    D. Paralytic ileus
    E. Sore throat
    F. Sedation

29. Which information will the nurse on a medical-surgical unit expect to be included in a client "handoff" report from a postanesthesia care unit (PACU) nurse? **Select all that apply**.
    A. Is Jewish
    B. Is drowsy but coherent
    C. Is allergic to strawberries
    D. Can have a progressive diet
    E. Had a left total hip replacement
    F. Was given 3 mg morphine IV 45 minutes ago
    G. Received 2 units of packed red blood cells in the PACU
    H. Weighs 280 lb (122.2 kg) and is 5 feet 11 inches (180 cm) tall

30. What is the nurse's best **first** action for a client who is 6 hours postoperative from abdominal surgery and now has profuse bleeding from the incision?
    A. Notify the surgeon.
    B. Apply pressure to the wound dressing.
    C. Assess the client's heart rate and blood pressure.
    D. Instruct the assistive personnel (AP) to get additional dressing supplies.

31. With which clients will the nurse remain especially vigilant for respiratory complications during the first 24 hours after surgery? **Select all that apply**.
    A. 21-year-old with opioid use syndrome
    B. 39-year-old with a 55–pack-year smoking history
    C. 55-year-old with type 2 diabetes mellitus
    D. 62-year-old with chronic obstructive pulmonary disease
    E. 70-year-old with early stage Alzheimer disease
    F. 80-year-old whose last influenza vaccination was 2 years ago

32. What is the nurse's **first** action when a client develops an abdominal wound evisceration after a hard sneeze?
    A. Call for help and stay with the client.
    B. Immediately take the client's vital signs.
    C. Leave the client to immediately call the surgeon.
    D. Attempt to reduce the evisceration by gently moving the contents back into the abdomen.

33. What is the nurse's **best** action to **prevent harm** for a client who arrives at the postanesthesia care unit (PACU) with a respiratory rate of 10 breaths/min and an SpO_2 an SpO_2 of 94% after receiving fentanyl during surgery?
    A. Monitor the client for the effects of anesthetic for at least 1 hour.
    B. Administer oxygen, maintain an open airway, and monitor pulse oximetry.
    C. Perform deep suction and stimulate the client by pinching the skin on the sternum.
    D. Closely monitor vital signs and pulse oximetry readings until the client is responsive.

34. Which action for care of a client after major abdominal surgery will the nurse perform to **prevent harm**?
    A. Use the knee gatch of the bed to bend the knees and relieve pressure.
    B. Gently massage the lower legs and calves to promote venous blood return to the heart.
    C. Encourage the client to request pain medication before the pain becomes too severe.
    D. Teach the client to splint the wound for support and comfort when getting out of bed.

35. Which assessment criteria indicate to the nurse that the client who had surgery 12 hours ago is experiencing respiratory difficulty? **Select all that apply**.
    A. Oxygen saturation drops from 98% to 96%.
    B. Use of accessory muscles during respiratory effort.
    C. Presence of a high-pitched crowing sound on exhalation.
    D. Blood pressure decreases from 120/80 to 110/78 mm Hg.
    E. Respiratory rate is 29/min.
    F. Hourly urine output decreases from 50 mL to 30 mL.

36. What is the nurse's **best** action/response when the family of an 89-year-old who had surgery yesterday states that they are concerned because although the client knew who everyone was, he was unable to tell them what day it is or the name of the vice president?
    A. Ask the family how long the client has had memory problems and whether any close relatives have been diagnosed with dementia or Alzheimer disease.
    B. Reassure the family that the drugs and anesthetics used in surgery often make the older adult need a little longer to return to his presurgical baseline.
    C. Go to the client's bedside and perform a mental status examination.
    D. Notify the surgeon and request a consultation with a geriatrician.

37. When assessing the hydration status of an older postoperative client, where will the nurse assess for skin dryness and tenting?
    A. Back of the hand
    B. Forearm
    C. Sternum
    D. Shin

38. With which client is the nurse most alert for postoperative nausea and vomiting (PONV)?
    A. 36-year old with a nasogastric tube
    B. 42-year-old with a history of motion sickness
    C. 50-year-old with a recent 50 lb (kg) weight loss
    D. 65-year-old who had cataract surgery under local anesthesia

39. Which assessment finding indicates to the nurse that a client's peristaltic activity has resumed after surgery?
    A. Presence of bowel sounds
    B. Client states he is hungry
    C. Passing of flatus or stool
    D. Presence of abdominal cramping

40. Which parameter is most important for the nurse to assess for the client admitted to the postanesthesia care unit (PACU) after surgery under epidural anesthesia?
    A. Determining the client's level of consciousness
    B. Checking for pain on dorsi and plantar flexion of the foot.
    C. Assessing the response to pinprick stimulation from the feet to mid-chest level
    D. Comparing blood pressure taken in the right arm to blood pressure taken in the left arm

41. What is the nurse's **best** action when assessment of a client's nasogastric tube drainage shows the presence of 140 mL of greenish-yellow drainage?
    A. Instruct the client to drink water until the drainage is clear.
    B. Reposition the tube to increase the drainage.
    C. Call and report this finding to the surgeon.
    D. Document the finding as the only action.

42. Which nonverbal manifestations in an older adult client indicate to the nurse that the client is likely having acute pain? **Select all that apply**.
    A. Restlessness
    B. Profuse sweating
    C. Difficult to arouse
    D. Confusion
    E. Increased blood pressure
    F. Decreased heart rate

43. What is the nurse's interpretation of a postoperative client's laboratory results that show an increase in band cells (immature neutrophils)?
    A. The client is developing an infection.
    B. The results reflect a normal laboratory value.
    C. The client is anemic and may need a transfusion.
    D. The clotting factors have been consumed, increasing the risk for bleeding.

44. Which drug does the nurse prepare to administer to a postoperative client who has received an overdose of a benzodiazepine?
    A. Hydromorphone
    B. Flumazenil
    C. Midazolam
    D. Naloxone

45. Which actions will the nurse take to prevent hypoxemia in the postoperative client? **Select all that apply**.
    A. Place the client in a supine position.
    B. Monitor the client's oxygen saturation.
    C. Encourage the client to cough and breathe deeply.
    D. Ambulate the client as early as the surgeon permits.
    E. Instruct the client to rest as much as possible.
    F. Remind the client to use incentive spirometry every hour while awake.

46. Which action does the nurse take to **prevent harm** from skin irritation, wound contamination, and infection for a postoperative client who has a Penrose drain?
    A. Keeps a sterile safety pin in place at the end of the drain
    B. Places absorbent pads under and around the exposed drain
    C. Offers pain medication 30 to 45 minutes before advancing (shortening) the drain
    D. Shortens the drain by pulling it out a short distance and trimming off the excess external portion

47. The nurse is about to give the prescribed pain medication to a client 30 minutes before a scheduled dressing change. The client states that the drug makes him feel sick and he would rather "tough it out." What is the nurse's best first response?
    A. "Tell me more about the sick feeling."
    B. "That's fine. You have the right to refuse any drug."
    C. "Your surgeon would not have prescribed the drug if it wasn't needed."
    D. "Remember that the pain of the dressing change would be worse than feeling sick."

48. What is the nurse's **best** action when crusting on about half of the suture line and oozing of a small amount of serosanguinous drainage is present during the dressing change of client's abdominal dressing on the second postoperative day?
    A. Loosen the sutures or staples in the area where crusts have formed.
    B. Clean the suture line with sterile saline and apply new dressings.
    C. Gently remove the crusts and culture the material beneath.
    D. Apply pressure over the incision and notify the surgeon.

49. Which precaution or issue will the nurse reinforce to the postoperative client about correct use of the patient-controlled analgesia (PCA) device?
    A. "Push the button when you feel the pain beginning rather than waiting until the pain is at its worst."
    B. "Push the button every 15 minutes whether you feel pain at that time or not."
    C. "Instruct your family or visitors to press the button for you when you are sleeping."
    D. "Try to go as long as you possibly can before you press the button."

50. Which action will the nurse take next after emptying 80 mL of sanguineous drainage from the Jackson-Pratt drain in the client's hip after hip surgery?
    A. Flush the tubing with urokinase to assure patency.
    B. Compress and close the drain to assure suction.
    C. Advance the tubing one-half inch from the insertion site.
    D. Clamp the drain for 2 hours and release the clamp for 2 hours.

Chapter 9 Answer Key

1. B, D, E
   The preoperative period begins when the client is scheduled for surgery and ends at the time of transfer to the surgical suite. During this period, the client receives preparatory education, as well as testing to establish a baseline and correct any abnormalities.

2. A
   While all of these concerns are important when caring for a preoperative client, the priority concern is client safety. This is true throughout the perioperative (before, during, and after) period to protect clients against mistakes.

3. A, D, E, F
   Advantages of same-day (outpatient) surgery centers include cost-effective care, service-oriented processes, and a high degree of client satisfaction. A case manager is used to coordinate post-discharge care for the client to ensure follow-up treatments and avoid postoperative hospital admission. Anesthesia is still needed for most surgical procedures, and increased client responsibility after the procedure would likely be considered a disadvantage of this type of surgery.

4. C
   Reconstructive surgery is performed on abnormal or damaged body structures to improve functional ability. Examples include hip and knee replacements. See Table 9.1 in your text.

5. B
   Diagnostic surgery is performed to determine the origin and cause of a disorder by taking a

tissue sample with the intention of diagnosing (and staging, if applicable) a condition. Examples include breast biopsy after an abnormal finding on a mammogram and joint arthroscopy. See Table 9.1 in your text.

6. D
Palliative surgery is performed to increase the quality of life (often to reduce pain) while reducing stressors on the body; non-curative in nature. Examples include ileostomy creation, stent placement to alleviate obstruction, and thoracentesis to drain fluid to reduce pain. See Table 9.1 in your text.

7. B
Curative surgery is performed to resolve a health problem by repairing or removing the cause. Examples include removal of cancerous tumor and removal of gallbladder or appendix (as long as the appendix has not ruptured and the surgery is uncomplicated). See Table 9.1 in your text.

8. C
An elective surgery is performed to correct a nonacute problem. Examples include cataract removal, hernia repair, hemorrhoidectomy, and total joint replacement. See Table 9.2 in your text.

9. B
An emergent surgery requires immediate intervention because of life-threatening consequences. Examples include a gunshot or stab wound, severe bleeding, abdominal aortic aneurysm, compound fracture, and appendectomy that is ruptured or at risk of rupture. See Table 9.2 in your text.

10. C
A minimally invasive approach to surgery is performed in a body cavity or body area through one or more endoscopes; it can correct problems, remove organs, take tissue for biopsy, reroute blood vessels and drainage systems; it is a fast-growing and ever-changing type of surgery. Examples include arthroscopy, tubal ligation, hysterectomy, lung lobectomy, coronary artery bypass (MIDCAB), and cholecystectomy. See Table 9.2 in your text.

11. D
Communicate this information to operative personnel to ensure that electrocautery pads, which could cause an electrical burn, are not placed on or near the area of the prosthesis. Other areas to **avoid** when placing electrocautery pads include on or near bony prominences, pacemakers, scar tissue, hair, tattoos, weight-bearing surfaces, pressure points, and metal piercings.

12. A, C, D, E, F
With MH, serum calcium and potassium levels are increased. Symptoms include tachycardia, dysrhythmias, muscle rigidity of the jaw and upper chest, hypotension, tachypnea, skin mottling, cyanosis, and myoglobinuria (muscle proteins in the urine due to rhabdomyolysis).

13. A, E
The most sensitive indications of MH are an unexpected rise in the end-tidal carbon dioxide level with a decrease in oxygen saturation, and tachycardia. All of the other signs and symptoms are indications of MH but not the most sensitive. Extremely elevated temperature, as high as 111.2°F (44°C), is a **late** sign of MH.

14. A, B, E, F
Table 9.3 in your text gives a long list of risk factors for complications during the perioperative period. Walking every day would not be a risk factor, nor would a history of hernia repair surgery.

15. D
ASA Class IV clients have severe systemic disease that is a constant threat to life. Examples include recent (less than 3 months) MI, CVA, TIA, or CAD/stents; ongoing cardiac ischemia or severe valve dysfunction; severe reduction of ejection fraction; sepsis; and DIC, ARD, or ESRD not undergoing regularly scheduled dialysis. See Table 9.4 in your text.

16. B
When a client expresses fear of a blood transfusion reaction, a possible alternative is that the client can donate his or her own blood (autologous) a few weeks before the scheduled surgery. This procedure eliminates transfusion reactions

and reduces the risk for acquiring bloodborne disease. A special tag is placed on the blood bag when an autologous blood donation has been made to ensure that clients receive only their own donated blood. Options A, C, and D do not respond to the client's stated fears.

17. B, C, D, E

Common preoperative laboratory tests include: urinalysis; blood type and screen; complete blood count (or hemoglobin and hematocrit); clotting studies (prothrombin time [PT], international normalized ratio [INR], activated partial thromboplastin time [aPTT], platelet count); metabolic panel (including serum glucose, serum electrolytes, kidney function, liver function, and serum proteins); and pregnancy test for the female client.

18. A, C, E, F

Informed consent implies that the client has sufficient information to understand: the nature of and reason for surgery; who will be performing the surgery and whether others will be present during the procedure (e.g., students, vendors); all available treatment options, and the benefits and risks associated with each option; the risks associated with the surgical procedure and its potential outcomes; the risks associated with the use of anesthesia; and the risks, benefits, and alternatives to the use of blood or blood products during the procedure.

19. C

It is the surgeon's responsibility to provide a complete explanation of the planned surgical procedure and to have the consent form signed before sedation is given and before surgery is performed. The perioperative nurse is **not** responsible for providing detailed information about the surgical procedure. The nurse's role is to clarify facts that have been presented by the surgeon and dispel myths that the client or caregiver may have about the surgical experience. The nurse must verify that the consent form is signed, dated, and timed, and he or she may serve as a witness to the signature, **not** to the adequacy of the client's understanding (which is the surgeon's responsibility).

20. A

After the client is prepared for surgery and just before transport into the surgical suite, the nurse would ask the AP to assist the client to the bathroom to empty his or her bladder. This action prevents incontinence or overdistention and is a starting point for intake and output measurement. Most facilities have clients remove their clothes and wear a hospital gown to surgery.

21. A, C, D, E

An essential responsibility of the preoperative nurse is to teach clients about postoperative procedures that will prevent complications after surgery including respiratory procedures such as splinting the incision to cough and deep breath as well as incentive spirometry. Range-of-motion exercises are important to prevent loss of range or motion. Clients should be taught how to perform these exercises and given opportunities to practice. Massaging lower extremities would be avoided to prevent DVT. Clients should not wait to ask for pain medication until the pain is severe.

22. C

A blind client may sign his or her own consent form, which will need to be witnessed by two people. Clients who cannot write may sign with an X, which must be witnessed by two people, one of whom can be the nurse.

23. B, D

Drugs for cardiac disease, respiratory disease, seizures, and hypertension are commonly allowed with a sip of water before surgery. Some antihypertensive or antidepressant drugs are withheld on the day of surgery to reduce adverse effects on blood pressure during surgery. Usual drug schedules are individualized so the nurse would be sure to check with the surgeon regarding which drugs should be given and which should be held.

24. A

Indications of poor fluid or nutrition status include: brittle nails; muscle wasting; dry or flaky skin, decreased skin turgor, and hair changes (e.g., dull, sparse, dry); orthostatic (postural) hypotension; and decreased serum protein levels and abnormal serum electrolyte values.

25. C
This client's BP is low, HR is high, and oral temperature is elevated. These changes in vital signs may indicate that the client is at risk for an infection which must be treated before the client can have surgery. Options A, B, and D may be included in the care of this client, but at this time, the priority action is to notify the surgeon.

26. A
Phase I care occurs immediately after surgery and requires ongoing monitoring of the airway, vital signs, and evidence of recovery that varies from every 5 to 15 minutes. Phase II care focuses on preparing the client for care in an extended-care environment and may last only 15 to 30 minutes, although 1 to 2 hours is more typical. Phase III care is less intense and occurs on a hospital unit or in the home, with frequency of vital sign monitoring ranging from several times daily to just once daily. There is no official phase IV level of client care after surgery.

27. D
Although all vital signs and client parameters are important to assess on arrival at the PACU, the most important is the client's respiratory status and adequacy of gas exchange. Problems with gas exchange can lead to death and require immediate action.

28. A, C, D
Although most clients have a slightly below core body temperature after surgery, it should not be more than 2 degrees lower than normal. The temperature cited is bordering on hypothermia and should be addressed. A pulmonary embolism is never a normal response to surgery. Although a paralytic ileus is a relatively common occurrence, it is considered a surgical complication. Most clients have pain initially at the surgical site and are usually sedated to some degree, even if local anesthesia or a nerve block

was used for anesthesia. Sore throat is common for clients who have been intubated.

29. B, E, F, G
The list of expected information is not all-inclusive, but the relevant pieces include level of consciousness and cognition, the surgical procedure, exact timing of the last dosage of pain medication, and the fact that the client received two units of blood products while in the PACU. Information not relevant to the hand-off report includes religion, an allergy that is not drug-related or likely to be immediately encountered on the medical-surgical unit, or that a progressive diet is permitted. Although the client's height and weight are not totally irrelevant, this information is not something needed for immediate action at this time.

30. B
Profuse bleeding from a fresh incision site is an emergency and could lead to exsanguination. Halting blood loss by applying pressure to the wound is the priority. Someone else can call the surgeon. Although assessment of heart rate and blood pressure can provide information about the severity of the hemorrhage, it is less important than slowing or stopping the bleeding. Application of additional dressing materials without applying pressure does not do anything to stem the bleeding.

31. B, D, F
Clients at greatest risk for respiratory complications after surgery are older adults, those who smoke, and those with a history of lung disease or obesity and require more frequent respiratory assessment. Diabetes alone and early stage Alzheimer disease do not increase the risk for respiratory complications (and 70 years is not terribly old). The client who is 80 is at greater age-related risk, but the lack of an influenza vaccination does not increase the postoperative respiratory complication risk.

32. A
The priority action is to stay with the client to ensure the evisceration does not extend and to reassure him or her through this emergency.

Call for help and have someone else call the surgeon and assemble supplies for covering the evisceration with saline-saturated dressings. Vital signs are not a priority at this time. Only the surgeon repositions abdominal contents, usually in an operating room.

33. B

Fentanyl is an opioid that can cause respiratory depression and significant sedation. Although the client's oxygen saturation is a little low, just applying the oxygen (standard in all PACUs) is likely to bring it up even with a slow respiratory rate. However, the client does require close monitoring of pulse oximetry to determine the effectiveness of this action. Monitoring only does not prevent harm. Deep suctioning is only needed when indications of ineffective airway clearance are evident. Pinching the client does not increase his or her overall wakefulness, which requires either that the drug wear off or that the client be given an opioid antagonist.

34. D

Splinting the wound when moving or getting out of bed supports the tissues and reduces the risk for wound dehiscence or evisceration. It also reduces pain in the area. Massaging the legs and using the knee gatch can interfere with venous return and increases the risk for venous thromboembolism. Taking pain medication, while increasing comfort, does not physically prevent harm.

35. B, C, E

The oxygen saturation is within normal limits Use of accessory muscles during respiratory effort and crowing on exhalation are not normal and indicate some degree of respiratory distress. The respiratory rate is high, which may indicate shallow breaths that could be less effective. The changes in blood pressure and urine output are not influenced by the presence or absence of respiratory difficulty.

36. B

The older adult has a slower metabolism and clears anesthesia and other drugs that can alter cognition much more slowly than a younger adult. Thus, return to his or her presurgical level of orientation takes longer. Often the older client, on waking from anesthesia does not know how long he or she was "out" and has some confusion about what day it is. There is no indication of dementia in this situation and asking the family about it will only increase their concerns.

37. C

The skin on the back of the hand, the forearm, and the shin of an older adult can be very dry and form a tent even when the client is well hydrated. The best location for hydration assessment of an older adult is on the sternum or the forehead.

38. B

Clients at greatest risk for PONV are those who have motion sickness, those who are obese, and those with abdominal surgery. Much of PONV is related to the anesthetic agents and not age. Risk is not increased when a nasogastric tube is in place or when under local, rather than general anesthesia.

39. C

The best indicators of return of peristalsis is the passage of flatus or stool. The presence of bowel sounds alone is not sufficient as clients may continue to have some bowel sounds even when a paralytic ileus is present. Abdominal cramping can occur as a result of trapped bowel contents and does not necessarily indicate movement. Hunger is also not an indicator of peristaltic return.

40. C

Epidural anesthesia blocks both motor and sensory function of spinal nerves from at least the level of injection down. The agent can climb higher in the epidural space and affect function above the level of injection. The motor and sensory responses must be assessed for the return of function. Moving the extremities is an indication of return of motor function. Sensory function is assessed by the ability of the client to feel. The most common method of sensory assessment is to lightly prick the client's skin with a needle or pin and having the client indicate when the sensation feels sharp rather than dull or just pressure. Blood pressure can fall as a result of the vasodilation from epidural anesthesia but the anesthesia does not cause a difference in blood pressure from one arm to the other. The level of consciousness is not affected by epidural anesthesia.

41. D
Both the amount and color of the fluid draining from the nasogastric tube are normal and expected for this point in the postoperative period. It is not necessary to notify the surgeon, nor should the tube be repositioned. The client remains NPO while the NG tube is in place. Moreover, the fluid would not be expected to ever be clear.

42. A, B, D, E
Common physical and emotional signs of acute pain in adults include increased pulse and blood pressure and increased respiratory rate (as a result of activating the stress response of the sympathetic nervous system), profuse sweating, and restlessness. Often acute pain will cause confusion in the older adult. Other indicators include wincing, moaning, and crying. Difficulty arousing the client is not an indication of acute pain.

43. A
Increased release of immature neutrophils (bands) (also known as a "left-shift" or "bandemia") is an indication of an ongoing infection that has outpaced the client's immune defenses. It is not a normal white blood cell finding and has nothing to do with anemia or the clotting factors.

44. B
Flumazenil is a benzodiazepine antagonist and can help reverse a benzodiazepine overdose. Midazolam is a benzodiazepine and would only worsen the overdose. Hydromorphone is an opioid that would make respiratory depression worse and do nothing for the overdose. Naloxone reverses an opioid overdose but has no effect on a benzodiazepine overdose.

45. B, C, D, F
Coughing, deep breathing, ambulating, and using the incentive spirometer all promote maximum tidal volume and prevent both fluid accumulation and atelectasis. These actions enhance gas exchange. Monitoring oxygen saturation allows the nurse to know when gas exchange is less than adequate and take early action to increase it. Staying in a supine rather than an upright position reduces gas exchange. Resting rather than moving and ambulating promotes fluid accumulation.

46. B
Drainage on the skin poses a risk for irritation, wound contamination, and infection. Using absorbent padding under and around the exposed drain reduces skin contact with the drainage. The safety pin only prevents the drain from slipping back into the body and does not block drainage. Pain medication would not prevent drainage from coming into contact with the skin. (Most of the time shortening a Penrose drain does not induce pain.) Shortening the drain also does not prevent skin contact with drainage.

47. A
Although the client does have the right to refuse any medication, the "sick feeling" is only a vague description. He may mean nausea but he could also mean some other response that could indicate a possible adverse reaction to the drug. It is important to gather more information. Also, by acknowledging the client's feelings, the nurse is using therapeutic communication before implementing the next step.

48. B
Serosanguinous drainage and a small amount of crusting are normal incision findings on the second postoperative day and do not represent infection. No culture is needed. The nurse does not loosen the sutures or staples without a surgeon's order.

49. A

Clients should be instructed to push the button to release medication when pain begins rather than waiting until the pain becomes so great that the dose limited by the pump cannot control the pain. Only the client should push the button as only he or she really knows his or her level of pain.

50 B

The Jackson-Pratt drain removes fluid from the wound through closed suction. The drain must be compressed and closed to create suction as it slowly re-expands. It is in a fixed position and not advanced until removal and is neither flushed nor clamped.

10 CHAPTER

Concepts of Emergency and Trauma Nursing

1. Which **first** action would the triage nurse take for a client who comes to the ED with blurred vision, difficulty speaking, left extremity weakness, and difficulty walking?
   A. Send the client immediately for a head CT scan.
   B. Notify the ED health care provider.
   C. Delegate the assistive personnel (AP) to stay with the client.
   D. Categorize the client as emergent.

2. Which information would the ED nurse be sure to include in a Situation, Background, Assessment, Recommendation (SBAR) report to be given to the medical nurse regarding a client admitted for bacterial meningitis? **Select all that apply.**
   A. "Client is currently alert and oriented × 2; speech is clear but rambling."
   B. "Client is very demanding and has used call bell repeatedly in the ED."
   C. "IV normal saline is infusing into the left anterior forearm."
   D. "Client has received the first dose of IV ceftriaxone at 07:00 a.m."
   E. "Client reports severe headache with high fever which started 4 days ago."
   F. "Lumbar puncture results are pending, but meningococcal meningitis is suspected."
   G. "Client has male characteristics but prefers to be called Ms. Jenny Jones."
   H. "Cardiac monitor shows normal sinus rhythm with occasional PAC."

3. What is the nurse's **best** response when a client with a sprained ankle complains that several clients who arrived later have been admitted before him or her?
   A. "I understand your frustration, but please sit down and wait until we call you."
   B. "We must attend to the clients who are unstable with life-threatening conditions first."
   C. "This is a system problem and if you wish to complain, I can call a supervisor."
   D. "Other clients have problems more serious than yours."

4. Which are among the most common reasons that clients seek care in the ED? **Select all that apply.**
   A. Chest pain
   B. Breathing problems
   C. Vaccinations and shots
   D. Injuries such as falls in older adults
   E. Headache
   F. Homelessness

5. What is the ED nurse's **best** response when the surgical nurse answers the phone and says, "You people always dump admissions on us during shift change"?
   A. "I apologize for the timing. How much time do you need for shift change?"
   B. "I apologize. We just now received this bed assignment."
   C. "I'm sorry. I realize you are busy, but we are busy too."
   D. "I'm also trying to finish a hand-off report. Should I call the supervisor?"

6. Which are vulnerable populations that often seek care in the ED? **Select all that apply.**
   A. Clients with substance use problems
   B. Clients who are pregnant
   C. Clients with mental health needs
   D. Clients who are older adults
   E. Clients with small children
   F. Clients who are poor

7. For which situation would the ED nurse, who is working alone, in triage activate the panic button?
   A. Emergency medical services call on their way to the ED with a client in full arrest.
   B. Several clients who have been in the waiting room for a long time begin to complain.
   C. The line for clients waiting to be triaged becomes overwhelmingly long.
   D. A person walks in and starts threatening the registration staff with a weapon.

8. Which strategies would the ED nurse use to conduct an interview with a client who has been verbally aggressive for the past couple of hours? **Select all that apply.**
   A. Sit at eye level with the client in a secluded room.
   B. Attempt de-escalating strategies before harm is done.
   C. Notify security and supervisory staff of the situation.
   D. Conduct the interview near the door in a quiet room.
   E. Ask the family members to sit in while the interview is completed.
   F. Request a security guard to stand by the client during the interview.

9. What is the **first priority** concern for nurses providing care for homeless clients in the ED setting?
   A. Assessing for substance use problems
   B. Providing clients with adequate nutrition
   C. Attending to their needs for personal safety
   D. Referring to social services related to economic hardship

10. Which actions would the nurse use to promote trust with a homeless client? **Select all that apply.**
    A. Make eye contact.
    B. Speak calmly.
    C. Be patient.
    D. Show care by listening.
    E. Instruct the client at all times.
    F. Follow through on promises.

11. What is the **best** procedure for client identification when caring for an unconscious admission with no known identification or family, and the ED nurse must administer a medication to the client?
    A. The client is designated as John/Jane Doe (based on gender) and the nurse uses two unique identifiers.
    B. Emergent conditions prevent identification, so the nurse gives the medication as prescribed.
    C. The nurse administers the medication, and identification of the client is made as soon as possible.
    D. The nurse validates the order with another nurse and both verify that the client is unidentified.

12. Which statement would the nurse use **first** when giving a hand-off report to the next shift nurse using the SBAR method?
    A. "The client's vital signs are T 98.6°F (37°C), HR 80/min, RR 16/min, BP 160/80 mm Hg."
    B. "The client is a 65-year-old who came to the ED for a severe headache."
    C. "The client is very uncomfortable and we should get him admitted as soon as possible."
    D. "The client has a history of hypertension but stopped taking medications 3 months ago."

13. For which client is the forensic nurse examiner **most likely** to be consulted?
    A. Client who accidentally received a large dose of opioid medication
    B. Older adult client who died under mysterious circumstances in the ED
    C. Client who was injured by a police officer while resisting arrest
    D. Client who was gang-raped by a group of fraternity students

14. Which ED clients, who are currently on stretchers and waiting for discharge or transfer to an inpatient bed, are at **greatest** risk for falls? **Select all that apply.**
    A. Young client with heavy vaginal bleeding secondary to a miscarriage
    B. Client with chronic pain who received 10 mg oxycodone orally for myalgia
    C. Middle-aged adult with severe nausea and vomiting and frequent watery stool over 3 days
    D. Opioid-naïve teenager with a fracture who received morphine sulfate 3 mg IV for pain
    E. Old adult client with acute dementia secondary to an infection
    F. Younger adult with gastroesophageal reflux disease.

15. Which actions are within the scope of practice for an emergency medical technician (EMT) as a prehospital care provider? **Select all that apply.**
    A. Cardiac monitoring
    B. Oxygen application
    C. Endotracheal intubation
    D. Splinting
    E. Establishing IV lines
    F. Basic life support (CPR)

16. What type of personal protective equipment (PPE) or attire would the nurse wear to provide care for a motor vehicle crash victim with severe chest trauma who is coughing up blood and has a crush injury to the right leg?
    A. No PPE is needed because the nurse is only recording and not giving direct care.
    B. The client situation must be assessed before determining what type of PPE would be worn.
    C. Gloves only, but handwashing is required before and after all emergency care.
    D. Impervious cover gown, gloves, eye protection, face mask, cap, and shoe covers are required.

17. Which intervention in the ED is **least likely** to be covered by a standing protocol for the nurses when the health care provider is not readily available?
    A. Insert a peripheral IV line with normal saline at 125 mL/hr.
    B. Give 50% dextrose IV push for low blood sugar.
    C. Ventilate with bag-valve-mask at 100% oxygen and intubate client.
    D. Initiate pulse oximetry monitoring and start oxygen therapy.

18. Which client would the triage nurse categorize as urgent?
    A. 35-year-old with chest pain and diaphoresis
    B. 44-year-old with a dislocated elbow
    C. 65-year-old with redness and swelling on the forearm due to a bee sting
    D. 83-year-old with new confusion and very elevated blood pressure compared with his baseline

19. Which instruction would the nurse give to the assistive personnel (AP) after giving a client with a migraine headache medication for the pain?
    A. Check the client frequently to make sure of arousal and that the headache is not getting worse.
    B. Wait 45 minutes and then assess the client to find out if the pain has been relieved.
    C. Help the client out of bed, sit them up slowly and dangle the feet, then assist them to stand.
    D. Ask the client if they need a ride home and if so, call a family member to arrange for client pickup.

20. Which technique would the nurse use to estimate the systolic blood pressure for a client who was transported to the ED on a stretcher in a resuscitation situation?
    A. Place the client on a cardiac monitor and count heart rate.
    B. Palpate the client for the presence of a radial pulse.
    C. Check the client for the presence of capillary refill.
    D. Apply and use an automated blood pressure cuff.

21. Which actions would the nurse take to **prevent harm** from the risk of injuries to clients in the ED? **Select all that apply.**
    A. Keep rails up on the stretcher.
    B. Keep the stretcher at a level for easy client access by staff.
    C. Frequently reorient any client who is confused.
    D. Ask a family member to remain with a confused client.
    E. Allow family members to escort client to the bathroom.
    F. Reposition any client who is at risk for skin breakdown every 1 to 2 hours.

22. What does the nurse expect will be the appearance of a client when the hand-off report states that the client has a Glasgow Coma Scale of 3?
    A. Client will withdraw from painful stimuli.
    B. Client will be completely unresponsive.
    C. Client will open eyes spontaneously.
    D. Client will moan but speech will be incoherent.

23. Which actions would the nurse take to reduce the potential for medical errors or adverse events in the ED? **Select all that apply.**
    A. Contact the family by phone to get an accurate medical history.
    B. Look for a medical alert necklace or bracelet when a client has altered mental status.
    C. Perform a two-person search of belongings looking for a medication list or containers.
    D. Search among belongings for the name of the client's health care provider or pharmacy.
    E. Try to find out the name of the person who provides in-home care for the client.
    F. Check client's belongings for drugs or drug paraphernalia as well as weapons.

24. Which **priority** question must the nurse be sure to ask the paramedics when an older adult is brought to the ED alert, but with lower left leg swelling and deformity and an air splint in place?
    A. "What time was the air splint applied?"
    B. "Does the client normally walk independently?"
    C. "How did the client describe the level of pain?"
    D. "What was the mechanism of injury?"

25. When the nurse collaborates with the ED health care provider, which procedures must he or she be prepared to assist with? **Select all that apply.**
    A. Lumbar puncture
    B. Wound closure by suturing
    C. Chest tube insertion
    D. Colonoscopy
    E. Central line insertion
    F. Bronchoscopy

26. Which is the **most** essential component of the emergency nurse's skill base?
    A. Communication
    B. Establishing IV access
    C. Interpreting cardiac monitor rhythms
    D. Providing pain relief

27. Which nursing action would be **incorrect** when a client is likely to be the subject of a forensic investigation?
    A. Nurse declines to give information to friends of the deceased client.
    B. Nurse invites the family to spend time with the deceased client.
    C. Nurse gives the client's clothes and belongings to the family of the deceased.
    D. Nurse leaves intravenous lines and indwelling tubes in place.

28. Which clients would the triage nurse classify as emergent, needing to be seem immediately? **Select all that apply.**
    A. Client with crushing substernal chest pain and shortness of breath
    B. Client with a generalized skin rash who had shellfish for dinner yesterday
    C. Client with active hemorrhage after a motor vehicle crash
    D. Client with back pain and hematuria with a history of kidney stones
    E. Client with a dislocated shoulder
    F. Client with dysuria from a long-term care facility

29. What would the nurse do **first** when the provider has written a discharge order for an older adult client who cannot walk independently and has no family?
    A. Speak with the provider about the client's self-care abilities.
    B. Consult social services for nursing home placement.
    C. Ask the client if a friend could come to the hospital.
    D. Obtain a taxi voucher for the client.

30. What would the ED nurse do when a family arrives and wants to see the client, after death due to multiple injuries from an aggravated assault?
    A. Remove any tubes and debris that are near the client's face, then cover the rest of the body with a blanket.
    B. Explain what the family will see, dim the lights, leave the client's face exposed, and cover the rest of the body with a blanket.
    C. Suggest that the family could spend time with their loved one at the morgue after the medical examiner is finished.
    D. Explain that viewing the body would be too traumatic because all the tubes must remain in place for the forensic exam.

31. What is the **best** way for the emergency health care provider and nurse to inform a family that their family member has died of extensive injuries despite resuscitation efforts?
    A. "We're sorry to inform you that your loved one died due to extensive injuries."
    B. "We did everything we could but your loved one expired."
    C. "Your loved one never woke up, but we are sure that they passed without discomfort."
    D. "We want to extend our sympathies because your loved one is not with us anymore."

32. Which actions would the ED nurse expect to perform as a member of the ED bereavement committee?
    A. Assign a staff nurse to sit with the family during resuscitation efforts for the client.
    B. Provide grief counseling and group support for nurses who care for dying clients.
    C. Attend funerals, send sympathy cards and make follow-up calls to the family.
    D. Advocate that one or two family members be allowed at the bedside during resuscitation.

33. Which injuries would the ED nurse categorize as intentional injuries? **Select all that apply.**
    A. Motor vehicle crash
    B. Suicide
    C. Fracture due to fall
    D. Assault
    E. Homicide
    F. Near-drowning

34. When would the nurse working in a large urban hospital **most** likely refer to the ED's automated electronic tracking system?
    A. When seeking complete records of previous admissions for a client
    B. When needing a medication for a client that should have come from the pharmacy
    C. When desiring to know if the client's CT scan has been completed
    D. When believing the client frequently visits the ED for opioids prescriptions

35. What is the **most important** action for the ED nurse to take for a client admitted with repeated kicks to the abdomen, and for whom testing currently reveals no life-threatening damage?
    A. Assign vital signs every 4 hours to the assistive personnel (AP).
    B. Place the client in a quiet place to assure he or she can rest.
    C. Initiate serial abdominal assessments every hour.
    D. Administer pain medication in a timely manner.

36. What is the **primary** focus for client care at a Level III trauma center?
    A. Offer advanced life support in rural or remote areas
    B. Provide care for majority of injured clients; may not meet needs of complex multisystem injury management
    C. Focus on initial injury stabilization and emergent client transfer
    D. Regional resource facility capable of providing leadership and total collaborative care for every aspect of injury

37. Which are the key elements when the nurse performs a primary survey on a client brought into the emergency department? **Select all that apply.**
    A. Airway/cervical spine
    B. Breathing
    C. Circulation
    D. Disability
    E. Exposure
    F. Functional ability

38. What is the one exception to the ABCDE primary survey?
    A. Total cardiac and respiratory arrest
    B. Uncontrolled external bleeding
    C. Fifty percent total body surface burns
    D. Client with HIV and active AIDS (HIV-III)

39. What important information does the Disability (D) portion of the primary survey provide for the emergency department staff?
    A. A rapid baseline assessment of the neurological status of the client
    B. A look at the client's body searching for additional injuries
    C. An estimate of the likelihood that the client will need to be intubated
    D. An estimate of blood loss during the injuries that led to admission

40. Which signs of trafficking would the ED nurse watch for when interviewing and assessing an 18-year-old? **Select all that apply.**
    A. Headache and dizziness
    B. Missing patches of hair
    C. Vaginal or rectal trauma
    D. Smiling and friendly
    E. Burns and bruises
    F. Unusual tattooing

Chapter 10 Answer Key

1. D

    This client's symptoms suggest a possible stroke which would be classified as emergent (life-threatening) and requires immediate treatment. The HCP would need to be notified immediately and the stroke team or protocol activated immediately. A head CT scan is likely to be ordered and someone would likely stay with the client. These actions would happen very quickly, almost simultaneously, but the triage nurse would first recognize the stroke and categorize it emergent.

2. A, C, D, E, F, G, H

    All of the options are appropriate for an SBAR report, except for option B. Option B includes a judgmental statement by the ED nurse.

3. B

    Based on the severity of the patient's condition, a well-known triage scheme is the three-tiered model of "emergent, urgent, and nonurgent". Clients who are classified as emergent need to be seen immediately in the ED. When clients are classified as urgent, they should be treated quickly but an immediate threat to life does not exist. A client with a sprain would be classified as nonurgent and would likely tolerate waiting for hours without great risk of deterioration. In option B, the nurse explains this in clear, simple terms to the complaining client.

4. A, B, D, E

    The most common reasons clients seek ED care include: abdominal pain, breathing difficulties, chest pain, fever, headache, injuries (especially falls in older adults), and pain (the most common symptom. Vaccinations and shots would be sought from a primary HCP, clinic, or pharmacy. Homeless clients do seek care in the ED, but this is not one of the most common reasons.

5. A

    ED nurses and inpatient unit nurses need to understand the unique aspects of their two practice environments to prevent conflicts. Nurses on inpatient units may be critical of the push to move patients out of the ED setting quickly, particularly when their unit activity is high such as at change of shift. Effective interpersonal communication skills and respectful negotiation can optimize teamwork and collaboration between the emergency nurse and the inpatient unit nurse. Option A gives an example of understanding and effective communication regarding the ED admission.

6. A, C, D, F

    Vulnerable populations who visit the ED include the homeless, clients with mental health needs, clients with substance use problems, and older adults. While pregnant clients and clients with small children do sometimes use the ED, they more often seek care from obstetricians and pediatricians.

7. D

    Panic buttons and remote door access controls allow staff to get help and secure major entrances. The triage reception area, a particularly vulnerable access point into the ED, is often designed to serve as a security barrier with bullet-proof glass and staff-controlled door entry into the treatment area. The situation in option D poses danger for staff and clients, so the nurse would use the panic button to get help from security for the safety of everyone. Options A, B, and C require help but do not require security at this time.

8. B, C, D

    In volatile situations where clients demonstrate aggressive or violent tendencies through verbal or nonverbal behaviors, follow the hospital security plan, including identifying the nearest escape route, attempting de-escalation strategies before harm can occur, and notifying security and supervisory staff of the situation. Do not go to a secluded area. Family should not be part of the interview unless a client is unable to speak for himself or herself. Having a security guard present would not foster trust or rapport.

9. C

    To provide best care for homeless clients in the ED setting, nurses must first maintain their situational awareness and attend to their own needs for personal safety. Substance use problems and economic hardship are factors that contribute to homelessness. Homeless clients often seek a safe place to go for food, medical care, pain relief, and human interaction. The ED represents that safe place.

10. A, B, C, D, F

The nurse must demonstrate behaviors that promote trust with homeless clients. These actions include making eye contact (if culturally appropriate), speaking calmly, avoiding any prejudicial or stereotypical remarks, being patient, showing genuine care and concern by listening, following through on promises, and exercising caution when there is a need to enter into the client's personal space. Option E, instructing the client at all times is very directive, taking decision-making from the client and likely would not inspire trust.

11. A

For clients with an unknown identity and those with emergent conditions that prevent the standard identification process (e.g., unconscious client without identification, emergent trauma client), hospitals commonly use a "Jane/John Doe" or other system of identification. Always verify the client's identity using two unique identifiers before each intervention and before medication administration per The Joint Commission's (TJC) 2018 National Patient Safety Goals. Examples of appropriate identifiers include the client's name, birth date, agency identification number, home telephone number or address, and/or Social Security number. For this client, name and agency ID number would likely be the identifiers.

12. B

The SBAR method (Situation, Background, Assessment, Response) or some variation of that method is used to ensure complete and clearly understood communication. Option B best covers the situation which is the first element of SBAR.

13. D

Forensic nurse examiners (RN-FNEs) are educated to obtain patient histories, collect forensic evidence, and offer counseling and follow-up care for victims of rape, abuse, and domestic violence—also known as intimate partner violence (IPV). Forensic nurses who specialize in helping victims of sexual assault are called sexual assault nurse examiners (SANEs) or sexual assault forensic examiners (SAFEs).

14. A, C, D, E

Clients can enter the ED without fall risk factors, but because of interventions such as pain medication, and sedation, they can develop a risk for falls. Falls can also occur in clients with medical conditions or drugs that cause syncope ("blackouts"). Some older adults experience orthostatic (postural) hypotension as a side effect of cardiovascular drugs. In this case, patients become dizzy when changing from a lying or sitting position. Option A has heavy bleeding. Option C is likely dehydrated. Option D is a client who has not used morphine before, and option E is an older adult with dementia. All four are at increased risk for falls. Option B has chronic pain and chronic use of pain medications so this dose of oxycodone is not likely to increase risk for a fall. Option F has GERD which is not at risk for falls.

15. B, D, F

EMTs offer basic life support (BLS) interventions such as oxygen, basic wound care, splinting, spinal motion restriction, and monitoring of vital signs. Some units carry automatic external defibrillators (AEDs) and may be authorized to administer selected drugs such as an epinephrine autoinjector, intranasal naloxone (Narcan), or nitroglycerin based on training and established protocols. Intubation, cardiac monitoring, and establishing IV lines are functions in the scope of practice for paramedics.

16. D

Before engaging in trauma resuscitation as a nurse member of the trauma team, keep in mind that there is a high risk for contamination with blood and body fluids. For this reason, use Standard Precautions in all resuscitation situations and at other times when exposure to blood and body fluids is likely. Proper attire consists of an impervious cover gown, gloves, eye protection, a facemask, surgical cap, and shoe covers. This client has severe chest trauma, is coughing up blood, and has a crush injury to the right leg and the nurse is at high risk for contamination with blood.

17. C

While most EDs have health care providers available around the clock who are physically located within the unit, nurses often initiate collaborative interprofessional protocols for lifesaving interventions such as cardiac monitoring, oxygen therapy, insertion of IV catheters, and infusion of appropriate parenteral solutions. In many EDs, nurses function under clearly defined medical protocols that allow them to initiate drug therapy for emergent conditions such as anaphylactic shock and cardiac arrest. Emergency care principles extend to knowing which essential laboratory and diagnostic tests may be needed and, when necessary, obtaining them. Nurses often assist health care providers with procedures such as intubation, but do not perform this skill independently.

18. B

In the three-tiered system, the urgent category includes clients with a new onset of pneumonia (as long as respiratory failure does not appear imminent), renal colic, complex lacerations not associated with major hemorrhage, displaced fractures or dislocations, and temperature greater than 101°F (38.3°C). Options A and D would be classified as emergent and option C with the bee sting could be nonurgent as long as the client is not allergic to bee stings.

19. C

Administering pain medication often increases the risk for a client fall. Checking for arousal and assessing for pain relief require additional training as with the professional nurse. The AP could ask if the client needed a ride home, but the unit clerk would likely call family to arrange for someone to pick up the client when ready for discharge.

20. B

In a resuscitation situation, the nurse can estimate the client's systolic blood pressure by palpating for peripheral and central pulses. Presence of a radial pulse: BP at least 80 mm Hg systolic; presence of a femoral pulse: BP at least 70 mm Hg systolic; and presence of a carotid pulse: BP at least 60 mm Hg systolic. During resuscitation, BP cuffs usually cannot detect blood pressure. Cardiac monitoring gives information about the heart's rhythm, and checking capillary refill provides information about peripheral circulation to small vessels, not systolic blood pressure.

21. A, C, D, F

To prevent injuries, nurses should use these actions: keep rails up on stretcher; keep stretcher in lowest position (not in position of comfort for staff); remind the client to use call light for assistance; reorient the confused patient frequently; if patient is confused, ask a family member or significant other to remain with him or her; and implement measures to protect skin integrity for patients at risk for skin breakdown.

22. B

The GCS is a method of determining and documenting consciousness. It measures eye opening, verbal response, and motor response. The lowest score is 3, which indicates a totally unresponsive patient; a normal GCS score is 15. If the GCS is less than 8, the client is at risk for airway compromise.

23. B, C, D, E, F

The only questionable option is A. If possible, the nurse obtains the client's history from the client first. If the client has altered mental status, the nurse will rely on alternative sources of information such as family, care providers, HCP's, and pharmacists. Safety is always a concern which is why it is essential to search the client's belongings for dangerous equipment, as well as drug lists, bottles, and names of health care providers.

24. D

The mechanism of injury (MOI) describes how the client's traumatic event occurred (e.g., motor vehicle crash, fall). The MOI details can provide insight into the energy forces involved and may help trauma care providers predict injury types, and in some cases, client outcomes. Prehospital care providers report the MOI as a communication standard when handing off care to ED and trauma personnel. Clients who present to the ED for medical care will often relate the MOI by describing the particular chain of events that caused their injuries.

25. A, B, C, E

Common ED procedures include: central line insertion; chest tube insertion; endotracheal intubation and initiation of mechanical ventilation; fracture management; foreign body removal; lumbar puncture; paracentesis; pelvic examination; and wound closure by suturing. Colonoscopy and bronchoscopy are usually performed in special labs by specialty physicians.

26. A

The most essential component of the emergency nurse's skill base is communication. Because the ED setting is complex, there are many possible barriers to effective communication between staff and with clients and family or caregivers. Respect for each other and for each client's beliefs is essential, and communication in a nonjudgmental manner is key. A solid set of nursing skills is important also, but first and most important is communication.

27. C

When a case is forensic, the forensic nurse collects physical and photographic evidence. This can include clothes as well as any other physical evidence (e.g., hair, skin under fingernails). ED staff may not be able to remove IV lines and indwelling tubes or clean the patient's skin if these actions could potentially damage evidence. When this happens, cover the body with a sheet or blanket while leaving the client's face exposed and dim the lights before family viewing.

28. A, C

Clients with chest pain or severe bleeding are at risk for life-threatening consequences and should be seen immediately. The client with severe bleeding would likely go into a trauma room with a trauma team providing care.

29. A

If discharge from the ED to home is possible, ensure that safety issues are considered. In this case the client has no family and cannot walk independently, making the ability to perform self-care doubtful. The nurse must collaborate with the provider to evaluate possible solutions for the safety of this client. It may be necessary to involve the social services or a case manager.

If the client has a friend who provides the role of caregiver, that person should be contacted and involved. If the patient does not have a reliable caregiver to perform ongoing neurologic checks in that 12- to 24-hour window, the patient may need admission for observation.

30. B

If the client dies before family members arrive, ED staff members should prepare the body and the room for viewing by the family. However, certain types of ED deaths may require forensic investigation or become medical examiner's cases. ED staff may not be able to remove IV lines and indwelling tubes or clean the client's skin if these actions could potentially damage evidence. Trauma deaths, suspected homicides, or cases of abuse always fall into this category. In these situations, tell the family what to expect, cover the body with a sheet or blanket while leaving the client's face exposed, and dim the lights before family viewing.

31. A

When dealing with family members in crisis, simple and concrete communication is best. Words such as death or died, although seemingly harsh, create less confusion than terms such as expired or passed away.

32. C

Some EDs have developed bereavement committees. These focus on meeting the needs of grieving families. Actions such as sending sympathy cards, attending funerals, making follow-up phone calls, and creating memory boxes are common. These actions facilitate communication of caring and compassion after the moment of crisis.

33. B, D, E

Injuries such as assault, homicide, and suicide are intentional. Unintentional injuries include accidents such as motor vehicle crashes, fractures due to falls, and near drownings.

34. C

Automated electronic tracking systems are available in some EDs and help staff to identify the location of clients at any given time as well as monitor the progress of care delivery during the visit. These valuable safety measures are very important in large or busy EDs with a high population of older adults.

35. C
While the client has no life-threatening symptoms at the moment, he or she may develop abdominal symptoms later, so the nurse should initiate repeated abdominal assessments in case this happens. Do not put the client in a quiet place and forget to check for symptoms. Two or four hours may be too long.

36. C
Initial stabilization and emergent transfer (option C) is the focus of a Level III trauma center. Offering advanced life support in remote areas fits with a Level IV trauma center (option A). Providing care for majority of clients, but may not meet needs of complex, multisystem injury management (option B) refers to Level II trauma center, and serving as a regional resource with capability to care for every aspect of injury (option D) best describes a Level I trauma center.

37. A, B, C, D, E
The initial assessment of the trauma client is called the primary survey, which is an organized framework used to rapidly identify and effectively manage immediate threats to life. The primary survey is typically based on a standard "ABC" mnemonic plus a "D" and "E" for trauma patients: airway/cervical spine (**A**); breathing (**B**); circulation (**C**); disability (**D**); and exposure (**E**).

38. B
There is one notable exception to the standard ABCDE trauma resuscitation approach; that is

the presence of massive, uncontrolled external bleeding. Hemorrhage control techniques are the highest priority intervention and the sequence of priorities shifts to CAB (circulation, airway, breathing). The initial focus of resuscitation is to effectively stop the active bleeding.

39. A
The disability examination provides a rapid baseline assessment of neurologic status. A simple method to evaluate level of consciousness is the "AVPU" mnemonic: A: **A**lert, V: Responsive to **v**oice, P: Responsive to **p**ain, and U: **U**nresponsive.
Another common way of determining and documenting level of consciousness is the **Glasgow Coma Scale (GCS)**, an assessment that scores eye opening, verbal response, and motor response. The lowest score is 3, which indicates a totally unresponsive client; a normal GCS score is 15.

40. A, B, C, E, F
The ED nurse must be alert to signs and symptoms of human trafficking. Physical signs of trafficking include headaches, dizziness, back pain, missing patches of hair (where it has been pulled out), burns, bruises, vaginal or rectal trauma, jaw problems, and head injuries. The victim may also have unusual tattooing or "branding" marks, which are a sign of trafficker ownership. Psychosocial symptoms experienced by victims include stress, paranoia, fear, suicidal ideation, depression, anxiety, shame, and self-loathing.

11

CHAPTER

Concepts of Care for Patients with Common Environmental Emergencies

1. Which are the most common **environmental** factors that cause heat-related illnesses? **Select all that apply.**
   A. Temperature (above 95° F [35° C])
   B. Homelessness
   C. Drugs such as angiotensin-converting enzyme (ACE) inhibitors
   D. High humidity (above 80%)
   E. Use or abuse of substances
   F. Infectious illnesses

2. What is the nurse's **best** response when the spouse of an older adult asks why it is so important to avoid situations where the client would be at risk for a heat-related illness?
   A. "Your spouse might get a blistery sunburn."
   B. "Your spouse has less body fluid and can become easily dehydrated."
   C. "Your spouse avoids drinks containing caffeine and alcohol."
   D. "Your spouse has a low sodium level and should take salt tablets when going outside."

3. Which client will the nurse consider to have the **most** predisposing factors that increase the risk for a heat-related injury?
   A. Middle-aged female with hypothyroidism, living in the southern United States
   B. Older adult male with iron-deficiency anemia who does not drink alcohol
   C. Overweight older adult male who drinks beer during an afternoon baseball game
   D. Malnourished young female with an eating disorder who exercises in the early morning

4. Which factors will help an older adult client to avoid a heat-related injury? **Select all that apply.**
   A. Use a sunscreen with an SPF of at least 30.
   B. Limit activity at the hottest time of day.
   C. Wear lightweight, light-colored, and loose-fitting clothing.
   D. Take hot baths or showers to help cool the body's temperature.
   E. Pay attention to personal physical limitations.
   F. Take breaks from being in a hot environment.

5. Which is the **priority** action for the nurse when providing care for an older adult with weakness, nausea, vomiting, and dizziness, who was outside during a period when the temperature was 110°F (43.4°C) but forgot to drink water?
   A. Assess if client takes medications that increase risk for heat stroke.
   B. Observe for skin turgor and other signs of dehydration.
   C. Assess the size and responsiveness of the client's pupils.
   D. Check the client for orthostatic hypotension and tachycardia.

6. Which signs and symptoms support the nurse's suspicion that a client has developed heat stroke? **Select all that apply.**
   A. Oliguria
   B. Bradycardia
   C. Hypotension
   D. Acute confusion
   E. Decreased respiratory rate
   F. Body temperature of 104°F (40°C)

7. Which are appropriate actions for the nurse to take when a client with heat stroke has been admitted to the ED? **Select all that apply.**
   A. Administer cooled normal saline solution.
   B. Give aspirin or another antipyretic drug as prescribed.
   C. Place client on oxygen by nasal cannula as prescribed.
   D. Insert an indwelling urinary catheter.
   E. Stop cooling efforts when body temperature is 100°F (37.8°C).
   F. Obtain baseline lab tests (e.g., CBC, electrolytes, cardiac enzymes, liver enzymes).

8. Which laboratory test would predict severity of organ damage for a homeless client found confused, with severe sunburn on exposed skin and with a core body temperature of 106°F (41.1°C)?
   A. Cardiac troponin I
   B. Creatine kinase
   C. Complete blood count
   D. Clotting studies

9. What is the **next priority** for the nurse in the ED caring for a client with a heat injury after airway, breathing, and circulation are ensured?
   A. Apply oxygen at 2 L/min by nasal cannula.
   B. Establish a second large bore IV line.
   C. Monitor for seizure activity.
   D. Use methods of rapid cooling.

10. What guidance would the nurse be sure to give the assistive personnel (AP) when caring for a client with a heat injury who started shivering and received an IV dose of propofol?
    A. Keep the client on strict bedrest in the prone position.
    B. Check the client's blood pressure before allowing them out of bed.
    C. Watch for any signs of confusion.
    D. Report any signs that might be seizure activity.

11. What is the **first priority** for the nurse when walking in the woods with a friend who is bitten by a snake?
    A. Call 911 for emergency assistance.
    B. Suck the venom from the fang marks.
    C. Move the person to a safe area.
    D. Attempt to capture the snake.

12. Which first-aid measure will the nurse apply to a client who was bitten by a pit viper on the lower left leg, while waiting for transportation to the hospital?
    A. Incise the fang marks with a pocket knife.
    B. Apply a constricting band proximal to the fang marks.
    C. Elevate the left leg and apply cool packs to the site.
    D. Immobilize the leg with a splint in a functional position.

13. Which is the **most** significant risk for any snakebite victim?
    A. Airway compromise and respiratory failure
    B. Gangrene and loss of limb
    C. Breakdown of human tissue proteins and altered tissue integrity
    D. Nerve and muscle toxins block neurotransmission

14. Which common sense actions to avoid being bitten by a poisonous snake would the nurse teach to a group of clients in the community setting? **Select all that apply.**
    A. Be extremely careful in locations where snakes may hide.
    B. Wear protective clothes such as boots, heavy pants, and leather gloves.
    C. Inspect suspicious areas before placing hands and feet in them.
    D. Striking distance can be up to two thirds the length of the snake.
    E. Newly dead or decapitated snakes can inflict a bite for up to an hour after death.
    F. Do not transport the snake; take a digital photo of the snake at a safe distance.

15. What is the nurse's **best** response when a client calls the emergency department (ED) to ask what should be done immediately for a brown recluse spider bite on the hand?
    A. Apply a snug constricting band at the level of the wrist.
    B. Apply cold compresses and rest as much as possible.
    C. Scrub the bite area several times with soap and warm water.
    D. Apply a warm pack and elevate the extremity.

16. Which complications will the nurse expect that are related to a black widow spider bite? **Select all that apply.**
    A. Muscle rigidity and spasms
    B. Hypertension
    C. Severe abdominal pain
    D. Acute confusion
    E. Severe tinnitus
    F. Nausea and vomiting

17. Which disorder has clinical signs and symptoms that may cause a black widow spider bite to be misdiagnosed?
    A. Thromboembolism
    B. Acute renal failure
    C. Myocardial infarction
    D. Acute abdomen

18. Which assessment technique would the nurse use to confirm a scorpion sting on the right hand of a client?
    A. Observe for the stinger embedded in the skin
    B. Raise the right arm and observe for blanching in the hand
    C. Central bite mark, which may appear as a bleb or vesicle with edema and erythema
    D. Gentle tapping at the site of sting usually causes increased pain

19. What is the **priority** action for the nurse to take at a picnic when an adult who is alert, has no difficulty breathing, and is not allergic to wasps is stung by a wasp?
    A. Apply a warm pack to the area and elevate.
    B. Place a tourniquet proximal to the sting.
    C. Gently scrape the stinger off with the edge of a credit card.
    D. Observe for signs of inflammation before taking any action.

20. Which instructions will the nurse give to a group of community-dwelling adults preparing for a field trip to a farm, to prevent wasp and bee stings? **Select all that apply.**
    A. Wear protective clothing in areas where wasps and bees can be found.
    B. Keep leftover food in covered containers.
    C. Do not try to run from swarms of bees or wasps.
    D. Inspect clothes and shoes for insects before putting them on.
    E. Do not swat at bees or wasps that are close to you.
    F. Carry a prescription epinephrine autoinjector if you are allergic to bee and wasp stings.

21. For which signs and symptoms does the nurse monitor when a client comes in to the emergency department (ED) with an anaphylactic reaction to a bee sting? **Select all that apply.**
    A. Bronchospasm
    B. Hypertension
    C. Laryngeal edema
    D. Respiratory distress
    E. Hypoglycemia
    F. Cardiac dysrhythmias

22. For which statement by a client who experienced a bee sting would the nurse recommend the client go to the emergency department (ED)?
    A. "I am not having shortness of breath but I am a little anxious."
    B. "The affected area is red, swollen, and somewhat painful."
    C. "I was stung by at least 40 to 50 bees all over my belly."
    D. "I don't think it was those 'killer bees' that stung me."

23. When the nurse is teaching clients about lightning injuries, which person would be cited as **most** at risk for injury from a lightning strike?
    A. Deer hunter walking in the woods in the evening during late October
    B. Golfer on the green in the late afternoon in mid-June
    C. Jogger in the park at mid-morning during early December
    D. Camper walking on the beach during early morning in early April

24. Which key points would the nurse include when presenting information about lightning injuries in a community setting? **Select all that apply.**
    A. A lightning strike is imminent if your hair stands on end, you see a blue halo around objects, and hear high-pitched or crackling noises.
    B. Do not stand under an isolated tall tree or structure in an open area such as a field, ridge, or hilltop; lightning tends to strike high points.
    C. If you are caught out in the open and cannot seek shelter, attempt to move to higher ground.
    D. If inside a building, stay away from open doors, windows, fireplaces, metal fixtures, and plumbing.
    E. If inside a tent, stay away from the metal tent poles and wet fabric of the tent walls.
    F. Avoid metal objects such as chairs or bleachers; put down tools, fishing rods, garden equipment, golf clubs, and umbrellas.

25. Which is the **most important** assessment tool for a nurse to use when assessing a client struck by lightning, who was brought to the emergency department (ED) who is alert, but confused and reports pain in his right hand and foot with fern-like marks?
    A. Glasgow coma scale
    B. Rule of nines chart
    C. Pulse oximeter
    D. Cardiac monitor

26. What would the nurse suspect when caring for a client who had a cardiac and respiratory arrest after being struck by lightning when the client is now alert and appears to be recovering, but urine in the drainage bag is now decreased in volume and is dark and tea-coloured?
    A. Dehydration
    B. Urinary tract infection
    C. Rhabdomyolysis
    D. Renal failure

27. Which information will the nurse be sure to include when teaching a client about how to avoid cold injury during cross-country skiing? **Select all that apply.**
    A. Wear layered clothing so it can easily be added or taken off as the temperature changes.
    B. Inner layers of clothing should be cotton which will keep you warmer.
    C. Keep water, extra clothing, blankets, food, and essential personal medications in your car when driving in cold climates.
    D. Body heat is lost through the head, so a hat should always be worn.
    E. Wear synthetic clothing because it moves moisture away from the body and dries fast.
    F. Use sunscreen (minimum sun protection factor [SPF] 10) to protect skin from the sun's harmful rays.

28. Which are common predisposing factors that the nurse knows can cause hypothermia in a client exposed to prolonged cold? **Select all that apply.**
    A. Immobilization
    B. Traumatic injury
    C. Chronic illness
    D. Occasional alcohol use
    E. Use of phenothiazines or barbiturates
    F. Malnutrition

29. Which signs and symptoms does the nurse expect when assessing a client admitted to the emergency department (ED) with mild hypothermia?
    A. Shivering, slurred speech, and mental slowness
    B. Acute confusion, apathy, and incoherence
    C. Bradycardia, hypotension, and acid-base imbalance
    D. Bradypnea, ventricular fibrillation, and decreased neurological reflexes

30. Which treatment does the nurse **most likely** expect for a client admitted with severe hypothermia?
    A. Application of external heat with heating blankets
    B. Extracorporeal rewarming methods such as cardiopulmonary bypass
    C. Heated oxygen or inspired gas to prevent further heat loss via the respiratory tract
    D. Core rewarming by using heated intravenous fluids

31. Which signs and symptoms would the nurse recognize in a client with the **most** severe (grade 4) frostbite?
    A. Hyperemia of the area with edema formation
    B. Small blisters that contain dark fluid and an affected body part that is cool, numb, blue, or red and does not blanch
    C. Large clear-to-milky fluid-filled blisters develop with partial-thickness skin necrosis
    D. Blisters over the carpal or tarsal (instead of just the digit) and the body part is numb, cold, and bloodless

32. Which actions will the nurse use when rewarming a client who has deep frostbite of the right lower leg? **Select all that apply.**
    A. Apply a heating pad with the temperature at the lowest setting.
    B. Administer a tetanus immunization for prophylaxis.
    C. Elevate the extremity above the heart for rewarming.
    D. Administer an opioid analgesic for pain associated with rewarming.
    E. Briskly rub the area to speed the warming process by increasing perfusion.
    F. Use rapid rewarming in a 104 to 106°F (40 to 42°C) water bath.

33. What does the nurse do for a client who has white, waxy skin on the nose, cheeks, and ears?
    A. Seek shelter immediately and warm the body parts using body heat.
    B. Seek medical attention and place the body parts on the car heating vents on the way to the hospital.
    C. Seek shelter immediately and massage the body parts briskly.
    D. Seek medical attention and put cool water compresses on the nose, cheeks, and ears.

34. What condition does the nurse suspect when a client admitted with high-altitude sickness develops apathy and refuses to perform ADLs the next morning, then later in the day is unable to move in bed or to sit up independently?
    A. Acute mountain sickness
    B. Severe hypothermia
    C. High-altitude cerebral edema
    D. Severe hypoxemia

35. Which signs and symptoms indicates to the nurse that a client has developed high-altitude pulmonary edema (HAPE)? **Select all that apply.**
    A. Bradycardia at rest
    B. Tachypnea at rest
    C. Cyanotic lips and nail beds
    D. Abdominal pain and cramping
    E. Waxy appearance around nose and mouth
    F. Persistent dry cough

36. Which assessment findings would indicate to the nurse that the administered acetazolamide treatment given to a client for acute mountain sickness was effective?
    A. Decreased heart rate and decreased urine output
    B. Decreased sleep disturbance and decreased respiratory rate
    C. Increased urine output and increased respiratory rate
    D. Periodic decrease in respirations during sleep and decreased heart rate

37. When a rescue team's descent is delayed by weather from taking a client to the hospital for symptoms of high-altitude pulmonary edema (HAPE), what is the **most important** immediate treatment for this client during the delay?
    A. Oxygen administration
    B. Dexamethasone administration
    C. Keep the client as warm as possible
    D. Plan rapid descent when weather breaks

38. Which are **essential** teaching points when a nurse instructs a community group about prevention of drowning? **Select all that apply.**
    A. Watch people who can't swim and who are in or around the water.
    B. Never dive in shallow water.
    C. Swim alone only if you are a strong swimmer.
    D. Make sure that water rescue equipment is available.
    E. Minimize the use of alcohol or any other substance when swimming.
    F. Test water depth before diving in head first.

39. Which responses caused by the diving reflex may help save the life of a drowning victim? **Select all that apply.**
    A. Metabolic acidosis
    B. Tachypnea
    C. Bradycardia
    D. Increased blood flow into the peripheral circulation
    E. Decreased cardiac output
    F. Vasoconstriction of vessels in the intestines and kidneys

40. Which task would the nurse assign to the assistive personnel (AP) when the emergency department (ED) team is giving emergency care to a drowning victim?
    A. Insert the nasogastric tube and attach to suction.
    B. Advice the victim's family of the resuscitation status.
    C. Assist with the bag-valve-mask device during intubation.
    D. Take, report, and record vital signs every 15 minutes.

Chapter 11 Answer Key

1. A, D
   The most common environmental factors causing heat-related illnesses are high environmental temperature (above 95°F [35°C]) and high humidity (above 80%). Conditions related to this problem with thermoregulation include heat exhaustion and heat stroke. At-risk population factors include older adults, homeless people, people with substance use problems, people with mental health/behavioral health conditions, those who work outside, athletes who engage in outdoor sports, and military members stationed in hot climates. Some prescribed drugs (e.g., ACE inhibitors) increase the risk of heat-related injuries.

2. B
   Older adults have less body fluid volume, can easily become dehydrated, and are a vulnerable at-risk population for heat-related injuries. The client may get sunburned, but that is not why an older adult is at risk for this type of injury.

   Salt tablets should be avoided. Avoiding drinks with caffeine and alcohol will help reduce the risk for heat-related injuries.

3. C
   The client in option C has three risk factors (overweight, alcohol intake, and out in the heat of the day). In each of the other three options (A, B, and D), the client has only two risk factors.

4. A, B, C, E, F
   All of the options are appropriate for avoiding heat-related injuries in older adults, except option D. A client must be taught to take cool baths or showers to help bring the body temperature down.

5. D
   The client is exhibiting flulike symptoms and may be suffering from heat exhaustion, which is primarily due to dehydration. Clients should be assessed for orthostatic hypotension and

tachycardia, especially the older adult who can become dehydrated quickly.

6. A, C, D, F

Options A, C, D, and F are correct. A client with heat stroke would have tachycardia (not bradycardia) and tachypnea (not bradypnea). Additional findings would include warm and dry skin (client may or may not be diaphoretic), electrolyte abnormalities (sodium and potassium), mental status changes, pulmonary edema, and coagulopathy (abnormal clotting).

7. A, C, D, F

Options A, C, D, and F are appropriate. Aspirin and other antipyretics should be avoided. Cooling functions should be stopped when the core body temperature reaches 102°F (39°C).

8. A

Cardiac troponin I (cTnI) is frequently elevated during nonexertional heat-related illnesses when the myocardium releases it in response to damage. Research indicates that this test can be used to cost effectively predict severity and organ damage at the beginning of heat stroke, even in a remote setting.

9. D

After ensuring airway, breathing, and circulation, the next priority is rapid cooling of the client by implementing methods including removing clothing; placing ice packs on the neck, axillae, chest, and groin; immersing the client or wetting the client's body with cold water; and fanning rapidly to aid in evaporative cooling.

10. B

Propofol increases the client's risk for hypotension but does not increase the risk for delirium or seizures. If the client's BP is low, the AP should check for orthostatic BP and tachycardia, then report the findings to the nurse. Clients are unlikely to be kept in the prone position on bedrest. Midazolam has an increased risk for delirium, and benzodiazepines are used to treat seizures.

11. C

When a snakebite occurs, the first priority is to move the person to a safe area away from the snake and encourage rest to decrease venom circulation. Remove jewelry and constricting clothing before swelling worsens. Call for immediate emergency assistance. Do not attempt to capture or kill the snake, but do take digital photographs at a safe distance (if possible) to aid in snake identification.

12. D

While waiting for transportation, the nurse would immobilize the affected extremity in the position of function, and maintain at the level of heart. Do not incise or suck wound, apply ice, or use a tourniquet. Remove jewelry and constrictive clothing.

13. A

The most significant risk to the snakebite victim is airway compromise and respiratory failure. The nurse must make sure that IV lines are patent and that resuscitation equipment is immediately available. The nurse should also contact Poison Control in collaboration with the health care provider to receive guidance for possible antivenom administration and client management.

14. A, B, C, D, E, F

All of these options are appropriate actions for snakebite prevention. Do not harass any snakes encountered. Snakes are most active on warm nights. Venomous snakes should not be kept as pets.

15. B

First-aid or prehospital care for a client with a brown recluse spider bite includes: apply cold compresses over the site of bite to reduce swelling and induce some degree of vasoconstriction that will help reduce systemic spread of the venom; do not apply heat because it increases enzyme activity and potentially worsens the wound; elevate the affected extremity, provide local wound care, and rest.

16. A, B, C, E, F
All of these options are correct except option D. Acute confusion is not a complication of a black widow spider bite.

17. D
A black widow spider bite has symptoms very similar to an acute abdomen and this may be initially incorrectly diagnosed.

18. D
Gentle tapping at the site of sting usually causes an increase in pain to confirm a scorpion bite. Sting sites are often not reddened. Symptoms occur immediately after the sting, reaching crisis level within 12 hours.

19. C
Remove stinger with tweezers or by gently scraping or brushing it off with the edge of a knife blade, credit card, or needle (if available). Then apply an ice pack to decrease swelling.

20. A, B, D, E, F
All options except C are appropriate to teach the students. When a swarm of bees or wasps attack someone, they should try to outrun the swarm.

21. A, C, D, F
When a client has an allergic reaction to a bee or wasp sting, monitor for anaphylaxis, which is a true medical emergency, evidenced by respiratory distress with bronchospasm, laryngeal edema, hypotension, decreased mental status, and cardiac dysrhythmias.

22. C
Any client who has sustained multiple stings (especially if more than 50) should be observed in an emergency care setting for several hours to monitor for the development of toxic venom effects. A critical care admission may be prescribed.

23. B
Most lightning-related injuries occur in the summer months during the afternoon and early evening because of increased thunderstorm activity and greater numbers of people spending time outside. Anyone without adequate shelter, including golfers, hikers, campers, beach-goers, and swimmers, is at risk.

24. A, B, D, E, F
All of these options are correct teaching points except option C. If a client is caught out in the open and cannot seek shelter, he or she should attempt to move to lower ground (not higher ground).

25. D
The most lethal initial effect of massive electrical current discharge on the cardiopulmonary system is cardiac arrest. However, these victims can have serious myocardial injury, which may be indicated by electrocardiogram (ECG) and myocardial perfusion abnormalities such as angina and dysrhythmias.

26. C
Rhabdomyolysis is a serious syndrome due to a direct or indirect muscle injury. It results from the death and breakdown of muscle fibers and release of their contents into the bloodstream. The symptoms of rhabdomyolysis include: muscle weakness, low urine output, fatigue, soreness, bruising, dark, tea-colored urine, infrequent urination, and fever.

27. A, C, D, E
Options A, C, D, and E are appropriate for helping to prevent cold injuries. Cotton clothing holds moisture, becomes wet, and contributes to the development of hypothermia. It should be strictly avoided in a cold outdoor environment; this rule applies to gloves and socks as well because wet gloves and socks promote frostbite in the fingers and toes. Sunscreen should have a minimum sun protection factor (SPF) of 30 to protect the skin from the sun's harmful rays.

28. A, B, E, F
Common predisposing conditions that promote hypothermia include: cold-water immersion, acute (not chronic) illness such as sepsis, traumatic injury, shock states, immobilization, cold weather (e.g., homeless and people working outdoors), older age, selected medications such as phenothiazines or barbiturates, inappropriate

(not occasional) alcohol and substance use, malnutrition, hypothyroidism, and inadequate clothing or shelter (as with the homeless population or people who work outside).

29. **A**

Shivering, slurred speech (dysarthria, decreased muscle coordination, mental slowness (impaired cognition), and diuresis are signs of mild hypothermia. Muscle weakness, increased loss of coordination, acute confusion, apathy, incoherence, possibly stupor, and decreased clotting are signs of moderate hypothermia. Bradycardia, severe hypotension, decreased respiratory rate, cardiac dysrhythmias, including possible ventricular fibrillation or asystole, decreased neurologic reflexes to coma, decreased pain responsiveness, and acid-base imbalance are signs of severe hypothermia.

30. **B**

The treatment of choice for severe hypothermia is to use extracorporeal rewarming methods such as cardiopulmonary bypass or hemodialysis. Application of external heat with heating blankets, heated oxygen, or inspired gas to prevent further heat loss via the respiratory tract, and core rewarming by using heated intravenous fluids are active external and core (internal) rewarming methods. With severe hypothermia, avoid active external rewarming with heating devices because it is dangerous and contraindicated in these clients due to rapid vasodilation.

31. **D**

Blisters over the carpal or tarsal, instead of just the digit, and the body part is numb, cold, and bloodless are characteristic of grade 4 frostbite (the most severe). Grade 1 frostbite (least severe) typically has hyperemia of the area with edema formation. Grade 2 frostbite has large clear-to-milky fluid-filled blisters develop with partial-thickness skin necrosis. Grade 3 frostbite appears as small blisters that contain dark fluid and the affected body part is cool, numb, blue or red, and does not blanch.

32. **B, C, D, F**

Options B, C, D, and F are appropriate rewarming strategies for a victim of deep frostbite.

Recognize that dry heat (e.g., heating pad) or massage (e.g., briskly rubbing) should not be used as part of the warming process for frostbitten areas because these actions can produce further damage to tissue integrity.

33. **A**

When a client has white, waxy appearing body parts, the indication is early frostbite. In this case, the priority action is to seek shelter from the wind and cold, and to warm the affected body parts. Superficial frostbite is easily managed using body heat to warm the affected area(s).

34. **C**

When acute mountain sickness (AMS) progresses to high-altitude cerebral edema (HACE), the client cannot perform ADLs and has extreme apathy. An important sign of HACE is the development of ataxia (defective muscular coordination). The client also experiences a change in mental status with confusion and impaired judgment. Cranial nerve dysfunction and seizures may occur. If untreated, a further decline in the client's level of consciousness can occur. Stupor, coma, and death can result from brain swelling and the subsequent damage caused by increased intracranial pressure over the course of 1 to 3 days.

35. **B, C, F**

Important signs and symptoms of HAPE include a persistent dry cough, and cyanosis of the lips and nail beds. Tachycardia and tachypnea occur at rest. Crackles may be auscultated in one or both lungs. Pink, frothy sputum is a late sign of HAPE.

36. **C**

Acetazolamide is a carbonic anhydrase inhibitor diuretic and is commonly prescribed to prevent or treat AMS. It acts by causing a bicarbonate diuresis, which rids the body of excess fluid and causes metabolic acidosis. The acidotic state increases the respiratory rate and decreases the occurrence of periodic respiration during sleep at night. It also increases urine output by ridding the body of excess fluid.

37. A

The most important intervention to manage serious altitude-related illnesses is descent to a lower altitude. In this case that is not feasible, so the most important treatment while waiting to descend is to administer oxygen to treat the symptoms of AMS. Remember that descent from high altitude should always be slow.

38. A, B, D, F

When providing health teaching, include these points: constantly observe people who cannot swim and are in or around water, do not swim alone, test the water depth before diving in head first; never dive into shallow water, avoid alcoholic beverages and substance use when swimming and boating and while in proximity to water, and ensure that water rescue equipment such as life jackets, flotation devices, and rope is immediately available when around water.

39. C, E, F

The diving reflex is a physiologic response to asphyxia when a person drowns. It produces bradycardia; a reduction in cardiac output; and vasoconstriction of vessels in the intestine, skeletal muscles, and kidneys. These physiologic effects are thought to reduce myocardial oxygen use and enhance blood flow to the heart and cerebral tissues. Survival is thought to be linked to some combination of the effects of hypothermia and the diving reflex.

40. D

The nurse must be familiar with the scope of practice for an AP, which includes checking, reporting, and recording vital signs. Reporting on the victim's status, inserting the nasogastric tube, and assisting with the bag-valve-mask device would require additional training and education and would be within the scope of the nurse, the health care provider, and the respiratory therapist.

12

CHAPTER

Concepts of Disaster Preparedness

1. Which are examples of external disasters? **Select all that apply.**
   A. Loss of critical utility such as electricity
   B. Malfunction of a nuclear reactor with radiation
   C. A violent active shooter situation
   D. Ebola virus crisis
   E. Fire in a long-term care facility
   F. Terrorist act using explosive advice

2. Which statement about The Joint Commission Mandates for Emergency Preparedness Plans for maintenance of ongoing disaster preparedness is true?
   A. All facilities must prepare to become trauma centers in the event of any disaster.
   B. The emergency preparedness plan must be tested through drills or actual participation in a real event at least twice a year.
   C. Both drills or events must involve community-wide resources and influx of actual or simulated clients to assess the ability of collaborative and command structures.
   D. Long-term care facilities are required to take an "all-hazards approach" to disaster planning.

3. What information would be **most** important for the nurse to get in order to determine the potential for a multi-casualty event versus a mass casualty event at a local high school?
   A. "Have emergency medical services been notified?"
   B. "What are school officials saying about the event?"
   C. "What are the number and the severity of injuries?"
   D. "How long ago did the event occur?"

4. Which **priority** would be included in the emergency management plan for a small community hospital in a suburban area of a large city?
   A. Plan for transporting patients to other hospitals
   B. Method for contacting the National Disaster Medical System
   C. Stockpiling postexposure prophylactic antibiotics
   D. Plan for evacuation routes out of the city

5. Which clients would the triage nurse designate as black-tagged? **Select all that apply.**
   A. Client with massive head trauma
   B. Client with airway obstruction
   C. Client with an open fracture
   D. Client with extensive full-thickness burns
   E. Client with multiple abrasions and contusions
   F. Client with sprained wrist who can walk

6. During a disaster drill, which action would be **most** appropriate to assign to an assistive personnel (AP) who usually works in labor and delivery?
   A. Care for and support the green-tagged clients.
   B. Stay with the black-tagged clients in the holding area.
   C. Answer questions for the families of the red-tagged clients.
   D. Obtain and record vital signs for the yellow-tagged clients.

7. What must a nurse based in Texas, who is a member of a Disaster Medical Assistance Team (DMAT) and has been asked to serve in Colorado, do when he or she does not hold an active Colorado nursing license?
   A. Discover whether Colorado has reciprocity with Texas before accepting deployment.
   B. Prepare for deployment because he or she will be considered a federal employee with valid licensure.
   C. Decline deployment because his or her nursing license will not allow him or her to practice in Colorado.
   D. Delay deployment until he or she has reviewed the Nurse Practice Act that is specific to Colorado.

8. Which is the personnel function of the hospital incident commander?
   A. Person who serves as liaison between the health care facility and the media
   B. Physician or nurse who rapidly evaluates each client to determine priority of treatment
   C. Physician who decides the number, acuity, and resource needs of clients
   D. Physician or administrator who assumes overall leadership for implementing the emergency plan

9. What is the nurse's **best** response when a local news station calls the hospital ED to verify the number of victims and details of a local disaster?
   A. "Hold and I will connect you with the emergency command center."
   B. "Please hold and I will connect you with the community relations officer."
   C. "We have many stable victims but so far no one has died."
   D. "Don't bother us because we are trying to care for the disaster victims."

10. Which actions are appropriate for the ED charge nurse of a large suburban hospital who is informed at 3:00 a.m. that a commercial airplane just crashed outside the city limits? **Select all that apply.**
    A. Activate the hospital's emergency management plan.
    B. Initiate the staff telephone tree.
    C. Collaborate with the triage officer.
    D. Alert the critical incident stress debriefing team.
    E. Organize nursing and ancillary services.
    F. Collaborate with the medical command physician.

11. What is an appropriate project for nurses serving on a committee that is to develop tools and aids for the medical command physician to use during a disaster event?
    A. Create a telephone tree for contacting the nursing and ancillary staff.
    B. Design a triage algorithm that addresses different types of disaster events.
    C. Make a list that includes contact information for all trauma and orthopedic surgeons.
    D. Create an algorithm for contacting the Federal Emergency Management Agency.

12. Which action would the nurse include in her or his personnel emergency preparedness plan?
    A. Teach family members about radiation and bioterrorism safety issues.
    B. Stockpile antibiotics, first-aid supplies, and resuscitation equipment.
    C. Resolve all ethical conflicts of family and professional obligations.
    D. Create a disaster supply kit with clothing and basic survival supplies.

13. What is the **priority** action for a nurse when a client comes to the ED worried that he has been exposed to an infectious bioterrorism agent?
    A. Escort the client to a quarantined area.
    B. Call the local police and Department of Public Health.
    C. Take a comprehensive history and assess for any symptoms.
    D. Activate the emergency preparedness plan.

14. Which basic supplies will the nurse include in his or her personal disaster kit? **Select all that apply.**
    A. Cell phone and charger
    B. Towel, washcloth, soap, hand sanitizer
    C. Battery-powered radio
    D. Sturdy footwear
    E. Toiletry articles
    F. One gallon water per day for at least 3 days
    G. Sleeping bag and pillow
    H. Duct tape and plastic sheeting

15. Which responsibility is appropriate for the nurse assigned to assist the hospital incident commander during a disaster drill?
    A. Contact the security department and instruct them to control the number of people who attempt to enter the hospital.
    B. Call all nursing units to determine the number of patients who could potentially be discharged.
    C. Call the physical therapy department and direct the therapists to assist in the operating room and the intensive care unit.
    D. Go to the emergency department and assist with the triage of disaster victims to appropriate clinical areas.

16. Which situation describes the **most** appropriate reassignment of nursing staff?
    A. Intensive care nurse is reassigned to care for clients with massive head injuries and black tags.
    B. Physical therapist is reassigned to take and record vital signs on medical-surgical clients.
    C. Medical staff nurses are reassigned to provide care for stable emergency room clients.
    D. Operating room nurse is reassigned to the emergency room to assist with triage.

17. Which is the **best** example of the "greatest good for the greatest number of people"?
    A. Twenty victims infected by a bioterrorism agent are placed on life support with mechanical ventilation.
    B. Elderly community members are treated with prophylactic antibiotics for a bioterrorism agent.
    C. The city's supply of antibiotics is sent to one hospital that has 25 victims with exposure to a bioterrorism agent.
    D. Thirty people with possible exposure to a bioterrorism agent are quarantined, including five children who are asymptomatic.

18. After a mass casualty disaster, what is the purpose of conducting the postplan administrative review?
    A. To identify employees who need financial help or reimbursement
    B. To provide all employees the opportunity to express positive and negative comments
    C. To establish a system of networking and support for employees
    D. To focus on errors that were made and things that went wrong during the plan

19. Which actions or behaviors by a nurse who was involved in a mass casualty event are most consistent with practices recommended to reduce the risk for development of posttraumatic stress disorder (PTSD)? **Select all that apply**.
    A. Drinking two to four glasses of wine before bed daily
    B. Interacting with a crisis intervention specialist weekly
    C. Hugging a fellow nurse when he or she bursts into tears at the sound of an alarm
    D. Bringing a fruit basket to work and sharing the contents with all co-workers for snacks
    E. Changing his or her work schedule from two 16-hour shifts per week to four 8-hour shifts per week
    F. Wearing headphones at breaks to avoid sharing thoughts and feelings with co-workers who also experienced the event

20. What must be the **initial** action of first responders in a community-based disaster?
    A. Provide first aid.
    B. Triage the victims.
    C. Remove people from danger.
    D. Notify the local hospital.

21. Which element of a long-term care facility's emergency preparedness plan must be resolved to meet the guidelines of the Life Safety Code published by the National Fire Protection Association?
    A. Many residents are unwilling or unable to participate in fire drills.
    B. Fire extinguishers are heavy and difficult to use.
    C. Fire safety training is difficult to keep current because of high staff turnover.
    D. The building has one main front door and the side doors are sealed shut.

22. Which actions are part of the nurse's role in responding to health care facility fires? **Select all that apply.**
    A. Remove any client or staff from immediate danger from fire or smoke.
    B. Direct ambulatory clients to walk to a safe location.
    C. Continue oxygen on all clients who have it prescribed by the HCP.
    D. Ask ambulatory clients to push wheelchair clients out of danger if possible.
    E. When everyone is out of danger, contain the fire by closing doors and windows.
    F. Move bedridden clients out of danger in beds, on stretchers or wheelchairs.

23. When a mass casualty event occurs, which group of victims is **most** likely to require the largest amount of physical space?
    A. Green-tagged victims
    B. Yellow-tagged victims
    C. Red-tagged victims
    D. Black-tagged victims

24. Which client is correctly triaged and marked with the appropriate color tag?
    A. A teenager with profuse bleeding from a severe arm laceration: black tag
    B. An older adult woman with a fractured ankle: yellow tag
    C. A child who has died from severe injuries: green tag
    D. An older adult male with shortness of breath and a pneumothorax: red tag

25. What would the nurse do **first** when gunshots are heard in the waiting room?
    A. Grab a resuscitation box and hurry to the waiting area.
    B. Assist ambulatory clients to leave through the back entrance.
    C. Assess the level of threat to self and others then call for help.
    D. Alert the ED health care provider that additional trauma clients will need care.

26. What is the best action for the nurse to take after using the Impact of Event Scale-Revised (IES-R) with an assistive personnel (AP) who works in a long-term care facility that was devastated by a fire when the IES-R scores are high on all subscales?
    A. Suggest coping strategies that the AP can use to decrease stress.
    B. Refer the AP to a psychiatrist or clinical psychologist for additional evaluation.
    C. Reinforce the coping strategies that the AP is using successfully.
    D. Refer the AP to a social worker or a support group for survivors of disasters.

27. Which situation constitutes an internal disaster?
    A. Two nurses losing consciousness while providing care to an unconscious client suffering a fentanyl overdose
    B. Regional power failure after a snow storm requiring a hospital to continue services while using emergency generators
    C. Broken water pipe in the service level of a nursing home causing a total loss of electricity for two days
    D. Waste-basket fire in an emergency department from an inadequately extinguished client cigarette

28. Which actions would be useful when the nurse is helping people after a mass casualty event? **Select all that apply.**
    A. Establish rapport through active listening and honest communication.
    B. Allow survivors to talk about their experiences.
    C. Offer resources to help survivors gain a sense of personal control.
    D. Provide a sense of safety and security.
    E. Give complete and complex responses to all questions from survivors.
    F. Request crisis counselors respond to assist survivors and families by providing compassionate support.

Chapter 12 Answer Key

1. B, D, F
   An external event or disaster occurs outside the health care facility or campus, but requires activation of the facility's emergency management plan. Examples include options B, C, and F. Other examples include hurricanes, earthquakes, and tornadoes. Options A, D, and E are internal disasters that occur inside a health care facility or campus and endanger clients and staff.

2. B.
   The emergency preparedness plan for all hospitals must be tested through drills or actual participation in a real event at least twice a year. All facilities are not expected to become trauma centers, though many small hospitals will likely send seriously injured clients to larger facilities. One of the drills or events must involve community-wide resources and influx of actual or simulated clients. Accredited health care organizations are required to take an "all-hazards approach" to disaster planning.

3. C
   Multi-casualty and mass casualty (disaster) events are not the same. The main difference is based on the scope and scale of the incident considering the number and severity of victims or casualties involved. Multi-casualty events can be managed by a hospital using local resources, but a mass casualty event overwhelms local medical capacities and may require state, regional, or national resources to support the event. The nurse would need to know the number and nature of injuries to determine which type of event had occurred.

4. A
   Hospitals that are heavily impacted by a disaster event will need to evacuate clients to other facilities. In smaller hospitals with limited specialty resources, it is often necessary to determine if and when clients should be transported out of the facility to a higher level of care or to a specialty hospital (e.g., burn center, critical care unit).

5. A, D
   Black-tagged clients are expected (and permitted) to die or are dead. Examples are options A and D. The client with an airway obstruction would be red-tagged and needs to be seen emergently. Green-tagged clients have minor injuries that can be managed in a delayed manner. Examples include clients with closed fractures, sprains, strains, abrasions, and contusions. A green-tagged client ("walking wounded") is nonurgent and in many cases can evacuate him or herself from the mass casualty scene to the hospital.

6. D
   To respond to this question, the nurse must be familiar with the scope of practice for an AP which includes taking and recording vital signs.

Although this AP usually works in labor and delivery, he or she would be familiar and skilled with this task. Answering questions requires additional skills of the licensed nurse. Green-tagged clients do not require treatment at this time. Black-tagged clients are those who are dead or are dying.

7. B

Licensed health care providers (e.g., nurses) act as federal employees when they are deployed, so their professional licenses are recognized as valid in all states. The nurse should prepare for deployment.

8. D

The hospital incident commander assumes overall leadership for implementing the situational plan. It is usually a physician in the ED or a hospital administrator. The community relations officer is liaison between the facility and the media. The triage officer rapidly evaluates clients and determines priorities for treatment. The medical command physician decides the number, acuity, and resource needs of clients.

9. B

The community relations officer serves as liaison between the hospital facility and the media. He or she should be contacted to respond to any questions from the media. The nurse should not give out information about the victims, and the emergency command center is not responsible for communications with the media.

10. B, C, E, F

Options B, C, E, and F are appropriate actions for the ED charge nurse to take when notified of a potential disaster, especially since the time is 3:00 a.m., when hospitals usually have the fewest staff. Activating the emergency management plan is the role of the hospital incident commander and alerting the critical incident stress debriefing team involves provision of sessions for small groups of staff in which teams are brought in to discuss effective coping strategies (critical incident stress debriefing), which usually occurs after the disaster stand-down.

11. C

The role of the medical command physician is to decide the number, acuity, and resource needs of clients. A list of orthopedic and trauma surgeons would be of use in contacting these types of surgeons if it were determined that clients had need of these resources.

12. D

A personal emergency preparedness plan is developed in advance of a disaster by each individual nurse and can help in such situations. It should include creation of a disaster supply kit ("go bag") with a 3-day supply of clothes and basic survival supplies and can be kept in the home or car. It should also outline the pre-planned specific arrangements that are to be made for child care, pet care, and older adult care if the need arises, especially if the event prevents returning home for an extended period.

13. A

This client was able to self-transport to the ED. A danger of these clients is that they may unknowingly carry contaminants from nuclear, biologic, or chemical incidents into the hospital. The priority action for the nurse is to quarantine the client to stop the spread of the bioterrorism agent to others, and then appropriate decontamination measures must be taken.

14. A, B, C, D, E, F, G, H

All of these options are included in a personal preparedness kit. See Table 12.3 in your text for additional options to include.

15. B

An appropriate responsibility for a nurse assisting the hospital incident commander is to check with all nursing units to determine how many clients can possibly be discharged. The hospital commander is the overall leader for implementing the disaster drill and would direct departments to cancel their usual operation to convert space into treatment areas. If the nurse went to help with triage, he or she would not be available to assist the hospital incident commander.

16. C

General medical staff nurses would collaborate with ED nurses to provide care for stable clients, allowing ED nurses to focus on triage and caring for disaster victims. ICU nursing skills would be wasted on black-tagged clients who are dead or dying. Taking and recording vital signs is not in the scope of practice for physical therapists. OR nurses' skills do not focus on triage.

17. D

The greatest good for the greatest number of people is still the organizing principle when considering roles and responsibilities in mass casualty events. Option D gives an example of the highest number of clients treated or the "greatest good for the greatest number of people."

18. B

The administrative review is a type of debriefing that focuses on staff and system performance during the event and determines whether opportunities for improvement in the emergency plan exist. The goal of this debriefing is to discover what went right and what could be improved during activation and implementation of the emergency preparedness plan so needed changes can be made. Usually, representatives from all groups who were involved in the incident come together soon after plan activation has been discontinued. They are each given an opportunity to hear and express positive and negative comments related to their experiences with the event.

19. B, C, D, E

The best practices shown to help reduce the risk for PTSD are:
Use available counseling.
Encourage and support co-workers.
Monitor each other's stress level and performance.
Take breaks when needed.
Talk about feelings with staff and managers.
Drink plenty of water and eat healthy snacks for energy.
Keep in touch with family, friends, and significant others.
Do not work more than 12 hours per day.
Drinking alcohol for sleep often does not produce a restful sleep and can lead to excess alcohol usage.

20. C

The first initial action of first responders in a disaster is to remove injured and uninjured people from danger. After removal from danger, victims should be triaged by health care personnel. After triage, nurses can provide first aid and emergency care. Nurses would supervise and teach volunteers. The hospital should be notified to expect victims who will need additional care.

21. D

The facility has only one exit. Part of the response plan must include a method for evacuation of residents from the facility in a timely and safe manner in the event of a disaster. This is not acceptable and makes evacuation of residents in a timely, safe manner very difficult.

22. A, B, D, E, F

Oxygen can be removed if a client can breathe without it. The other options are all appropriate to the nurse's role in response to health care facility fires. For additional options, see the box labeled Best Practices for Patient Safety and Quality Care – Nurse's Role in Responding to Health Care Facility Fires in your text.

23. A

Green-tagged patients usually make up the greatest number of victims in most large-scale multi-casualty situations. They can overwhelm the system if provisions are not made to handle them as part of the disaster plan. They are also called the "walking wounded" because they may actually evacuate themselves from the mass casualty scene and go to the hospital in a private vehicle.

24. D

A client with a red tag has an immediate threatening condition such as airway obstruction or shock and requires immediate attention like option D. The child who died should have a black tag. The teenager with profuse bleeding should have a yellow tag. The older woman with a fractured ankle should have a green tag.

25. C

Gunshots in the waiting room is a disaster occurring within a facility (internal disaster). The most important outcome for any internal disaster is to maintain client, staff, and visitor safety. The core components of the nursing process apply in the overall assessment of the emergency situation. Assessing the threat to staff and clients would be the first action the nurse would take in this active shooter setting.

26. B
All of the subscales for the AP have high scores. Depending on the client's presentation and the results of the nurse's assessment, remember that behavioral health evaluation and referral to counseling may be appropriate. This AP would likely benefit for further evaluation and counseling to cope with living through the fire disaster.

27. C
An internal disaster is one that occurs inside a health care facility that requires the evacuation of clients for safety. Anything that causes a total loss of electricity for 2 days would definitely endanger nursing home clients, requiring their evacuation from the facility. The other situations do not require evacuation, only slight relocation within the facility, if at all.

28. A, B, C, D, F
All options are correct except option E. Survivors should be helped to adapt to their new surroundings and routines by way of simple, concrete explanations.

13

CHAPTER

Concepts of Fluid and Electrolyte Balance

1. Which adult would normally be expected to have the highest total body water volume?
   A. 25-year-old woman
   B. 25-year-old man
   C. 75-year-old woman
   D. 75-year-old man

2. Which body fluid compartment is considered the "third space?"
   A. Extracellular fluid
   B. Intracellular fluid
   C. Interstitial fluid
   D. Blood (plasma)

3. Which symptom does the nurse expect to see **first** in a client whose plasma volume has an increased hydrostatic pressure?
   A. Dependent edema
   B. Decreased urine output
   C. Poor skin turgor with "tenting"
   D. Greatly increased sensation of thirst

4. Plasma is part of which body fluid space compartments? **Select all that apply**.
   A. The intracellular compartment
   B. The extracellular compartment
   C. All fluid within the cells
   D. Interstitial fluid
   E. Intravascular fluid
   F. Fluid within joint capsules

5. What **immediate response** does the nurse expect as a result of infusing 1 liter of an isotonic intravenous solution into a client over a 3-hour time period if urine output remains at 100 mL per hour?
   A. Extracellular fluid (ECF) osmolarity increases; body weight increases
   B. Extracellular fluid (ECF) osmolarity decreases; body weight decreases
   C. Extracellular fluid (ECF) osmolarity is unchanged; body weight increases
   B. Extracellular fluid (ECF) osmolarity is unchanged; body weight decreases

6. Ankle and foot edema in a nurse who has been standing for 12 hours is a result of which type of pressure, force, or influence?
   A. Filtration from the plasma volume to the interstitial space as a result of increased capillary hydrostatic pressure
   B. Filtration from the plasma volume to the interstitial space as a result of decreased capillary hydrostatic pressure
   C. Osmosis from the interstitial space to the plasma volume as a result of increased osmotic pressure because the nurse also was dehydrated as well as overworked
   D. Osmosis from the plasma volume to the interstitial space as a result of decreased cellular osmotic pressure because tissues damaged from standing released intracellular fluid

7. What is the minimum amount of urine output per day needed to excrete toxic waste products?
   A. 200 to 300 mL
   B. 400 to 600 mL
   C. 500 to 1000 mL
   D. 1000 to 1500 mL

8. Which IV fluid does the nurse expect to administer to a client who is prescribed to receive **hypotonic** fluids?
   A. 9% saline
   B. 3% saline
   C. 0.9% saline
   D. 0.45% saline

9. What sign or symptom does the nurse expect to see in a client whose blood osmolarity is 310 mOsm/L (mOsm/kg)?
   A. Body temperature below normal
   B. Increased thirst
   C. Pitting edema
   D. Diarrhea

10. For which indication of a fluid balance problem will the nurse assess in an older client at risk for fluid and electrolyte problems?
    A. Fever
    B. Elevated blood pressure
    C. Poor skin turgor
    D. Mental status changes

11. Which types of fluid loss are considered "insensible fluid loss?" **Select all that apply.**
    A. Sweat
    B. Salivation
    C. Urine
    D. Diarrhea
    E. Vomit
    F. Wound drainage

12. Which client factors affect the amount and distribution of body fluids? **Select all that apply**.
    A. Race
    B. Age
    C. Gender
    D. Height
    E. Body fat
    F. Muscle mass

13. Which potential problems does the nurse assess for when caring for a client whose urine output is less than what is needed as the obligatory urine output? **Select all that apply**.
    A. Lethal electrolyte imbalances
    B. Alkalosis
    C. Urine becomes diluted
    D. Toxic buildup of nitrogen
    E. Increased infection risk
    F. Acidosis

14. With which client does the nurse remain most alert for an electrolyte imbalance?
    A. 49-year-old with intermittent asthma who also uses an albuterol inhaler PRN
    B. 60-year old with a sprained wrist who also takes acetaminophen for pain
    C. 72-year-old with diabetes mellitus who also takes a diuretic daily
    D. 80-year-old anemia who also take an iron supplement

15. Which electrolyte change does the nurse expect to see in a client who produces excessive amounts of aldosterone?
    A. Low serum sodium level
    B. High serum potassium level
    C. Low serum calcium level
    D. High serum sodium level

16. Which serum electrolyte finding on a newly admitted client does the nurse report immediately to the health care provider? **Select all that apply**.
    A. Potassium 2.8 mEq/L (mmol/L)
    B. Sodium 143 mEq/L (mmol/L
    C. Calcium 9.9 mg/dL (2.59 mmol/L)
    D. Chloride 101 mEq/L (mmol/L)
    E. Chloride 98 mEq/L (mmol/L)
    F. Magnesium 1.2 mEq/L (0.7 mmol/L

17. With which client condition will the nurse remain most alert for insensible water loss?
    A. Continuous GI suctioning
    B. Deep respirations
    C. Receiving oxygen therapy
    D. Hypothermia

18. What response does the nurse expect to see in the blood volume and blood osmolarity of a client whose secretion of antidiuretic hormone (ADH) is extremely low?
    A. Decreased blood volume; decreased blood osmolarity
    B. Decreased blood volume; increased blood osmolarity
    C. Increased blood volume; decreased blood osmolarity
    D. Increased blood volume; increased blood osmolarity

19. Which health problems are most likely to activate the renin-angiotensin-aldosterone system (RAAS)? **Select all that apply?**
    A. Shock
    B. Urinary tract infection
    C. Constipation
    D. Dehydration
    E. Severe asthma
    F. Hypertension

20. Which electrolyte plays the largest role in maintaining blood osmolarity?
    A. Calcium
    B. Chloride
    C. Potassium
    D. Sodium

21. The electrolyte magnesium is responsible for which functions? **Select all that apply**.
    A. Formation of hydrochloric acid
    B. Carbohydrate metabolism
    C. Contraction of skeletal muscle
    D. Regulation of intracellular osmolarity
    E. Vitamin activation
    F. Blood coagulation

22. Clients with which problems will the nurse assess most frequently for dehydration? **Select all that apply**.
    A. Fever of 103°F (39.4°C)
    B. Extensive burns
    C. Thyroid crisis
    D. Water intoxication
    E. Continuous fistula drainage
    F. Diabetes insipidus

23. What is the main reason a nurse caring for a postoperative surgical client in the recovery room carefully monitoring the client's urine output?
    A. Decreasing urine output indicates poor kidney function.
    B. Increasing urine output can indicate excessive IV fluid during surgery.
    C. Decreasing urine output may mean hemorrhage and risk for shock.
    D. Increasing urine output may mean that kidney function is returning to normal.

24. What change in respiratory function does the nurse expect to find in a client who is dehydrated from severe diarrhea and vomiting?
    A. No changes, because the respiratory system is not involved
    B. Increased respiratory rate, because the body perceives dehydration as hypoxia
    C. Hypoventilation, because the respiratory system is trying to compensate for low pH
    D. Normal respiratory rate, but a decreased oxygen saturation

25. Which is the best technique to use for assessing the skin turgor of an 80-year-old client?
    A. Observing the skin for a dry, scaly appearance and compare it to a previous assessment.
    B. Pinching the skin over the back of the hand and observe for tenting; count the number of seconds for the skin to recover position.
    C. Observing the mucous membranes and tongue for cracks, fissures, or a pasty coating.
    D. Pinching the skin over the sternum and observe for tenting and resumption of skin to its normal position after release.

26. What is the nurse's interpretation of a client's urine specific gravity of 1.039?
    A. Overhydration
    B. Dehydration
    C. Normal value for an adult
    D. Renal disease

27. Which actions will the nurse teach to the spouse of a client with reduced cognition who has been treated twice in the emergency department for dehydration to prevent this condition? **Select all that apply.**
    A. Avoid offering fluids after 6:00 p.m.
    B. Weigh the client daily to check fluid status.
    C. Offer frequent snacks of gelatins and ice cream.
    D. Give the client salty crackers to increase his or her sensation of thirst.
    E. Offer four ounces of the client's favorite fluids every hour while awake.
    F. Watch the client while he or she drinks any liquids to ensure it is ingested.
    G. Estimate or measure the number of liquid ounces ingested daily to ensure an intake of at least 1500 mL.

28. Which findings indicate to the nurse that a client may have hypervolemia (fluid overload)? **Select all that apply**.
    A. Increased, bounding pulse
    B. Jugular venous distention
    C. Presence of crackles
    D. Excessive thirst
    E. Elevated blood pressure
    F. Orthostatic hypotension

29. For which client problem will the nurse question a prescription for a diuretic?
    A. Pulmonary edema
    B. Heart failure
    C. End-stage renal disease
    D. Ascites

30. Which possible imbalance does the nurse suspect when assessment findings on a newly admitted client include pitting dependent edema, engorged neck and hand veins, and headache?
    A. Dehydration
    B. Hypervolemia
    C. Fluid volume deficit
    D. Hemoconcentration

31. How many milliliters will the nurse record as being lost by a client with pulmonary edema who initially weighed 178 lb and now weighs 161.6 lb?
    A. 1000
    B. 3000
    C. 5000
    D. 7000

32. Which specific discharge instruction will the nurse provide to **prevent harm** in a client with advanced heart failure who is at continued risk for fluid volume overload?
    A. Greater than 3 lb gained in a week or greater than 1 to 2 lb gained in a 24-hour period
    B. Greater than 5 lb gained in a week or greater than 1 to 2 lb gained in a 24-hour period
    C. Greater than 15 lb gained in a month or greater than 5 lb gained in a week
    D. Greater than 20 lb gained in a month or greater than 5 lb gained in a week

33. The nurse will monitor which clients for development of hyponatremia? **Select all that apply**.
    A. Postoperative client who has been NPO (nothing by mouth) for 24 hours with no IV fluid infusing
    B. Client with decreased fluid intake for 3 days
    C. Client receiving excessive intravenous fluids with 5% dextrose in water
    D. Client with diabetes who has a blood glucose of 250 mg/dL
    E. Client with overactive adrenal glands
    F. Tennis player in 100°F (37.7°C) weather who has been drinking water

34. Which serum value indicates to the nurse that the client has hyponatremia?
    A. Sodium 129 mEq/L (mmol/L)
    B. Chloride 98 mEq/L (mmol/L)
    C. Sodium 144 mEq/L (mmol/L)
    D. Chloride 103 mEq/L (mmol/L)

35. Which assessment findings would indicate to the nurse that the client may have hyponatremia? **Select all that apply**.
    A. Hyperactive bowel sounds on auscultation
    B. Acute-onset confusion
    C. Muscle weakness
    D. Decreased deep tendon reflexes
    E. Abdominal cramping
    F. Nausea

36. Which drug therapy does the nurse expect the health care provider to prescribe for a client with low serum sodium and signs of hypervolemia?
    A. Conivaptan
    B. Furosemide
    C. Hydrochlorothiazide
    D. Bumetanide

37. Which symptom in a client with psychiatric issues who is continuously drinking water will the nurse monitor as an indicator of potential hyponatremia?
    A. Insomnia
    B. Pitting edema
    C. Tremors
    D. Decreased cognition

38. Which serum value indicates to the nurse that the client has hypernatremia?
    A. Potassium 3.9 mEq/L (mmol/L)
    B. Chloride 103 mEq/L (mmol/L)
    C. Sodium 149 mEq/L (mmol/L)
    D. Potassium 4.9 mEq/L (mmol/L)

39. A client is talking to the nurse about sodium intake. Which statement by a client indicates to the nurse a correct understanding of high-sodium food sources?
    A. "I have bacon and eggs every morning for breakfast."
    B. "We never eat seafood because of the salt water."
    C. "I love Chinese food, but I gave it up because of the soy sauce."
    D. "Pickled herring is a fish, and my doctor told me to eat a lot of fish."

40. The nurse observes clients with which of the following conditions for potential hypernatremia? **Select all that apply.**
    A. Chronic constipation
    B. Heart failure
    C. Severe diarrhea
    D. Decreased kidney function
    E. Profound diaphoresis
    F. Cushing's syndrome

41. Which sign or symptom does the nurse expect to see in a client who has mild hypernatremia?
    A. Muscle twitching and irregular muscle contractions
    B. Inability of muscles and nerves to respond to a stimulus
    C. Muscle weakness occurring bilaterally with no specific pattern
    D. Reduced or absent bilateral deep tendon reflexes

42. Which intervention does the nurse anticipate for a client who has hypernatremia caused by reduced kidney sodium excretion?
    A. IV administration of 0.9% sodium chloride solution
    B. IV administration of Ringer's lactate solution
    C. Administration of convaptan
    D. Administration of furosemide

43. Which common signs and symptoms will the nurse be sure to assess for in the older client whose serum sodium level is 152 mEq/L? **Select all that apply**.
    A. Intact recall of recent events
    B. Increased pulse rate
    C. Weight loss
    D. Hypertension
    E. Muscle weakness
    F. Difficulty palpating peripheral pulses

44. Which precaution is **most important** for the nurse to teach a client at continued risk for hypernatremia?
    A. Avoid salt substitutes.
    B. Avoid aspirin and aspirin-containing products.
    C. Read labels on canned or packaged foods to determine sodium content.
    D. Increase daily intake of caffeine-containing foods and beverages.

45. Which serum laboratory value does the nurse expect to see in the client with hypokalemia?
    A. Sodium less than 8.0 mEq/L (mmol/dL)
    B. Potassium less than 3.5 mEq/L (mmol/dL)
    C. Chloride less than 100.0 mEq/L (mmol/dL)
    D. Calcium less than 9.0 mg/dL (2.25 mmol/dL)

46. Which effect on respiratory effort does the nurse expect to find in a client with severe hypokalemia?
    A. Shallow respirations and low oxygen saturation
    B. Deep, rapid respirations with high oxygen saturation
    C. Deep, slow respirations with high oxygen saturation
    D. No specific change in respiratory rate or effectiveness

47. Which GI complication will the nurse monitor for in a client who has a serum potassium level of 2.4 mEq/L (mmol/L)?
    A. Hyperactive bowel sounds
    B. Paralytic ileus
    C. Esophageal reflux
    D. Excessive flatus

48. Which conditions or health problems increase a client's risk for hypokalemia? **Select all that apply.**
    A. Liver failure
    B. Metabolic alkalosis
    C. Cushing syndrome
    D. Hypothyroidism
    E. Paralytic ileus
    F. Kidney failure

49. For which serious complication will the nurse administering an IV potassium solution to a client carefully monitor to **prevent harm**?
    A. Pulmonary edema
    B. Cardiac dysrhythmia
    C. Postural hypotension
    D. Kidney failure

50. Which IV potassium solution can the nurse safely administer to a client with severe hypokalemia?
    A. KCl 5 mEq in 20 mL NS
    B. KCl 10 mEq in 100 mL NS
    C. KCl 15 mEq in 50 mL NS
    D. KCl 20 mEq in 100 mL NS

51. Which action is **most important** for the nurse to perform to **prevent harm** before starting an IV infusion of potassium to a client who has a low serum potassium level?
    A. Determine IV line patency and blood return.
    B. Assess oxygen saturation level with pulse oximetry.
    C. Evaluate baseline mental status.
    D. Check the apical pulse for a full minute.
    E. Check deep tendon reflexes.
    F. Measure intake and output.

52. Which client statement indicates to the nurse a correct understanding of the management of hypokalemia?
    A. "My wife does all the cooking. She shops for food high in calcium."
    B. "When I take the liquid potassium in the evening, I'll eat a snack beforehand."
    C. "I will avoid bananas, orange juice, and salt substitutes."
    D. "If I switch to a vegetarian diet, I can stop taking the liquid potassium."

53. The pharmacy sends a 250-mL IV bag of dextrose in water with 40 mEq of potassium, marked "to infuse over 1 hour" for a client with hypokalemia. What is the nurse's **best** action?
    A. Obtain a pump and administer the solution.
    B. Double-check the prescription and call the pharmacy.
    C. Recheck the client's potassium level to ensure the IV is safe to administer.
    D. Recalculate the rate so that it is safe for the client.

54. Which foods does the nurse teach a client to include in his or her diet to help prevent future episodes of hypokalemia? Select all that apply.
    A. Soybeans
    B. Bananas
    C. Cantaloupe
    D. Potatoes
    E. Peaches
    F. Lettuce

55. Which serum potassium value indicates to the nurse that a client has hyperkalemia?
    A. 2.9 mEq/L (mmol/L)
    B. 3.9 mEq/L (mmol/L)
    C. 4.9 mEq/L (mmol/L)
    D. 5.9 mEq/L (mmol/L)

56. In reviewing a client's electrocardiogram (ECG), which finding does the nurse associate with hyperkalemia?
    A. Tall peaked T waves
    B. Narrow QRS complex
    C. Tall P waves
    D. Elevated ST segment

57. Which medication or class of drugs taken regularly at home does the nurse associate with a newly admitted client's laboratory finding of hyperkalemia?
    A. Insulin
    B. Beta blocker
    C. Cephalosporin antibiotic
    D. Spironolactone

58. Which assessment findings does the nurse expect to see in a client who has mild hyperkalemia? **Select all that apply**.
    A. Wheezing on exhalation
    B. Numbness in hands, feet, and around the mouth
    C. Hyperactive bowel sounds
    D. Irregular heart rate
    E. Skeletal muscle twitching
    F. Excessive skin dryness

59. Which additional laboratory changes does the nurse anticipate in a client who has hyperkalemia resulting from dehydration?
    A. Increased hematocrit and hemoglobin levels
    B. Decreased serum electrolyte levels
    C. Increased urine potassium levels
    D. Decreased serum creatinine levels

60. Which foods does the nurse recommend to a client who remains at continued risk for hyperkalemia? **Select all that apply**.
    A. Avocados
    B. Butter
    C. Cranberries
    D. Lettuce
    E. Eggs
    F. Dried beans
    G. Grapefruit
    H. Strawberries

61. Which serum calcium level in a client laboratory findings does the nurse interpret as normal?
    A. 3.7 mEq/L (1.05 mmol/L)
    B. 1.05 mEq/L (3.75 mmol/L)
    C. 9.5 mEq/L (2.38 mmol/L)
    D. 2.38 mEq/L (9.5 mmol/L)

62. By which mechanisms does parathyroid hormone (PTH) increase serum calcium levels? **Select all that apply**.
    A. Releasing free calcium from the bones
    B. Increasing calcium excretion in the urine
    C. Stimulating kidney reabsorption of calcium
    D. Activating vitamin D
    E. Increasing calcium absorption in the GI tract
    F. Pulling calcium out of muscle cells

63. Which measure put into place by the nurse while caring for a client with severe hypocalcemia is most likely to **prevent harm**?
    A. Urge the client to eat foods high in calcium content.
    B. Instruct the client to increase his or her intake of water.
    C. Instruct assistive personnel (AP) to avoid taking blood pressures.
    D. Use a lift sheet to move or reposition the client.

64. Which is the correct technique for the nurse to use when assessing the client for a positive Chvostek sign?
    A. Client flexes arms against the chest and the nurse attempts to pull the arms away from the chest.
    B. The nurse inflates a blood pressure cuff around the upper arm to higher than the client's systolic pressure.
    C. The nurse taps the client's face just below and in front of the ear.
    D. The nurse lightly taps the client's patellar tendon with a reflex hammer and measures the movement.

65. With which client conditions does the nurse remain alert for potential hypocalcemia? **Select all that apply**.
    A. Crohn disease
    B. Acute pancreatitis
    C. Removal or destruction of parathyroid glands
    D. Immobility
    E. Use of beta-adrenergic inhalers
    F. GI wound drainage

66. Which client assessment findings are related to hypercalcemia? **Select all that apply**.
    A. Increased heart rate
    B. Paresthesia
    C. Decreased deep tendon reflexes
    D. Hypoactive bowel sounds
    E. Shortened QT interval
    F. Profound muscle weakness

67. Which action does the nurse anticipate in the management of a client who has mild hypercalcemia?
    A. Administering IV normal saline (0.9% sodium chloride)
    B. Massaging calves to encourage blood return to the heart
    C. Providing vitamin D supplementation
    D Monitoring for tetany

68. Which system is most important for the nurse to monitor closely for a client who has severe hypomagnesemia?
    A. Autonomic nervous system
    B. Gastrointestinal
    C. Cardiovascular
    D. Renal/urinary

69. How does the nurse prepare to administer the prescribed magnesium sulfate (MgSO4) for a client with severe hypomagnesemia?
    A. Orally
    B. Subcutaneously
    C. Intramuscularly
    D. Intravenously

70. Which assessment findings does the nurse expect to see in a client who has severe hypermagnesemia?
    A. Bradycardia and hypotension
    B. Tachycardia and weak palpable pulse
    C. Hypertension and irritability
    D. Irregular pulse and deep respirations

Chapter 13 Answer Key

1. B
Men have a higher percentage of total body water at any age because they have more muscle mass than women and muscle cells contain a high concentration of water. Women have more body fat than men, and fat cells contain practically no water. As adults age, their total body water volume decreases because both older men and older women lose muscle mass with aging.

2. C
The extracellular fluid includes both the blood (plasma) volume and the interstitial fluid. Another term for the interstitial fluid is the third space, which is between the cells rather than inside the cells or in the blood (plasma).

3. A
Hydrostatic pressure is a "water pushing" pressure and will move water from an area of higher hydrostatic pressure to an area of lower hydrostatic pressure. When the plasma volume hydrostatic pressure increases, the water will first move into the interstitial space and cause edema formation.

4. B, E
The extracellular fluid includes both the blood (plasma) volume (also known as the intravascular volume) and the interstitial fluid. Although the interstitial fluid comes from the plasma, it is not considered part of it.

5. C
Isotonic solutions have the same tonicity as plasma and other extracellular fluids. Therefore, the intravenous fluid would not change the ECF osmolarity. When 1000 mL is infused within 3 hours and the client only urinates 300 mL, the extra fluid would increase the client's weight. Remember that 1 liter of fluid is equal to 2.2 lb.

6. A
Gravity affects hydrostatic pressure in capillaries. When in the standing position, hydrostatic pressure increases in the dependent areas of the ankles and feet. This increased capillary hydrostatic pressure forces fluid to leave the ankle and feet capillaries into the interstitial spaces

resulting in the formation of visible edema in these dependent areas.

7. B
Much of the body's waste products, especially nitrogen, is excreted in the urine. Depending on body size, 400 to 600 mL/day of urine must be generated to ensure waste product excretion. This is known as the *obligatory urine output.* Less than this amount of urine will result in retained waste products that could lead to toxic levels.

8. D
Isotonic saline is 0.9%. The options of 9% saline and 3% saline are hypertonic. Only 0.45% saline is a hypotonic solution.

9. B
The normal blood osmolarity is 270 to 300 mOsm/L (mOsm/kg). The value of 310 is hyperosmolar, which will cause cells to move water into the extracellular fluid compartment and shrink slightly. When the osmoreceptor cells in the hypothalamus shrink, the thirst center is stimulated so the client will drink more to dilute the hyperosmolarity.

10. D
Although all of the assessment findings listed may appear with a fluid balance problem, the first indication in older clients is a change in mental status.

11. A, B, D, E, F
Of all these fluid loss routes, the only one that adjusts or is regulated is urine output. The others represent fluid loss that has no regulatory or control mechanisms, also known as insensible.

12. B, C, E, F
Total body water in adults varies by age, gender, degree of muscle mass, and percent of body fat. Water makes up about 55% to 60% of total weight for younger adults and 50% to 55% of total weight for older adults. Women of all ages usually have a lower percentage of body water than do men of the same ages because of greater muscle mass. Fat cells contain little or no water. The higher the percentage of body fat,

the lower the percentage of total body water. Neither race nor height affect total body water.

13. A, D, F
The kidney is the main way excess waste products and electrolytes are eliminated from the body. It must cause a 500 to 600 mL output daily for adequate elimination of these products daily. When these products are retained, the consequences include lethal levels of electrolytes, toxic buildup of nitrogen, and retention of hydrogen ions causing acidosis.

14. C
This client has three risk factors for an electrolyte imbalance: older adult, endocrine disorder, and takes a diuretic daily, which alters fluid and electrolyte excretion. Although the 80-year-old has an increased risk because of age, he or she has no other specific risk factors listed.

15. D
Aldosterone increases sodium and water reabsorption in the kidney. Higher than normal levels of this hormone usually result in high serum sodium levels.

16. A, F
The serum potassium and serum magnesium levels are both lower than normal (potassium = 3.5 to 5.0 mEq/L or mmol/L; magnesium = 1.8 to 2.6 mEq/L or 0.74 to 1.07 mmol/L). Low levels of these electrolytes can have profound effects on heart function. All other electrolytes listed are within the normal range.

17. A
Continuous gastric suctioning removes fluid before it is absorbed into the body, which decreases fluid intake by the oral route. This ongoing fluid loss, if not measured as replaced by another route, can result in a fluid volume deficit.

18. B
The normal action of ADH is making kidney nephrons more permeable to water and increasing water reabsorption that is returned to the blood. With less ADH available, the client excretes more water in the urine leading to decreased blood volume and the osmolarity of the blood is increased.

19. A, D
The RAAS system is activated by any condition that causes reduced blood volume, hypotension, or reduced serum sodium levels, such as could happen with shock and dehydration. When activated, RAAS increases sodium and reabsorption to increase blood volume and serum sodium levels. It also increases vasoconstriction to help increase blood pressure. Asthma, urinary tract infection, hypertension, and constipation do not induce symptoms of shock or dehydration.

20. D
Sodium is the electrolyte with the highest concentration in the blood. This high concentration keeps more of the chloride ions in the blood. As a result, sodium keeps the blood osmolarity within the normal range. Both calcium and potassium have low blood levels.

21. B, C, E, F
Magnesium is important for skeletal muscle contraction, carbohydrate metabolism, generation of energy stores, vitamin activation, blood coagulation, and cell growth. Adequate amounts of intracellular magnesium are particularly essential for the health and maintenance of cardiac muscle.

22. A, B, C, E, F
Common causes or risk factors for dehydration are those that increase fluid loss or interfere with fluid intake, including: hemorrhage, vomiting, diarrhea, profuse salivation, fistulas, ileostomy, profuse diaphoresis, burns, severe wounds, long-term NPO status, diuretic therapy, GI suction, hyperventilation, diabetes insipidus, difficulty swallowing, impaired thirst, unconsciousness, fever, and impaired motor function. Water intoxication is related to over hydration, not dehydration.

23. C
Because urine output is related to blood pressure remaining high enough to perfuse the kidneys, urine output is a sensitive indicator of adequate fluid volume. When blood volume starts to decrease, the body attempts to conserve volume by decreasing urine output. Although decreasing output can be reflective of poor kidney function,

that is not the reason it is measured so carefully after surgery when clients have an increased risk for hemorrhage.

24. B

Blood pressure decreases with dehydration because of a low blood volume. This condition is perceived by the body as hypoxia and impending shock. The respiratory rate increases to ensure adequate oxygenation even when blood pressure is low.

25. D

The skin of an older adult is usually dry and scaly. Thinning skin and loss of subcutaneous tissue on the back of the hand makes assessing skin turgor here unreliable because this skin may tent even when hydration is good. Observing mucous membranes is not assessing skin turgor. The skin on the forehead and sternum are recommended for assessing turgor on an older adult.

26. B

With dehydration, the urine is usually concentrated, with a specific gravity greater than 1.030 and has a dark amber color and a strong odor. A urine specific gravity is reflective of dehydration. Overhydration (fluid overload) usually is associated with a very low specific gravity. Renal disease is based on parameters other than urine specific gravity.

27. B, C, E, F, G

Options B, C, E, F, and G are recommended to help clients drink more fluids throughout the day and prevent dehydration. Avoiding fluids after early evening, a technique some families believe will reduce the risk for night time incontinence, does not reduce incontinence and may result in a lower daily intake of fluids. Salty food may not increase the sensation of thirst, especially in an older adult, and may induce an electrolyte imbalance.

28. A, B, C, E

Common symptoms and problems associated with fluid overload first appear in the cardiopulmonary systems. These include: increased pulse rate, bounding pulse quality, elevated blood pressure, decreased pulse pressure, elevated central venous pressure, distended neck and hand veins, engorged varicose veins, weight gain, increased respiratory rate, shallow respirations, shortness of breath, and moist crackles on auscultation. Excessive thirst and hypotension are associated with dehydration.

29. C

Diuretics are a common and effective drug for the fluid overload associated with pulmonary edema, heart failure, and ascites. They are only used when kidney function is normal or at least adequate. In end-stage kidney disease kidney function is greatly and perhaps totally impaired.

30. B

The client's assessment findings are consistent with hypervolemia (fluid overload) and opposite of dehydration (fluid volume deficit). Hemoconcentration is a manifestation of dehydration, not a type of fluid imbalance.

31. D

1 kg = 2.2 lb. 1 kg of water = 1 L (1000 mL) of water. 16.6 lb divided by 2.2 = 7000 g (7000 mL).

32. A

Rapid weight gain is a good and reliable indicator of fluid retention, which would indicate worsening of heart failure that requires intervention. Usually only 0.5 lb of weight gain in a day represents true weight gain. Any amount above that is fluid retention.

33. A, C, D, F

Without sodium intake, hyponatremia can develop. Although dextrose 5% in water is technically isotonic, as soon as it is infused the dextrose is metabolized and the fluid is very hypotonic, capable of diluting blood and causing it to be hyponatremic. The high blood glucose level makes the blood hyperosmotic, which then pulls fluid from the interstitial and intracellular spaces into the plasma volume, diluting both the glucose and the sodium levels. Heavy sweating results in both water and sodium losses. Replacing the loss with only water can cause hyponatremia.

34. A

    Normal serum sodium ranges between 136 and 145 mEq/L (mmol/L). Hyponatremia is a serum sodium value lower than 136 mEq/L (mmol/L). The other values are within their normal ranges.

35. A, B, C, D, E, F

    Low serum sodium levels reduce membrane excitability and result in confusion, muscle weakness, and decreased deep tendon reflexes. GI changes include nausea, increased motility, and cramping.

36. A

    The drug therapy should increase water loss without causing sodium loss. Furosemide, hydrochlorothiazide, and bumetanide all promote sodium loss as well as water loss.

37. D

    Hyponatremia increases intracranial pressure and decreases central nervous system excitability. Behavioral and cognitive changes are often the first changes apparent in a person who develops hyponatremia because of excessive water consumption in a short period of time.

38. C

    Normal serum sodium ranges between 136 and 145 mEq/L (mmol/L). Hypernatremia is a serum sodium value higher than 145 mEq/L (mmol/L). The other electrolyte values are within their normal ranges.

39. C

    Soy sauce is a source of sodium because 1 tablespoon (15 mL) has nearly 900 mg of sodium. Clients who are to restrict sodium intake should be taught to avoid foods that contain significant amounts of soy sauce. Seafood itself does not contain high concentrations of sodium. Bacon and pickled herring do contain higher concentrations of sodium.

40. C, D, E, F

    Severe diarrhea and profound diaphoresis cause both water loss and some sodium loss. However, water loss is greater than sodium loss and can result in a relative hypernatremia. Cushing syndrome with increased levels of cortisol causes an increased reabsorption of sodium from the kidneys leading to hypernatremia. Decreased kidney function reduces the normal amount of sodium that is excreted in the urine leading to hypernatremia. Constipation has no effect on loss or reabsorption of sodium. Heart failure is affected by excess sodium but does not lead to excess sodium.

41. A

    Movement of sodium into the intracellular fluid from the extracellular fluid is a trigger for depolarization of excitable membranes. Higher than normal sodium levels increase muscle twitching and contractions with a lower stimulus and sometimes even without a stimulus.

42. D

    Both IV solutions contain isotonic levels of sodium chloride and would not significantly reduce the hypernatremia. The fluid may be problematic if the client's kidney function is low. Convaptan would increase water excretion and not induce sodium excretion, which would make the sodium level even higher. Furosemide increases both water and sodium excretion, along with other electrolytes.

43. B, D, E, F

    Elevated sodium levels increase vascular volume "where sodium goes, water follows," increasing heart rate and blood pressure. With increased edema associated with hypernatremia, pulses may be difficult to palpate. Although mild hypernatremia increases the irritability of excitable membranes causing muscle twitching and irregular contraction, higher levels of sodium dehydrate excitable tissues, including muscle cells, to the extent that they may not be able to contract. Confusion and weight gain are associated with hypernatremia, especially when it is accompanied by hypervolemia.

44. C

    Most canned and prepared packaged foods contain high levels of sodium and their intake should be limited. Salt substitutes have a much lower sodium content than standard table salt and is recommended for clients who need to limit sodium intake. Aspirin has no influence on serum sodium levels. Caffeinated food and beverages can increase water excretion without increasing sodium excretion and lead to higher serum sodium levels.

45. B
Hypokalemia refers to a lower than normal serum potassium level, not sodium, chloride, or calcium. The normal serum potassium level is 3.5 to 5.0 mEq/L or mmol/L.

46. A
Severe hypokalemia causes profound skeletal muscle weakness. Because skeletal muscle contraction is absolutely required for the ventilation of respiration, muscle weakness reduces respiratory depth and effectiveness, leading to low oxygen saturation. The most common cause of death with severe hypokalemia is respiratory failure.

47. B
Hypokalemia reduces GI motility and greatly increases the risk for a paralytic ileus.

48. B, C
Metabolic alkalosis causes a relative hypokalemia by increasing movement of potassium ions from the extracellular fluid into the intracellular fluid in exchange for hydrogen ions. Cushing syndrome involves higher than normal levels of cortisol, which increases potassium loss resulting in an actual hypokalemia. Paralytic ileus is caused by hypokalemia and does not cause it. Kidney failure causes hyperkalemia. Potassium levels are not affected directly by hypothyroidism or liver failure.

49. B
If the potassium solution raises the serum potassium level too rapidly, hyperkalemia can result. Higher-than-normal serum potassium levels delay electrical conduction through the heart and can cause a variety of dysrhythmias, including asystole.

50. B
Intravenous potassium is a high-alert dangerous drug that can lead to death if administered too rapidly or at a high concentration. It must

always be diluted. The maximum allowable concentration of the drug is 1 mEq (mmol) per 10 mL of solution.

51. A, D
Potassium is a severe tissue irritant and can cause damage (as well as pain) if the IV line extravasates or infiltrates. The nurse must ensure the line is patent and has a good blood return before administering IV fluids containing potassium. Elevated serum potassium levels can cause bradycardia and dysrhythmias. Therefore, it is best to establish the client's baseline heart rate and rhythm before administering any IV potassium solution.

52. C
In option A, the client is confusing calcium with potassium. Foods with more potassium include bananas, orange juice, and organ meats. Salt substitutes are about 50% potassium.

53. B
Intravenous potassium is a high-alert dangerous drug that can lead to death if administered too rapidly or at too a high concentration. The maximum allowable infusion rate is 5 to 10 mEq (mmol) per hour. The rate of 40 mEq (mmol) in 1 hour is completely unsafe even if it is administered with a pump or controller. Whether or not the label matches the health care provider's prescription, the rate of infusion is wrong and both the prescription and label must be clarified. The nurse is not the prescriber and cannot change the prescribed infusion rate.

54. A, B, C, D
Soybeans, bananas, cantaloupe, and potatoes are good sources of potassium. Peaches and lettuce contain little, if any potassium.

55. D
The normal range for serum potassium level is 3.5 to 5.0 mEq/L (mmol/L). Hyperkalemia is a serum potassium level higher than 5.0 mEq/L (mmol/L).

56. A
Hyperkalemia has deleterious effects on electrical conduction through the heart and can cause death. Some earlier changes in the ECG reflecting

a rising potassium level include tall, peaked T waves, prolonged PR intervals, flat or absent P waves, and wide QRS complexes.

57. D

Spironolactone is a potassium-sparing diuretic that increases its reabsorption in the kidney. Taking it daily can lead to hyperkalemia. Insulin is associated with hypokalemia. The beta blocker and antibiotic are not associated with disturbances of potassium.

58. B, C, D, E

Hyperkalemia increases GI motility and changes electrical conduction through the heart, which induces an irregular heart rate. In the early stages of hyperkalemia (mild potassium elevations), paresthesias are present as is skeletal muscle twitching. The respiratory muscles are not affected until potassium levels are very high. Potassium excesses do not result in skin manifestations.

59. A

In dehydration-associated hyperkalemia, the amount of total potassium is not increased but water loss from the plasma fluid increases the concentration of all electrolytes and blood cells.

60. B, C, D, E, G, H

Avocados and dried beans are a rich source of potassium and should be avoided by clients requiring potassium restriction. Many clients believe that all fruit contains high levels of potassium. This is not true. The fruits listed are all low in potassium as are butter and eggs.

61. C

The normal range for serum calcium levels is 9.0 to 10.5 mEq/L (or 2.25 to 2.75 mmol/L).

62. A, C, D, E

When more calcium is needed, parathyroid hormone (PTH) is released from the parathyroid glands and increases serum calcium levels by releasing free calcium from bone storage sites, stimulating vitamin D activation to help increase intestinal absorption of dietary calcium, inhibiting kidney calcium excretion, and promoting kidney calcium reabsorption.

63. D

With hypocalcemia, calcium leaves bone storage sites, causing a loss of bone density. Bones are less dense, more brittle and fragile, and may break easily with slight trauma. Using a lift sheet rather than pulling the client helps prevent harm. Eating a high-calcium diet can help the hypocalcemia but does not directly prevent harm. Hypocalcemia is not caused by water loss, and increasing fluid intake may dilute the already low serum calcium level. Clients with hypocalcemia are at risk for hypotension and orthostatic hypotension. Blood pressure still needs to be measured and does not pose a risk to safety.

64. C

To test for Chvostek sign, the nurse taps the face just below and in front of the ear to trigger facial twitching of one side of the mouth, nose, and cheek (a positive response). Option A is a test of muscle strength. Option B describes correct technique for measuring Trousseau sign. Option D describes correct technique for assessing a deep tendon reflex.

65. A, B, C, D, F

Many conditions lead to an actual or relative hypocalcemia, especially GI conditions that interfere with calcium absorption or increase calcium loss, and anything that impairs parathyroid activity. Immobility causes bone resorption of calcium causing a whole body reduction of calcium. Beta-adrenergic drugs do not affect calcium metabolism.

66. A, C, D, E, F

Hypercalcemia at first causes increased heart rate and blood pressure and later causes depressed electrical conduction, slowing heart rate and shortening the QT interval. Deep tendon reflexes and GI motility are decreased. Paresthesias are associated with hypocalcemia. The excess calcium stabilizes skeletal muscle membranes slowing or preventing depolarization, which leads to severe muscle weakness.

67. A

Often the cause of hypercalcemia is dehydration. Increasing fluids, especially IV normal saline, can bring the serum calcium level back to normal. Hypercalcemia promotes excessive clot formation. Calves are not massaged to prevent movement of any existing clot. Vitamin D supplementation would increase calcium absorption and potentially worsen hypercalcemia. Tetany is associated with hypocalcemia.

68. C

Cardiovascular changes associated with hypomagnesemia are serious. Low magnesium levels increase the risk for hypertension, atherosclerosis, hypertrophic left ventricle, and a variety of dysrhythmias. The dysrhythmias include premature contractions, atrial fibrillation, ventricular fibrillation, and long QT intervals.

69. D

Magnesium sulfate is a severe irritant and is no longer administered subcutaneously or intramuscularly. Oral administration takes too long to achieve the desired outcome and would cause severe diarrhea.

70. A

Magnesium is a membrane stabilizer that decreases depolarization of all excitable membranes. As a result, heart rate is slower and the client can become hypotensive.

14 CHAPTER

Concepts of Acid-Base Balance

1. Which pH value indicates the highest concentration of free hydrogen ions in the blood and other extracellular fluids?
   A. 7.57
   B. 7.47
   C. 7.37
   D. 7.27

2. Which client arterial blood gas results would the nurse interpret as within normal limits?
   A. pH 7.28, $PaCO_2$ 24, bicarbonate 15, PaO_2 95
   B. pH 7.45, $PaCO_2$ 41, bicarbonate 25, PaO_2 97
   C. pH 7.35, $PaCO_2$ 24, bicarbonate 15, PaO_2 95
   D. pH 7.30, $PaCO_2$ 66, bicarbonate 38, PaO_2 70

3. Which arterial blood pH level can be fatal?
   A. 7.22
   B. 7.11
   C. 7.05
   D. 6.85

4. By which mechanism do buffers help maintain arterial blood pH within the normal range?
   A. Binding excess free hydrogen ions
   B. Increasing kidney excretion of free hydrogen ions
   C. Triggering increased bicarbonate production in the pancreas
   D. Stimulating respiratory neurons to increase the rate and depth of ventilation

5. What changes in body functions does the nurse anticipate in a client who has lower than normal blood pH levels? **Select all that apply**.
   A. Decreased serum potassium levels
   B. Increased effectiveness of drugs
   C. Reduced function of hormones
   D. Increased function of enzymes
   E. Decreased electrical conduction in the heart
   F. Decreased skeletal muscle strength

6. The continuous normal function of which organs is most critical for acid-base balance? **Select all that apply.**
   A. Adrenal glands
   B. Bladder
   C. Heart
   D. Kidneys
   E. Liver
   F. Lungs

7. Which statement most accurately describes the relationship between the hydrogen ion concentration and carbon dioxide concentration in extracellular fluids?
   A. Because carbon dioxide is a gas and hydrogen ions are electrolytes, these two substances have no relationship in extracellular fluids.
   B. The concentrations of hydrogen ions and carbon dioxide are directly related, with an increase or decrease in one always resulting in a corresponding increase or decrease in the other.
   C. Carbon dioxide buffers hydrogen ions, thus these two concentrations are inversely related to each other. The greater the carbon dioxide concentration, the fewer hydrogen ions present in that fluid.
   D. Hydrogen ions and carbon dioxide ions exist in a balanced relationship as a result of their charges. The positively charged hydrogen ions are attracted to the negatively charged carbon dioxide ions, forming an electrically neutral substance.

8. Which statement about compensation for acid-base imbalance is accurate?
   A. The respiratory system is less sensitive to acid-base changes.
   B. The respiratory system can begin compensation within seconds to minutes.
   C. The renal system is less powerful than the respiratory system.
   D. The renal system is more sensitive to acid-base changes.

9. Which condition or response is an example of physiologic compensation to maintain acid-base balance?
   A. Increasing rate and depth of respiration when running 2000 feet
   B. Increasing urine output when blood pressure increases during heavy exercise
   C. Drinking more fluids when spending an extended period of time in a dry environment
   D. Shifting body weight when pain occurs as a result of remaining in one position for too long

10. Which statements correctly apply to acid-base balance in the body? **Select all that apply**.
    A. Renal mechanisms are stronger in regulating acid-base balance but slower to respond than respiratory mechanisms.
    B. The immediate binding of excess hydrogen ions occurs primarily in the red blood cells.
    C. Combined acidosis is less severe than either metabolic acidosis or respiratory acidosis alone.
    D. Respiratory acidosis is caused by a patent airway.
    E. Acid-base balance occurs through control of hydrogen ion production and elimination.
    F. Buffers are the third-line defense against acid-base imbalances in the body.

11. Which alteration in acid-base balance does the nurse expect to see as a compensatory response in a client who has a long-term severe respiratory impairment?
    A. Decreased arterial blood pH
    B. Increased arterial blood oxygen
    C. Increased arterial blood bicarbonate
    D. Decreased arterial blood carbon dioxide

12. Which specific type of medication reported as taken daily by an older client will cause a nurse to assess for indications of an acid-base imbalance?
    A. Antilipidemics
    B. Hormonal therapy
    C. Diuretics
    D. Antidysrhythmics

13. Which client does the nurse anticipate will have acidosis because of a decreased arterial bicarbonate level?
    A. Client with pancreatitis
    B. Client with hypoventilation
    C. Client who is vomiting
    D. Client with emphysema

14. Which arterial blood gas (ABG) results would the nurse expect for a client admitted to the hospital for diabetic ketoacidosis? **Select all that apply**.
    A. pH 7.32
    B. $PaCO_2$ 50 mm Hg
    C. Bicarbonate 18 mEq/L (mmol/L)
    D. pH 7.46
    E. Bicarbonate 29 mEq/L (mmol/L)
    F. PaO_2 98 mm Hg

15. What type of acid-base problem does the nurse expect in a client who is being insufficiently mechanically ventilated for the past 4 hours and whose most recent arterial blood gas results include a pH of 7.29?
    A. Metabolic acidosis with an acid excess
    B. Metabolic acidosis with a base deficit
    C. Respiratory acidosis with an acid excess
    D. Respiratory acidosis with a base deficit

16. What cause does the nurse expect to see for a client's arterial pH of 7.28 after he has been NPO for 5 days and receiving only dextrose 5% in lactated Ringer's solution (4 liters daily)?
    A. Acidosis in response to the presence of excessive ketoacids
    B. Acidosis in response to the presence of excessive lactic acid
    C. Alkalosis in response to the excessive loss of carbonic acid
    D. Alkalosis in response to the excessive loss of sulfuric acid

17. Which acid-base imbalance will the nurse expect in a client who has chronic kidney disease?
    A. Respiratory acidosis
    B. Metabolic acidosis
    C. Respiratory alkalosis
    D. Metabolic alkalosis

18. Which laboratory value indicates to the nurse that a client has acidosis as a result of a metabolic problem?
    A. $PaCO_2$ = 43 mm Hg
    B. HCO_3^- = 17 mEq/L (mmol/L)
    C. Lactate = 2.5 mmol/L
    D. pH = 7.32

19. Overdose of which drug or drug category could cause metabolic acidosis?
    A. Acetaminophen
    B. Antihistamines
    C. Antacids
    D. Aspirin

20. For which client will the nurse remain **most** alert for the possibility to develop respiratory alkalosis?
    A. Client who is anxious and breathing rapidly
    B. Client who has multiple rib fractures
    C. Client receiving IV Ringer's lactate
    D. Client who has diarrhea

21. Which laboratory value will the nurse check immediately to prevent harm for a client with metabolic acidosis who now has tall, peaked T waves on his or her ECG?
    A. Serum glucose
    B. Serum sodium
    C. Serum potassium
    D. Serum magnesium

22. Which clients would the nurse assess for problems of inadequate chest expansion that may increase the risk for respiratory acidosis? **Select all that apply**.
    A. 87-year old with osteoporosis and severe kyphoscoliosis
    B. 27-year-old client in the first trimester of pregnancy
    C. 44-year-old severely obese client on prolonged bedrest
    D. 67-year-old 2 days postoperative from arthroscopic surgery
    E. 37-year-old with ascites
    F. 56-year-old with end-stage emphysema

23. Which laboratory values indicate to the nurse that a client's acid-base imbalance is specifically a respiratory acidosis? **Select all that apply**.
    A. pH 7.31
    B. $PaCO_2$ 58 mm Hg
    C. Bicarbonate 17 mEq/L (mmol/L)
    D. PaO_2 75 mm Hg
    E. Serum potassium 5.5 mEq/L (mmol/L)
    F. $PaCO_2$ 31 mm Hg

24. Which signs and symptoms would the nurse expect to find in a client with severe metabolic acidosis? **Select all that apply**.
    A. Kussmaul respirations
    B. Increased urine output
    C. Warm, flushed skin
    D. Skin pale to cyanotic
    E. Elevated $PaCO_2$
    F. Decreased bicarbonate

25. Which findings on lower limb assessment indicates to the nurse that the client has acidosis? **Select all that apply.**
    A. No change from baseline
    B. Bilateral weakness
    C. Muscle twitching without weakness
    D. Weakness on the dominant side
    E. Hypoactive patellar reflex
    F. Tetany of the great toe on the left foot

26. Which client conditions does the nurse assess for as a cause of the underproduction or overelimination of bicarbonate? **Select all that apply.**
    A. Heavy exercise
    B. Kidney failure
    C. Liver failure
    D. Seizure activity
    E. Dehydration
    F. Diarrhea

27. Which arterial blood gas changes indicates to the nurse that a client may have respiratory alkalosis?
    A. High pH; normal bicarbonate; low PaO_2
    B. High pH; normal bicarbonate; low $PaCO_2$
    C. High pH; high bicarbonate; high PaO_2
    D. High pH; low bicarbonate; high $PaCO_2$

28. Which alterations in acid-base balance does the nurse expect to see in a client who has acute pancreatitis with severe pain and is hyperventilating? **Select all that apply**.
    A. Overproduction of hydrogen ions
    B. Metabolic acidosis
    C. Low or normal $PaCO_2$
    D. Underproduction of bicarbonate
    E. Metabolic alkalosis
    F. Respiratory acidosis

29. Which statement made by the client suggests to the nurse that an alkaline condition may be present?
    A. "I am more and more tired and can't concentrate."
    B. "I have tingling in my fingers and toes."
    C. "My feet and ankles are swollen."
    D. "My knee joints ache."

30. With which client will the nurse remain most alert for respiratory alkalosis?
    A. Hypoxic client
    B. Morbidly obese client
    C. Client with a tight body cast
    D. Fearful client having a panic attack

31. Which type(s) of electrolyte imbalance does the nurse expect to see in a client with metabolic alkalosis? **Select all that apply**.
    A. Hyperkalemia
    B. Hypokalemia
    C. Hypercalcemia
    D. Hypocalcemia
    E. Hypernatremia
    F. Hyponatremia

32. Which client ABG results would the nurse interpret as metabolic alkalosis?
    A. pH 7.30, $PaCO_2$ 66, bicarbonate 38, PaO_2 70
    B. pH 7.38, $PaCO_2$ 36, bicarbonate 15, PaO_2 95
    C. pH 7.48, $PaCO_2$ 24, bicarbonate 20, PaO_2 95
    D. pH 7.50, $PaCO_2$ 45, bicarbonate 36, PaO_2 95

33. Which client will the nurse observe **most closely** for development of a base excess metabolic alkalosis?
    A. 26-year-old who received a massive blood transfusion
    B. 36-year-old who is having nasogastric suction
    C. 56-year-old who has vomited for 2 days
    D. 76-year-old taking thiazide diuretics

34. Which alteration will the nurse expect in client who has taken antacids for the past 3 days to relieve "heartburn?"
    A. Respiratory alkalosis (acid deficit)
    B. Metabolic alkalosis (acid deficit)
    C. Respiratory alkalosis (base excess)
    D. Metabolic alkalosis (base excess)

35. What would the nurse expect to see **first** as compensation in a client who has a decreased amount of hydrogen ions and a decreased amount of carbon dioxide in the body to restore acid-base balance?
    A. Decreased rate and depth of respirations
    B. Decreased renal absorption of hydrogen ions
    C. Increased rate and depth of respirations
    D. Decreased renal excretion of bicarbonate

36. Which acid-base and electrolyte changes would the nurse monitor for in a client who has had diarrhea for the past 2 days? **Select all that apply**.
    A. Overelimination of bicarbonate
    B. Respiratory alkalosis
    C. Metabolic acidosis
    D. Underelimination of hydrogen ions
    E. Overproduction of hydrogen ions
    F. Hyperkalemia
    G. Hyponatremia

Chapter 14 Answer Key

1. D
   The blood level of free hydrogen ions is calculated in negative logarithm units. This calculation makes the value of pH inversely related (negatively related) to the concentration of free hydrogen ions. Thus, the lower the pH value of a fluid, the higher the level of free hydrogen ions in that fluid.

2. B
   The normal arterial pH range is 7.35-7.45.
   The normal $PaCO_2$ range is 35-45 mm Hg.
   The normal PaO_2 range is 80-100 mm Hg.
   The normal arterial bicarbonate range is 21-28 mEq/L (mmol/L).

3. D
   An arterial pH below 6.85 is considered incompatible with life because all vital organ functions would be inhibited.

4. A
   Buffers in body fluids act like hydrogen ion "sponges," soaking up hydrogen ions when too many are present and squeezing out hydrogen ions when very few are present. Buffers have no mechanism to change kidney, pancreas, or neuronal function.

5. C, E, F
   Higher concentration of hydrogen ions (reflected by a lower pH) increases (not decreases) serum potassium levels, decreases effectiveness of drugs, reduces function of hormones, reduces function of enzymes, slows electrical conduction through the heart (because of the elevated potassium levels) and decreases muscle strength.

6. D, F
   The kidneys are critical in retaining and eliminating hydrogen ions and bicarbonate to maintain acid-base balance. The lungs are the organs that control carbon dioxide elimination. Normal functioning of both these organs are necessary for acid-base balance. A problem interfering with the function of either of them can lead to life-threatening acid-base imbalances. The heart, liver, and bladder have no role in acid-base balance. Although specific adrenal gland problems are indirectly associated with acid-base imbalances, they do not directly affect acid-base balance.

7. B
   Through the action of the carbonic anhydrase reaction, the concentration of hydrogen ions is directly related to the concentration of carbon

dioxide in the blood. Any condition that increases the concentration of one also increases the concentration of the other. Carbon dioxide is not a buffer.

8. B
    The healthy respiratory system can compensate for acid-base imbalances from other causes. It represents the second line of defense to prevent an imbalance and can begin to compensate within seconds to minutes after a change in hydrogen ion concentration (reflected as a corresponding change in carbon dioxide). The central chemoreceptors controlling rate and depth of ventilation are extremely sensitive to changes in carbon dioxide levels.

9. A
    The respiratory system increases its activity by "blowing off" excess carbon dioxide that developed as a result of lactic acidosis occurring in skeletal muscle when blood flow and oxygenation were insufficient to meet the increased demand for oxygen (oxygen debt) created during increased skeletal muscle metabolism.

10. A, B, E
    Acid-base balance is maintained by controlling the body's hydrogen ion production with mechanisms to eliminate hydrogen ions at the same rate they are produced. Renal mechanisms for control of acid-base balance are the most powerful but are slow to start, usually requiring that an acid-base disturbance be present for at least 24 hours before becoming active. The first line of defense against acid-base changes are the buffers in the blood, other extracellular fluids, and inside cells. Red blood cells in particular can reduce excess hydrogen ions by having them enter the cells and then binding them to buffers and hemoglobin. Respiratory acidosis is caused by problems that interfere with effective ventilation. A patent airway never causes respiratory acidosis. When conditions that cause respiratory acidosis are present at the same time as conditions that cause metabolic acidosis, the severity of the imbalance increases, not decreases.

11. C
    Because kidneys regulate pH by controlling bicarbonate concentration and the lungs regulate pH by controlling carbon dioxide loss, a loss of one function can be at least partially compensated by the other function. When pulmonary function is decreased so that adequate amounts of carbon dioxide are not excreted, the pH drops, stimulating the kidneys to reabsorb more bicarbonate to balance the increased acid production.

12. C
    Of all the drug categories listed, only the diuretics induce the excretion of specific electrolytes and hydrogen ions, leading to the development of acid-base imbalances.

13. A
    The pancreas produces bicarbonate, which is a base. Pancreatitis inhibits this function resulting in underproduction of bicarbonate. This would lead to a relative acidosis. Vomiting would cause loss of hydrogen ions and alkalosis. Emphysema would increase carbon dioxide and hydrogen ion production, as would hypoventilation.

14. A, B, E, F
    Diabetic ketoacidosis results from the excessive production of ketoacids as a byproduct of fat breakdown. These ketoacids release hydrogen ions which lower, not raise the pH. The excess hydrogen ions also increase the blood level of CO_2 which is what stimulates deep and rapid respirations that try to decrease the hydrogen ion concentration. Bicarbonate is not lowered or increased because there has not been enough time for kidney compensation to start. Oxygen levels are normal because ventilation is not impaired.

15. C
    When a person being mechanically ventilated is insufficiently ventilated, respiratory acidosis occurs with retention of carbon dioxide. The retained carbon dioxide is converted to hydrogen ions resulting in an acid excess. Bases have neither been lost or retained in an acute

respiratory acidosis. Insufficient ventilation does not cause any form of metabolic acidosis.

16. A
Clients who are NPO and receiving only crystalloid solutions (including glucose) are in a condition of starvation. Each liter of 5% dextrose contains only a little over 170 calories. Four liters daily provides approximately 700 calories, not nearly enough to support adult metabolic needs. These clients are breaking down body fat for fuel, which increases production of ketoacids.

17. B
Clients with chronic kidney disease are unable to excrete sufficient hydrogen ions or to reabsorb sufficient bicarbonate to maintain acid-base balance. This results in a metabolic acidosis. Although an increased rate of ventilation may also occur, it is not great enough to cause a respiratory alkalosis.

18. B
Option D is incorrect because the question already states that the client has acidosis and is asking which laboratory value indicates the acidosis is metabolic in origin. The hallmark of a metabolic origin acidosis is a lower than normal bicarbonate level coupled with a normal carbon dioxide level and a low pH.

19. D
Although aspirin overdose initially causes a respiratory alkalosis by stimulating an increased respiratory rate, at the cellular level it results in a true metabolic acidosis that, untreated, can cause death. Antacid overdose can lead to alkalosis. Acetaminophen causes liver toxicity, not acidosis. Antihistamines are not associated with development of acidosis.

20. A
Clients who hyperventilate can exhale excessive amounts of carbon dioxide which leads to a decreased blood level of free hydrogen ions and acidosis of respiratory origin. A client with multiple rib fractures may have poor gas exchange from shallow breathing because of pain

and because the rib fractures may inhibit adequate chest expansion. Ringer's lactate does not cause a respiratory problem. The client with diarrhea is at risk for metabolic acidosis from loss of bicarbonate ions in the stool.

21. C
During acidosis, the body attempts to bring the pH closer to normal by moving free hydrogen ions into cells in exchange for potassium ions. This exchange can cause hyperkalemia, which can block electrical conduction through the heart and cause severe bradycardia and even cardiac arrest. A hallmark of hyperkalemia is tall, peaked T waves on the ECG. Although other electrolytes are affected to some degree, the most important one to assess is the serum potassium level.

22. A, C, E, F
Severe kyphoscoliosis, severe obesity, ascites, and emphysema all make chest expansion more difficult and can lead to respiratory acidosis. Arthroscopic surgery and early pregnancy do not impinge on the chest cavity or interfere with chest expansion.

23. B, D
The hallmarks of a respiratory acidosis are high $PaCO_2$ and low PaO_2 coupled with a low pH. However, a low pH is also associated with a metabolic acidosis and is not specific to a respiratory acidosis. The elevated potassium level is associated with both metabolic and respiratory acidosis. The low bicarbonate level is associated with a metabolic acidosis. The low $PaCO_2$ is associated with respiratory alkalosis, not with acidosis.

24. A, C, F
Regardless of the cause of a severe metabolic acidosis, the greatly increased hydrogen ion concentration results in high CO_2 levels (through the carbonic anhydrase reaction) that trigger the central nervous system to increase the rate and depth of breathing (Kussmaul respirations). These deep and rapid breaths help "blow off" the excessive CO_2 and bring down the hydrogen

ion level. The high CO_2 level causes widespread vasodilation, which results in warm, flushed, and dry skin. Blood pressure is low, which decreases urine output. Bicarbonate is decreased either as a cause of the acidosis or because it is binding to hydrogen ions forming carbonic acid to help buffer the low pH.

25. **B, E**
Skeletal muscle changes occur in acidosis because of the accompanying hyperkalemia. Muscles are weak and deep tendon reflexes, including the patellar reflex, are hypoactive. In the lower limbs, the muscle weakness is bilateral and can progress to paralysis.

26. **B, C, E, F**
The kidney, pancreas, and liver are responsible for much of the body's production of bicarbonate. Any problem with these organs interferes with its production. In dehydration, bicarbonate may continue to be produced but does not leave the producing organ. With diarrhea, bicarbonate is lost from the body.

27. **B**
The hallmarks of respiratory alkalosis are a pH above normal coupled with a normal bicarbonate level and a low $PaCO_2$. The client's gas exchange is unimpaired but more rapid, leading to an excessive loss of CO_2. Because gas exchange is unimpaired, oxygen levels are normal and cannot go higher on normal atmospheric air.

28. **B, C, D**
The pancreas is an important producer of bicarbonate. With pancreatitis, bicarbonate is underproduced, leading to a relative metabolic acidosis (hydrogen ion production is normal, not excessive). The $PaCO_2$ can be normal because gas exchange is not impaired and may be lower than normal because the client is hyperventilating as a result of the severe pain.

29. **B**
A condition resulting in alkalosis usually also causes hypocalcemia, which increases the sensitivity of excitable membranes, often seen as tingling of the fingers, toes, and around the mouth. Edema and joint pain are not indicators of an acid-base balance problem. With increased nerve sensitivity, tiredness and difficulty concentrating are not common with alkalosis.

30. **D**
Hypoxia is associated with respiratory acidosis. Morbid obesity and a tight body cast can restrict chest movements and result in respiratory acidosis. Clients in a panic attack tend to hyperventilate, blowing off excessive amounts of carbon dioxide, leading to respiratory alkalosis.

31. **B, D**
Alkalosis of any type causes hypokalemia as a compensatory response. Hydrogen ions move out of cells, especially red blood cells, in exchange for potassium from the blood moving into the cells in order to maintain electroneutrality. A rising blood pH promotes ionized calcium to bind to plasma proteins, decreasing the amount of ionized (free calcium) ions in the blood, resulting in hypocalcemia.

32. **D**
Alkalosis has a pH above 7.45, which would make options A (partially compensated respiratory acidosis) and B (metabolic acidosis) incorrect. Metabolic alkalosis has normal carbon dioxide and oxygen levels because breathing is not affected. Elevated bicarbonate levels (or acid losses) cause metabolic alkalosis.

33. **A**
Base excesses are caused by excessive intake of bicarbonates, carbonates, acetates, and citrates. Citrates are products used to preserve blood components for transfusion therapy. A massive blood transfusion would increase citrate levels and cause a base excess acidosis. Development of base excess alkalosis is not age-related. Thiazide diuretics, nasogastric suctioning, and prolonged vomiting lead to acid-deficit metabolic alkalosis.

34. **D**
Antacids buffer the hydrochloric acid in the stomach, which causes heartburn, by adding more base, usually in the form of bicarbonate.

Thus, excessive antacid use leads to a base-excess metabolic alkalosis.

35. A

The respiratory compensation for acid-base derangements is the second line of defense (buffers in body fluids are first) but begins within minutes of changes. For decreased carbon dioxide and hydrogen ion levels, respiratory compensation would be to decrease the rate and depth of respiration so that more carbon dioxide would be retained, which would also increase the hydrogen ion concentration.

Renal compensation takes much longer (at least 24 hours) to initiate.

36. A, C, F

Bicarbonate is a base that is lost with excessive diarrhea leading to a base-deficit metabolic acidosis. In addition, bicarbonate that is produced may not get into body fluids if the diarrhea was severe enough to cause dehydration. The acidosis would cause hydrogen ions to move into cells in exchange for potassium moving from the cells into the extracellular fluid to maintain electroneutrality, resulting in hyperkalemia.

15 CHAPTER

Concepts of Infusion Therapy

1. Which are among the **most common** reasons for a nurse to administer infusion therapy to a client? **Select all that apply.**
    A. Keep a line open for surgery
    B. Administer medications
    C. Maintain electrolyte or acid-base balance
    D. Maintain fluid balance or correct fluid imbalance
    E. Chemotherapy for cancer clients
    F. Correct electrolyte or acid-base imbalance

2. Which activities would be performed by infusion nurses for clients requiring infusion therapy? **Select all that apply.**
    A. Provide education about infusion therapy for staff, families, and clients.
    B. Monitor client outcomes with infusion therapy.
    C. Develop evidence-based policies and procedures.
    D. Consult on product selection and purchasing decisions.
    E. Develop new products for more effective infusion therapy.
    F. Insert and maintain peripheral, midline, and central venous catheters.

3. What is the RN generalist's role for a client in need of infusion therapy?
    A. Placement of a peripherally inserted central catheters (PICC)
    B. Changing dressing on all intravenous sites every 48 hours
    C. Insertion of short peripheral catheters (SPC)
    D. Providing services such as hypodermoclysis and intraosseous infusions

4. Which intravenous (IV) fluid would the nurse infuse for a client when the health care provider prescribes a hypotonic solution?
    A. 0.9% NaCl
    B. 0.45% NaCl
    C. Lactated Ringer's solution
    D. 5% dextrose with 0.9% saline

5. Which type of intravenous (IV) access would the nurse use to administer a client's chemotherapy treatment? **Select all that apply.**
    A. Intra-arterial catheter
    B. Peripherally inserted central catheter (PICC)
    C. Implanted port
    D. Short peripheral catheter
    E. Dialysis catheter
    F. Midline catheter

6. What is the nurse's **first** action(s) when a client who is receiving IV chemotherapy through a PICC line develops infiltration into the tissue and redness is observed?
    A. Stop the infusion and disconnect the IV line from the administration set.
    B. Apply pressure and elevate the site of swelling and redness.
    C. Aspirate the drug from the intravenous access device.
    D. Check vital signs, monitor the client, and document the incident.

7. Which grade of infiltration (based on Infusion Nurses Society [INS] criteria) would the nurse document after observing a client's IV site to have skin that is blanched and translucent, gross edema more than 6 inches in any direction, area cool to touch, moderate pain, and site numbness?
   A. Grade 1
   B. Grade 2
   C. Grade 3
   D. Grade 4

8. What information must the nurse know before giving any IV drug to a client? **Select all that apply.**
   A. Indications and proper dosage
   B. Contraindications and precautions
   C. Percentage of adverse events for the drug
   D. Compatibility with other IV medications
   E. Rate of infusion and osmolarity
   F. Potential for irritant and vesicant effects

9. What information must be included with each prescription for IV therapy for the nurse to administer it safely to a client? **Select all that apply.**
   A. Frequency of drug administration
   B. Specific type of administration equipment
   C. Rate of administration
   D. Specific type of solution
   E. Method for diluting drugs for the solution
   F. Specific drug to be added to the solution

10. Where would the nurse insert an IV short peripheral catheter (SPC) in an active client with a prescription for IV therapy?
    A. Wrist
    B. Hand
    C. Antecubital area
    D. Forearm

11. What would the nurse's **first action(s)** be when a client's IV site demonstrates slowed flow rate, skin tightness, discomfort at the site (e.g., burning, tenderness), and leakage around the site?
    A. Apply a cold pack and elevate the extremity.
    B. Place a sterile dressing over the site if weeping from the tissue occurs.
    C. Stop the solution and remove the intravenous access.
    D. Insert a new IV catheter above the site of the old one.

12. When the nurse is providing care for a client with a midline catheter, which key points are true? **Select all that apply.**
    A. Midline catheters are inserted in the upper arm, most commonly in the median antecubital vein.
    B. Midline catheters are used for hydration and for IV drug therapy up to 14 days.
    C. Strict sterile techniques are used for insertion and for dressing changes for midline catheters.
    D. Midline catheters can be used for the infusion of vesicant medications.
    E. All parenteral nutrition formulas may be infused through a midline catheter.
    F. When using a double-lumen midline catheter, do not administer incompatible drugs.

13. Which criteria must the nurse follow **before** using a newly established peripherally inserted central catheter (PICC) to start IV therapy for a client?
    A. Wait for the results of a chest x-ray indicating that the tip resides in the lower superior vena cava (SVC).
    B. Check the client's chart to ensure that sterile technique is used for insertion to reduce the risk for catheter-related bloodstream infection (CRBSI).
    C. Review the purpose of the PICC line and check the pH or osmolality of fluids to be infused through the line.
    D. Check patency of the PICC line by flushing with 20 mL of sterile normal saline.

14. Which statement by a client to a nurse indicates the need for additional teaching regarding care of a PICC line?
    A. "My PICC line has a lumen size 4 French so blood samples can be drawn from it."
    B. "I will be able to rejoin my soccer team as long as I protect the PICC with padding."
    C. "My PICC line will work for IV antibiotics even up to 14 days."
    D. "I will be careful to use sterile technique when I change the dressing."

15. Which major components and precautions of the catheter-related bloodstream infection (CRBSI) prevention bundle must the specially trained nurse follow when inserting a PICC line into a client? **Select all that apply.**
    A. Measuring upper arm circumference as a baseline before insertion
    B. Betadine skin antisepsis
    C. Proper aseptic hand hygiene
    D. Maximal barrier precautions on insertion
    E. Optimal catheter site selection
    F. Daily review of line necessity with prompt removal of unnecessary lines

16. Which technique is recommended by the Infusion Nurses Society (INS) for the nurse to maintain a PICC line for a client receiving IV antibiotic therapy every 4 hours?
    A. Flush the catheter with 10 mL heparinized saline after each dose of antibiotic.
    B. Flush the catheter every 12 hours using a 5-mL syringe.
    C. Avoid flushing the catheter with heparinized saline more than twice a week.
    D. Use 10 mL of sterile saline to flush before and after each dose of antibiotic.

17. Which client condition influences the nurse's choice of right versus left forearm placement when a short peripheral catheter (SPC) needs placement?
    A. Myocardial infarction with pain radiating down the left arm
    B. Pneumothorax with a chest tube on the right side
    C. Regular renal dialysis with a shunt on the left forearm
    D. Right hip fracture with immobilization and traction in place

18. What is the nurse's **priority** action when attempting to insert a short peripheral catheter (SPC) and the client reports a feeling of "pins and needles"?
    A. Ask the client to wiggle the fingers to stimulate circulation.
    B. Stop immediately, remove the catheter, and choose a new site.
    C. Change to a short-winged butterfly needle.
    D. Pause the procedure and gently massage the fingers.

19. Which type of equipment **decreases** the risk of disconnection or leakage when a nurse attaches an administration set to a client's central venous catheter?
    A. Slip lock connector
    B. Extension set
    C. Luer-Lok connector
    D. Needleless connector

20. Which client is the nurse **most** likely to teach about placement of a tunneled central venous catheter?
    A. Client in wheelchair to receive IV antibiotics for 16 weeks
    B. Client with trauma from a motor vehicle crash
    C. Client in need of fluid replacement for dehydration
    D. Client with acute renal failure and decreased urine output

21. Which nursing actions are implemented when caring for a client with an implanted port? **Select all that apply.**
   A. Before giving a drug through the port, always check for a blood return.
   B. De-access the port using a 5-mL syringe and 5 mL of heparin 5 units/mL.
   C. Before puncturing a port, palpate the port and locate the septum.
   D. Use a noncoring needle to access the implanted port.
   E. Flush the implanted port at least once monthly between courses of therapy.
   F. Use a topical anesthetic cream to decrease the pain of accessing the port.

22. What complication does the nurse suspect when a client receiving IV antibiotic therapy over the past 3 days develops chills, headache, and an elevated temperature?
   A. Fluid volume overload
   B. Allergic reaction to antibiotics
   C. Phlebitis with infiltration
   D. Catheter-related bloodstream infection (CRBSI)

23. What is the minimum gauge of short peripheral catheter (SPC) through which a nurse can infuse a unit of packed RBCs for a client?
   A. 18 gauge
   B. 20 gauge
   C. 22 gauge
   D. 24 gauge

24. Which substances does the nurse understand are not compatible with plastic containers when administering IV therapy to clients? **Select all that apply.**
   A. Insulin
   B. Nitroglycerin
   C. Propranolol
   D. Lorazepam
   E. Furosemide
   G. Fat emulsion

25. What would the nurse do when caring for an older adult client receiving IV fluids through a central line at 150 mL/hr, who becomes short of breath, develops puffiness around the eyes, and now has a cough?
   A. Place the client in an upright position, administer oxygen, slow the IV fluids, and notify the health care provider.
   B. Notify the health care provider, place the client in Trendelenburg position, and administer urokinase to unclot the catheter.
   C. Assess for patency of the central line catheter, change the tubing, and resume the IV fluids.
   D. Remove the central line, apply pressure, notify the health care provider, and place the client in a semi-Fowler's position.

26. Which technique will the nurse use to access a client's implanted port for chemotherapy?
   A. Palpate the port, scrub the skin, and access port with a butterfly needle.
   B. Scrub the port with alcohol and access the port with a needleless device.
   C. Palpate the port, scrub the skin, and access the port with a noncoring needle.
   D. Scrub the port with betadine and flush using saline in a 10-mL syringe.

27. What is the best place for the nurse to add a filter to a client's IV administration set?
   A. As close as possible to the catheter hub
   B. Immediately below the infusion pump
   C. As close to the solution container as possible
   D. At any convenient connection point unlikely to be disconnected

28. Which teaching would the nurse provide for the client and family on prevention of catheter-related bloodstream infection (CRBSI) before the IV catheter was inserted? **Select all that apply.**
   A. The type of catheter to be inserted
   B. Hand hygiene
   C. Aseptic technique for care of the catheter
   D. Activity limitations
   E. Signs and symptoms of complications
   F. Alternatives to catheter and therapy

29. What is the **priority** nursing responsibility when a client is receiving IV therapy through an infusion pump?
    A. Monitor the client's infusion site and rate.
    B. Program the correct amount of fluid into the pump.
    C. Position the container for gravity flow.
    D. Check the equipment at the end of the infusion.

30. Which instruction will the nurse be sure to give the assistive personnel (AP) when checking the blood pressure of a client receiving IV therapy?
    A. "Avoid taking blood pressure in an extremity with any type of IV catheter in place."
    B. "Put the pump on hold while you take the client's blood pressure, then restart it."
    C. "Remind the phlebotomist to draw blood from the extremity without an IV catheter."
    D. "You can check blood pressure with a short peripheral catheter, but not with a midline catheter."

31. Which intervention would the nurse use to reduce the risk of infection when a client is receiving IV drugs by way of a needleless system?
    A. Always use a hand scrub when entering a client's room.
    B. Clean all needleless system connections with an antimicrobial agent for 10-15 seconds before connecting infusion sets.
    C. Use tape to assure that secondary IV sets remain attached to primary IV sets.
    D. Disconnect secondary IV sets after each dose of IV drug is completed.

32. Which specific actions will the nurse take when assessing a client's IV site? **Select all that apply.**
    A. Look for redness, swelling, hardness, or drainage.
    B. Check integrity of the dressing to make sure it is clean, dry, and adherent to the skin on all sides.
    C. Ensure that all connections are taped to prevent disconnection and leaking of fluids.
    D. Check the rate and amount of fluid that has infused.
    E. Be sure that the correct type of fluid is being infused.
    F. Check the skin around the dressing for medical adhesive–related skin injury (MARSI).

33. How often would the nurse routinely change the transparent dressing on a client's central venous IV site?
    A. Every 24 hours
    B. Every 48 hours
    C. Every 3 days
    D. Every 5 to 7 days

34. Which techniques will the nurse use to prevent air emboli when changing the IV administration set or connectors for a client with a central venous catheter? **Select all that apply.**
    A. Placing the client flat or in Trendelenburg so that the catheter site is below the heart
    B. Using sterile technique when handling the IV set and connectors
    C. Asking the client to perform the Valsalva maneuver by holding his or her breath and bearing down
    D. Timing the IV set change to the expiratory cycle if the client is spontaneously breathing
    E. Having an assistive personnel (AP) apply pressure at the insertion site
    F. Timing the IV set change to the inspiratory cycle when the client is receiving positive-pressure mechanical ventilation

35. What solution and volume does the nurse typically use to flush a client's short peripheral catheter IV saline lock?
    A. 3 mL heparinized saline
    B. 5 mL bacteriostatic saline
    C. 3 mL normal saline
    D. 5 mL heparin solution

36. Which actions must the nurse follow to remove a short peripheral catheter (SPC) when a client is ready for discharge to home? **Select all that apply.**
    A. Flush the SPC before removal.
    B. Remove the SPC dressing.
    C. Explain the procedure to the client.
    D. Rapidly withdraw the catheter from the skin.
    E. Immediately cover the puncture site with dry gauze.
    F. Hold pressure until hemostasis is achieved.
    G. Assess the catheter tip to ensure it is intact and completely removed.
    H. Document catheter removal and appearance of site.

37. Which nursing action is essential when a client is receiving infusion therapy through an intra-arterial catheter placed in the carotid artery?
    A. Monitor respirations for rate and regularity.
    B. Perform frequent neurologic and cognitive status assessments.
    C. Assess the extremities for sensation and peripheral pulses.
    D. Place antiembolic stockings on client's lower extremities.

38. Which factor increases the likelihood that a client who comes into the emergency department (ED) after a serious motor crash is a candidate for intraosseous (IO) therapy?
    A. Endotracheal intubation is difficult to accomplish.
    B. IV access cannot be established within a few minutes.
    C. Client is an older adult and very thin.
    D. Client has a history of chronic renal failure.

39. Which key points would the nurse teach a client about intraosseous (IO) therapy? **Select all that apply.**
    A. The only absolute contraindication is fracture in the bone to be used as a site.
    B. The IO route is for short term use and should not be used for more than 24 hours.
    C. The most common site accessed for IO therapy is the distal femur.
    D. The same fluids and drugs given IV can be given IO.
    E. During the IO procedure, most clients rate the pain as a 2 or 3 on a scale of 0 to 10.
    F. For access, 12- or 14-gauge needles specifically designed for IO therapy are preferred.

40. Which statements does the nurse recognize as true when providing care for a client receiving intraperitoneal (IP) infusions? **Select all that apply.**
    A. IP infusion therapy involves the administration of chemotherapy agents into the peritoneal cavity.
    B. An IP catheter has large internal lumens with multiple side-holes along the catheter length to allow for delivery of large quantities of fluid.
    C. Clean techniques are used when handling IP access and supplies.
    D. IP therapy is used for clients who are receiving medications for diagnostic tests.
    E. IP therapy includes three phases: the instillation phase; the dwell phase, usually 1 to 4 hours; and the drain phase.
    F. Strict aseptic techniques are used when handling the IP access and supplies.

41. What is the nurse's **best** action when a client receiving IP therapy reports nausea and vomiting?
    A. Reduce the IP flow rate and administer antiemetics.
    B. Help the client move from side to side to distribute the fluid evenly.
    C. Flush the catheter with normal saline after the fluid has drained.
    D. Notify the health care provider and obtain a prescription for abdominal x-ray.

42. Which site will the nurse choose for a client who is to receive hypodermoclysis treatment for palliative care?
    A. Anterior forearm
    B. Lateral aspect of the upper arm
    C. Area under the clavicle
    D. Posterior tibial area

43. For which conditions does the nurse consider intrathecal infusion appropriate for a client? **Select all that apply.**
    A. Traumatic brain injury
    B. Leukemia
    C. Multiple sclerosis
    D. Cancer of the central nervous system
    E. Cerebral palsy
    F. Chronic pain

44. For which potential problem does the nurse assess the client after receiving epidural therapy when symptoms of headache, stiff neck, or temperature higher than 101°F (38.3°C) develop?
    A. Allergic reaction
    B. Leakage of cerebrospinal fluid
    C. Meningitis
    D. Catheter migration

45. At what rate would the nurse set the infusion when a client is to receive 0.45% normal saline, 1000 mL over 15 hours?
    A. 50 mL/hr
    B. 67 mL/hr
    C. 75 mL/hr
    D. 83 mL/hr

46. Which **priority** concept concerns the nurse when performing infusion therapy for any client?
    A. Fluid and electrolyte balance
    B. Tissue integrity
    C. Acid-base imbalance
    D. Perfusion

Chapter 15 Answer Key

1. B, C, D, F
   The most common reasons for using infusion therapy with clients are to: maintain fluid balance or correct fluid imbalance; maintain electrolyte or acid-base balance or correct electrolyte or acid-base imbalance; administer medications; and replace blood or blood products.

2. A, B, C, D, F
   Infusion nurses may perform any or all of these activities: develop evidence-based policies and procedures; insert and maintain various types of peripheral, midline, and central venous catheters and subcutaneous and intraosseous accesses; monitor client outcomes of infusion therapy; educate staff, clients, and families regarding infusion therapy; consult on product selection and purchasing decisions; provide therapies such as blood withdrawal, therapeutic phlebotomy, hypodermoclysis, intraosseous infusions, and administration of medications.

3. C
   The registered nurse (RN) generalist is taught to insert peripheral IV lines; most institutions have a process for demonstrating competency for this skill (e.g., demonstrate successful placement a specified number of times on clients with a preceptor watching). Options A and D are specialty actions not usually performed by a generalist nurse. Option B is wrong because of the time frame which varies depending on the type of IV line and dressing.

4. B
   A hypotonic solution has a lower than normal blood plasma osmolarity (fluids less than 270 mOsm/L). An example of a hypotonic solution is half-strength saline (0.45% NaCl).

5. A, B, C

Use of an intra-arterial catheter for infusion therapy is not common and is generally used for direct treatment of tumor sites. Chemotherapy agents administered arterially allow infusion of a high concentration of drug directly to the tumor site. With a PICC line, there are no limitations on the pH or osmolality of fluids that can be infused. Clients requiring lengthy courses (more than 14 days) of antibiotics, chemotherapy agents, parenteral nutrition formulas, and vasopressor agents can benefit from a PICC. Implanted ports are used most often for clients receiving chemotherapy.

6. A

The IV insertion site should be assessed carefully for early signs of infiltration, including swelling, coolness, tingling, or redness. If any of these symptoms are present, discontinue the drug immediately and notify the infusion therapy team and/or primary health care provider per agency policy when complications like this occur.

7. C

According to INS criteria, Grade 3 infiltration includes the following symptoms: skin blanched, translucent, gross edema more than 6 inches in any direction, cool to touch, mild-to-moderate pain, and possible numbness.

8. A, B, D, E, F

For all drug administration, nurses must be knowledgeable about drug indications, proper dosage, contraindications, and precautions. IV administration also requires knowledge of appropriate dilution, rate of infusion, pH and osmolarity, compatibility with other IV medications, appropriate infusion site (peripheral versus central circulation), potential for vesicant/irritant effects, and specific aspects of client monitoring because of its immediate effect.

9. A, C, D, F

A drug prescription should include: drug name, preferably by generic name; specific dose and route; frequency of administration; time(s) of administration; length of time for infusion (number of doses/days); purpose (required in some health care agencies, especially nursing homes). The specific type of equipment to be used is not a requirement for a valid prescription. The pharmacy determines the correct diluent based on manufacturer's recommendations or requirements.

10. D

Short peripheral catheters are most often inserted into superficial veins of the forearm. In emergent situations, these catheters can also be used in the external jugular vein of the neck. The areas in options A and C are over joints, which would then have to be immobilized. The back of the hand contains little subcutaneous tissue and is easily damaged. Option B, the hand is not appropriate for older patients with a loss of skin turgor and poor vein condition or for active patients receiving infusion therapy in an ambulatory care clinic or home care. Use of veins on the dorsal surface of the hands should be reserved as a last resort for short-term infusion of nonvesicant and nonirritant solutions in young patients.

11. C

First, stop infusion and remove short peripheral catheter immediately. After this, a sterile dressing can be applied if there is weeping from the tissue. Next, the extremity can be elevated and cold or warm compresses applied. A new catheter should be inserted in the opposite (not the same) extremity. Finally, the nurse would rate the infiltration using the INS Infiltration Scale and document the event.

12. A, B, C, F

Options A, B, C, and F are correct statements about midline catheters. Midline catheters should not be used to infuse vesicant solutions. Vesicant solutions can cause severe tissue damage if they escape into the subcutaneous tissue (**extravasation**). When using a double-lumen midline catheter, do not administer incompatible drugs simultaneously through both lumens because the blood flow rate in the axillary vein is not high enough to ensure adequate hemodilution and prevention of drug interaction in the vein.

13. A

Before the PICC line can be used for infusion, a chest x-ray indicating that the tip resides in the lower SVC is required when the catheter is not placed under fluoroscopy or with the use of the electrocardiogram tip-locator technique. Sterile technique is used with all IV insertions. The PICC line is placed in a vein with high flow that can handle hyperosmolar fluids and those in various pH ranges. Flushing the catheter should be done before each use to assess patency of the catheter and after each use to ensure that occlusion from blood that backflows into the lumen does not occur.

14. B

Option B indicates that the client needs additional teaching about the PICC line. While clients will be able to perform their usual activities of daily living (ADLs), they should avoid excessive physical activity (e.g., playing soccer) because of the increased risk for catheter dislodgment and possible lumen occlusion. Options A, C, and D indicate understanding of care for PICC lines.

15. A, C, D, E, F

All options are appropriate and part of the catheter-related bloodstream infection (CRBSI) prevention bundle, except option B which should be chlorhexidine skin antisepsis (not betadine).

16. D

The INS recommends that PICC lines not actively in use be flushed with 5 mL of heparin (10 units/mL) in a 10-mL syringe at least daily when using a nonvalved catheter and at least weekly with a valved catheter. Use 10 mL of sterile saline to flush before and after medication administration; 20 mL of sterile saline to flush after drawing blood. Always use 10-mL barrel syringes to flush any central line because the pressure exerted by a smaller barrel poses a risk for rupturing the catheter.

17. C

Mastectomy, axillary lymph node dissection, lymphedema, paralysis of the upper extremity, and the presence of dialysis grafts or fistulas alter the normal pattern of blood flow through the arm. Using veins in the extremity affected by one of these conditions requires a primary health care provider's order.

18. B

Reports of tingling, feeling "pins and needles" in the extremity, or numbness during the venipuncture procedure can indicate nerve puncture. If any of these symptoms occur, stop the IV insertion procedure immediately, remove the catheter, and choose a new site.

19. C

A Luer-Lok connection has an end with a threaded collar that requires twisting onto the corresponding threads of the catheter hub. All connections, including extension sets, should have a Luer-Lok design to ensure that the set remains firmly connected. A slip lock has a male end that slips into the female catheter hub but does not have the threaded collar. An extension set lengthens the tubing but does not protect against disconnection or leakage. A needleless connection protects against needlesticks but does not stop disconnection or leakage.

20. A

Tunneled catheters are used primarily when the need for infusion therapy is frequent and long term. Tunneled catheters are chosen when several weeks or months of infusion therapy are needed and a PICC is not a good choice (e.g., wheelchair bound, paraplegic).

21. A, C, D, E, F

All options are appropriate for the care of an implanted port except option B. The INS recommendation for locking or de-accessing a port is the use of a 10-mL syringe with either heparin 10 units/mL or preservative-free 0.9% normal saline.

22. D

With catheter-related bloodstream infection (CRBSI), early symptoms include fever, chills, headache, and general malaise. Later symptoms include tachycardia, hypotension, and decreased urinary output.

7. C

Clients with cirrhosis of the liver have a decreased production of clotting factors, including prothrombin, causing them to be at an increased risk for bleeding.

8. A

A deep vein thrombosis is a clot formation in either superficial or deep (most often) veins. If a thrombus becomes dislodged or broken into smaller clots, it is known as an embolus. Emboli may travel to the brain (causing a thrombotic stroke) or to the lung (causing a pulmonary embolus). An embolus does not cause a hemorrhagic stroke. A myocardial infarction (MI) occurs when one or more clots form in a coronary artery. Clots formed elsewhere in the body do not result in an MI. Superficial phlebitis is caused by vein irritation or inflammation, and not deep vein thrombosis.

9. A, C, D, F

Signs and symptoms of decreased clotting include purpural lesions such as ecchymosis (bruising), and petechiae (pinpoint purpura). Bleeding may be prolonged as a result of injury or trauma. Check urine and stool for the presence of occult or frank blood. Observe for frank bleeding from the gums or nose.

10. A

Prevention strategies when there is an increased risk for clotting include:
- Drink adequate fluids to prevent dehydration.
- Avoid crossing the legs.
- Ambulate frequently and avoid prolonged sitting.
- Explore smoking cessation programs as needed.
- Call the primary health care provider if redness, pain, swelling, and warmth occur in a lower extremity.

11. A

Delirium is an acute, fluctuating confusional state with a fast or sudden onset and lasting only a short time (days to hours). It is reversible when the conditions causing it can be eliminated. Dementia is a chronic, progressive cognitive decline occurring over months to years. Some forms of dementia can be temporarily helped by specific medications, but the progression continues and the dementia is permanent. Amnesia is a loss of memory but the person often can learn new facts. Although delirium can have an intermittent component, no such condition is described in the question.

12. B, D, E

Providing a safe environment and observing for associated behaviors such as delusions and hallucinations are important nursing actions. Helping the family to know what home environment areas can pose a danger to the client and how to reduce the risk for harm are critical for client safety. Reorienting the client seldom is successful and may anger him or her. Often clients cannot tell the difference between what is real and what is not real. Correcting such statements again does not help and may anger the client. Although clients with dementia may be able to assent to treatment, they cannot sign an informed consent statement because it is extremely unlikely they can truly comprehend the meaning of consent.

13. D

Adults who experience urinary incontinence need frequent toileting every 1 to 2 hours. This routine can prevent incontinence and train the bladder to empty at more regular intervals. Assisting clients with toileting is within the scope of practice for an AP and appropriately delegated to an AP by the nurse. Although the AP may report any redness or skin breakdown, the nurse must assess the client for this change. The AP is not expected to have the knowledge of physiology or pathophysiology related to electrolyte imbalance. Although the AP may notice a change, it is the nurse rather than the AP who must monitor for physiologic/pathophysiologic changes.

14. B

Clients with fluid excess (overload) usually have an increase in blood pressure due to increased blood volume. Peripheral pulses are often strong, bounding, and rapid. Many clients experience peripheral edema due to fluid excess, not decreased skin turgor.

15. A, C, D, E

Infection prevention actions (e.g. handwashing), smoking cessation to prevent COPD, and getting immunizations as recommended to prevent influenza and pneumonia are the most appropriate actions. Drugs used to treat respiratory health problems include antihistamines, decongestants, glucocorticoids, bronchodilators, mucolytics, and antimicrobials. Chest expansion is improved when the client is sitting or is in a semi-Fowler's position, not a flat, side-lying position. Teach the client about the need for deep breathing and coughing to further enhance lung expansion and decrease breathing effort. Teach him or her how to correctly use incentive spirometry and inhalers if indicated. Oxygen is a drug that must be prescribed at a specific rate (dose). The client should not be instructed to change the rate without consulting his or her respiratory health care provider.

16. B, E, F

Traditional cancer chemotherapy greatly reduces inflammation and immunity by reducing the number of circulating leukocytes. Clients undergoing cancer chemotherapy are at increased infection risk regardless of age. Corticosteroids reduce the immune response and increase the risk for infection. Older clients are always at risk for infection because of age-related declines in immunity. When a chronic illness, especially a respiratory ailment, is also present, the risk is even greater. Although going without an influenza vaccination does increase the risk for acquiring this disease, it does not increase general infection risk or require special actions.

17. A, C

The temperature elevation and the higher-than-normal total leukocyte count are indications of a systemic infection. Wound redness, pain, and exudate are associated with a localized infection. A localized infection can be present for weeks without becoming a systemic infection.

18. A, C, F

Allergic rhinitis is not caused by an invasion of pathogens but by airborne irritants such as pollens. Rheumatoid arthritis is a chronic autoimmune disease in which autoantibodies damage the joint tissues and generate a chronic inflammatory response, which leads to more tissue damage. In most instances, cholecystitis (gall bladder disease and inflammation) does not involve the presence of pathogens (although the gall bladder can become infected).

19. C

Chronic inflammatory responses are overall tissue damaging when they are prolonged, resulting in excessive scar tissue formation and reduced function. Inflammation does not lead to or cause immunosuppression or autoimmune disorders, nor does it convert to an infection. However, autoimmune disorders usually result in chronic inflammation. Chronic inflammation does not cause immunosuppression although many treatments for chronic inflammation cause some degree of immunosuppression.

20. A

Clients who have dysfunction of the musculoskeletal or nervous system are at highest risk for decreased mobility or immobility. For example, a client with a fractured hip is not able to walk because of pain and hip joint instability until the hip is surgically repaired and healed. Any person who is bedridden or on *prolonged* bedrest is at risk for immobility issues.

21. A, D, E, F, G

The common physiologic complications of decreased mobility include:
- Pressure injuries (pressure on the skin over bony prominences)
- Disuse osteoporosis (increased bone resorption)
- Constipation (decreased gastrointestinal [GI] motility)
- Weight loss or gain (decreased appetite and movement)
- Muscle atrophy (catabolism)
- Atelectasis/hypostatic pneumonia (decreased lung expansion)
- Venous thromboembolism (e.g., deep venous thrombosis and pulmonary embolus [decreased blood circulation])
- Urinary system stones (urinary stasis)

22. A, B, E

    For a client with bulimia and low weight, common interventions include high-protein oral supplements, enteral supplements (either oral or by feeding tube), or parenteral nutrition. Obtain the client's height and weight and calculate body mass index (BMI). Assess the client's skin, hair, and nails because poor nutrition often causes very dry skin and brittle hair and nails. The most common assessment for generalized malnutrition is prealbumin and albumin measurement. Albumin is a major serum protein that is below normal in clients who have had inadequate nutrition for weeks. Prealbumin assessment is preferred because it decreases more quickly when nutrition is not adequate. Monitor and interpret these laboratory data to assess the client's nutritional status. Although nutrition is poor and weight is low, excessive intake of high-fat foods is not therapeutic. Bariatric surgery is designed to increase weight loss and is not appropriate for clients with bulimia. Excessive strenuous exercise leads to weight loss, not gain, and should be avoided.

23. A, C, D, E

    Signs and symptoms of inadequate central perfusion include dyspnea, dizziness or syncope, and chest pain. Signs and symptoms of decreased cardiac output include hypotension, tachycardia, diaphoresis, anxiety, decrease in cognitive function, and dysrhythmias.

24. A

    Persistent pain tends to be diffuse rather than confined to any single area associated with a known injury. All other reports are most often associated with acute pain.

25. C

    The most common cause of changes in smell and taste (impaired sensory perception) for adults is a dry mouth, which is a frequent side effect of drug therapy. Examples of drugs that can cause dry mouth include antidepressants, chemotherapeutic agents, antihistamines, and antiepileptic drugs (AEDs). When the causative drug is discontinued, the problem usually subsides.

4 CHAPTER

Common Health Problems of Older Adults

1. Which newly admitted client is **most likely** to need assessment by the nurse for geriatric frailty?
   A. 72-year-old with mild heart failure who lives alone independently
   B. 80-year-old with a pacemaker and hearing aid who uses a cane
   C. 73-year-old with bilateral total hip replacements
   D. 91-year-old with unintentional weight loss, weakness, and slowed activity

2. What are the **best** interventions for the nurse to use to help reduce relocation stress in an older adult client? **Select all that apply.**
   A. Explain all procedures to the client before they occur.
   B. Reorient the client frequently to his or her location.
   C. Initially, encourage family and friends to keep their visits to a minimum.
   D. Provide opportunity and time for the client to participate in decision making.
   E. Arrange for familiar keepsakes to be at the client's bedside.
   F. Change room assignment several times and assess for client's preferred choice.
   G. Early on establish a trusting relationship with the client.
   H. Teach the client to expect limited food selection and a set schedule for bathing.

3. Which question would the nurse ask to identify an **immediate** physiologic consequence when an older adult's teeth are in poor condition and the client says that he or she only eats soft foods?
   A. "Do you have any problems with your bowel movements?"
   B. "Have you lost any weight recently?"
   C. "Do you take any over-the-counter vitamin supplements?"
   D. "Would you like me to help you make an appointment with the dentist?"

4. Which exercise will the nurse **most likely** suggest to a client who is homebound?
   A. During the winter months, go to the mall and walk around.
   B. Attend an exercise class at a senior citizens' center.
   C. Walk on a treadmill three to five times per week for 60 minutes.
   D. Maintain independent performance of ADLs.

5. Which older adult has the **greatest** risk for falls?
   A. A 73-year-old who takes frequent walking excursions
   B. A 90-year-old who frequently calls for help to change position
   C. An 80-year-old who uses a cane when ambulating
   D. A 68-year-old who has decreased sensation in the lower extremities

6. Which home modifications will the nurse recommend to the family of a client at risk for falls before discharge to home? **Select all that apply**.
   A. Placement of handrails
   B. Install grab bars in the bathroom
   C. Lowered toilet seats
   D. Remove clutter from all rooms
   E. Assure adequate lighting in the home
   F. Remove scatter rugs
   G. Use nonslip bathmats

7. Which actions will the nurse take for a client who requires physical restraints? **Select all that apply**.
   A. Check the patient every 30 to 60 minutes
   B. Encourage family members to go home at night
   C. Release the restraints every 1 to 2 hours for turning, repositioning, and toileting
   D. Provide soft, calming music
   E. Turn the television on if the client is agitated
   F. Cover tubes and lines with roller gauze if the client pulls at them
   G. Place the client in an area where he or she can be supervised

8. Based on the Beers Criteria for Potentially Inappropriate Medication Use in Older Adults, which drug(s) would the nurse question when prescribed for an older adult client? **Select all that apply**.
   A. Promethazine
   B. Diazepam
   C. Amitriptyline
   D. Diphenhydramine
   E. Oxycodone
   F. Ticlopidine
   G. Chlorpropamide

9. Which action will the nurse take for an older client whose creatinine clearance (CrCl) is 70 mL/min?
   A. Consult the pharmacy to determine if the patient's drugs are harmful to the liver.
   B. Notify the health care provider because serum drug levels could become toxic.
   C. Notify the health care provider because drug doses will need to be increased.
   D. Document the level in the patient's record as within the normal range.

10. Which action will the nurse **avoid** using for the older adult with delirium?
    A. Talking to the patient using a calm voice.
    B. Sedating the client to prevent self-harm.
    C. Assessing the client for possible causes of delirium.
    D. Reorienting the client to place and person frequently.

11. Which screening tool should the nurse use when an older adult reports early morning insomnia, excessive daytime sleeping, poor appetite, lack of energy, and unwillingness to participate in social or recreational activities?
    A. Confusion Assessment Method (CAM)
    B. Geriatric Depression Scale-Short Form (GDS-SF)
    C. CAGE questionnaire
    D. Brief Abuse Screen for the Elderly

12. Which are health-protective behaviors? **Select all that apply**.
    A. Using over-the-counter medications that are acceptable for treating symptoms
    B. Getting an annual influenza vaccination
    C. Wearing seat belts when in an automobile
    D. Installing grab bars in showers and tubs
    E. Having a pneumococcal vaccination as recommended by the HCP
    F. Consuming alcohol only on weekends
    G. Avoiding smoking and never smoking in bed
    H. Putting up smoke detectors and changing the batteries regularly

13. What instructions will the nurse give the assistive personnel (AP) who reports that an older adult gentleman was wearing a bra and panties when admitted to the unit?
    A. "Show me the bra and panties, and then I will confront the patient."
    B. "Store the bra and panties away, and I'll talk to the family later on."
    C. "Pretend like you never saw the lingerie, and treat the patient like a male."
    D. "Assist the patient to dress, and allow him to select his own clothing."

14. What is the most important action for the nurse to take when a client is both confused and agitated?
    A. Place the patient in a quiet, supervised area.
    B. Check the patient every 2 hours.
    C. Sedate the patient using IV medication.
    D. Apply soft wrist restraints for a limited time.

15. Which tasks can the nurse delegate safely to an assistive personnel (AP) caring for an older adult? **Select all that apply.**
    A. Assist the client with tray preparation and feeding at mealtimes.
    B. Check and record vital signs every shift.
    C. Accurately record intake and output.
    D. Remind the client to consume at least 2 liters of fluids each day.
    E. Help the client out of bed to the bathroom.
    F. Teach the client about healthy foods and a balanced diet.
    G. Assess the client's skin every 2 hours during repositioning.
    H. Send a referral to physical therapy to evaluate client's ability to walk.

16. Which actions should nurses take for all clients to prevent fall regardless of risk for falls? **Select all that apply**.
    A. Monitor client's activities and behavior as often as possible.
    B. Teach clients and ok families about fall prevention to become safety partners.
    C. Help the incontinent client to the toilet at least once each shift.
    D. Remind the client to wear glasses and hearing aid.
    E. Clean up spills immediately.
    F. Remind clients to call for help before getting out of bed or a chair.
    G. Teach clients to use grab bars when walking in the hall without assistive devices.
    H. Assist clients to ambulate to the bathroom with a walker or cane as needed.

Chapter 4 Answer Key

1. **D**
Frailty is a geriatric syndrome with signs including unintentional weight loss, weakness and exhaustion, and slowed physical activity including walking. The client described in option D meets these criteria. Mild heart failure and bilateral total hip replacements do not alone make an older adult frail. Although multiple health issues as in option C can increase frailty, the client who is most likely to be frail is described in option D.

2. **A, B, D, E, G**
Family and friends should be encouraged to visit often. Unnecessary room changes should be avoided. Clients should be assessed for usual lifestyle, daily activities, food likes and dislikes, and preferred time for bathing. All of the other selections will help minimize relocation stress for older adults.

3. **A**
Older adults with poor dentition often eat soft and high-calorie foods such as ice cream, mashed potatoes, and macaroni with cheese. These foods lack roughage and fiber which can lead to constipation. Additionally, unless older adults choose nutritious foods, they may develop vitamin deficiencies. Although vitamin deficiency can develop, altered bowel elimination is more immediate.

4. **D**
Clients who are homebound must focus on maintaining functional abilities such as performing activities of daily living (ADLs). The nurse teaches clients who are not homebound about the importance of regular exercise.

5. **D**
Changes in sensory perception create challenges for older adults regardless of age. Decreased sense of touch leads to decreased sense of body orientation and an older adult may not be able to determine exactly where his or her feet are in relation to steps, resulting in a fall.

6. **A, B, D, E, F, G**
All responses are appropriate except option C. Raised toilet seats would be more appropriate, especially for a client with hip or knee arthritis, because this type of toilet seat facilitates sitting and rising from the toilet.

7. **A, C, D, F, G**
Family members or friends should be asked or encouraged to stay with the patient at night. When the client is agitated, the television should be turned off to avoid excessive stimulation, **not** on. The remaining responses are all appropriate for the care of a patient who requires restraints. Before restraints are applied, alternative should be tried and restraints applied only if the alternatives are ineffective.

8. **A, B, C, D, E, F, G**
All of these drugs are examples of potentially inappropriate medication use for older adults. Digoxin (dose greater than 0.125 mg) and ferrous sulfate (dose greater than 325 mg daily) are also on this list. These drugs have been proven to have more significant side effects/adverse effects in older adults and should be avoided. Many of these drugs have exaggerated effects on the level of alertness and other central nervous system activity that would increase the risk for falls and alteration in judgment.

9. **B**
Age-related changes in the kidneys can result in high plasma concentrations of drugs. These changes include decreased renal blood flow and reduced glomerular filtration rate (as indicated by this client's abnormal creatinine clearance), which can lead to a decreased CrCl. Serum drug levels can become toxic and the client can become very seriously ill or die. The nurse must notify the primary health care provider so that he or she can take this information into consideration for medication type and dosage when prescribing drug therapy.

10. B

Delirium includes client inattentiveness, disorganized thinking, and altered level of consciousness. To help manage a client with delirium, use a calm voice when speaking with the client and frequently reorient them. Playing soothing music can also be calming to a client. Sedating the client may worsen, not improve the delirium.

11. B

The signs and symptoms this older adult client reports are classic for depression, so the Geriatric Depression Scale would be the best assessment tool to use. In older adults, the CAM tool measures confusion; the CAGE questionnaire measures alcoholism; and the Brief Abuse Screen for the Elderly looks at risk for elder abuse.

12. B, C, D, E, G, H

OTC drugs should be approved by the health care provider. Alcohol should be consumed in moderation or avoided. The remaining options are all appropriate health-protective behaviors.

13. D

Teach direct care givers such as assistive personnel to not be offensive or judgmental. Not all older adults are heterosexual. It's important to establish a trusting relationship with any client.

The nurse may discuss sexual orientation and gender identity with the UAP in a private setting and must be sure to emphasize confidentiality for the client.

14. A

When a client is both confused and agitated, the best action is to place him or her in a quiet, supervised area. Two hours is too long to wait to check the client. Sedation with IV medication may cause increased confusion and soft restraints should only be used after alternative strategies have failed.

15. A, B, C, D, E

To delegate to an assistive personnel (AP), the nurse must be familiar with their scope of practice which includes direct client care, vital signs, intake and output, assisting to the bathroom, and reminding clients about what has already been taught by the nurse. Teaching, assessing, and sending referrals require additional education and are actions appropriate to the scope of professional nursing practice.

16. A, B, D, E, F, G, H

Incontinent clients should be helped to the toilet every 1 to 2 hours. All of the other options are appropriate actions to implement with all older adult clients regardless of risk for falls.

23. C
Using a 22-gauge SPC is adequate for most therapies and blood can infuse without damage. Needles with a smaller gauge can damage blood cell membranes, making them useless in transfusion therapy.

24. A, B, D, G
A problem with using some plastic containers is that they are not compatible with substances such as insulin, nitroglycerin, lorazepam, fat emulsions, and lipid-based drugs. Nitroglycerin and insulin adhere to the walls of the polyvinyl chloride (PVC) container, making it impossible to know exactly how much medication the client is receiving.

25. A
The client's symptoms point to circulatory overload, not a clot or other obstruction within the catheter. Key interventions at this time would include: slow the IV rate and notify the health care provider; raise client to an upright position; monitor vital signs and administer oxygen as prescribed; administer diuretics as prescribed. When breathing difficulties are present, lying flat or in Trendelenburg position makes breathing harder.

26. C
Port access should be done only by formally trained health care professionals using a mask and aseptic technique. Before puncture, palpate the port to locate the septum. Carefully palpate to feel the shape and depth of the port body to ensure puncture of the septum. Scrub the skin over the port with alcohol. Implanted ports are accessed by using a noncoring needle (a common brand name is *Huber*) that is specially designed with a deflected tip. This design slices through the dense septum without coring out a small piece of it, thus preserving the integrity of the septum.

27. A
The purpose of filters is to remove particulate matter, microorganisms, and air from the infusion system. Filters should be placed as close to the catheter hub as possible to prevent particulate matter (e.g., rubber pieces, glass particles, cotton fibers, drug particles, paper, and metal fibers) from becoming trapped in the small circulation of the lungs. A red blood cell is about 5 microns in diameter and is the largest size that can pass through the pulmonary capillary bed; IV fluids may contain particles larger than 5 microns. For patients receiving infusion therapy for long periods, a significant number of particles could block the blood flow through the pulmonary circulation. Microcirculation in the spleen, kidneys, and liver could also be affected.

28. A, B, C, D, E, F
All options are correct responses to essential teaching that the nurse should provide for the client and family before an IV catheter is inserted for therapy.

29. A
The use of pumps does not decrease the nurse's responsibility to carefully monitor the client's infusion site and the infusion rate. Smart pumps (infusion pumps with dosage calculation software) have been promoted to reduce adverse drug events (ADEs). Incorrect programming of pumps without this feature is one of the most common types of drug errors, especially in hospitals.

30. A
Remind assistive personnel (AP) to avoid taking blood pressures in an extremity with any type of catheter in place. If a short peripheral catheter is being used for continuous infusion, the compression while taking the blood pressure can increase venous pressure, causing fluid to overflow from the puncture site and infiltration. When a midline catheter or PICC is being used, compression from the blood pressure cuff could increase vein irritation and lead to phlebitis.

31. B
Clean all needleless system connections vigorously with an antimicrobial agent (usually 70% alcohol or alcohol and 2% chlorhexidine swabs) for 10-15 seconds before connecting infusion sets or syringes, paying special attention to the small ridges in the Luer-Lok device. The "scrub the hub" technique suggests generating friction

by scrubbing the connection hubs in a twisting motion.

32. A, B, D, E

Options A, B, D, and E are appropriate to assessing a client's IV site. Connections should not be taped. The skin *under* the dressing (not around) should be checked for medical adhesive–related skin injury (MARSI).

33. D

For central IV lines, when a transparent dressing (e.g., Tegaderm) is used, the dressing is routinely changed every 5 to 7 days. If the dressing does not adhere to the skin or is loose, it may need to be changed sooner.

34. A, C, D, F

Techniques used to increase the intrathoracic pressure and prevent air embolism during IV set change include: placing the client in a flat or Trendelenburg position to ensure that the catheter exit site is at or below the level of the heart; asking the client to perform a Valsalva maneuver by holding his or her breath and bearing down; timing the IV set change to the expiratory cycle when the client is spontaneously breathing; and timing the IV set change to the inspiratory cycle when the client is receiving positive-pressure mechanical ventilation. Intravenous sets and connectors are not sterile except for where they connect together. The AP would not be asked to apply pressure at the insertion site during an IV set change.

35. C

For short peripheral catheters, usually 3 mL normal saline is adequate to flush the catheter. For all other catheters, 5 to 10 mL of preservative-free normal saline is needed. Flush catheters immediately after each use. A saline lock should be flushed at least once each shift. Research has shown that for SPCs, 3 mL of saline is just as effective at maintaining patency of the catheter without the risks associated with the use of heparin flushes.

36. B, C, E, F, G, H

All options are appropriate actions for removal of an SPC, except A and D. It is not necessary

to flush the catheter before removing it. The catheter should be slowly (not rapidly) withdrawn from the skin.

37. B

When the carotid artery is used for intra-arterial infusion, perform neurologic and cognitive assessments to determine adequate blood flow to the brain. When a femoral catheter is used, the client will have very limited movement so apply antiembolic stockings or other measures to prevent deep vein thrombosis.

38. B

Adult victims of trauma benefit from IO therapy because health care providers often cannot access these clients' vascular systems for traditional IV therapy.

39. A, B, D, E

Options A, B, D, and E are appropriate for the nurse to teach a client about IO therapy. The most commonly used site is the proximal tibia (not the distal femur). The preferred access needles are 15- or 16-gauge needles specifically designed for IO therapy.

40. A, B, E, F

Options A, B, E, and F are correct statements about IP therapy. Microbial peritonitis and inflammation of the peritoneal membranes from the invasion of microorganisms is a complication of IP therapy, so it is essential to use aseptic technique (not clean) to decrease the risk of this occurrence. IP therapy is used for administration of chemotherapy agents into the peritoneal cavity and to treat intra-abdominal malignancies such as ovarian and GI tumors, not for diagnostic purposes.

41. A

Reducing the flow rate and treatment with antiemetic drugs can reduce symptoms of nausea and vomiting. Option B will evenly distribute the IP fluid but will not relieve nausea and vomiting. Option C ensures patency of the catheter but does not relieve nausea and vomiting. With option D, the nurse would notify the health care provider for something to relieve nausea and vomiting, but the abdominal x-ray would not do this.

42. C

When choosing the infusion site, consider the client's level of activity. The area under the clavicle or the abdomen prevents difficulty with ambulation. In general, extremities are avoided for hypodermoclysis because other sites provide larger surface areas for absorption and the client's use of upper extremities is not restricted.

43. A, C, D, E, F

Intrathecal infusion of chemotherapy is used for treating central nervous system (CNS) cancers and postoperative pain. It can also be used to manage chronic pain and treat spasticity of neurologic diseases such as cerebral palsy, multiple sclerosis, reflex sympathetic dystrophy, and traumatic brain injuries. It is not an appropriate therapy for the treatment of leukemia in adults.

44. C

The client may also exhibit neurologic and systemic signs of infection (e.g., meningitis) such as headache, stiff neck, or temperature higher than 101°F (38.3°C). Report any neurologic change to the primary health care provider immediately!

45. B

1000mL / 15 hr = 66.6 rounded up to 67 mL/hr

46. A

The priority concept for when a nurse is providing infusion therapy for any client is fluid and electrolyte balance. The interrelated concept for infusion therapy is tissue integrity.

16
CHAPTER

Concepts of Inflammation and Immunity

1. Which statement regarding a temporary reduction of a client's immunity response is true?
   A. The client's health is at risk for the duration of the reduction.
   B. The reduction has little, if any effect, on the client's overall health.
   C. The client's microbiome can take over this function for several weeks.
   D. The temporary reduction increases the likelihood for development of autoimmune disease.

2. Which cells, actions, or characteristics are components of nonspecific general immunity? **Select all that apply**.
   A. Antibody production
   B. Can be transferred from one person to another
   C. Inflammation
   D. Intact mucous membranes
   E. Macrophages
   F. Microbiome
   G. Neutrophils
   H. NK-cells
   I. Provides long-lasting immunity
   J. Self-tolerance

3. Which white blood cell types are involved in the development of antibody-mediated immunity? **Select all that apply**.
   A. Basophils
   B. B-lymphocytes
   C. Cytotoxic T-cells
   D. Helper T-cells
   E. Macrophages
   F. Natural killer cells
   G. Neutrophils

4. Which client conditions will the nurse recognize as factors that may reduce immune function? **Select all that apply**.
   A. A severely limited diet for several weeks to quickly lose weight
   B. Homelessness and use of large public shelters during cold weather
   C. Daily use of corticosteroids and an NSAID
   D. Family history of hypertension and high cholesterol
   E. Age over 80 years and living alone in own home
   F. Well-controlled type 2 diabetes mellitus

5. Which client situation indicates self-tolerance to the nurse?
   A. Chemotherapy eradicates the client's cancer cells.
   B. Antibiotic medication cures the client's urinary tract infection.
   C. Skin from the client's thigh is successfully grafted to a burn wound.
   D. Client receives an uneventful blood transfusion during surgery.

6. Which adaptations in care will the nurse anticipate as specifically appropriate for an 85-year-old client? **Select all that apply**.
   A. Carefully assessing all open skin areas daily
   B. Encouraging annual influenza immunization
   C. Administering IV antibiotics before a colonoscopy
   D. Using sterile technique during all invasive procedures
   E. Observing for diarrhea as a result of overgrowth of the microbiome
   F. Asking when the client last received a tetnus booster immunization

7. Which client health problems will the nurse identify as most commonly an infectious process along with inflammation rather than inflammation alone? **Select all that apply**.
   A. Cholecystitis
   B. Conjunctivitis
   C. Contact dermatitis
   D. Rheumatoid arthritis
   E. Streptococcal pneumonia
   F. Sciatica

8. Why does a white blood cell count with differential **not** provide information about macrophages?
   A. Macrophage is the less common name for an eosinophil.
   B. Macrophages mature in the tissues and circulate as monocytes.
   C. The normal blood level of macrophages is too low to be measured.
   D. These cells mature in the bone marrow and are released as monocytes.

9. Which responses does the nurse expect to see as a direct result of inflammation with a severely sprained knee in a client who has no other health problems?
   A. Edema at the site of injury
   B. Elevated monocyte count
   C. Increased risk for embolism formation
   D. Localized warmth and redness
   E. Pain
   F. Purulent drainage
   G. Reduced range of motion

10. Which specific action of phagocytosis occurs as a result of chemotaxins?
   A. Attraction
   B. Adherence
   C. Recognition
   D. Degradation

11. Which response does the nurse expect as a result in the client who has a chemically-induced scar occupying the entire upper right lung lobe?
   A. Trapping of antibody-mediated immunity in that area
   B. Increased resistance to lung infections
   C. Reduction of pulmonary gas exchange
   D. Initiation of tissue repair

12. Which increased health problem risks will the nurse expect as a result of a client's decreased cell-mediated immunity? **Select all that apply**.
   A. Autoimmune disorders
   B. Cancer development
   C. Allergic reactions
   D. Parasitic infestations
   E. Urinary tract infections
   F. Need for solid organ transplantation

13. Which family member would the nurse expect to be a perfect human leukocyte antigen (HLA) match with the client considering a kidney transplant?
   A. Sister who is 12 years older than the client
   B. Identical twin
   C. Stepmother
   D. Father

14. Which client does the nurse expect to be immunocompetent?
   A. 79-year-old who lives independently, exercises daily, and eats balanced meals
   B. 25-year-old who drinks alcohol daily and stays out late every night
   C. 50-year-old who has had type 1 diabetes for 35 years
   D. 45-year-old who runs 5 miles daily and eats a well-balanced diet

15. Which finding in a client's laboratory report of white blood cell count with differential indicates to the nurse that the client has a serious ongoing bacterial infection?
   A. Total white blood cell count is 9,000/mm^3 (9 x 10^9/L)
   B. Lymphocytes outnumber the basophils
   C. "Bands" are equal to the "segs"
   D. Monocyte count is 600/mm^3 (0.6 x 10^9/L)

16. Which information will the nurse include when teaching a client about the swelling and pain resulting from a severe ankle sprain?
    A. The amount of pain and swelling is directly related to the severity of the injury.
    B. If the client had received a vaccination, these symptoms could have been prevented.
    C. These symptoms indicate that inflammation is present and treatment for infection is advised.
    D. The symptoms indicate that long-term protection against inflammation is being developed so that the symptoms will be less severe with the next sprain injury.

17. Which client circumstance indicates to the nurse an increased risk for infection as a result of exposure to microorganisms?
    A. A sanitation worker who forgets to wear gloves when picking up a garbage can
    B. Confused older adult who stays 8 hours twice weekly at an adult day care facility
    C. Spouse who performs dressing changes on his or her partner's infected leg wound
    D. An animal care technician who gives vaccinations and draws blood from cats and dogs

18. Which are actions of leukocytes that provide protection against invading organisms? **Select all that apply**.
    A. Phagocytic destruction of foreign invaders and unhealthy or abnormal cells
    B. Lytic destruction of foreign invaders and unhealthy cells
    C. Stimulation of maturational pathway of stem cells
    D. Production of antibodies directed against invaders
    E. Production of cytokines that decrease specific leukocyte growth and activity
    F. Increased growth and differentiation of platelets

19. In which conditions is the inflammatory response present? **Select all that apply.**
    A. Allergic rhinitis
    B. Appendicitis
    C. Myocardial infarction
    D. Sprain injuries to joints
    E. Contact dermatitis
    F. Esophagitis

20. Which white blood cell types have the greatest role in phagocytosis?
    A. Neutrophils and eosinophils
    B. Macrophages and neutrophils
    C. Macrophages and eosinophils
    D. Eosinophils and basophils

21. Which assessment will the nurse perform **first** when a client's laboratory results indicate a left shift (bandemia)?
    A. Indications of bleeding, such as bruising and petechiae
    B. Indications of inflammation, such as swelling and discomfort
    C. Indications of infection, such as purulent sputum or foul-smelling urine
    D. Indications of anemia, such as pallor, slow capillary refill, and tachycardia

22. Which client laboratory response indicates to the nurse that erythropoietin therapy is successful?
    A. Increased platelets
    B. Increased lymphocytes
    C. Increased red blood cells
    D. Increased white blood cells

23. What is the nurse's **best** response to a client undergoing cancer chemotherapy who asks why the absolute neutrophil count (ANC) is so important?
    A. A higher count indicates you have more resistance to infection."
    B. A higher count indicates the chemotherapy is eradicating the cancer."
    C. A higher count indicates you may be allergic to the chemotherapy drugs"
    D. A higher count indicates you need to start taking antibiotics immediately."

24. Which clinical symptom(s) will the nurse expect to find in a client who is experiencing the release of histamine and kinins by basophils?
    A. Excessive bleeding
    B. Foul-smelling urine
    C. Swelling and edema
    D. Diarrhea and abdominal cramping

25. Which situation is an example of innate-native immunity?
    A. Nurse obtains hepatitis B series before starting a new job abroad.
    B. Client, bitten by wild rabid animal, receives four doses of rabies vaccine.
    C. New mother decides to breastfeed her infant for first several months.
    D. Nurse has intact healthy skin on hands and healthy mucous membranes.

26. What action will the nurse take to **prevent harm** for a client who has a negative tuberculosis (TB) skin test result even though he has been treated for tuberculosis in the distant past and now has a productive, bloody cough?
    A. Re-apply the skin test on the opposite arm.
    B. Assume the client has incorrect recall about previous TB.
    C. No particular additional actions are required beyond documenting the report.
    D. Initiate Airborne Precautions until definitive testing also indicates TB is not present.

27. Why are mast cells not listed in the differential of a white blood cell count?
    A. Mast cells are reported officially as basophils.
    B. These cells are not myeloid- or lymphoid-derived cells.
    C. Mast cells have no role in either inflammation or immunity.
    D. Immature monocytes circulate briefly and then move into tissues where they mature into mast cells.

28. Which outcome does the nurse expect for a client who experienced a myocardial infarction (MI) 6 months ago in which 25% of the left ventricle was damaged and replaced by scar tissue?
    A. The client will have permanently reduced left ventricular contraction function.
    B. The right side of the heart will adapt and the client will have no loss of cardiac function.
    C. After full healing, left ventricular function will return to the same level as before the MI.
    D. Over time, the scar tissue will gradually take on the activity of healthy myocardial tissue.

29. Which precaution is a **priority** for the nurse to teach a client to **prevent harm** after a splenectomy was performed?
    A. "Be sure to take antibiotics before you have any dental work because you have fewer white blood cells and a greater risk for infection."
    B. "Look for other indications of infection such as redness or foul-smelling drainage because you will not have a fever."
    C. "Be sure to get an influenza vaccination early every year because it will take longer for your body to make antibodies."
    D. "Have chest x-ray annually because you will no longer have an accurate response to a skin test for tuberculosis."

30. Which substances are or could be considered antigens in the body of client with a healthy immune system? **Select all that apply**.
    A. Pollen
    B. Blood transfusion
    C. Client's own Tregs
    D. Intravenous immunoglobulin
    E. Medications
    F. Tetanus toxoid vaccine

31. An immunosuppressed client who has many serious health problems has just been heavily exposed to hepatitis B. Which type of protection does the nurse explain the client will have after receiving an injection with serum that has a high concentration of antihepatitis antibodies?
    A. Naturally acquired active immunity
    B. Artificially acquired active immunity
    C. Naturally acquired passive immunity
    D. Artificially acquired passive immunity

32. What is the nurse's interpretation of a laboratory result that indicates a client has a high blood concentration of IgM directed against the herpes simplex virus?
    A. The client is in the midst of his or her first response to herpes simplex infection.
    B. The client is at risk for major hypersensitivity reactions to attenuated vaccines.
    C. The client is mounting an appropriate response to a recurrent exposure to the virus.
    D. The client is at increased risk for becoming ill from opportunistic infectious organisms.

33. Which cells interact in the presence of an antigen to start antibody production? **Select all that apply.**
    A. Platelets
    B. B-lymphocytes
    C. Macrophages
    D. Neutrophils
    E. T–helper cells
    F. Red blood cells

34. Which type of immunity is the only one that can be transferred from one person to another?
    A. Innate immunity
    B. Nonspecific immunity
    C. Cell-mediated immunity
    D. Antibody-mediated immunity

35. A client who developed hepatitis A 6 weeks after eating contaminated food asks why his wife, who ate the same food and was sick with hepatitis A 2 years ago, did not develop the infection this time. What is the nurse's **best** response?
    A. "Women are more likely to wash their hands after using the bathroom than are men."
    B. "It is likely you ate more of the contaminated food than your wife, so your exposure to the virus was greater."
    C. "The scar tissue from the last infection in your wife's intestinal tract makes her more resistant to heptitis."
    D. "Your wife's infection 2 years ago caused her to produce antibodies to this infectious virus, making her immune to it."

36. Which type of immunity will the nurse initiate by administering an influenza vaccination to a client?
    A. Natural active immunity
    B. Artificial active immunity
    C. Natural passive immunity
    D. Artificial passive immunity

37. What is the nurse's best response to a client who asks what type of health problems could be expected as a result of having a lower than normal number of regulatory T-cells?
    A. "You will need to receive booster vaccinations more often because your ability to make antibodies is reduced."
    B. "Try to avoid crowds and people who are ill because you are now more susceptible to bacterial and viral infections."
    C. "You will be more prone to allergic reactions when exposed to allergens or drugs."
    D. "Your risk for cancer development is increased."

38. The nurse expects that production of immune cells will be **most** jeopardized by which client condition or event?
    A. Thymus gland atrophy from the aging process
    B. Splenectomy removed because of trauma
    C. Liver failure secondary to alcohol abuse
    D. Bone marrow failure

Chapter 16 Answer Key

1.   A
     Any time a client's immunity response is reduced the client has an increased risk for infection. Allergic responses and autoimmune disorders are also reduced when immune responses are reduced or impair. Although the microbiome influences immunity, it cannot take over immune functions.

2.   C, D, E, F, G, J
     Neutrophils, macrophages, and the microbiome are all components of nonspecific immunity, as are intact mucous membranes. Cells involved in nonspecific immunity are able to recognize normal self cells (self-tolerance) to prevent attacking normal, healthy body cells. Inflammation is a nonspecific response rather than an adaptive response. General, nonspecific immunity does not provide long-lasting immune protection and is not responsible for antibody production (a B-cell function). General nonspecific immunity cannot be transferred from one person to another.

3.   B, D, E
     Basophils, cytotoxic T-cells, natural killer cells, and neutrophils have no role in antibody production, which is the basis of antibody-mediated immunity. Antibody production requires the interaction of macrophages, helper T-cells, and B-lymphocytes. The macrophages initially recognize and process the antigen. The helper/inducer T-cell presents to and assists the unsensitized B-lymphocyte to recognize the antigen as an invader. The B-lymphocyte then becomes sensitized to the antigen and begins producing antibodies against it.

4.   A, B, C, E, F
     Eating a limited diet rather than a balanced diet can reduce immunity by not including substances critical for immune cell function. Clients who are homeless and using public shelters have reduced immunity and greater exposures to pathogenic microorganisms in close quarters, as well as generally poor hygiene. Use of corticosteroids reduces all areas of immune function and NSAIDs reduce inflammation. Diabetes mellitus, regardless of type, always increases infection risk even

when well-controlled. General and specific immunity decreases with age. Hypertension and high cholesterol levels do not have a direct impact on immune function.

5.   C
     Self-tolerance is the ability of the immune system to recognize normal self cells and not mount tissue-damaging actions against them. If the client had received a skin graft from another person, the immune system would have caused rejection of the graft. Cancer cells, microorganisms, and blood cells from another person are not considered normal, healthy body cells that are tolerated by immune system cells.

6.   A, B, F
     Older clients have age-related reductions in immunity and inflammation and are more at risk for infection when exposed to any microorganism. The nurse encourages annual influenza immunization as well as obtaining "booster" immunizations to infectious disorders to which the client had been previously vaccinated (secondary antibody responses are slower and lower with aging). Open skin areas reduce the natural barrier and provide an entry for microorganisms. IV antibiotics as prophylaxis are not standard for clients of any age. Aging may change the microbiome but does not contribute to its overgrowth, In addition, a reduced microbiome (not an overgrowth) is more likely to result in diarrhea. Using sterile technique during all invasive procedures should be performed for all clients, not just older adults.

7.   B, E
     Streptococcal pneumonia is a bacterial infection. Both tonsilitis and conjunctivitis are commonly caused by bacterial and viral infections. Most types of cholecystitis do not have an infectious cause. Contact dermatitis is an irritant/allergic reaction, not an infection. Rheumatoid arthritis is an inflammatory autoimmune disorder, not an infection. Sciatica is an inflammatory response to irritation of the sciatic nerve from pressure or injury.

8. B
   The immature form of macrophages is released from the bone marrow as monocytes, which circulate briefly and move into various tissues. Once in the tissues, monocytes mature into macrophges, which do not circulate in the blood.

9. A, D, E, G
   The five cardinal symptoms of inflammation, including that caused by injury, are edema, redness, and warmth (from increased capillary leak); pain from bradykinin release from damaged tissues; and reduced function. The monocyte count does not increase. Purulent drainage only occurs as a result of infection. The inflammation does not directly increase the risk for embolism formation, although being sedentary while recovering from the injury does increase the risk for development of thrombosis in the veins below the injury.

10. A
    Attraction is the second step and brings the WBC into direct contact with the target (antigen, invader, or foreign protein). Damaged tissues secrete chemotaxins that act like chemical magnets drawing the neutrophils and macrophages to the site of invading organisms or proteins so that phagocytosis can occur.

11. C
    The replacement of normal lung alveolar tissue with scar tissue results in reduced lung function because the scar tissue does not behave like normal alveolar tissue and does not permit gas exchange. Antibody-mediated immunity cannot be "trapped." With scar tissue formation, the resistance to infection would either be unaffected or reduced, not increased. Microorganisms could still enter the area but reduced blood flow in scar tissue would reduce access of immune system cells and products to the area. Scarring is the result of some types of tissue repair; however, its formation does not cause tissue repair.

12. B, D
    Cell-mediated immunity responses are important in cancer prevention and reducing the risk for parasitic infestations. Loss of cell-mediated immune responses would only help reduce the risk for both autoimmune disorders or allergic reactions by reducing the body's ability to produce IgE. Protection against urinary tract infections is provided largely by innate or general immunity, not cell-mediated immunity. Cell-mediated immune responses are the ones that induce rejection of solid organ transplants. These responses have no role in causing organ damage leading to the need for solid organ transplants.

13. B
    An identical twin would have all HLAs identical to the client. A sister would be expected to share between less than 100% of the client's HLAs. A parent would only contribute 50% of his or her HLAs to the client, although he or she may share some of the same HLAs contributed by the other parent. A step-parent is unlikely to have more than 20% of the same HLAs as the client.

14. D
    All older adults have some immunity reduction as a result of normal aging. Although the 25-year-old should have a more intact immune system than the other clients, lifestyle choices of alcohol consumption and inadequate rest can reduce immune function. Long-standing diabetes and its management reduces immune function. Keeping physically active and maintaining good nutrition contribute to adequate immune function.

15. C
    The segmented neutrophils are normally the largest population of circulating leukocytes (55% to 70%) and provide immediate protection against infection. The percentage of circulating band neutrophils should be much lower (about 5%). The greatly increased band population with a decrease in the segmented neutrophil population indicates an ongoing infection in which bone marrow production of fully functional neutrophils is failing. This is known as a "left shift." Even though the total white blood cell count is within the normal range (making option A an incorrect response), the client is losing the infection battle and is a risk for sepsis. Option B is incorrect because the

normal lymphocyte count is greatly higher than the basophil count. Option D is incorrect because the monocyte count is within the normal range.

16. A

Inflammation is a nonspecific response to injury and the severity of symptoms is related to the extent of the injury. No vaccination or immunization prevents or reduces injury-related inflammation. Because the process is nonspecific, inflammation does not result in long-term protection. Unless infection is present, inflammation is not treated as an infectious event.

17. B.

The other adults can choose to wash their hands or take other precautions after exposure to microorganisms. The confused older adult in a day care setting shares toileting facilities, food utensils, as well as entertainment objects such as cards, puzzles, and games with other people who may have lost the ability to use proper infection control measures.

18. A, B, C, D

Leukocytes that can provide protection against invading organisms include neutrophils, macrophages, and lymphocytes. The neutrophils and macrophages are phagocytes. The lymphocyes can generate antibodies and cause lytic destruction of invading organisms and unhealthy cells. They also trigger cytokine production that increases maturation of stem cells and and contributes to *increased* growth and activity of other leukocytes. They do not increase platelet growth and differentiation.

19. A, B, C, D, E, F

Inflammation is nonspecific response to tissue injury, irritation, and invasion by organisms or allergens. All of the options have tissue injury, irritation, or invasion as the pathophysiologic mechanism causing the response.

20. B

Of the cells on this list, only neutrophils and macrophages are capable of phagocytosis. Eosinophils and basophils secrete inflammatory mediators that intensify or continue the inflammatory response.

21. C

A left shift occurs in response to the presence of a prolonged infection. It indicates the body is no longer able to respond to the continuing infection by stimulating the bone marrow to produce mature neutrophils capable of fighting off invading microorganisms. A left shift does not indicate an increased risk for bleeding, inflammation, or anemia.

22. C

Erythropoietin is a growth factor made by the kidneys that increases the rate of production for red blood cells (erythrocytes). Although other blood cell types may also increase somewhat, the main effect (and desired effect) is increasing the circulating red blood cell count.

23. A

The absolute neutrophil count includes the number of circulating mature neutrophils (segs) and the number of circulating slightly less mature neutrophils (bands) that will mature within a few hours. The ANC represents how well the client's nonspecific defenses can provide protection against infection. The higher the number, the greater the protection. The ANC does not indicate anything about allergies or whether the chemotherapy is effective.

24. C

Histamines and kinins cause capillary leak syndrome by increasing the size of the capillary pores, which causes fluid to leave the capillaries and collect in the interstitial space with edema and swelling.

25. D

Innate-native immunity is nonspecific and not acquired. Having intact skin and healthy mucous membranes is part of innate-native immunity. Obtaining any type of vaccination is artificial, not innate. Although the transference of antibodies from mother to infant by breastfeeding is natural, it provides acquired, not innate, immunity to the infant.

26. D

As immunity declines with age, clients who have had TB in the past or who have active disease now may have a false-negative response to a skin TB test, a condition termed *anergy*. Because TB is a contagious infectious disease, Airborne Precautions should be used with the client until more definitive testing indicates the client does not have active TB.

27. B

Although mast cells have major roles in the inflammatory responses, they are not true white blood cells derived from either the myeloid or lymphoid white blood cell lines. They do act in a similar manner to basophils but do not circulate in the blood. They are not mature monocytes.

28. A

Although damaged tissue can heal and often recover some function, myocardial tissue that is replaced by scar tissue does not recover the function of normal healthy cardiac muscle cells. It is a permanent change. The right and left sides of the heart have different functions and one cannot take over the function of the other (unlike the kidneys).

29. C

The spleen is an important site for B-lymphocyte storage and antibody production. Clients who have a splenectomy have a lower and slower response to vaccinations and require more time for development of antibody-mediated responses, which makes them at higher risk for viral infections. Cell-mediated immunity (tuberculosis skin test response) and general nonspecific immunity responses (indications of infection) are unimpaired. The microbiome is unimpaired.

30. A, B, D, E, F

All of the substances in this list, with the exception of the client's own Treg cells, are synthesized outside of the client's body and are considered non-self antigens. Any of them could potentially stimulate the client to produce antibodies against them.

31. D

The hepatitis B antibodies were not actively made by this client. He or she is receiving them passively. Because they were generated by another person(s), they will be viewed as "foreign" by the client's immune system and eliminated over time.

32. A

When naive B-cells become sensitized to a specific microorganism, they divide forming plasma cells and memory cells, both of which retain the antigen sensitization. The plasma cell immediately begins to secrete antibodies in the form of immunoglobulin M (IgM) against the microorganism. Upon later re-exposure to the same antigen, memory cells will secrete immunoglobulin G (IgG) against it. Therefore the presence of specific IgM in the blood indicates a normal immune response to an initial infection with a virus or other antigen. Option B is incorrect because IgM does not mediate hypersensitivity reactions. Option C is incorrect because a recurring exposure would be indicated by increased IgG levels against the microorganism, not IgM. Option D is incorrect because the presence of high levels of IgM does not indicate the client's immune status.

33. B, C, E

Antibody formation in response to the presence of an antigen requires the interaction of B-lymphocytes, macrophages, and T-helper cells, even though only B-lymphocytes produce antibodies. First the macrophage recognizes and binds the antigen, and then "present" the bound antigen to the helper T-cell. Then the helper T-cell and the macrophages together process the antigen to expose the antigen's recognition sites (universal product code), and then bring the antigen into contact with the B-cell so that the B-cell can recognize the antigen as non-self and begin to produce antibodies against it.

34. D

Innate immunity, nonspecific immunity, and cell-mediated immunity all require direct interaction with invaders or antigens. When cells are transferred from one person to another, they are reconized as non-self by the receiving person and destroyed too rapidly to provide immunity. Antibodies are produced by B-lymphocytes and secreted into the blood and other body fluids. This makes transferring antibodies to another person easier and they last long enough (usually several weeks) to provide the person with short-term immunity.

35. D

A previous illness with a viral-induced infectious disease causes the person to develop an anamnestic antibody response in which on re-exposure to the same organism, the person produces so many antibodies against the organism that it is cleared from the body before the person becomes ill again. Scar formtion in the GI tract is unrelated. Although handwashing is important, if the food itself is contaminated, hand-washing will not help prevent the infection of a food or water-borne disease. The degree of exposure can make a difference in development of an infectious disease, but the predeveloped immunity to the organism is much more likely to play a role in the wife's response to the exposure.

36. B

The client will be making his or her own antibodies to influenza, this immunity he or she develops will be active. Because the client is making the antibodies in response to an injection (vaccination) rather than in response to actually being sick with influenza, the immunity is artificial.

37. C

Regulatory T-cells have the opposite action of helper T-cells. For optimal CMI, then, a balance between helper T-cell activity and regulatory T-cell activity must be maintained. This balance occurs when the helper T-cells outnumber the regulatory T-cells by a ratio of 2:1. When this ratio increases, indicating that helper T-cells vastly outnumber the regulatory T-cells, in this case because of way too few regulatory T-cells, overreactions can occur. These include allergies to almost anything, including drugs. Some of these overreactions are tissue damaging and dangerous, as well as unpleasant.

38. D

All conditions or events listed can result in some degree of immunosuppression, actual production of white blood cells occurs in the bone marrow.

17
CHAPTER

Concepts of Care for Patients with HIV Disease

1. Which factors increase the efficiency of infection by the human immune deficiency virus (HIV)?
   A. Is activated by contact with antibodies
   B. Is activated by normal human enzymes
   C. Contains the enzyme reverse transcriptase
   D. Has DNA similar to human DNA as its genetic material

2. Which change in laboratory immune indicators does the nurse expect to find in a client whose HIV disease is at stage HIV-III (AIDS)?
   A. Leukocytosis
   B. Lymphocytopenia
   C. High plasma macrophage count
   D. Increased functional antibody production

3. When educating women clients about HIV prevention, which route does the nurse emphasize as the most common way women acquire the disease?
   A. Prenatal transmission during the birth process
   B. Sex with an infected female partner
   C. Sex with an infected male partner
   D. Injection drug use

4. What is the nurse's **best** response to a client considering pre-exposure prophylaxis who asks why HIV testing must be performed every 3 months while on this therapy?
   A. "If you should become HIV positive while taking this therapy, your disease may become drug resistant."
   B. "Continued monitoring of your HIV status allows us to calculate the lowest effective dose you need."
   C. "The protection prophylaxis provides is effective against HIV but not against other infections."
   D. "If you are not monogamous, you could transmit the disease to your other partners."

5. Which client conditions experienced over the past year indicates to the nurse that the client's HIV status may have progressed to HIV-III (AIDS)? **Select all that apply**.
   A. Had influenza 2 months ago
   B. Diagnosed with invasive cervical cancer
   C. Lost his long-term partner to heart disease 6 months ago
   D. Had two episodes of bacterial pneumonia in the past year
   E. Developed hepatitis A during a vacation to South America
   F. Had an abscessed tooth that required treatment by root canal

6. Which symptoms reported by a client who has HIV-III (AIDS) indicates to the nurse possible infection with *Pneumocystis jiroveci*?
   A. Chronic diarrhea and weight loss
   B. Severe headache and neck stiffness
   C. Persistent dry cough and breathlessness
   D. Pain behind the sternum and difficulty swallowing

7. Which noninfection-related health promotion behavior is a **priority** for the nurse to teach a client with HIV disease at stage II?
   A. Exercise regularly and maintain a healthy weight.
   B. Avoid salt substitutes and foods high in potassium.
   C. Do not travel to countries outside of North America.
   D. Avoid using acetaminophen and any type of NSAID.

8. Which assessment findings in a client who is HIV positive and has new-onset acute confusion will the nurse report immediately to the immunity health care provider? **Select all that apply**.
   A. Alopecia
   B. Substernal pain
   C. Unequal pupil size
   D. Reduced grip strength
   E. Numbness of the fingers and toes
   F. Dry mouth with sticky tongue coating

9. Which actions does the nurse recommend for a night shift co-worker, who just experienced a sharps injury from a known HIV-positive source client, to take immediately? **Select all that apply**.
   A. Go to the emergency department immediately for a tetanus booster vaccination.
   B. Immediately use an alcohol-based handrub on the injured area.
   C. Notify employee health tomorrow morning when it opens.
   D. Ask your sex partner to have HIV testing as soon as possible.
   E. Wash the injured area immediately for at least 1 minute with soap and water.
   F. Make an appointment with the nursing department and request a transfer to an area where direct physical contact with a client is not expected.

10. The client with HIV-III (AIDS) and pain is refusing to take the newly prescribed antidepressant amitriptyline, stating that depression is not a problem. What is the nurse's **best** response?
    A. "Depression is common in adults with AIDS and can make pain worse."
    B. "In addition to helping depression, this drug can reduce neuropathic pain."
    C. "Your primary health care provider knows all the latest drugs and would only have prescribed this one if it were needed."
    D. "I will notify your primary health care provider to check whether a drug with a similar sounding name is what should have been prescribed."

11. Which factors or problems in an HIV-positive client does the nurse know increases the risk for HIV transmission? **Select all that apply**.
    A. Diarrhea
    B. High viral load
    C. Chronic confusion
    D. HIV positive partner
    E. Pneumocystis pneumonia
    F. Nonadherence to the drug regimen

12. Which personal protective equipment does the nurse assemble for use when giving oral and parenteral drugs care to an HIV-positive client who has amoebic diarrhea? **Select all that apply**.
    A. Air-purifying respirator
    B. Eye goggles
    C. Gloves
    D. Gown
    E. Hair cover
    F. Surgical mask

13. A nurse who is HIV positive and is now a client on a surgical unit the day after abdominal surgery asks a nurse colleague to keep her HIV status from the rest of the nursing staff. What is the unit nurse's **best** response?
    A. "Of course, there is no need for anyone else here to know."
    B. "Unless you require a blood transfusion, this should not be a problem."
    C. "I will only inform the person who is assigned to change your dressing."
    D. "I cannot promise that because I have an ethical obligation to protect everyone who works here."

14. Which part of the HIV infection process is disrupted by the antiretroviral drug class of CCR5 antagonists?
    A. Activating the viral enzyme "integrase" within the infected host's cells
    B. Binding of the virus's gp120 protein to one of the CD4+ co-receptors
    C. Clipping the newly generated viral proteins into smaller functional pieces
    D. Fusing of the newly created viral particle with the infected cell's membrane

15. With which activities does the nurse teach assistive personnel (AP) caring for a client who is HIV positive to wear gloves to prevent disease transmission? **Select all that apply**.
    A. Applying lotion during a back rub
    B. Brushing the client's teeth
    C. Emptying a Foley catheter reservoir
    D. Feeding the client
    E. Filing the client's fingernails
    F. Providing perineal care

16. A client diagnosed with HIV-III (AIDS) who is receiving combination antiretroviral therapy (cART) now has a CD4+ T-cell count of 525 cells/mm³. How will the nurse interpret this result?
    A. The client can reduce the dosages of the prescribed drugs.
    B. The virus is resistant to the current combination of drugs.
    C. The client no longer has AIDS.
    D. The drug therapy is effective.

17. A young male client who has just been diagnosed as HIV positive suspects that he contracted the virus from a sex worker several weeks ago and is worried because he had sex with his girlfriend several days ago. What is the nurse's **best** response?
    A. "The virus needs time to replicate, so your girlfriend is not at risk unless you have symptoms."
    B. "Even in the early phase, it is possible to transmit the HIV virus and your girlfriend should be told and tested."
    C. "HIV always progresses to AIDS. You and your girlfriend need to start antiviral medication right away."
    D. "This is a reportable disease and you need to contact the health department so that both women can be informed."

18. The rate of new HIV infection in North America is highest among which groups people?
    A. White homosexual men and women
    B. Older non-monogamous heterosexual men and women
    C. Asian women who have sex with men
    D. Black and Hispanic men and women

19. Which findings would the nurse expect when assessing a client with HIV disease at HIV-I classification? **Select all that apply**.
    A. Multiple Kaposi's sarcoma lesions
    B. One or more opportunistic infections
    C. Emaciation from AIDS wasting syndrome
    D. No indications of an AIDS-defining illness
    E. HIV antibody negative and undetectable viral load
    F. CD4+ T-cell count of greater than 500 cells/mm³ (0.5 × 10⁹/L)

20. Which conditions, all present in a female client, alert the nurse to the possibility of HIV infection? **Select all that apply**.
    A. Chronic vaginal candidiasis
    B. Pelvic inflammatory disease
    C. Spontaneous abortion
    D. Chronic sinus infection
    E. Mononucleosis
    F. Genital herpes

21. Which HIV-positive client does the nurse expect will progress to HIV-III (AIDS) the most quickly?
    A. Adult female who has one-time sex with an HIV-positive partner
    B. Older male who has vaginal sex with an HIV-positive female
    C. Adult male who is transfused with HIV-contaminated blood
    D. Older nurse who is stuck with an HIV-contaminated needle at work

22. Which routes are the most common means of HIV transmission? **Select all that apply**.
    A. Airborne
    B. Enteral
    C. Oral
    D. Parenteral
    E. Perinatal
    F. Sexual

23. What is the most common route by which nurses and other health care workers or providers are exposed to the HIV virus when caring for HIV-positive clients?
    A. Getting blood on exposed skin of hands or arms
    B. Touching infected body fluids with bare hands
    C. Having urine splashed on mucous membranes
    D. Sharps injuries with contaminated needles

24. Which factor does the nurse consider most likely to be responsible for promoting infection development in an older adult client after an HIV exposure?
    A. Decline in the overall efficiency of the immune system
    B. Belief that HIV is not an issue for older people
    C. Reluctance to discuss sexual activity with a health care professional
    D. Mistaking signs/symptoms as normal part of aging

25. Based on the concept of "Treatment as Prevention," which outcome statement indicates to the nurse that the goal of combination antiretroviral therapy for an HIV-positive client is being met?
    A. Client states understanding of the prescribed medication regimen.
    B. Client's disease stage is classified as unknown.
    C. Opportunistic infections are not present.
    D. Viral load is at an undetectable level.

26. Which assessment is a **priority** for the nurse caring for a client with HIV-III (AIDS) who has an exacerbation of cryptosporidiosis?
    A. Assess breath sounds and respiratory status.
    B. Assess neurologic status and presence of headache.
    C. Assess for signs of dehydration and electrolyte imbalance.
    D. Assess for difficulty in swallowing and pain behind the sternum.

27. Which precautions (in addition to Standard Precautions) will the nurse initiate for the newly admitted client who has HIV-III and symptoms that include cough, dyspnea, chest pain, fever, chills, night sweats, weight loss, and anorexia?
    A. Airborne Precautions
    B. Enteric Precautions
    C. Contact Precautions
    D. Droplet Precautions

28. Which type of focused assessment is a priority for the nurse to perform for an HIV-positive client who has toxoplasmosis encephalitis? **Select all that apply**
    A. Performing a mental status examination
    B. Assessing heart rate and rhythm
    C. Asking about headache presence
    D. Palpating the abdomen for tenderness
    E. Listening for bowel sounds
    F. Assessing neck movement

29. What is the nurse's best response to an assistive personnel (AP) who is upset because "Some of the client's spit got on my arm when I was helping him with oral hygiene, and he is HIV positive?"
    A. "Don't worry about it. A little bit of saliva is no big deal."
    B. "Wash your arm; saliva is not infectious with HIV unless it is bloody."
    C. "Use alcohol-based handrub on your arm and go to employee health for HIV testing."
    D. "Next time, wear a gown and stand back during the swish and spit."

30. Which items will the nurse tell family members living with a client who is HIV positive to avoid sharing to prevent the spread of HIV? **Select all that apply**.
    A. Safety razor
    B. Dishes
    C. Towels
    D. Toilet
    E. Shoes
    F. Toothbrushes

Chapter 17 Answer Key

1. C
   HIV is a type of retrovirus, which is a family of viruses that use RNA as their genetic material instead of DNA and have three special enzymes to ensure infection. These viruses can insert their RNA into a human cell's DNA with the enzyme reverse transcriptase to exert control over the human cell's actions. Thus, the HIV retrovirus is very efficient at infecting host cells.

2. B
   At stage HIV-III, the immune system is profoundly suppressed with decreased numbers of all immune system cell types, especially lymphocytes. Leukocytosis is an increase in the total white blood cell count, not a decrease. Macrophages do not circulate in the blood. Although antibody production may be increased, the antibodies produced are incomplete and nonfunctional.

3. C
   In North America and worldwide, the most common route of HIV transmission to women is by having sex with an infected male partner.

4. A
   If pre-exposure prophylaxis is used in clients who become infected with HIV-1, the risk for developing drug resistance greatly increases. Thus, clients on this therapy must adhere to an every-3-month HIV testing schedule. The best dose for this therapy is generally established and is not modified individually. It is true that the therapy does not protect against other sexually transmitted infections, but that is not the reason HIV status must be monitored, nor is the fact that if the client becomes HIV positive, he or she could transmit the disease to another person.

5. B, D
   Invasive cervical cancer and two or more episodes of bacterial pneumonia within a 12-month period are AIDS-defining illnesses. Anyone, even a person with a healthy immune system can get influenza, an abscessed tooth, or hepatitis A (when exposed to the virus). Having a partner who died from heart disease is not in itself an indicator that the partner had late-stage HIV disease.

6. C
   Infection with *Pneumocystis jiroveci* causes a form of pneumonia resulting in persistent dry cough and breathlessness. Infection with *Candida albicans* causes pain behind the sternum and difficulty swallowing. Severe headache and neck stiffness is associated with *Toxoplasma gondii* infection. Chronic diarrhea and weight loss have many causes, some of which are infectious; however, *Pneumocystis jiroveci* does not cause these symptoms.

7. A
   With appropriate antiviral therapy, HIV stage II can last decades. However, the disease itself and many of the drugs used for its management increase the risk for diabetes and coronary artery disease, which are common causes of death for an HIV-positive client. A healthy weight

and regular exercise help reduce the risks for these problems. Unless kidney impairment is present, potassium is not restricted. Infection risk is not great at this stage and there are no specific travel restrictions related to the client's health. There is no specific recommendation to avoid acetaminophen or NSAIDs during this stage of HIV disease.

8. C, D
    New-onset acute confusion is associated with several serious central nervous system problems that can increase intracranial pressure (ICP). Increased ICP requires immediate intervention to prevent brain impairment. Indicators include unequal pupil size or reactivity and reduced grip strength. Numbness of the fingers and toes is a peripheral nerve problem, not a CNS problem and is not associated with increased ICP. Alopecia, substernal pain, and dry mouth are not CNS problems indicating possible increased ICP.

9. E
    The first step with a sharps injury from a known HIV-positive source is to wash the hands thoroughly with soap and water for at least 1 minute. Using an alcohol-based handrub is not sufficient for this purpose. Although the co-worker should go immediately to the emergency department, the purpose is to initiate postexposure prophylaxis and begin documentation, not to get a tetanus booster (irrelevant to this situation). Notifying employee health to continue documentation and prophylaxis is important but cannot be done immediately. The co-worker's sex partner should have HIV testing relatively soon, but not immediately, to determine his or her current status. There is no legal, ethical, or medical reason for the co-worker to avoid direct physical contact with clients.

10. B
    The client has the right to refuse any drug but should only do so when adequately informed about the reason the therapy was prescribed and all of its side effects. Although amitriptyline is an antidepressant, it is effective in reducing neuropathic pain for many clients.

11. B, C, F
    The higher the viral load, the greater the risk for transmission. Chronic confusion often reduces the client's adherence to drug therapy, which may cause inadequate suppression of viral replication and a higher viral load. Also, a confused client may not use other transmission prevention techniques. Diarrhea does not increase the transmission of HIV. Pneumocystis pneumonia is an opportunistic infection and does not increase HIV transmission risk. Having an HIV-positive partner does not increase the client's risk for transmitting the disease to anyone else.

12. C, D
    When performing the action of giving either oral or parenteral drugs to any client with diarrhea, including those who are HIV positive, only Contact Precautions are needed.

13. A
    The consistent use of Standard Precautions is sufficient to prevent HIV transmission from an infected client to a health care worker. Standard Precautions are universally applied and, thus, the client's HIV status does not need to be disclosed regardless of whether a blood transfusion is needed or dressing changes are needed. Although the nurse does have an obligation to ensure safety for all personnel, there is no ethical, legal, or other reason to not comply with the client's wishes.

14. B
    CCR5 antagonists work by binding to and blocking the CCR5 receptors on CD4+ T-cells, the main target of HIV. In order to successfully enter and infect a host cell, the virus must have its gp120 protein attach to the CD4 receptor and have its gp41 bind to the CD4+ T-cell's CCR5 receptor. Viral binding to both receptors is required for infection. By blocking the HIV's attachment to the CCR5 receptor, infection is inhibited.

15. B, C, F
    Standard Precautions for preventing the spread of any type of infection including HIV requires wearing gloves when coming into contact with

mucous membranes, including oral and peri-neal membranes, as well as secretions and excretions. Although saliva has a low concentration of HIV unless frank blood is present, gloves are used for this task because of potential contact with the moist mucous membranes of the mouth.

Standard Precautions require that gloves be worn when contact with urine is possible, including during such tasks as emptying a Foley catheter reservoir.

Perspiration is not considered a body fluid with risk for transmission and neither is contact with the client's intact skin.

Feeding the client should not result in direct contact with transmissible fluids, nor should clipping finger nails.

16. D

When a client diagnosed with HIV-III (AIDS) has a CD4+ T-cell count increase as a result of therapy, the diagnosis of AIDS remains. The fact that the T-cell count has risen indicates the combination of drugs used for therapy are effective; however, the dosages are not decreased.

17. B

It is possible to transmit the disease even in the early stages of the disorder. Also, the client does not know for sure when he acquired the disorder. His girlfriend is at risk and should be told so that she has options for testing. HIV disease does not always progress to AIDS and only those who are found to be HIV positive should be taking life-long therapy. Although all states require that new cases of HIV-III (AIDS) be reported, not all states require reporting of HIV-positive status.

18. D

Although the prevalence of HIV infection in North America is highest among men who have sex with men, the incidence of new cases is highest among Black and Hispanic men and women. Another emerging population of HIV-positive individuals is transgender females.

19. D, F

HIV-I classification is applied to clients who are HIV antibody positive, have no AIDS-defining illnesses, and have an immune profile in which the CD4+ T-cell count is greater than 500 cells/mm^3 (0.5 × 10^9/L). Their viral load may be undetectable but their antibody test is positive. The immune function is sufficient to prevent any opportunistic infection or AIDS-defining illness.

20. A, B, F

Although any one of these conditions may occur in any client, when chronic vaginal candidiasis occurs in a woman who has genital herpes and a history of pelvic inflammatory disease (most often caused by a sexually transmitted infection), the client may have HIV disease. Spontaneous abortion, sinus infection, and mononucleosis are not associated with HIV disease either as a cluster of problems or as an individual problem.

21. C

The development of HIV disease and its course of progression depends on transmission route and degree of viremia. A client who receives HIV-contaminated blood has a much higher risk for development of HIV disease and more rapid progression to HIV-III than the other listed exposures. Even having sex once with an HIV-positive partner has only a 10% to 20% risk to result in infection. An uninfected male having sex with an infected female has a lower risk for successful infection. Even being stuck with an HIV-contaminated needle once is less likely to result in HIV disease than is receiving a blood transfusion with HIV-contaminated blood.

22. D, E, F

Infected body fluids with highest HIV concentrations are semen, blood, breast milk, and vaginal secretions. HIV is transmitted most often by these routes: 1) sexual (genital, anal, or oral sexual contact with exposure of mucous membranes to infected semen or vaginal secretions), 2) parenteral (sharing of needles or equipment contaminated with infected blood or receiving contaminated blood products), and 3) perinatal (across the placenta, from contact with maternal blood and body fluids during birth, or through breast milk from an infected mother to child).

23. D

Needlestick sharps injuries remain common in health care settings even though new equipment and action rules (i.e., do not recap needles) have reduced their incidence.

24. A

A major part of susceptibility for developing HIV infection after an exposure is the efficiency of the client's immunity. All immunity decreases with age, placing the older adult client more at risk for infection after any type of infectious exposure, including HIV.

25. D

Understanding the medication regimen is not sufficient. When it is followed and the client's viral load is undetectable, the goal of treatment as prevention has been met. An unknown disease stage is dangerous and does not help in prevention. Absence of opportunistic infection is a positive sign and may indicate the disease has not progressed, but does not indicate the goal of prevention has been met.

26. C

Cryptosporidiosis is an intestinal infection caused by *Cryptosporidium* organisms with problems ranging from a mild diarrhea to a severe wasting with electrolyte imbalance and dehydration. Oral and esophageal candidiasis causes difficulty swallowing and pain behind the sternum. Severe headache and neurologic changes are associated with *Toxoplasma gondii* infection. Respiratory problems are associated with *Pneumocystis jiroveci* infection.

27. A

The client's symptoms are consistent with tuberculosis (TB), which is common in HIV-III and can be difficult to diagnose because standard TB skin testing may not be accurate and also takes 48 to 72 hours, during which time the client is contagious. Airborne precautions are most appropriate for TB because the organism is suspended in the air for long periods of time and does not form heavy droplets.

28. A, C,

Infection with *Toxoplasma gondii* causes encephalitis with symptoms of headache and acute confusion. Neck stiffness is associated with meningitis, not encephalitis. Heart rhythm changes and GI disturbances are not part of the toxoplasmosis encephalitis.

29. B

Intact skin is not a portal of entry for HIV even if contaminated blood is in contact with it. The correct procedure is just to wash the area with soap and water. HIV testing is not necessary. Helping the AP to calm down is a nursing responsibility and the nurse does not just dismiss the AP's concern. A gown would not be needed according to the information provided in this question.

30. A, F

Anyone living with a client who is HIV positive is taught to avoid sharing items that might have the client's blood on them, which include safety razors and toothbrushes. Dishes and eating utensils do not pose an HIV transmission risk to the family (although family infections could be transmitted to the client). Sharing of towels, toilets, and shoes pose no HIV transmission risk to anyone living with an HIV-positive client.

18
CHAPTER

Concepts of Care for Patients with Hypersensitivity (Allergy) and Autoimmunity

1. Which statement best describes allergy or hypersensitivity?
   A. Excessive response to the presence of an antigen
   B. Excessive response against self cells and their products
   C. Failure of the immune system to recognize self cells as normal
   D. Failure of the immune system to recognize pathogenic organisms as non-self

2. Which statement(s) regarding hypersensitivity reactions is/are accurate? **Select all that apply**.
   A. The predisposition to develop hypersensitivity is genetic.
   B. Allergies to specific antigens (allergens) are directly inherited.
   C. Hypersensitivity symptoms are triggered by excessive inflammation.
   D. Avoidance of an antigen (allergen) reduces an adult's existing sensitivity to it.
   E. A client may have more than one type of hypersensitivity reaction at the same time.
   F. A person can develop hypersensitivity to almost any substance at any time during the lifespan.

3. Which assessment findings does the nurse expect in a client who is having a localized reaction to an environmental allergen?
   A. Hypotension
   B. Blood clotting
   C. Persistent constipation
   D. Redness and swelling in contact areas

4. Which immunoglobulin elevation does the nurse expect to see in the laboratory report of a client who is having a type I hypersensitivity response?
   A. Immunoglobulin A (IgA)
   B. Immunoglobulin E (IgE)
   C. Immunoglobulin G (IgG)
   D. Immunoglobulin M (IgM)

5. Which vasoactive amine is **most** responsible for the initial symptoms of inflammation during an allergic response?
   A. Leukotriene
   B. Bradykinin
   C. Histamine
   D. Prostaglandins

6. Which statement made by a client who is scheduled to undergo diagnostic testing with use of contrast dye requires the nurse to take action to **prevent harm**?
   A. "Both diabetes and high blood pressure run in my family."
   B. "My sister is allergic to the dye that they use for x-ray procedures."
   C. "I have a lot of seasonal allergies, and they make me pretty miserable."
   D. "Last year I had a test with dye and my face got so swollen I could not see."

7. Which statement(s) regarding type II hypersensitivity (cytotoxic) reactions is/are true? **Select all that apply.**
   A. Responses always occur within minutes of exposure to the allergen.
   B. Hemolytic transfusion problems are an example of type II hypersensitivity.
   C. Type II responses are usually directed against self cells attached to non-self cells and the response destroys the self cells.
   D. Susceptibility for developing a type II hypersensitivity response follows an autosomal dominant pattern of inheritance.
   E. Rashes and blister formation from poison ivy exposure are a typical response for this type of hypersensitivity reaction.
   F. The major mechanism of the reaction is the release of mediators from sensitized T-cells that trigger antigen destruction by macrophages.
   G. An effective management strategy may include plasma filtration to remove specific substances.

8. When taking the history of a client being treated for angioedema, which information does the nurse consider **most relevant** to the situation? **Select all that apply.**
   A. Has long time known allergy to penicillin
   B. African American
   C. Has severe hypertension
   D. Is 52 years old
   E. Has well-controlled type 2 diabetes mellitus
   F. Has taken an angiotensin-converting enzyme inhibitor for 8 months
   G. Takes a beta blocker daily
   H. Eats a vegan diet

9. Which questions are **most important** for the nurse to ask **first** to **prevent harm** for a client who comes to the emergency department with signs of severe angioedema? **Select all that apply.**
   A. "Are you able to swallow?"
   B. "When did you last eat or drink?"
   C. "Do you have an allergy to cortisone?"
   D. "What drugs do you take on a daily basis"?
   E. "Is there any possibility that you may be pregnant?"
   F. "Do any members of your family also have allergies?"

10. Which change in a client with angioedema indicates to the nurse that immediate action is needed to **prevent harm**?
    A. Systolic blood pressure decrease from 136 mm Hg to 120 mm Hg
    B. Presence of stridor on inhalation and exhalation
    C. Mouth breathing because of nasal swelling
    D. Inability to sip liquids through a straw

11. Which precaution has the highest **priority** for the nurse to teach a client taking an angiotensin-converting enzyme inhibitor (ACEI) to **prevent harm**?
    A. Go to the emergency department or call 911 if you develop tongue and lip swelling or have difficulty breathing.
    B. Avoid touching this drug with your bare hands to prevent absorbing it through direct skin contact.
    C. Stop taking the drug immediately if you develop a runny nose, itchy eyes, or a persistent cough.
    D. Take this drug with food or milk at the same time every day.

12. What is the nurse's **best** response when client recovering from drug-induced angioedema caused by an ACEI asks why it took 6 months before a reaction occurred?
    A. "As your blood pressure was reduced, less drug was needed and the excess triggered an allergic response."
    B. "Possibly when you took your most recent dose you held it in your mouth too long instead of swallowing it, causing a local response."
    C. "It takes time for the main body chemical causing the reaction to build-up enough to cause symptoms."
    D. "If you took this drug with grapefruit juice, the two substances together are much more likely to result in an allergic reaction."

13. Which action does the nurse perform **first** to **prevent harm** when a client receiving IV penicillin reports difficulty breathing and feeling dizzy about 15 minutes after the infusion is started?
    A. Stop the infusion.
    B. Initiate the Rapid Response Team.
    C. Assess the client's blood pressure.
    D. Ask whether the client is allergic to penicillin.

14. Which client symptoms that started after IV administration of a newly prescribed drug prompts the nurse to initiate the Rapid Response Team for possible anaphylaxis? **Select all that apply**.
    A. Facial flushing
    B. Bradycardia
    C. Oxygen saturation of 88%
    D. Wheezing on exhalation
    E. Increased deep tendon reflexes
    F. Hives at the IV site spreading upward

15. Which drug does the nurse expect to administer **first** to a client with anaphylaxis?
    A. Oral diphenhydramine
    B. Parenteral epinephrine
    C. Albuterol via high-flow nebulizer
    D. Intravenous corticosteroids

16. Which action is a **priority** for the nurse to perform before giving the first dose of any drug or therapeutic agent to a client?
    A. Ask the patient about allergies to drugs or other substances.
    B. Be aware of types of drugs that are likely to cause allergic reactions.
    C. Check the medication administration record for allergic response to drugs.
    D. Make sure that emergency medications are readily available.

17. Which nursing response is most likely to **cause harm** to a client who has anaphylaxis?
    A. Failing to inform the family about a change in the client's condition
    B. Using a nonrebreather mask to administer oxygen
    C. Delaying the administration of epinephrine
    D. Increasing the IV saline flow rate

18. While waiting for the Rapid Response Team to arrive and assist a client with anaphylaxis, which nursing actions will the nurse take to help manage the situation? **Select all that apply**.
    A. Obtain IV access.
    B. Apply oxygen.
    C. Place the client in Trendelenburg position.
    D. Stay with the client.
    E. Ask the client whether he or she has a specific drug allergy.
    F. Ask the client whether other family members have ever had an allergic reaction.
    G. Arrange for arterial blood to be drawn for blood gas evaluation.
    H. Elevate the head of the bed.

19. Which prescription will the nurse question for a client who has an allergy to penicillin?
    A. Acetaminophen 650 mg every 4 hours for pain
    B. Angiotensin-converting enzyme inhibitor (ACEI) daily for hypertension
    C. Cephalosporin to treat a chronic sinus infection
    D. Decongestant as needed for rhinorrhea

20. Which statement(s) about autoimmunity is/are accurate? **Select all that apply**.
    A. The basic pathophysiologic changes result in immunosuppression.
    B. Autoimmune disorders are most common among men over 60 years of age.
    C. With early and appropriate management, autoimmune disorders are highly curable.
    D. Clients who have allergies as children usually develop autoimmune disorders as adults.
    E. Autoimmune disorders are caused by excessive or overactive immune and inflammatory responses.
    F. Clients who are most susceptible to developing autoimmune disorders are those who have human leukocyte antigen types DR2, DR3, DRB, DQA, DQB, and Cw6.

21. Which adult-onset disorders have an autoimmune component? **Select all that apply**.
    A. Asthma
    B. Cardiovascular disease
    C. Colorectal cancer
    D. Diabetes mellitus type 2
    E. Pernicious anemia
    F. Psoriasis
    G. Rheumatoid arthritis
    H. Systemic lupus erythematosus

22. What role do T-regulatory lymphocytes (Tregs) have in the development of autoimmune disease?
    A. Reduced numbers of Tregs lead to loss of self-tolerance.
    B. The presence of Tregs inhibit secretion of tumor necrosis factor (TNF).
    C. Tregs secrete autoantibodies directed against one or more types of normal self cells.
    D. Increased numbers of Tregs stimulate excessive amounts of cytokines that damage normal healthy tissues.

23. Which factor for a client who has type 1 diabetes mellitus indicates to the nurse that the disorder most likely has an autoimmune origin rather than a lifestyle basis?
    A. Is a vegetarian whose diet is high in soy-based proteins
    B. Works in a large chemical manufacturing plant
    C. Has an identical twin with Graves disease
    D. Has a parent with a severe peanut allergy

24. Which client assessment finding indicates to the nurse the possibility of systemic lupus erythematosus (SLE)?
    A. Use of penicillin prophylactically before dental examinations and procedures
    B. Intermittent fever and fatigue with no other symptom of infection
    C. Joint and muscle pain without swelling after exercise
    D. Oily skin and increased facial acne

25. Which client statement indicates to the nurse that more teaching about systemic lupus erythematosus is needed?
    A. "During flares, I may need higher doses of my corticosteroid."
    B. "I will take walks and stretch my muscles daily even when my joints hurt."
    C. "If I do not have a flare in over a year, I can stop taking my anti-inflammatory drugs."
    D. "If my urine becomes bloody or foamy, I will call my rheumatology health care provider immediately."

26. What precaution is **most important** for the nurse to teach the client with systemic lupus erythematosus (SLE) prescribed to take 40 mg of a corticosteroid daily for 2 weeks to manage an SLE flare?
    A. "Take this drug at bedtime to avoid nausea and vomiting."
    B. "Avoid crowds and anyone who is ill because this drug reduces your immunity."
    C. "Drink at least 3 liters of fluid per day because this drug can cause kidney damage."
    D. "If you are vomiting and cannot take the oral drug, contact your health care provider immediately."

27. Which actions will the nurse recommend to the client who has systemic lupus erythematosus (SLE) for relief of general joint and muscle pain?
    A. Warm, moist heat
    B. Medical marijuana
    C. Avoidance of all exercise
    D. Application of ice packs

28. Which precautions are **most important** for the nurse to teach a client newly diagnosed with systemic lupus erythematosus (SLE) to **prevent harm**? **Select all that apply**.
    A. Avoiding direct sunlight
    B. Monitoring urine output
    C. Keeping open lesions clean and covered
    D. Avoiding the use of make-up
    E. Wearing a medical alert bracelet
    F. Avoiding any form of aerobic exercise
    G. Being immunized yearly against influenza
    H. Avoiding the use of hair dyes and having permanents

29. Which client laboratory test results will the nurse identify as supporting a diagnosis of systemic lupus erythematosus (SLE)? **Select all that apply**.
    A. Increased erythrocyte sedimentation rate (ESR)
    B. Decrease erythrocyte sedimentation rate (ESR)
    C. Increased complement C3 protein levels
    D. Increased basophils
    E. Decreased eosinophils
    F. Increased extractable nuclear protein antibodies

30. Which client symptom appearing 2 weeks after an extended camping trip does the nurse associate with the possibility of Lyme disease?
    A. Acute confusion
    B. Sudden onset of difficulty swallowing
    C. Sudden onset of painful, swollen joints
    D. Persistent watery diarrhea and weight loss

Chapter 18 Answer Key

1. A
   A hypersensitivity or allergy is an overactive immunity with excessive inflammation occurring in response to the presence of an antigen to which the patient usually has been previously exposed. Although inflammation and immunity are generally protective, they can cause uncomfortable and serious responses when excessive. With hypersensitivity reactions, the immune system very much recognizes self cells as normal. The responses are directed against nonself but are excessive.

2. A, C, E, F
   The predisposition to develop hypersensitivity is inherited as a polygenic trait although hypersensitivities to specific substances is not inherited, making option B incorrect.
   The symptoms associated with hypersensitivity are caused by excessive inflammation in response to degranulation of basophils, eosinophils, and mast cells with release of a variety of vasoactive amines.
   Once a hypersensitivity to a specific substance develops, avoiding that allergen can prevent an episode of responses but does not reduce the adult's sensitivity to the allergen.
   Allergies can develop to almost any substance across the lifespan and can trigger more than one type of hypersensitivity response at the same time.

3. D
   Local reactions to an allergen involve only the tissues in direct contact with the specific allergen,
   such as redness and swelling in contacted areas. Hypotension blood clotting are systemic symptoms or manifestations. Allergic responses with inflammation in the GI tract to a swallowed allergen result in diarrhea, not constipation.

4. B
   The immunoglobulin type associated with hypersensitivity reactions is excessive production of IgE. Acute inflammation occurs when IgE responds to an antigen, such as pollen, by binding to the membranes of basophils, eosinophils, and mast cells, causing the release of many pro-inflammatory vasoactive amines.

5. C
   The initial inflammatory response is triggered by histamine, often within 10 minutes of exposure to an allergen. It is also a very prevalent vasoactive amine. The other amines are secreted later, causing the secondary phase and prolonging the allergic reaction.

6. D
   The most important concern to prevent immediate harm is the potential hypersensitivity to contrast medium. The client has clearly had some type of adverse reaction during a test using "dye" previously and may be at great risk for a severe reaction to the contrast medium for the scheduled procedure. The nurse must notify the radiologist and primary health care provider to explore this potential risk immediately. Although the client also has seasonal allergies, these are not associated with hypersensitivity to contrast

medium. The sister's allergies are not relevant to the client's condition, and education for lifestyle changes to reduce the risk for diabetes and high blood pressure, although important, should not be the immediate focus.

7. B, C, G

    Type II cytotoxic reactions occur when the body makes autoantibodies directed against self cells that have some form of foreign protein attached to them. The autoantibody binds to the self cell and forms an immune complex and destroys the self cell along with the attached protein.

    Examples of this type of hypersensitivity reaction include hemolytic transfusion reactions, hemolytic anemias, immune thrombocytopenic purpura, and drug-induced hemolytic anemia.

    Poison ivy and T-cell-mediated responses are associated only with type IV hypersensitivities.

    No hypersensitivities follow an autosomal dominant pattern of inheritance because they are not inherited as single gene traits.

    Although hemolytic transfusions often occur within 15 minutes of exposure, most type II cytotoxic reactions occur many hours after exposure.

    An effective management strategy may include plasma filtration to remove specific substances, especially when the problem is identified early.

8. B, F

    Although, in theory, any drug can cause angioedema, the main risk factor for drug-induced angioedema is taking an angiotensin-converting enzyme inhibitor (ACEI). This response to ACEIs is more common among African Americans. Therefore, these two factors are **most relevant** to the situation.

    Age is not an issue nor is having type 2 diabetes mellitus.

    The fact that the client is hypertensive, although an indication for the drug, does not itself increase the risk for this reaction.

    Neither beta blockers nor penicillin are likely to cause this reaction.

    A vegan diet is also an unlikely cause of the reaction.

9. A, D

    The client has severe angioedema that can progress rapidly to laryngeal edema and loss of the airway. The very first question should be to assess symptom severity. Asking whether the client can swallow provides an indication of severity. If the client can still swallow, an immediate intubation or tracheotomy is not needed. Asking what drugs he or she takes can help establish the diagnosis and the cause. It is not necessary to know when the last food or drink were taken. Also, regardless of whether the client is pregnant, interventions for angioedema must be started. It is not helpful during this emergency to know whether other family members also have allergies. This information can be obtained at a later time or from family members. Cortisone is used to treat allergies and does not cause them.

10. B

    Stridor on inhalation and exhalation indicates a severe partial obstruction of the airway from edema. Steps must be taken to maintain the airway with either immediate endotracheal tube placement or performance of an emergency tracheostomy to prevent death. The systolic blood pressure decrease is not associated with worsening of the angioedema. Facial and nasal swelling are expected and may be severe but, unless the airway is compromised, do not require additional immediate action.

11. A

    ACEIs are the most common cause of drug-induced angioedema, which can be life-threatening. Indications for emergency care include lip and tongue swelling and difficulty breathing. Other indicators are the sensation of a "lump in the throat" and itching of the oral mucous membranes.

    It does not matter if the client absorbs this drug through his or her skin, he or she is taking it. A persistent cough may occur as a side effect of any ACEI but is not an indicator of need for emergency care. Taking the drug with food is important as is taking it at the same time every day but does not have the highest priority to prevent harm.

12. C

    Bradykinin is the inflammatory mediator most responsible for ACEI-induced angioedema. This mediator is a strong vasodilator and promoter of deep-tissue inflammation. It is rapidly deactivated by angiotensin-converting enzyme (ACE). Drugs that inhibit ACE lead to increasing tissue accumulation of bradykinin over time, which is responsible for the delayed onset of ACEI-induced angioedema even though it is a type I hypersensitivity reaction. Angioedema is a systemic response, not a local one. Holding it in the mouth a little longer does not make angioedema occur. The drug does not become more likely to cause an allergic reaction if taken with grapefruit juice and the response does not appear to be dose-related.

13. A
The client is exhibiting more than one indication of anaphylaxis and time is critical. Stop the infusion of the likely offending substance to limit the amount of allergen entering the client and maintain the IV access. Then initiate the Rapid Response Team. The client may not know the names of the drugs he or she is allergic to or may not have had a severe enough response to an earlier exposure to understand that an allergy exists. Blood pressure assessment would provide additional substantiation of the problem but does nothing to help prevent harm.

14. C, D, F
Wheezing on exhalation is an indication of bronchoconstriction, which occurs during anaphylaxis. The bronchoconstriction is severe enough to result in some degree of hypoxia. Hives are an indicator of an allergic reaction, especially if they are spreading. Bradycardia does not occur with anaphylaxis; clients become tachycardic with a weak and thready pulse as a result of sympathetic nervous system compensation for shock. Skin becomes cyanotic, not flushed. Increased deep tendon reflexes are not associated with anaphylaxis.

15. B
Although all drugs listed have some utility in managing anaphylaxis, only parenteral epinephrine is an effective first-line therapy that can save the client's life. Although diphenhydramine is a second-line drug, it also would be administered parenterally to be most effective.

16. A
Although some drugs are more commonly associated with an allergic reaction, the response can occur to any drug. Therefore, always ask clients about *any* allergy or other problem they have ever had with *any* drug before giving the first dose of a newly prescribed drug. It is better to rely on the client's report of a drug allergy or adverse reaction than to depend on the client's chart or record. All nursing units where drugs are administered should have an emergency cart with appropriate drugs to manage an allergic or other adverse reaction.

17. C
According to the Centers for Disease Control and Prevention, the single most harmful action during anaphylaxis is delaying the administration of epinephrine. It is safer to give the drug when it is not needed than it is to not give it when it is needed. When oxygen is applied, the recommendation is to use a nonrebreather mask to increase oxygen delivery. Increasing the IV flow rate (when the IV is not the source of anaphylaxis) can help support circulation and blood pressure. Informing the family, although a good action, is not the priority action during management of anaphylaxis.

18. A, B, D, H
Actions that would be immediately helpful to promote perfusion and gas exchange are to apply oxygen, obtain IV access, and elevate the head of the bed. It is also important to stay with the client. Trendelenburg position is NOT recommended and could impinge on ventilation. Asking the client questions at this time is not helpful. Arterial blood gas values are not needed to identify and manage anaphylaxis.

19. C
Cephalosporins have the same basic chemical structure as penicillin. A client with a penicillin allergy is very likely to have cross-reactivity and also have an allergic reaction to a cephalosporin. None of the other drugs are cross-reactive with penicillin.

20. **E, F**
Autoimmune disorders represent a failure of the immune system to tolerate self cells and make antibodies directed against normal cells. These antibodies then initiate excessive inflammatory responses that damage and sometimes destroy normal tissues. Women are 5 to 20 times more likely to develop an autoimmune disease. Autoimmunity is much more common among adults who have the human lymphocyte antigen subtypes of DR2, DR3, DRB, DQA, DQB, and Cw6. The basis of autoimmunity is immune system excess, not immunosuppression. At the current time, autoimmune disorders are chronic, progressive, and not curable. The presence of childhood allergies does not appear to increase the risk for development of autoimmunity.

21. **E, F, G, H**
Pernicious anemia, psoriasis, rheumatoid arthritis, and systemic lupus erythematosus are all autoimmune disorders in which one or more tissues are attacked by autoantibodies and cytokines. Asthma, cardiovascular disease, colorectal cancer, and type 2 diabetes mellitus do not have autoimmunity as a basis for the pathophysiology of the disease although some have a strong genetic component and asthma has a major inflammatory component.

22. **A**
During infancy and childhood, Tregs are able to remove the clones of lymphocytes that are prone to attack self cells. An individual with reduced numbers of Tregs develops greater numbers of immune system cells that cannot distinguish between normal healthy cells and non-self cells. Thus, self-tolerance is lost or reduced, which allows immune cells and their products to inappropriately attack normal body cells and tissues.

23. **C**
Twin studies have confirmed a strong link between genetic inheritance and autoimmunity. For monozygotic twins (identical twins), when one twin is diagnosed with an autoimmune disease, development of an autoimmune disorder (but not necessarily the same disorder) in the other twin is about 50%. Susceptible tissue types, known as human leukocyte antigens (HLAs), include DR2, DR3, DRB, DQA, DQB, and Cw6.

24. **B**
The most common recurrent symptoms presenting in clients with SLE are unexplained intermittent fever and fatigue (often with swollen, painful joints) with no other indicators of infection. These occur even when other members of the household do not have these symptoms. Penicillin is not a drug that causes manifestations of SLE. Joint and muscle pain after exercise usually just results from the exercise, especially when joint swelling is not present, not SLE. Although skin lesions may be present on the face and elsewhere on the body, the skin is not oily and the lesions are not acne.

25. **C**
Although the disorder is intermittent and flares may be avoided for a relatively long period, anti-inflammatories are needed to slow disease progression and permanent damage. There is no cure. Higher doses of all anti-inflammatories, including corticosteroids, may be needed during a flare. Low-impact exercises are needed on a regular basis, despite joint pain, to maintain muscle strength, joint function, and reduce the risk for cardiovascular problems associated with a sedentary lifestyle. Bloody or foamy urine can indicate kidney involvement and must be treated as early as possible to prevent chronic kidney disease.

26. **D**
The prescribed dose is relatively high and use for 2 weeks could cause some degree of adrenal suppression. Therefore, it should not be stopped suddenly. If the client cannot take an oral dose because of nausea or vomiting, he or she should have the dose administered parenterally and not "skipped." The drug is most effective when taken either in the morning or when doses are divided with two-thirds in the morning and one-third later in the day. Corticosteroids are not associated with kidney damage although they do increase the reabsorption of sodium and water, raising blood pressure. Although the

chronic use of corticosteroids decreases the inflammatory and immune responses, making the client more susceptible to infection, this drug is being prescribed on a short-term basis for a flare, not chronic use.

27. A

For the general joint and muscle pain of SLE, most clients achieve relief with applications of warm, moist heat, including baths. Medical marijuana has not yet been approved for use with SLE. Avoiding exercise does not reduce pain and will contribute to more loss of joint function. Ice and cold applications are recommended only when sprains or strains are present and not for general joint and muscle pain.

28. A, B, E, G

The UV light exposure exacerbates all aspects of SLE and must be avoided.

A common cause of death for clients with SLE is chronic kidney disease, which can be managed if identified earlier. Monitoring urine output and urine characteristics helps identify kidney changes.

Wearing a medical alert bracelet or other disease identifying objects is important in case the client is unable to communicate his or her disorder and therapies.

Management of SLE reduces the immune response and increases the risk for infection. Obtaining an annual influenza vaccination reduces the risk for this contagious disease.

Open lesions do not have to be covered.

Make-up is not contraindicated and neither is the use of hair dyes or other hair products.

Clients are urged to continue low-impact aerobic exercise to prevent complications.

29. A, C, F

The erythrocyte sedimentation rate is increased because of attached inflammatory proteins and debris.

Some complement levels, including C3, are increased as a result of the chronic inflammatory nature of the disease.

Basophils and eosinophil levels are not affected by the pathophysiology of the disorder.

Many of the autoantibodies present in a client with SLE are directed against parts of cellular nuclei, including extractable nuclear protein antibodies (anti-ENA).

30. C

In the early and localized stage I, the client appears with flulike symptoms, erythema migrans (round or oval, flat or slightly raised rash often in a bull's eye pattern), and pain and stiffness in the muscles and joints. Symptoms begin within 3 to 30 days of the bite of an infected tick, but most present in 7 to 14 days. Gastrointestinal problems are not usually associated with Lyme disease. Acute confusion is not present in stage I but can be a part of stages II and III.

19 CHAPTER

Concepts of Cancer Development

1. Which statements about development of neoplasms are correct? **Select all that apply**.
   A. Cancer cells are considered neoplasms.
   B. All neoplasms are considered abnormal.
   C. Neoplasms are derived from normal cells.
   D. Benign tumors are considered neoplasms.
   E. Neoplasms represent new tissue growth that is not needed for structure or function.
   F. Neoplasms occur when suppressor genes prevent normal growth factors from stimulating cell division.

2. Which body cells continue to undergo regular mitosis to maintain normal body function throughout the lifespan? **Select all that apply**.
   A. Bronchial lining
   B. Skeletal muscle
   C. Skin
   D. Bone marrow
   E. Neurons
   F. Intestinal lining

3. What factor or conditions make normal cells euploid?
   A. Are unable to migrate
   B. Retain contact inhibition
   C. Have the normal number of chromosome pairs
   D. Only undergo mitosis when new cells are needed

4. Which characteristic of a tumor indicates that it is benign rather than malignant?
   A. It does not cause pain.
   B. It is less than 2 cm in size.
   C. It is surrounded by a capsule.
   D. It causes the sensation of itching.

5. Which characteristics are most associated with malignant tumors rather than with benign tumors? **Select all that apply**.
   A. Have more or fewer than normal chromosomes
   B. Arise from normal parent tissues
   C. Have growth that is orderly with normal growth patterns
   D. Perform their differentiated function
   E. Invade other tissues
   F. Do not respond to signals for contact inhibition

6. What is the nurse's best response to a client who says that she has heard that the origin of most cancers is "genetic?"
   A. "The development of most cancers is predetermined and not affected by environmental factors."
   B. "Cancers arise in cells that have alterations in the genes."
   C. "Cancer is more common among males than females."
   D. "The majority of cancers are inherited."

7. Which feature/characteristic of benign tumors prevents them from invading other tissues and organs?
   A. Have a small nuclear-to-cytoplasmic ratio
   B. Perform specific differentiated functions
   C. Retain a specific morphology
   D. Are tightly adherent

8. Which tumor grade will the nurse interpret from the pathology report of a client's biopsy of a lymph node with the features of: "moderately differentiated; lung epithelial tissue; euploid?"
   A. Grade 1
   B. Grade 2
   C. Grade 3
   D. Grade 4

9. What is the nurse's best response when a client asks how does a chemical carcinogen cause cancer?
   A. By allowing cells to produce more than two cells when undergoing normal cell division
   B. By limiting the immune system from recognizing cancer cells
   C. By preventing normal cells from obtaining essential nutrients
   D. By damaging genes that control how and when cells divide

10. Which cancer type does the nurse interpret from a client's pathology report that indicates stage III osteogenic sarcoma?
    A. Bone
    B. Brain
    C. Breast
    D. Muscle

11. Which conditions does the nurse teach a client that are some of the seven warning signs of cancer? **Select all that apply**.
    A. Bleeding between periods
    B. Increasing size of a mole
    C. Hoarseness that lasts longer than 6 weeks
    D. Difficulty swallowing when eating dry foods
    E. Change in bowel habits that persist for several months
    F. Bleeding from the gums with tooth brushing or flossing

12. How will the nurse interpret the finding on a client's pathology report that a cancerous tumor has a mitotic index of 80%?
    A. The tumor is fast growing.
    B. Metastasis has already occurred.
    C. The tumor has not yet undergone carcinogenesis.
    D. The tumor has an abnormal number of chromosomes.

13. What effect does a "driver" mutation in a gene have on cancer development?
    A. Driver mutations are another term for suppressor gene mutations.
    B. These mutations protect against cancer development by reversing the effects of initiation.
    C. These mutations occur later in cancer progression and enhance cancer cell survival.
    D. The driver mutation increases an initiated cell's latency period, amplifying the effect of the carcinogen.

14. Which client report does the nurse interpret as a possible warning sign of cancer?
    A. Joint soreness and stiffness on arising after sleep
    B. Soreness under the tongue present for 4 months
    C. Wheezing and coughing with seasonal asthma
    D. Redness to skin with pain after sun exposure

15. Which statement made by a client who was treated for breast cancer 2 years ago indicates to the nurse that the client's cancer may have metastasized?
    A. "I seem to be hungry all the time."
    B. "My ribs hurt but I haven't had any injuries."
    C. "My skin is dry and it feels itchy and irritated."
    D. "I feel like I need to urinate all of the time."

16. Which actions or behaviors represent to the nurse that the client is engaging in **primary** cancer prevention practices?
    A. Reducing cigarette smoking
    B. Getting a mammogram annually
    C. Having a mole removed from the neck
    D. Obtaining a colonoscopy every 5 years
    E. Having a health checkup, including chest x-ray, annually
    F. Electing to have bilateral mastectomies in a person who has a *BRCA*1 mutation

17. Which client report prompts the nurse to create a three-generation pedigree to assess for the possibility of an increased risk for cancer?
    A. Has one first-degree relative and two second-degree relatives with lung cancer
    B. Has a father and paternal grandfather with colorectal cancer
    C. Has a history of cervical cancer treatment 5 years ago
    D. Worked as a chemical engineer for 20 years

18. How will the nurse respond to a client with cancer in the right breast who, when told she has a tumor in her left lung, says "How can I have lung cancer when I have never smoked in my life?"
    A. "Not all lung cancers are caused by smoking cigarettes."
    B. "Many of the same carcinogens that cause breast cancer also cause lung cancer."
    C. "This tumor may be breast cancer that has moved to your lungs and not a new cancer."
    D. "This is probably a result of the radiation treatment you received as cancer treatment."

19. Which information will the nurse tell a client, who has been diagnosed with cancer, that can be learned by surgery for staging even though the type of cancer is established? **Select all that apply**.
    A. Assessment of tumor size
    B. Number of tumors
    C. Sites of tumors
    D. Types of tumors
    E. Pattern of spread of tumors
    F. Sensitivity to cancer therapies

20. With which types of cancers would a nurse expect the client to have a T,N,M report? **Select all that apply**.
    A. Breast cancer
    B. Colorectal cancer
    C. Leukemia
    D. Lung cancer
    E. Lymphoma
    F. Melanoma

21. Which factors interact to increase the risk for cancer? **Select all that apply**.
    A. Advancing age
    B. Exposure to carcinogens
    C. Genetic predisposition
    D. Presence of allergies
    E. Reduced immunity
    F. Vaccination status for childhood illnesses and tetanus

22. Which cancer types are associated with human papilloma virus infection? **Select all that apply.**
    A. Breast cancer
    B. Cervical cancer
    C. Head and neck cancer
    D. Leukemia
    E. Penile cancer
    F. Primary brain cancer

23. Which comment made by a client with breast cancer indicates to the nurse a need for clarification regarding cancer causes and prevention?
    A. "I will eat a low-fat diet from now on."
    B. "I know that nothing I did or didn't do caused this cancer."
    C. "I hope my daughter doesn't have this problem when she grows up."
    D. "I will have regular mammograms on my other breast to prevent cancer."

24. Which possible problem does the nurse suspect when a client who has been treated for prostate cancer reports that he is now having a lot of pain in his lower back and legs?
    A. Arthritis
    B. Urinary retention
    C. Metastasis to the bone
    D. Muscle atrophy from inactivity

25. What possible role could estrogen play in cancer development?
    A. Estrogen, a female hormone, can cause cancer in males.
    B. Estrogen is a normal hormone that has no role in cancer development.
    C. Cancers that are estrogen dependent undergo mitosis more often in the presence of estrogen.
    D. It can be given to men with prostate cancer to help reduce the growth of prostate cancer cells.

26. Which cancer types are **most important** for a nurse to include when creating a cancer risk reduction pamphlet for the clients who come to a clinic that serves a large African-American population? **Select all that apply**
    A. Breast
    B. Bone
    C. Lung
    D. Prostate
    E. Esophageal
    F. Skin

Chapter 19 Answer Key

1. A, B, C, D, E
   Neoplasia is any new or continued cell growth not needed for normal development or replacement of dead tissues. Although all neoplastic cells are derived from (come from) normal cells, they are always considered abnormal even if they cause no harm (are benign). Thus, some neoplasias (or neoplastic cells) are benign and others are malignant (cancer cells), which means that normal cellular regulation has been disrupted. The major disruption is when suppressor genes are not able to do their functions of controlling cell growth. Suppressor genes prevent cell division from occurring when it is not needed. They do not suppress normal cell growth.

2. A, C, D, F
   The epithelial linings of glandular tissues (bronchial lining, intestinal lining) are often damaged and require continual replacement, as does the skin. Thus, these tissues undergo mitosis daily. The bone marrow makes more than a billion new cells daily. are the cell types Bone marrow cells undergo mitosis more often than any other normal cell type and retain this ability throughout the lifespan. The skin, being on the outside of the body, also continually loses cells that must be replaced. Skeletal muscle cells and neurons are considered nonmitotic tissue that seldom undergoes mitosis even when cell injury or death occurs.

3. C
   Euploid means that cells have the correct number of chromosomes (chromosome pairs) for the species. In the case of humans, all somatic body cells with a nucleus have 46 chromosomes (23 pairs).

4. C
   Benign tumors are made up of normal cells growing in the wrong place or growing at a time when they are not needed. They grow by expansion rather than invasion and often are encapsulated. The size and the fact that it is painless does not mean that the tumor is benign. Additionally, the presence of any sensation (such as itching) does not rule out malignancy.

5. A, E, F
   Malignant tumor cells are usually aneuploid, not contact-inhibited, and invade other tissues and organs. They do arise from normal parent tissues, like benign tumors, but do not have an orderly growth pattern and do not continue to perform their differentiated functions.

6. B
   Cancer development involves a change in the expression of normal genes. Usually this change is a result of gene damage to either oncogenes or suppressor genes. Thus, cancer is "genetic" in origin although this does not mean that cancers are directly inherited from one human generation to the next.

7. D
Tight adherence of benign tumor cells to each other occurs because they continue to make cell adhesion molecules. This prevents them from migrating or wandering into blood vessels or any other tissue or organ for metastasis.

8. B
Grade 2 tumor cells are moderately differentiated and still retain enough of the characteristics of normal cells to be able to identify the tissue from which it arose. In this case, the tumor in the lymph node is from lung tissue and still has normal chromosomes.

9. D
The main effect of chemical carcinogens is entering cells and damaging the DNA in the genes that control or regulate normal cell growth. Even cancer cells, when they divide, only produce two new cells at each cell division. Although the immune system may fail to recognize cancer cells as abnormal, this is not the action that changes normal cells to cancer cells, nor do the carcinogens prevent or interfere with normal cell's nutrition.

10. A
The term "osteo" refers to bone and "sarcoma" refers to connective tissue. Thus, an osteogenic sarcoma arises from actual bone tissue. Brain cancers are neurogenic or glial; breast cancer is a type of carcinoma; muscle cancer is a rhabdomyosarcoma.

11. A, B, C, E
The seven warning signs of cancer include persistent changes in bowel habits, unusual bleeding or discharge, obvious change in a wart or mole, nagging cough, or hoarseness. Although difficulty swallowing can be a warning sign of cancer, this means a persistent change regardless of what type of food is eaten. Most people have difficulty swallowing dry foods without drinking something at the same time. Bleeding from the gums with brushing or flossing is usually associated with poor hygiene and not cancer.

12. A
A mitotic index of 80% means that 80% of the cells within the tumor sample are actively dividing, which represents a very high cell division rate. The presence or absence of metastasis cannot be determined by the mitotic index. By definition, a cancerous tumor has already undergone carcinogenesis, which is not determined by the mitotic index. When a tumor has an abnormal number of chromosomes, it is aneuploid, which is not related to the mitotic index.

13. C
As tumor cells continue to divide, some of the new cells undergo further genetic mutations that change features from the original, initiated cancer cell and form different groups. Driver mutations provide these cell groups with specific selection advantages that allow them to live and divide no matter how the conditions around them change. These mutations are not protective, cannot reverse initiation, and do not increase latency.

14. B
A sore anywhere that does not heal within 2 to 3 weeks is not normal and should be examined by a health care provider. Wheezing and coughing limited to asthma attacks is not cause for concern nor is joint stiffness or pain after a period of not moving. Skin redness and pain after sun exposure does not indicate cancer although multiple sunburns increase the risk for later skin cancer development.

15. B
The most common sites of metastasis for breast cancer are the bone, brain, lungs, and liver. Skin, kidney, and bladder are rarely involved in breast cancer metastasis. A decreased appetite rather than an increased one is more common when metastasis occurs.

16. C, D, F
Reducing exposure to a carcinogen, rather than totally avoiding it, does not really represent primary prevention. Removal of at-risk tissue

or a precancerous lesion (such as a mole, colon polyp, or breasts when a person has a specific mutation in a BRCA1 gene) does represent primary cancer prevention. Mammograms and health checkups represent secondary prevention in the form of possible early detection.

17. B

Lung cancer and cervical cancers are from environmental or lifestyle causes and do not represent an increased genetic risk for the client to develop cancer. Exposure to chemicals would also be an environmental risk factor, not a genetic one. Colorectal cancer can occur sporadically and also has an association with specific inherited gene mutations. Having a father and paternal grandfather with a history of colorectal cancer warrants more investigation as a possible indicator of increased genetic risk.

18. C

Although it is true that not all lung cancers are caused by cigarette smoking, this client's lung cancer is most likely a metastatic tumor from the breast cancer. Most of the carcinogens known to cause lung cancer are not associated with breast cancer. Radiation therapy has resulted in cancer development, but this usually takes a long time and would occur only in the area treated with radiation, which was the right breast, not the left one.

19. A, B, C, E

Surgical staging provides information about the tumor size, number, sites, and possible spread that has occurred at the time of surgery. It is not required for establishment of tumor or cancer type after this has been determined by a biopsy. Surgical staging does not provide any information on the sensitivity of the cancer to any therapy.

20. A, D

The cancers for which the tumor, node, metastasis (TNM) system is commonly used to describe the anatomic extent include lung and breast cancer. This staging system is not useful for leukemia or lymphomas, and some other cancers have more specific staging systems, such as Dukes' staging of colorectal cancer and Clark's levels method of staging skin cancer.

21. A, B, C, E

Cancer is a disease of aging and advancing age represents an increased risk for cancer development, as does exposure to carcinogens. A genetic predisposition greatly increases the risk for cancer although relatively few people have this risk factor. Reduced immunity increases the risk for cancer development. Allergies do not increase cancer risk and, in fact, represents greater immunity, not reduced immunity. Vaccination for general childhood disorders and tetanus does not affect cancer risk. Obtaining a vaccination against the human papilloma virus reduces, not increases, the risk for cancer development.

22. B, C, E

The human papilloma virus (HPV) has several subtypes that are carcinogenic and known as oncoviruses. Specific cancers that have HPV as one cause include cervical cancer, vulvar cancer, penile cancer, anogenital carcinomas, and head and neck cancer. Some leukemias are associated with other types of viral infection, and primary brain cancer is not associated with any viral infection.

23. D

Regular mammography can help detect breast cancer at an early stage, it does not prevent breast cancer. High-fat diets have a slight connection to breast cancer development, as does obesity. For the most part, the cause of breast cancer is unknown. Breast cancer has familial and hereditary forms. Having a mother with breast cancer does increase a woman's overall risk.

24. C

The primary site of metastasis for prostate cancer is the bone of the spine and legs. Pain in these areas in a client with prostate cancer is highly suggestive of cancer progression and metastasis. Arthritis is generally a joint disorder. Urinary retention usually causes lower abdominal pain. Muscle atrophy is painless.

25. C
Estrogen is a natural hormone that is a growth factor for estrogen-dependent tissues, such as the endometrium and breast ductal cells. When cancer cells have estrogen receptors, such as some breast, uterine, and ovarian cancers, estrogen promotes growth of those cancer cells. It does not cause cancer. Although it is used as hormone therapy for some prostate cancer, that is a therapeutic use and does not describe its role in cancer development.

26. A, C, D
Both the incidence and death rates from lung and prostate cancers in the African-American population are greater than for any other racial group. Although the incidence of breast cancer is not higher among African Americans, it is usually found at a later stage, is more aggressive, and has a higher death rate than in other racial or ethnic groups. The incidence of lung cancer has been proven to be reduced by smoking cessation and deaths from prostate cancer, as well as breast cancer, can be reduced by early detection. Thus, targeting information for these three cancers specifically among an African-American population may have the greatest impact for reduction of cancer risks and cancer deaths.

20
CHAPTER

Concepts of Care for Patients with Cancer

1. Which signs and symptoms does the nurse expect in a client whose cancer has invaded the bone marrow? **Select all that apply**.
   A. Diarrhea and vomiting
   B. Fatigue and weakness
   C. Low white blood cell counts
   D. Confusion with memory loss
   E. Bruises or other bleeding signs
   F. Tachycardia and shortness of breath

2. For which problem will the nurse expect to prepare a client for palliative cancer surgery?
   A. Extensive scarring after treatment for head and neck cancer
   B. An intestinal obstruction and continuous vomiting
   C. Irritated mole rubbed continually by a bra strap
   D. A rapidly growing skin lesion with irregular borders

3. For which side effects will the nurse prepare the client who is to receive 6 weeks of external beam radiation therapy for uterine cancer? **Select all that apply?**
   A. Dry mouth
   B. Taste changes
   C. Scalp alopecia
   D. Bowel changes
   E. Increased fatigue
   F. Skin rash and redness
   G. Difficulty swallowing
   H. Numbness and tingling in fingers and toes

4. The client receiving brachytherapy with implanted radioactive "seeds" for prostate cancer asks the nurse when these seeds will be removed. What is the nurse's **best** response?
   A. "The half-life of radiation in these seeds is so short that it is not necessary to remove them."
   B. "They will only be removed if their presence is painful or leads to an enlarged prostate gland."
   C. "When we know for certain that all cancerous cells have been killed, the seeds will be removed."
   D. "The seeds are small enough to be absorbed by your body and excreted in the urine or stool."

5. Which statements regarding care of the client receiving radiotherapy in the form of unsealed radioactive isotopes guides the nurse's care? **Select all that apply**.
   A. The client may have restrictions on who can visit and for how long.
   B. The client must be in total isolation while the isotopes are in place.
   C. When "seeds" are used for prostate cancer therapy, the client must have them removed before he leaves the hospital.
   D. The client's urine and stool must be handled as radioactive material.
   E. The nurse must ensure that all personnel entering the client's room use appropriate precautions.
   F. Only those female nurses who are past menopause can be assigned to care for this client.

6. What is the nurse's **first** action to **prevent harm** when finding the sealed radiation implant for cervical cancer in the 74-year-old client's bed?
   A. Assess the client's mental status.
   B. Use tongs to place the implant in the radiation container.
   C. Notify the radiologist and move the client to a different room.
   D. Don gloves and attempt to reposition the implant and positioning device.

7. Which precautions are a **priority** for the nurse to teach a client undergoing 6 weeks of daily external beam radiation for breast cancer? **Select all that apply**.
   A. Do not remove the markings.
   B. Use lotions liberally to keep skin soft and moist.
   C. Avoid direct skin exposure to sunlight for up to a year.
   D. Wash the area with your hand using only mild soap and water.
   E. Apply a heating pad to treated areas to stimulate circulation.
   F. Avoid wearing a tight-fitting bra during treatment and when the area is irritated

8. Which side effects in a client receiving traditional chemotherapy will the nurse report to the oncologist for reduction of the chemotherapy dose? **Select all that apply**.
   A. Alopecia
   B. Bone marrow suppression
   C. Chemo brain
   D. Mucositis
   E. Nausea and vomiting
   F. Peripheral neuropathy

9. For which type of cancer is chemotherapy most beneficial?
   A. Brain tumors
   B. Superficial cancers on the outside of the body
   C. Cancers that are localized to one tissue or body area
   D. Cancers that are large with evidence of distant metastasis

10. The client receiving high-dose chemotherapy who has neutropenia asks the nurse whether he and his wife can have sexual intercourse while he is receiving chemotherapy. What is the nurse's best response?
    A. "No, this activity will increase the side effects of the chemotherapy."
    B. "No, the danger of impregnating your wife is too great."
    C. "Yes, as long as you feel like it and use a condom."
    D. "Yes, if you do not have an infection."

11. The client who received combination chemotherapy 7 days ago for breast cancer calls the oncology clinic to report a temperature of 100.5°F (38.6°C) and has no other symptoms of infection. What is the nurse's best response?
    A. "This is a normal immune-related response to the chemotherapy."
    B. "Please go to the nearest emergency room for a full workup for infection."
    C. "You are most likely dehydrated. Come to the clinic now for IV fluids."
    D. "There is no concern at this time but call if your temperature reaches 101.5°F (38.6°C)."

12. How will the nurse instruct a client who is prescribed to receive an oral chemotherapy agent for colorectal cancer to dispose of unused or expired drug to **prevent harm**?
    A. Place in a puncture-proof container and throw out with the regular trash.
    B. Crush the drugs and mix them with kitty litter before placing the zippered bag in the trash.
    C. Flush down the toilet, taking care to wear gloves while wiping up splash areas on the toilet or walls.
    D. Take them back to the oncology clinic in the container in which they were dispensed for disposal with other medical waste.

13. Which personal protective equipment (PPE) is the nurse required to use when administering intravenous chemotherapy to a client with cancer? **Select all that apply**.
    A. Head cover
    B. Eye protection
    C. Mask
    D. Gown
    E. Chemo-designated gloves
    F. Shoe coverings

14. Which precautions are a **priority** for the nurse to teach a client who has chemotherapy-induced peripheral neuropathy to **prevent harm**? **Select all that apply**.
    A. Avoid taking aspirin or any aspirin-containing products.
    B. Use a bath thermometer to check bath water temperature.
    C. Do not use mouthwashes that contain alcohol or glycerin.
    D. Bathe daily using an antimicrobial soap or gel.
    E. Use handrails when going up or down steps.
    F. Wear shoes with a firm sole.

15. Which actions will the nurse teach a client receiving chemotherapy who has myelosuppression and neutropenia to **prevent harm** from development of an opportunistic infection? **Select all that apply**.
    A. Avoid drinking cold or cool liquids.
    B. Bathe daily using an antimicrobial soap.
    C. Wear gloves when digging in the garden.
    D. Be sure to wear sufficient clothing in cold weather.
    E. Wash dishes in hot sudsy waster or in a dishwasher.
    F. Clean your toothbrush daily in the dishwasher or with bleach.
    G. Wear a medical alert bracelet indicating you are immunosuppressed.
    H. Get a yearly influenza vaccination and the recommended pneumonia vaccination.

16. Which instruction will the nurse emphasize to assistive personnel (AP) about the hygiene needs of a client who is neutropenic?
    A. Do not enter the room unless absolutely necessary and then minimize time spent in the room.
    B. Mouth care and washing of the axillary and perianal regions must be done during every shift.
    C. If the client seems very tired, assist with toileting but defer all other aspects of hygienic care.
    D. Be sure to soak the client's feet in warm sudsy water for at least 30 minutes daily.

17. What are the nurse's **priority** actions to **prevent harm** for a client receiving IV chemotherapy into a peripheral line with an agent that is an irritant, who says the site burns terribly at and around the IV site? **Select all that apply**.
    A. Check for a blood return.
    B. Slow the rate of infusion.
    C. Apply ice to the site.
    D. Discontinue the infusion.
    E. Call the pharmacist.
    F. Raise the arm above the level of the heart.

18. Which assessment is a **priority** for the nurse to perform for a client who is taking an antiemetic from the serotonin antagonist (5-HT3 receptor blocker) class of drugs?
    A. Urine output
    B. Serum calcium level
    C. Heart rate and rhythm
    D. White blood cell count

19. What is the nurse's **best action** when a client's spouse reports that the last time the client received lorazepam before receiving chemotherapy, the client didn't remember the drive home?
    A. Explain that this is a normal response to the drug and that the client shouldn't drive home.
    B. Perform a mental status exam and assess pupillary responses before giving the lorazepam.
    C. Hold the dose of lorazepam for this round of chemotherapy until the client is seen by the oncologist.
    D. Document the response in a prominent place in the client's electronic health record as the only action.

20. Which interventions are **most important** for the nurse to teach a client who is receiving chemotherapy with an agent that causes thrombocytopenia to **prevent harm**? **Select all that apply**.
    A. Use an electric shaver, not a safety razor.
    B. Avoid eating raw meat, fish, or poultry.
    C. Take your temperature daily.
    D. Use a soft-bristled toothbrush and do not floss.
    E. Do not use enemas or rectal suppositories.
    F. Be sure to get an annual influenza vaccination.

21. Which action is **most important** for the nurse to take to **prevent** extravasation in a client receiving IV chemotherapy infusion?
    A. Identify the specific antidote and make sure it is readily available.
    B. Frequently assess the site for a blood return and ease of infusion.
    C. Use an intravenous pump or controller to deliver the chemotherapy infusion.
    D. Avoid administering any drugs or fluids that are tissue irritants or vesicants.

22. Which statement by a client taking an oral cancer agent indicates to the nurse that more education is needed?
    A. "This drug is much more convenient than my old IV drugs."
    B. "I understand that not skipping doses is very important in controlling my cancer."
    C. "My husband wants to help me but I told him that only I should touch this drug."
    D. "I have been crushing the drug and putting it in my tea because it is hard to swallow."

23. Which actions does the nurse teach a client who has mucositis to reduce the discomfort? **Select all that apply**.
    A. Apply a water-based moisturizer to lips as often as you like.
    B. Brush teeth and tongue rigorously with a toothbrush every 8 hours.
    C. "Swish and spit" room-temperature tap water every 1 to 2 hours.
    D. Use commercial mouthwashes and glycerin swabs to refresh mouth.
    E. Avoid smoking while open sores are present.
    F. Limit your fluid intake to 1 liter or less daily.

24. What is the nurse's **priority action** for a client whose platelet count is 18,000/mm^3 (18 × 10^9/L)?
    A. Applying pressure after blood draws to prevent bleeding
    B. Placing the client in protective isolation
    C. Applying oxygen to reduce dyspnea
    D. Restricting fluid to prevent edema

25. Which client will the nurse assess most frequently for sepsis?
    A. 34-year-old who has received high-dose radiation to the left chest area
    B. 53-year-old with hypercalcemia and dehydration
    C. 66-year-old with small cell lung cancer and hyponatremia
    D. 72-year-old patient with neutropenia and a low-grade fever

26. Which normal tissue or organ will nurse assess for side effects in a client who is receiving cancer therapy with an epidermal growth factor receptor inhibitor (EGFRI)?
    A. Skin
    B. Joints
    C. Liver
    D. Kidney

27. Which assessment findings in a client who has neutropenia from cancer chemotherapy indicates to the nurse that severe disseminated intravascular coagulation (DIC) is present? **Select all that apply**.
    A. The client is bleeding from the nose, IV sites, and rectum.
    B. The client's temperature is 99°F (37.2°C).
    C. The client's pulse rate is 130 beats/min.
    D. The client's respiratory rate is 24 breaths/min.
    E. The client's white blood cell count is 3200/mm³ (3.2 × 10⁹/L).
    F. The client's hourly urine output is 100 mL.

28. Which change in health status indicates to the nurse that the client's superior vena cava syndrome is worsening?
    A. The client's systolic blood pressure is rising and the diastolic pressure is decreasing.
    B. The client's severe nausea and vomiting no longer responds to antiemetics.
    C. The client has experienced four nose bleeds in the past 2 days.
    D. Pedal edema is now present.

29. Which client report indicates to the nurse that spinal cord compression may be present?
    A. The client reports having a headache for the past 7 hours.
    B. The client has reduced breath sounds in the left lung.
    C. The client has worsening mid-thoracic back pain.
    D. Pedal edema is now present bilaterally.

30. Which laboratory test is a **priority** for the nurse to monitor when a client has advanced breast cancer with bone metastasis?
    A. Serum calcium level
    B. Serum blood glucose
    C. Serum potassium level
    D. Serum sodium level

Chapter 20 Answer Key

1. B, C, E, F
   Cancer that invades the bone marrow crowds out the stem cells responsible for generating all the blood cells. As a result, the client has low red blood cell counts leading to anemia, which causes fatigue, weakness, tachycardia, and shortness of breath; low platelets, which enhances bleeding tendencies and causes bruising and petechiae; and low white blood cell counts, which increases infection risk. Decreased blood cell formation does not cause vomiting and diarrhea nor does it result in confusion until the client is severely hypoxic.

2. B
   Palliative cancer surgery focuses on providing symptom relief and improving the quality of life but is not curative. Surgery to correct an intestinal obstruction meets these criteria. Revising

scars is reconstructive surgery and removing a precancerous lesion is prophylactic surgery. Removal of tissue with abnormal features is diagnostic surgery.

3. B, D, E, F
   Radiation therapy is local therapy, and most effects on normal tissues are those in the radiation path, which, in this case, is the lower abdomen. Changes in tissues in the radiation path are the skin and the bowel. Generalized side effects from radiation therapy include taste changes and intense fatigue over time, although the exact mechanisms responsible for these effects are not clear. Although skin in the radiation path is affected, scalp alopecia will not occur from abdominal external beam radiation. Dry mouth and difficulty swallowing do not occur because the salivary glands and esophagus

are not in the radiation path, nor are the fingers and toes.

4. A

The seeds are small and painless. The half-life of the radiation source is less than 2 weeks. Thus, it is not necessary for the seeds to be removed as they pose no health hazard to the client or anyone else. They are neither absorbed nor excreted by the body.

5. A, D, E

While the radioactive elements are within the client, he or she does emit radiation and is a hazard to others. Children and pregnant women may not visit. Other visitors are limited to 30 minutes or less daily. With an unsealed source, the isotopes enter body fluids and are excreted in the urine and stool as radioactive substances. Because the client does emit radiation, all personnel entering the room can be exposed and must use the appropriate precautions, regardless of how short a time period they are present in the room.

6. B

The implant does emit radiation and should not be touched directly. If the room has the proper equipment, the nurse uses long-handled tongs to move the implant to an appropriate lead-lined container. If the proper equipment is not available in the client's room, the radiation department must be notified. The second action is to assess the client's mental status because she may have removed the implant and positioning-fixing device as a result of acute confusion. Repositioning the implant is not within the scope of nursing practice. The client does not need to be moved to a different room.

7. A, C, D, F

The skin in the path of radiation is injured by the treatment. The degree of injury is related to the intensity and duration of treatments. Six weeks of daily radiation treatment is a large dose and usually results in skin redness, tenderness, and peeling during the treatment period and for weeks afterward. The area remains sensitive to sun damage, heat damage, and direct contact damage for up to a year after therapy is complete.

It is important for the client to avoid trauma to the area by using only mild soap and water to cleanse the area with hands rather than a cloth, as well as avoiding clothing that rubs. If markings are present, they must remain in place through the treatment to appropriately direct the radiation beam. Some lotions and other products can disrupt the direction of the radiation beam and are not to be used unless approved by the radiology department. Heat to the area will make the skin reaction worse.

8. B, D

Although doses can be reduced when requested by clients experiencing unpleasant side effects, the two side effects that require dose reduction are bone marrow suppression and mucositis. Bone marrow suppression greatly increases the client's risk for bleeding, sepsis, and death. The side effect of mucositis cannot be prevented nor are there any therapies to actually treat it. All that is available are some comfort measures. When mucositis is severe, the client may have inadequate food and fluid intake, leading to a variety of problems. The open sores also increase infection risk and the pain can be unbearable.

9. D

Chemotherapy is considered systemic therapy and is used as primary therapy or adjuvant therapy for cancers that may not be confined to a localized body area. Because chemotherapy is systemic, it circulates through many body areas and can harm cancer cells that may be some distance from the primary tumor. Many types of chemotherapy, however, are not able to cross the blood-brain barrier and are not useful for tumors that either develop in the brain or metastasize to the brain.

10. C

Many people do not feel well enough to have sexual intercourse during the months they are taking chemotherapy. This activity is fine as long as the client takes precautions to limit chemotherapy drug exposure to his partner and protects himself from infection or trauma. Wearing a condom reduces chemotherapy drug exposure to his partner (as a result of any drugs entering the seminal fluid or that are in the urethra from presence in the urine) and also reduces his risk for developing an ascending urinary tract infection.

11. B

Clients with neutropenia, and with this being the 7th day after chemotherapy for breast cancer, this client is very likely to be neutropenic, have so few white blood cells that they often do not have the typical symptoms of inflammation and infection. Anti-infective therapy is started when the client's temperature reaches 100°F (37.8°C) to prevent sepsis.

12. D

Oral chemotherapy agents pose a toxic hazard to others and cannot be thrown out in the trash or flushed down the toilet. Instruct the patient to bring them back to the hospital or clinic in the container in which they were dispensed, and the hospital or clinic will dispose of them as hazardous medical waste.

13. B, C, D, E

The purpose of PPE when administering (or preparing) IV chemotherapy agents is to prevent the nurse from having direct skin or mucous membrane contact with these drugs because they can be absorbed through intact tissue. The Oncology Nursing Society and governmental protection groups require eye protection, mask (over nose and mouth), gowns with long, cuffed sleeves, and either special chemotherapy gloves or double gloving with standard gloves. Head coverings and foot coverings are not needed to prevent skin and mucous membrane absorption of these drugs.

14. B, E, F

Peripheral neuropathy reduces the ability to discriminate temperature sensation. It is very easy for a person with neuropathy to be unaware or water temperature and to become injured as a result of water for bathing/showering being too hot. When peripheral neuropathy is present in the feet (which is often where it starts), clients are at high risk for foot injury and falling because they cannot determine subtle terrain changes, be certain of foot placement, or feel injuries to the feet. Aspirin, although important

to avoid when platelets are low, is not contraindicated with peripheral neuropathy. Alcohol or glycerin mouthwashes are contraindicated for mucositis, not peripheral neuropathy. Bathing with an antimicrobial soap helps prevent infection but does not prevent injury.

15. B, C, E, F

Opportunistic infections are those caused by overgrowth of the neutropenic client's normal flora. These infections also include exogenous microorganisms in the environment that usually cause no problems to adults with healthy immune systems.

Bathing daily and using an antimicrobial soap will help decrease the risk for opportunistic infections by reducing the number of normal flora bacteria found on the skin.

Soil contains many microorganisms that can cause opportunistic infections in an immunocompromised client. Wearing gloves when digging or working with soil helps reduce this risk. Washing dishes well prevents infection from exposure to residual microbiome organisms after eating.

Cleaning a toothbrush daily by either rinsing it with liquid bleach (and then rinsing out the bleach) or having it go through a dishwasher cycle reduces residual organisms.

Getting an influenza or pneumonia vaccination prevents pathogenic infections, not opportunistic infections.

Drinking cold or cool liquids does not promote opportunistic infection.

Wearing warm clothing in cold weather does not prevent opportunistic infection and neither would wearing a medical alert bracelet for immunosuppression.

16. B

The client with neutropenia is at high risk for developing an opportunistic infection from overgrowth of his or her own normal flora in the mouth, perineal area, and skinfold areas. Cleansing these areas every shift is vital for client safety and cannot be deferred. There is no need for a healthy AP to stay out of the client's room. Soaking the feet does not reduce the risk for developing an infection.

17. D, E

Irritants and vesicants can both cause tissue damage. Even if the IV has a good blood return, some of the chemotherapy can still be leaking into the tissues. Slowing the rate of infusion is not sufficient to prevent further leakage and damage. Applying ice may or may not be the correct action, depending on the specific agent; however, the application would only be done after the infusion has been discontinued. The pharmacist would know precisely what action or antidote should be used for the specific agent involved.

18. C

The serotonin antagonists can cause cardiac changes, especially a prolonged QT interval. These drugs are not known to have adverse effects on calcium balance or white blood cell count. Although urine output could be decreased if the client is dehydrated from excessive vomiting, this is not a side effect of the antiemetic therapy.

19. A

Lorazepam, a benzodiazepine, induces sedation and amnesia in addition to having antiemetic effects. Many clients have little if any memory about events occurring within a few hours after receiving lorazepam. This is an expected side effect and does not denote any permanent reduced cognition in the client. Both the client and the spouse should be aware of this effect so that the client is not at risk for injury. Driving, cooking, or operating mechanical equipment should not be performed until the drug's effects have worn off.

20. A, D, E

Thrombocytopenia means that the client's platelets are greatly decreased, increasing the client's risk for prolonged bleeding in response to even minor injury, especially from highly vascular areas, such as the gums or rectal tissues. Clients must avoid injury, such as using a safety razor, whenever possible. Taking temperature daily; avoiding raw meat, fish, and poultry; and getting an annual influenza vaccine help to prevent infection but not injury that could lead to excessive bruising or bleeding.

21. B

Frequent site assessment to ensure the access is in the vein and infusing well is the best action for prevention of extravasation. Using a pump or controller does not prevent extravasation nor does having the antidote available. Many traditional chemotherapies are either tissue irritants and vesicants and, if they are the prescribed therapy, must be given.

22. D

These drugs should not be crushed, cut, or chewed. Other actions that can make them easier to swallow include taking them with a spoonful of pudding, some other "slippery" food, or thick drink. The client is correct that missed doses can reduce therapy outcomes. These drugs can be absorbed through the skin and only the client should have direct contact with them.

23. A, C, E

Recommendations are to apply only water-based moisturizers as needed, use soft-bristled toothbrushes and brush gently, swish and spit with tap water, and avoid smoking. Increasing, not decreasing, fluid intake is helpful and comforting. Using commercial mouthwashes is avoided because they contain alcohol and other drying agents.

24. A

Excessive bleeding occurs when the platelet count is this low (thrombocytopenia). In addition to handling the client gently, pressure needs to be applied after injections, blood draws, and the discontinuing of an IV. The client who only has thrombocytopenia is not at increased risk for infection. Platelets do not carry oxygen and low platelet counts do not cause hypoxia or dyspnea. Edema formation is not a result of a low platelet count.

25. D

A client with neutropenia is always at risk for sepsis regardless of age. However, this risk is increased in older adults. In addition, this client already has a low-grade fever. Neutropenic clients often do not develop a fever with infection. The fact that this client has any temperature elevation is an indicator of more severe infection. Radiation to the left chest does not significantly impair bone marrow production of neutrophils. Neither dehydration nor hyponatremia increase the risk for sepsis.

26. A

The EGRFIs target and bind to epidermal growth factor receptors which, in addition to cancer cells, are strongly present in the skin. Thus, the skin is at high risk for rashes and even sloughing in clients who are receiving EGFRIs, and should be assessed at every clinic visit. Minimal EGFRs are present in the bones and joints, liver, or kidneys, which have few side effects with this drug category.

27. A, C, D

DIC is a condition in which widespread microthrombi form and use all available circulating clotting factors. When these factors are gone, clotting cannot occur and the client bleeds from any site of trauma, no matter how minor the trauma. Spontaneous bleeding can also occur.

The elevated pulse rate is consistent with the hypovolemic shock phase of DIC, as is the increased respiratory rate. Both are attempting to maintain oxygenation to vital organs.

28. C

With superior vena cava syndrome, blood flow through the vena cava is compromised as a result of tumor growth. As blood backs up in the venous system drained by the superior vena cave, pressure in the veins increases and nose bleeds (epistaxis) occur easily and frequently. The increased venous pressure would not increase systolic pressure. Response to antiemetics is not affected by superior vena cava syndrome. Pedal edema could occur in response to a blockage in the inferior vena cava but not the superior vena cava.

29. C

One of the first symptoms of spinal cord compression in a patient with cancer is new-onset or worsening back pain as the disintegrating bones press and compress spinal nerves. Headache is not associated with spinal cord compression.

30. A

Bone metastasis is a common complication of advanced breast cancer. It injures bone and releases calcium into the blood leading to hypercalcemia, which is a medical emergency that can lead to death. Bone metastasis does not elevate or change blood levels of sodium, potassium, or glucose.

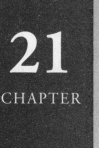

21 CHAPTER

Concepts of Care for Patients with Infection

1. Which circumstances are examples of colonization? **Select all that apply**.
   A. Health care provider contacts the Centers for Disease Control and Prevention because client has symptoms of smallpox.
   B. A nurse has a nasal swab that cultures out methicillin-resistant *Staphylococcus aureus* (MRSA) and remains asymptomatic.
   C. An 86-year-old client who is immunocompromised because of multiple chronic health problems lives in a long-term care facility.
   D. An assistive personnel chooses to use an alcohol-based hand rub rather than washing with soap and water after caring for a client with *Clostridium difficile*.
   E. A 55-year old client with fever and a productive cough has a sputum culture that is positive for *Streptococcus pneumonae*.
   F. A 64-year-old woman's urine culture is positive for *Escherichia coli* although the urine is clear and no symptoms of cystitis are present.

2. Which health behavior does the nurse teach a client who is immunocompromised to prevent infection from normal flora?
   A. Wiping perineal area from front to back after toileting for females
   B. Wearing insect repellent or long sleeves to avoid mosquito bites
   C. Washing fruit and vegetables first before eating them raw
   D. Receiving an annual influenza vaccination

3. Which situations are examples of an animate reservoir? **Select all that Apply**.
   A. Coronavirus (COVID-19) influenza was first transmitted to humans from infected bats and snakes.
   B. Escherichia coliform *(E. Coli)* bacteremia has been contracted from eating contaminated romaine lettuce.
   C. An immunocompromised client with HIV-III develops toxoplasmosis from changing a cat litter box daily.
   D. A 48-year-old man living in the tropics develops malaria after being extensively bitten by a swarm of mosquitoes.
   E. Health care personnel can transmit skin infections from one client to another by not cleaning stethoscope surfaces between clients.
   F. A 38-year-old client who is immunosuppressed from receiving chemotherapy develops aspergillus pneumonia while his 100-year-old house is renovated.

4. With which clients will the nurse use extra precautions to **prevent harm** from infection development as a result of medical or surgical intervention? **Select all that apply**.
   A. 27-year-old taking antirejection drugs after receiving a kidney transplant
   B. 36-year-old being mechanically ventilated
   C. 45-year-old with an indwelling urinary catheter
   D. 58-year-old with type 2 diabetes mellitus
   E. 60-year-old who had an artificial aortic valve replacement 4 years ago
   F. 65-year-old taking corticosteroids daily for chronic obstructive pulmonary disease (COPD)
   G. 80-year-old with mild chronic heart failure taking a diuretic daily

5. Which client factors does the nurse identify as increasing the risk for infection? Select **all that apply**.
   A. Drinking four to five alcoholic beverages daily
   B. Smoking two packs of cigarettes daily
   C. Using hormone-based contraceptives
   D. Eating a balanced vegetarian diet
   E. Serving a 5-year prison term
   F. Walking 2 miles daily

6. Which action will the nurse use during client care to **prevent infection** by mechanically disrupting biofilms?
   A. Washing hands with chlorohexidine for 15 seconds
   B. Cleaning the skin with alcohol prior to venipuncture
   C. Using sterile technique when inserting a urinary catheter
   D. Helping the client to floss and to brush teeth

7. Which is the **most important action** for the nurse to teach visitors to avoid acquiring influenza when visiting a client with the disease?
   A. Keeping windows open in rooms where the client spends the most time
   B. Remaining at least 6 feet away from the client
   C. Washing hands after touching the client
   D. Not sharing a toilet with the client

8. Which personal protective equipment (PPE) does the nurse assemble for use when giving oral and parenteral drugs to a client who has diarrhea from *Clostridium difficile* overgrowth? **Select all that apply**.
   A. Air-purifying respirator
   B. Eye goggles
   C. Gloves
   D. Gown
   E. Hair cover
   F. Surgical mask

9. Which action does the nurse take to prevent indirect contact transmission of microorganisms to a susceptible client?
   A. Wearing a high-efficiency particulate air filter mask when providing direct care to a client with a respiratory infection
   B. Placing the client on Airborne Precautions until a negative tuberculosis test is verified
   C. Cleaning the glucometer with disinfectant between testing clients
   D. Wearing gloves when obtaining blood for glucose testing

10. Which physical factors does the nurse assess for in an older adult client that are likely to increase the risk for infection? **Select all that apply**.
    A. Increased antibody production
    B. Thin, delicate skin
    C. Decreased gag reflex
    D. Increased gastrointestinal motility
    E. Decreased mobility
    F. Higher incidence of chronic disease

11. For which infectious diseases will the nurse recommend immunizations for older adult clients? **Select all that apply**.
    A. Influenza
    B. Pneumonia
    C. Human papilloma virus
    D. Herpes zoster (shingles)
    E. Measles, mumps, and rubella
    F. Tetanus, diphtheria, and pertussis

12. For which client care situation will the nurse teach assistive personnel to perform handwashing, rather than using alcohol-based hand rubs (ABHRs)?
    A. After removing gloves used when emptying a Foley catheter bag
    B. After setting up a basin and towels for a client's morning care
    C. After contact with a client who has had diarrhea for 3 days
    D. Before having direct contact with any clients

13. In addition to Standard Precautions, which type of transmission-based precautions will the nurse use to prevent infection transmission when caring for a client who has methicillin-resistant *Staphylococcus aureus* (MRSA)?
    A. Airborne Precautions
    B. Contact Precautions
    C. Cutaneous Precautions
    D. Droplet Precautions

14. For which clients does the nurse ensure placement in a private room? **Select all that apply**.
    A. 28-year-old client with influenza
    B. 36-year-old after a cholecystectomy who is HIV positive
    C. 48-year-old severely immunosuppressed client receiving cancer chemotherapy
    D. 59-year-old with active tuberculosis
    E. 63-year-old client with hepatitis C
    F. 84-year-old with methicillin-resistant *Staphylococcus aureus* (MRSA)

15. Which precaution is **most** important for the nurse to teach a client prescribed to take oral delafloxacin to treat a skin lesion infected with methicillin-resistant *Staphylococcus aureus* (MRSA)?
    A. Report any burning on urination to your primary health care provider immediately.
    B. Remain in an upright position for at least 1 hour after taking this drug.
    C. Take this drug 2 hours before or 6 hours after taking an antacid.
    D. Drink at least 3 L of fluid daily while taking this drug.

16. Which actions will the nurse take to prevent disease transmission when caring for a client who has an infection with a multidrug resistant organism? **Select all that apply**.
    A. Taking a prophylactic antibiotic daily
    B. Showering as soon as reaching home after work
    C. Remaining at least 6 feet away from infected clients
    D. Keeping work clothes separate from personal clothes
    E. Wearing scrubs and changing clothes before leaving work
    F. Wearing gloves while drawing blood for laboratory assessment

17. Which client is the nurse **most** likely to recommend for directly observed therapy (DOT)?
    A. Older client with poor dentition who requires liquid medications
    B. Homeless man with tuberculosis (TB) prescribed four anti-TB drugs daily
    C. College student prescribed oral antibiotics for a sexually transmitted infection
    D. Athlete with methicillin-resistant *Staphylococcus aureus* (MRSA) infection on the hand

18. Which action will the nurse take **first** to **prevent harm** when an assistive personnel (AP) reports that an 88-year-old client has a temperature of 100.2°F (37.9°C)?
    A. Administer prescribed acetaminophen.
    B. Assess the client for other indications of infection.
    C. Instruct the AP to recheck the temperature in 4 hours.
    D. Report the temperature elevation to the primary health care provider.

19. Which change in a client's white blood cell differential does the nurse interpret as associated with a severe or prolonged bacterial infection?
    A. Increased immature neutrophils
    B. Increased lymphocytes
    C. Increased eosinophils
    D. Increased monocytes

20. Which action performed during hand hygiene by an assistive personnel does the nurse need to correct?
    A. Wetting hands before applying soap
    B. Using hot water and a scrub brush
    C. Using friction under running water
    D. Washing for at least 15 seconds

21. Which actions will the nurse take when a client is placed on Droplet Precautions? **Select all that apply**.
    A. Using chlorhexidine for handwashing
    B. Wearing a disposable gown whenever entering the client's room
    C. Using a mask when within 6 feet of the client
    D. Putting a mask on the client whenever transport is necessary
    E. Double gloving before entering the client's room
    F. Prohibiting all visitors

22. When will the nurse draw blood from a client who has been ordered to have a serum trough level of the prescribed antibiotic measured?
    A. At the halfway interval between two scheduled doses
    B. 30 minutes before the next ordered dose
    C. 60 minutes after the next ordered dose
    D. Immediately after giving a scheduled dose

23. Which response during sponging of a client with a high fever indicates to the nurse that cooling may be occurring too quickly?
    A. Increased temperature
    B. Decreased urine output
    C. Acute confusion
    D. Shivering

24. What is the **priority action** for the nurse to take for a client who has just been diagnosed with scabies?
    A. Provide meticulous mouth care.
    B. Place the client on Contact Precautions.
    C. Give the client an antipyretic medication.
    D. Perform precise measurement of intake and output.

Chapter 21 Answer Key

1. B, F
   Colonization is the presence of microorganisms (often pathogenic) in the tissues of the host that do not cause symptomatic disease because of normal flora. Options B and F are consistent with this definition. Option A is incorrect because the client has disease symptoms although the organism remains unknown, and option E is incorrect because the client has infectious symptoms consistent with the organisms in the culture. In option C, the client is at increased risk for infection development but is not known to be harboring any pathogenic organisms. For option D, the client has an actual known infection and the assistive personnel is not using the recommended precautions to prevent spread.

2. A.
   Although all behaviors are appropriate actions for the client to take to reduce infection risk, only the action of option A helps reduce the risk of infection caused by normal flora of the intestinal tract from improperly entering the urinary tract (which should be a sterile site).

3. A, D
   Animate reservoirs include people, animals, and insects. COVID-19 influenza and mosquito-borne malaria are the examples in this list that meet the criteria. Romaine lettuce, kitty litter, stethoscopes, and aspergillus mold are inanimate reservoirs. Aspergillus is a newly designated inanimate reservoir of mold spores that

becomes environmental particulate matter when released into the atmosphere such as during extensive renovation of older buildings.

4.   A, B, C, E, F
Drug therapies that cause any degree of immunosuppression, such as corticosteroids or anti-rejection drugs, increase the risk for infection. Artificial (synthetic) medical devices also increase the risk for infection as do devices that provide a direct access to the client's internal environment and bypass normal protections, such as indwelling urinary catheters and endotracheal/tracheal tubes. Although diabetes mellitus increases a client's infection risk, this is not a medical or surgical intervention. Advancing age also increases a client's infection risk but is not a medical or surgical intervention. Diuretics do not increase infection risk.

5.   A, B, E
Client factors that increase infection risk include cigarette smoking and drinking substantial amounts of alcohol daily. Living in crowded conditions, especially in institutions, also increases the risk for infection transmission. Hormone-based contraceptives, eating a balanced vegetarian diet, and regular participation in low-impact exercise do not increase a client's susceptibility to infection.

6.   D
A biofilm is a complex of microorganisms that group together and form a gel-like coating (glycocalyx) that supports continued growth of the microorganisms. Effective treatment or prevention starts with disruption of biofilm. Human biofilms include plaque on teeth and gums, a coating on and in the crypts of tonsils, and as a layer of exudate in wounds. They do not usually form on normal skin or mucous membrane.

7.   B
Influenza is spread by droplets, which are heavy and do not travel far in the air. The CDC recommends prevention by remaining at least 6 feet away from the client, which is farther than the droplets travel when the client sneezes or coughs. Influenza is not spread from toilets. Keeping windows open would be helpful for airborne diseases but is of no value for preventing infections spread by droplets.

8.   C, D
When performing the action of giving either oral or parenteral drugs to any client with diarrhea, including those who have *Clostridium difficile*, only Contact Precautions are needed.

9.   C
Indirect contact transmission occurs when microorganisms are transmitted from a source to a host by passive transfer from a contaminated object. A commonly used object that can be contaminated is a glucose testing device such as a glucometer. Even if blood is not seen on the device, it should be disinfected appropriately between clients to prevent indirect contact transmission of infection. The use of Airborne Precautions, wearing of filter masks, and wearing gloves are examples of preventing direct transmission, not indirect transmission of infection.

10.   B, C, E, F
Thin, delicate skin is easily injured, reducing the barrier function and increasing the risk for infection. A decreased gag reflex increases the risk for aspiration and respiratory infection. Decreased mobility contributes to infection risk in many ways including venous stasis and loss of skin integrity. Increased age is associated with many chronic illnesses such as diabetes, chronic obstructive pulmonary disease, and neurologic impairment that also increase infection risk.

Increased antibody production reflects good immunity, which is not associated with aging. Increased intestinal motility also does not increase infection risk.

11.   A, B, D, F
The recommended immunizations for older adults include the following:
- Pneumococcal 13-valent conjugate vaccine (Prevnar 13) to prevent pneumonia
- Pneumococcal vaccine polyvalent vaccine (Pneumovax) to prevent pneumonia
- Yearly influenza vaccine (trivalent or quadrivalent) to prevent influenza (flu)

- Zoster vaccine recombinant (Shingrix) to prevent shingles (herpes zoster)
- Adult Tdap vaccine to prevent tetanus, diphtheria, and pertussis (whooping cough) (and Td booster every 10 years after Tdap)

Immunization against the human papilloma virus or against the childhood disorders of measles, mumps, and rubella are not recommended.

12. C

Handwashing is recommended instead of ABHRs when hands are visibly dirty or soiled or feel sticky and after toileting (including toileting clients). ABHRs are ineffective against spore-forming organisms such as *Clostridium difficile*, a common cause of health care-associated diarrhea, especially in older adults. A client with diarrhea may have spores in the fecal matter or on his or her body.

13. B

MRSA is an organism that is spread by direct and indirect transmission, not by the airborne or droplet route. The most appropriate type of precautions in addition to Standard Precautions are Contact Precautions. Cutaneous Precautions are not a designated category for protection.

14. C, D

Although all types of infections that can be transmitted by the direct contact, droplet, or the airborne routes are recommended to be cared for in private rooms, those that require private rooms are those clients who have airborne transmitted infections and those who are severely immunosuppressed and need a protected environment. HIV infection and hepatitis C are bloodborne infections and do not require separate private rooms to prevent transmission. Those clients who have infections spread by droplets, such as influenza, and those who have infections spread by contact (MRSA) can be cohorted with another client who has the same infection.

15. C

The drug can combine with any metal or divalent cation such as magnesium, reducing its effectiveness. Because many antacids contain magnesium, clients are taught not to take an antacid with or close to when delafloxacin is taken. There are no fluid requirements or position restrictions associated with the drug. Delafloxacin does not increase the risk for urinary tract infection.

16. B, D, E

To help prevent the transmission of an MDRO, nurses are expected to wear scrubs and change clothes before leaving work. Keeping work clothes separate from personal clothes, as well as taking a shower on reaching home helps rid the body of any unwanted pathogens. Taking prophylactic antibiotics can contribute to the development of MDRO and is most definitely not recommended. Remaining 6 feet away from infected clients is not possible during client care. Wearing gloves during blood draws is part of Standard Precautions and does not specifically address infection prevention for MDROs.

17. B

Tuberculosis is a highly contagious pulmonary infection transmitted by the airborne route that most commonly requires at least 6 months of daily drug therapy with four drugs. Failure to adhere to the drug regimen can result in disease progression, development of resistant organisms, and transmission to others. A homeless person is less likely to be adherent to the regimen for many reasons and would benefit most from directly observed therapy.

18. B

Although the client's temperature is not greatly above normal, older adults usually do not have high fevers even when infection is present. The most appropriate action is for the nurse to assess the client for other indications of infection before notifying the primary health care provider. Because this low-grade fever could represent a serious infection in an older client, administering acetaminophen is not performed before assessment to prevent masking the infection. Rechecking the temperature in 4 hours is not the first or priority action. The nurse will report the temperature elevation to the primary health care provider after gathering other pertinent assessment data.

19. A

A bacterial infection is usually associated with an increased total white blood cell count and an increase in the mature neutrophils. When a bacterial infection is severe or prolonged, the bone marrow increases the release of immature neutrophils, a phenomenon known as a "left shift." This change indicates that the body can no longer keep pace with the infection and the client is at increased risk for sepsis. An elevated lymphocyte count is associated with viral infections. An elevated eosinophil count is associated with allergic reactions. An elevated monocyte count is associated with mononucleosis.

20. B

Using hot water and scrub brushes can injure the skin surface and may cause open areas in which microorganisms can enter. Although friction is required for good hand hygiene, abrading the skin with a brush is not.

21. C, D

Infections spread by droplet transmission are heavy and released when the client sneezes or coughs. These droplets travel short distances, usually only 3 feet or less, and do not remain in the air. Wearing a mask within 6 feet of the client and having the client wear a mask whenever he or she is out of the room is all that is needed. Visitors are permitted but must remain at least 3 feet away from the client or wear a mask. Soap and water for handwashing is sufficient and gowns are not needed.

22. B

Peak and trough levels may be measured to determine the consistent blood levels of a prescribed antibiotic. A specimen for a trough level (lowest serum drug concentration) is drawn about 30 minutes before the next scheduled dose. Specimens for peak levels are drawn about 60 minutes after a dose is given.

23. D

Shivering during any form of external cooling usually indicates that the client is being cooled too quickly. A rising temperature indicates the cooling method is not effective. Neither acute confusion nor changing urine output indicate excessive or too rapid cooling.

24. B

Scabies is an infectious mite infestation of the skin that can be transmitted by both direct and indirect contact. This infection is not oral and does not cause fever. In addition, it has no deleterious effect on kidney function.

22
CHAPTER

Assessment of Skin, Hair, and Nails

1. What is the **priority** medical/surgical concept when the nurse assesses a client and finds reddened scratch marks on the right forearm?
   A. Infection
   B. Immunity
   C. Cellular regulation
   D. Tissue integrity

2. Which roles of a client's intact skin will the nurse consider **most important? Select all that apply.**
   A. Body temperature regulation
   B. Protection against infection
   C. Providing nutrition to underlying cells
   D. Maintaining fluid and electrolyte balance
   E. Sensory function to provide comfort
   F. Aid in elimination of excess CO_2

3. What is the **most** accurate method for the nurse to use when assessing cyanosis in a dark-skinned client admitted for pneumonia?
   A. Check the conjunctivae and nail beds for a bluish tinge color.
   B. Observe for asymmetrical skin color changes.
   C. Auscultate for decreased breath sounds in the lung fields.
   D. Inspect the palms and soles for a yellow-tinged color.

4. Which assessment technique would the nurse use to check the skin turgor of a client who is at risk for hypovolemia?
   A. Push on the skin with thumbs and observe for blanching.
   B. Gently pinch the skin on the back of the hand and observe for tenting.
   C. Brush the skin surface back and forth while observing for flaking.
   D. Push on the skin over the tibia and observe for depth of indentation.

5. What is the **best** site for the nurse to assess skin for dehydration in an older adult client?
   A. Forearm
   B. Mid-thigh
   C. Forehead
   D. Lower abdomen

6. What is the **best** method for the nurse to complete a client's skin assessment while effectively using time management?
   A. Examine the client's skin while bathing or assisting with hygiene
   B. Perform the examination when the client willingly consents and agrees
   C. Question the assistive personnel (AP) who has completed the client's bath
   D. Check the skin assessment from the previous shift and look for changes

7. Age-related changes in the integumentary system include **decreases** in which factors? **Select all that apply.**
   A. Rate of nail growth
   B. Thickness of epidermis
   C. Dermal blood flow
   D. Thickening of the nail
   E. Vitamin D production
   F. Epidermal permeability

8. Which skin changes does the nurse expect to see in an older adult client as a result of a decreased number of active melanocytes?
   A. Increased skin transparency
   B. Decreased skin firmness and elasticity
   C. Slowed and decreased healing
   D. Increased sensitivity to sun exposure

9. Which factors are included in the ABCDE features associated with skin cancer? **Select all that apply.**
   A. Evolving or changing of any feature
   B. Diameter greater than 5 mm
   C. Crusting, bleeding, or itching
   D. Color variation within a lesion
   E. Border regularity
   F. Asymmetry of shape

10. When regulating body temperature, how much evaporative water can the eccrine sweat glands lose in one day?
    A. 500-600 mL/day
    B. 700-900 mL/day
    C. 2-4 L/day
    D. 10-12 L/day

11. What area of a dark-skinned client would the nurse assess for petechiae when the client is at risk for thrombocytopenia?
    A. Palmar surface
    B. Anterior chest
    C. Oral mucosa
    D. Periorbital area

12. For a **decrease** in which integumentary factor would the nurse avoid taping the skin on an older adult client?
    A. Vitamin D production
    B. Dermal blood flow
    C. Thickness of epidermis
    D. Melanocyte activity

13. When caring for an older adult, what skin change would cause the nurse to keep the client's room warmer?
    A. Decreased number of active melanocytes
    B. Decreased layer of subcutaneous fat
    C. Decreased thickness or epidermis
    D. Decreased sebum production

14. Which questions would the nurse ask to determine if a client with a rash is having a new allergic reaction? **Select all that apply.**
    A. "Is your skin usually flakey or dry?"
    B. "Are you taking any new medications?"
    C. "Have you been using any different soaps, cosmetics, or lotions?"
    D. "Have you noticed any bruises or brownish discolorations?"
    E. "Have you been exposed to any new cleaning solutions?"
    F. "Have you had any recent changes in your diet?"

15. Which skin assessment finding in an older adult client is **most important** for the nurse to report to the primary health care provider (PHCP) for follow-up?
    A. Presence of cherry hemangiomas
    B. Multiple brownish liver spots on the arms
    C. Dry and flakey skin on the lower extremities
    D. Irregular light-brown macule (6.5 cm) on the right scapula

16. Which actions would the nurse take when a client has decreased eccrine and apocrine gland activity? **Select all that apply.**
    A. Instruct the client to use soap with a high fat content.
    B. Assess skin for size and shape of pores or comedones.
    C. Use the oral mucosa to assess for cyanosis
    D. Teach the client to avoid frequent bathing with hot water.
    E. Suggest wearing hats to prevent heat loss in cold weather.
    F. Encourage the client to apply moisturizers after bathing.

17. When the nurse takes a client's medication history after noting the presence of ecchymoses, which types of drugs are of concern? **Select all that apply.**
    A. Aspirin products
    B. Oral antidiabetic agents
    C. Anticoagulants
    D. Long-term corticosteroids
    E. Histamine blockers
    F. Short-term loop diuretics

18. Which question would the nurse ask when assessing a female client who reports an unusual increase in facial hair?
    A. "Does your skin seem unusually dry and flakey?"
    B. "Have you noticed any bruising or unusual bleeding?"
    C. "Are you having trouble with urination or moving your bowels?"
    D. "Have you noticed any deepening of your voice quality?"

19. Which is the **best** rationale for the nurse to use to encourage a client to seek treatment for dandruff?
    A. Dandruff is a cosmetic problem but appearance is important to self-esteem.
    B. Severe dandruff is caused by excessive oiliness and can cause hair loss.
    C. Dandruff flakes are caused by dry scalp and suggest possible dehydration.
    D. Brushing your hair everyday can prevent dandruff but may weaken hair follicles.

20. Which technique does the nurse use to assess the "...health of the nails of a client with very dark skin."
    A. Obtain a color chart to identify the normal color of nails for dark-skinned clients.
    B. Gently squeeze the end of the finger exerting downward pressure, then release it.
    C. Observe the nail bed for a pale pink color and a shiny, smooth surface
    D. Soak the fingertips in warm water, then gently push back cuticles.

21. Which assessment techniques would the nurse use when checking a client with dark skin for inflammation? **Select all that apply.**
    A. Compare affected area with nonaffected area for increased warmth.
    B. Examine the nail beds, palms, and soles for blue tinge.
    C. Compare the skin color of affected area with the same area on the opposite side.
    D. Examine the sclera nearest to the iris rather than the corners of the eye.
    E. Check the oral mucosa or conjunctive for petechiae.
    F. Examine the skin of the affected area to see if it is shiny, taut, or pits with pressure.

22. What does the nurse suspect when a client has skin that is tight and shiny over the lower extremities?
    A. Fluid retention and edema
    B. Early stage of infection
    C. Early signs of poor circulation
    D. Bleeding into the skin

23. What **priority** instruction would the nurse provide the assistive personnel (AP) who is to bathe a client with skin that is not intact and is draining?
    A. Save any fingernail clippings or hair samples for testing.
    B. Wear clean gloves and use Standard Precautions.
    C. Have a second AP assist you to get the client out of bed.
    D. Let the client soak in the tub for 15 minutes before rinsing.

24. For which conditions, which could contribute to overall hygiene, would the nurse assess when a client presents with matted hair, body odor, and soiled clothes? **Select all that apply.**
    A. Intact sensory functions (e.g., sight, smell)
    B. Range of motion and strength
    C. Access to shower and laundry
    D. Client's currently prescribed drugs
    E. Perception of his or her appearance
    F. Knowledge (memory) of hygiene care

25. What diagnostic test does the nurse prepare a client for when the PHCP prescribes a test to determine if the client has a fungal infection of the skin?
    A. Punch biopsy
    B. KOH test
    C. Shave biopsy
    D. Wood's light exam

26. What is the **best** place for the nurse to examine a fair-skinned client for yellow discoloration when jaundice is suspected?
    A. Palms
    B. Soles
    C. Sclera
    D. Nail beds

27. What is the **best** method for the nurse to collect a superficial specimen from a raised lesion for a suspected fungal infection in a client's groin?
    A. Express exudate from a lesion and use a sterile swab to collect fluid.
    B. Obtain a small sample of tissue from the groin using needle biopsy.
    C. Use a scalpel or razor blade and move it parallel to the skin surface to remove the tissue specimen.
    D. Have the PHCP do a deep excision with a scalpel followed by closure with sutures.

28. Which specimen would the nurse instruct the assistive personnel (AP) to **immediately** place on ice and transport to the lab as soon as possible?
    A. Vesicle fluid taken by sterile technique and placed in a viral culture tube
    B. Punch biopsy performed with sterile technique for collection of a tissue piece
    C. Exudate taken by sterile technique and swabbed on a bacterial culture medium
    D. Aspirate taken by sterile technique and placed in a bacterial culture tube

29. Which teaching points would the nurse be sure to share with a client scheduled for a punch biopsy? **Select all that apply.**
    A. A local anesthetic will be injected into the site.
    B. A circular instrument will cut out a tissue sample.
    C. The site will always require suturing after the procedure.
    D. You will have a scar similar to a healed surgical incision.
    E. Antibiotic ointment may be prescribed to reduce the risk for infection.
    F. Keep a dry dressing on the site until your sutures are removed.

30. Which equipment would the nurse obtain to assist the PHCP in examining a light-skinned client for evaluation of skin pigment changes?
    A. Glass slides
    B. Biopsy tray
    C. Bright nonfluorescent light
    D. Wood's lamp

31. Which skin disorder is most associated with a familial predisposition?
    A. Scabies
    B. Cellulitis
    C. Psoriasis
    D. Ringworm

32. Which preprocedural teaching will the nurse provide for a client suspected of a bacterial cellulitis?
    A. The primary health care provider will inject bacteriostatic saline, withdraw it, and send the aspirate to the lab for culture.
    B. The crusts will be removed with normal saline, then the underlying exudate will be swabbed for a specimen.
    C. A smear will be obtained from the base of the lesion and examined in the lab under a microscope.
    D. A cotton-tipped applicator will be used to obtain vesicle fluid from intact lesions.

33. What skin manifestations does the nurse expect to observe in a client during impending shock?
    A. Dry, flushed appearance
    B. Poor turgor with a rough texture
    C. Bluish color that blanches
    D. White, pale, cool skin

34. Which areas would the nurse give special attention to when assessing an obese older adult?
    A. Mucous membranes
    B. Skinfolds
    C. Scalp
    D. Nails

35. What changes in color does the nurse expect when assessing a client with polycythemia vera? **Select all that apply.**
    A. Brown localized skin areas
    B. Reddish blue generalized skin color
    C. Red color localized to area of involvement
    D. Dark red nail beds
    E. Diffuse blue discoloration of nails
    F. Yellow to brown nail beds

36. Which laboratory test would the nurse be sure to check when finding a large area of ecchymoses while assessing a client?
    A. Hemoglobin level
    B. White blood cell count
    C. Platelet count
    D. International normalized ratio (INR)

37. Which assessment finding does the nurse use as the **best** indicator of a client's healthy nails?
    A. Nail bed color is normal for the client.
    B. Nail bed blanches with gentle pressure.
    C. Nails are well groomed and nicely shaped.
    D. Nail surface is smooth and transparent.

38. For which client will the nurse instruct the assistive personnel (AP) to use a lift sheet when assisting with movement in bed?
    A. Older adult client on steroids with thin, fragile skin
    B. Client with type 2 diabetes and delayed wound healing
    C. Obese client with moisture in skin folds
    D. Client with a substance use problem

39. Which term would the nurse use to document a client's skin lesions that are widespread involving most of the body?
    A. Circumscribed
    B. Universal
    C. Linear
    D. Diffuse

40. Which terms would the nurse use to document a client's rash that is red, raised, and itching over most of his or her body?
    A. Red, macular, lichenified
    B. Cyanotic, annular, popular
    C. Red, universal, circinate
    D. Erythematous, diffuse, pruritic

Chapter 22 Answer Key

1. D
   This client has a break in the skin, which is the largest organ of the body. Skin tissue integrity plays a major role in protection by protecting the body against invasion of pathogenic organisms as the first, second, and third lines of defense. The question does not give indications of infection or immunity, nor does it suggest a problem with cellular regulation (the genetic and physiologic processes that control cellular growth, replication, differentiation, and function to maintain homeostasis).

2. A, B, D, E
   Skin tissue integrity plays a major role in protection by protecting the body against invasion of pathogenic organisms. Intact skin helps regulate body temperature and maintains fluid and electrolyte balance. The skin's sensory function allows the use of touch as an intervention to provide comfort, relieve pain, and communicate caring. The vascular system provides nutrients to cells and the lungs eliminate excess carbon dioxide (CO_2).

3. A
   In a dark-skinned client with cyanosis, the lips and tongue are gray; the palms, soles, conjunctivae, and nail beds have a bluish tinge. To support these findings, assess for other indicators of hypoxia, including tachycardia, hypotension, changes in respiratory rate, decreased breath sounds, and changes in cognition. These secondary findings are supportive but do not indicate cyanosis. Yellow-colored soles and palms are associated with jaundice.

4. B
   Turgor indicates the amount of skin elasticity. Gently pinch the client's skin between your thumb and forefinger and then release. If skin turgor is normal, the skin immediately returns to its original state when released. Poor skin turgor is seen as "tenting" of the skin, with a slower and more gradual return to the original state. Observing for flaking would be used to assess for dry skin; blanching for perfusion; and indentation for edema.

5. C
Older adult clients experience degeneration of elastic fibers in the skin which results in decreased tone (firmness) and elasticity. The best places to check skin turgor for older adults is the forehead or the chest. To avoid mistaking dehydration for dry skin in an older adult, assess skin turgor on the forehead or chest. Use of other sites may provide inaccurate findings.

6. A
A thorough assessment of the skin is best performed with the client undressed. Incorporate skin examination as a routine part of daily care during the bath or when assisting with hygiene. The nurse should not depend on information from the previous shift or the assistive personnel. While it is preferable that the client be willing and agreeable, this may not help with time management, which is the focus of this question.

7. A, B, C, E
Changes in the integumentary system related to aging include decreases in vitamin D production, thickness of epidermis, dermal blood flow, and rate of nail growth. There are increases in nail thickening and epidermal permeability.

8. D
Melanocytes are pigment-producing cells found at the basement membrane. Melanin protects the skin from damage by UV light, which stimulates melanin production. For this reason, people with dark skin (and thus more melanin) are less likely to experience sunburn than people with lighter skin. When there is a decrease in melanocytes, the client is more sensitive to sun exposure and is taught to wear protective clothing and a wide-brimmed hat.

9. A, D, F
The nurse assesses each lesion on a client for these ABCDE features that are associated with skin cancer: **A**symmetry of shape; **B**order irregularity; **C**olor variation within one lesion; **D**iameter greater than ¼ of an inch or 6 mm; and **E**volving or changing in any feature (shape, size, color, elevation, itching, bleeding, or crusting). A client who has a lesion with one or more of the ABCDE features should be evaluated by a dermatologist or surgeon.

10. D
Eccrine sweat glands arise from the epithelial cells. They are found over the entire skin surface and are not associated with the hair follicle. The odorless, colorless secretions of these glands are important in body temperature regulation. This sweat and the resultant water evaporation can cause the body to lose up to 10 to 12 L of fluid in a single day.

11. C
Petechiae are pinpoint, red spots on the mucous membranes, palate, conjunctivae, or skin. If a client has dark skin and thrombocytopenia, petechiae may be present on the oral mucosa or conjunctiva. Petechiae are rarely visible in dark skin.

12. C
For an older adult with decreased epidermal thickness, the nurse would avoid taping the client's skin; handle clients carefully to reduce skin friction and shear; and assess for excessive dryness or moisture. For decreased vitamin D production, the client would be encouraged to take a multiple vitamin or a calcium supplement with vitamin D. For decreased blood flow, the client is taught to apply moisturizers when the skin is still moist and to avoid agents that promote skin dryness. For decreased epidermal permeability, the client is instructed to avoid exposure to skin irritants.

13. B
A client with a decreased subcutaneous fat layer is at increased risk for hypothermia and is taught to dress warmly, as well as may need a warmer temperature in his or her room. Decreased melanocytes increase the risk of sun sensitivity. Decreased epidermal thickness causes skin transparency and fragility (these clients must be handled carefully and tape should be avoided). Decreased sebum production can lead to increased size of nasal pores.

14. B, C, E, F

   A new allergy would suggest that something has changed for the client such as new drugs, new products (soap, cosmetics, lotions, cleaning solutions), or changes in diet. Bruises or brownish discolorations suggest a bleeding problem. Flakey or dry skin suggests the need for something to moisturize the skin.

15. D

   A client's lesion that is evolving or changing in any feature (shape, size, color, elevation, itching, bleeding, or crusting) should be evaluated by a surgeon or dermatologist (remember ABCDE). Cherry hemangiomas are the result of proliferation of capillaries and are benign. Dry skin may require application of a moisturizer. Multiple liver spots are normal changes that occur with aging.

16. A, D, F

   Decreased eccrine and apocrine gland activity leads to increased susceptibility to dry skin. The nurse will: urge clients to use soaps with a high fat content; teach clients to avoid frequent bathing with hot water; and teach clients to apply moisturizers after bathing while skin is moist. Assessment of pores and comedones is done for decreased sebum secretion. Using the oral mucosa to assess for cyanosis is done for decreased nail bed blood flow, and suggesting a hat in cold weather would be done for decreased hair follicles and rate of hair growth.

17. A, C, D

   Certain drugs (e.g., aspirin, warfarin, corticosteroids) and low platelet counts lead to easy or excessive bruising. Anticoagulants and decreased numbers of platelets disrupt clotting action, resulting in ecchymosis. Anticoagulants, aspirin products, and long-term corticosteroids increase a client's risk for bleeding and ecchymoses (bruising). Oral antidiabetic agents are prescribed mainly for type 2 diabetes; short-term loop diuretics for excess fluid; and histamine blockers to decrease the production of acid in the stomach. None of these drugs are known to reduce blood clotting.

18. D

   Increased hair growth across the face and chest in women is a sign of hirsutism. It may occur on the face of a woman as part of aging, as a sign of hormonal imbalance, or as a side effect of drug therapy. If hirsutism is present, the nurse looks for changes in fat distribution and capillary fragility, which can occur in Cushing's disease, and for clitoral enlargement and deepening of the voice, which may indicate ovarian dysfunction.

19. B

   The flaking that occurs with dandruff causes many adults to mistakenly think the scalp is too dry; however, it is actually a problem of excessive oil production. Dandruff by itself is a cosmetic problem, but a very oily scalp can induce inflammatory changes with redness and itching. Severe inflammatory dandruff can extend to the eyebrows and the skin of the face and neck. If severe dandruff is not treated, alopecia (hair loss) can occur. The client is taught that dandruff is not caused by dryness and should be treated to prevent hair loss.

20. B

   Regardless of skin color, the healthy nail blanches (lightens) with pressure. Blanch the nail bed to see whether the color changes with pressure. The nurse gently squeezes the end of the finger or toe, exerting downward pressure on the nail bed, and then releases the pressure. Color changes caused by blood flow changes as pressure is applied and returns to the original state when pressure is released. Color caused by pigment deposits remains unchanged.

21. A, C, F

   To examine a dark-skinned client for inflammation, these techniques are used: compare the affected area with nonaffected area for increased warmth; examine the skin of the affected area to determine whether it is shiny or taut or pits with pressure; compare the skin color of the affected area with the same area on the opposite side of the body; and palpate the affected area and compare it with the unaffected area to determine whether texture is different (affected area may feel hard). Checking for bleeding includes if a client has thrombocytopenia, petechiae may be present on the oral mucosa or conjunctiva. Examining the nails, soles, and palms is used to assess for cyanosis. Assessing for jaundice includes examination of the sclera nearest to the iris rather than the corners of the eye.

22. A

Edema causes the skin to appear shiny, taut (tightly stretched), and paler than uninvolved surrounding skin. During skin inspection, the nurse documents the location, distribution, and color of areas of edema. Redness and swelling would be signs of infection. Decreased pulses and dry skin with flaking and scaling are typical of decreased circulation. Bleeding into the skin is abnormal and results in purpura (bleeding under the skin that may progress from red to purple to brownish-yellow), petechiae, and ecchymosis.

23. B

For a client with nonintact and draining skin, use of clean gloves and Standard Precautions is the standard of care. Gloves should be used to examine the skin, as well as to bathe the client and perform any dressing changes. Soaking in a bathtub would increase the risk of spreading infection from draining skin. Nail and hair samples would not be saved unless prescribed by the PHCP. The client would not be gotten out of bed without PHCP orders and when this is done, a lift would be used.

24. A, B, C, D, E, F

The nurse asks about living conditions and bathing practices. Information is collected about drug and substance use. Prescribed drugs, over-the-counter (OTC) drugs, herbal preparations or remedies, and tobacco use can cause skin reactions or affect skin appearance or function. Weakness and poor range of motion can interfere with self-care as can reduced access to a shower or laundry. A client's cognitive state and nonintact sensory functions can prevent recognition that there is a problem with his or her appearance to self or others.

25. B

Cultures for fungal infection are obtained by using a tongue blade and gently scraping scales from skin lesions into a clean container. The specimen is also treated with a potassium hydroxide (KOH) solution and examined microscopically. A positive fungal infection shows branched hyphae when viewed under a microscope after treatment with KOH and may eliminate the need for a culture. For a punch biopsy, a small circular cutting instrument, or "punch," ranging in diameter from 2 to 6 mm, is used. After the site is injected with a local anesthetic, a small plug of tissue is cut and removed. Shave biopsies remove only the part of the skin that rises above the surrounding tissue when injected with a local anesthetic. A scalpel or razor blade is moved parallel to the skin surface to remove the tissue specimen. For a Wood's lamp examination, a handheld, long-wavelength ultraviolet (black) light may be used during examination. Exposure of certain skin infections with this light produces a specific color, such as blue-green or red, that can be used to identify the infection.

26. C

To detect jaundice, the best place on the body to assess is: the sclera nearest to the iris rather than the corners of the eye; a second place to check for yellow tinge is the oral mucous membranes, especially the hard palate. The nail beds, palms, and soles would be examined for blue tinge if a client had cyanosis.

27. C

Shave biopsies remove only the part of the skin that rises above the surrounding tissue when injected with a local anesthetic. A scalpel or razor blade is moved parallel to the skin surface to remove the tissue specimen. Shave biopsies are usually indicated for superficial or raised lesions. Suturing is not needed.

28. A

Cultures for viral infection are indicated if a herpes virus infection is suspected. A cotton-tipped applicator is used to obtain vesicle fluid from intact lesions. Viral culture specimen tubes must be placed on ice **immediately** after specimens are obtained and are transported to the laboratory as soon as possible. None of the other specimens must be placed on ice.

29. A, B, E
For a punch biopsy, a small circular cutting instrument, or "punch," ranging in diameter from 2 to 6 mm, is used. After the site is injected with a local anesthetic, a small plug of tissue is cut and removed. The site may be closed with sutures or may be allowed to heal without suturing. After a punch, the client is taught that only a small amount of skin is removed and scarring is minimal. Antibiotic ointment may be prescribed to prevent infection. The dry dressing should be kept in place for at least 8 hours, and the site cleaned daily after the dressing is removed. Tap water or saline is used to remove any dried blood or crusts.

30. D
A handheld, long-wavelength ultraviolet (black) light or Wood's lamp may be used during examination. Exposure of certain skin infections with this light produces a specific color, such as blue-green or red, that can be used to identify the infection. Hypopigmented skin is more prominent when it is viewed under black light, making evaluation of pigment changes in lighter skin easier. This examination is carried out in a darkened room and does not cause discomfort.

31. C
Some skin problems (e.g., psoriasis, keloid formation, eczema) have a familial predisposition. Others are transmittable disorders (e.g., ringworm, scabies). Clients are asked about immediate family members' current health with regard to skin problems. Cellulitis is a deep bacterial infection.

32. A
A biopsy of deep bacterial infections may be needed to obtain a specimen for culture. If bacterial cellulitis is suspected, the primary health care provider can inject nonbacteriostatic

saline deep into the tissue and then aspirate it back; the aspirant is sent for culture.

33. D
When a client is going into shock from blood loss, the nurse would expect to assess skin that is pale, white, and cool. Skin temperature would be decreased. Nail beds would also be pale.

34. B
Depending on a client's degree of ability to perform ADLs, hard-to-reach areas (e.g., perirectal and inguinal skinfolds, axillae, feet) may be less clean than other skin surface areas. Clients are positioned to promote air circulation to skinfolds. Increased moisture is commonly found in skinfolds, especially for an obese client.

35. B, D
With polycythemia vera, the skin has a generalized reddish-blue tinge and the nail beds are dark red. Skin that is blue is related to increased deoxygenated blood and localized brown is associated with increased melanin. Blue nails (cyanosis) are commonly related to respiratory problems and yellow to brown nails to jaundice (See Table 22.2 and 22.5) for more information about alterations in skin and nail bed colors.

36. C
Ecchymoses (bruises) are larger areas of hemorrhage. In older adults, bruising is common after minor trauma to the skin. Certain drugs (e.g., aspirin, warfarin, corticosteroids) and low platelet counts lead to easy or excessive bruising. Anticoagulants and decreased numbers of platelets disrupt clotting action, resulting in ecchymosis.

37. B
Regardless of skin color, the healthy nail blanches (lightens) with pressure. During examination, the client's fingers and toes should be free of any surface pressure that interferes with local blood flow or alters the appearance of the digits. To differentiate between color changes from the underlying blood supply and those from pigment deposits, the nurse blanches the nail bed to see whether the color changes with pressure.

The end of the finger or toe is gently squeezed, exerting downward pressure on the nail bed, and then the pressure is released. Color changes caused by blood flow changes as pressure is applied and returns to the original state when pressure is released.

38. A

A client with decreased dermal thickness has very thin, transparent skin that is at risk for trauma. Steroids are known to induce skin thinning also. This client would be most at risk and in most need of use of a lift sheet when assisting him or her to move in bed to avoid shearing. All clients should be assessed regularly for risks to skin.

39. D

Diffuse lesions are widespread, involving most of the body with intervening areas of normal skin. Circumscribed lesions are well-defined with sharp borders. Universal lesions involve the entire body, and linear lesions occur in a straight line. (See Table 22.3).

40. D

Erythematous refers to redness of the skin; diffuse is widespread over most of the body; and pruritic refers to itching. (See Table 22.3 and key terms list).

23 CHAPTER

Concepts of Care of Patients with Skin Problems

1. Which medical-surgical concept would the nurse designate as the **highest** priority for a client with pressure injuries of both heels?
   A. Fluid and electrolyte balance
   B. Immunity
   C. Tissue integrity
   D. Cellular regulation

2. Which clients would the nurse understand are at risk for pressure injuries? **Select all that apply.**
   A. A middle-aged quadriplegic client who is alert and conversant
   B. An ambulatory client who has occasional urinary incontinence
   C. A very thin client who sits for long periods in a chair and refuses meals
   D. An obese client who must be assisted to move and turn in the bed
   E. An older adult who is bedridden and in late stage of Alzheimer's disease
   F. A client who is slightly confused but can use the bathroom with assistance

3. What **collaborative** action would the nurse take to promote wound healing for a thin, malnourished client who had emergency abdominal surgery?
   A. Encourage the client to be out of bed as soon as possible.
   B. Consult with the registered dietitian nutritionist (RDN) about a high-protein diet.
   C. Instruct the client and his or her caretaker about appropriate dressing changes.
   D. Delegate complete morning care including a bed bath to the assistive personnel (AP).

4. Which technique would the nurse use to check for tunneling when assessing a large pressure injury on a client's hip with a small opening in the skin draining purulent material?
   A. Use a sterile cotton-tipped applicator to probe gently for the tunnel.
   B. Using gloves, palpate the surface of the wound for spongy areas.
   C. Flush the wound with sterile saline and watch the flow of the fluid.
   D. Press around the edges of the wound and observe for erythema.

5. Which interventions would the nurse use to **prevent harm** from development of a pressure injury in a client with a prolonged coma? **Select all that apply.**
   A. Use pillows or padding devices to keep the client's heels free from pressure.
   B. When positioning a client on his or her side, position at a 30-degree tilt.
   C. Use donut-shaped pillows under the coccyx when elevating the head of the bed 90 degrees.
   D. Turn and reposition the client at least every 2 hours during all shifts.
   E. Place pillows or foam wedges between two bony surfaces or between bony surfaces and the bed.
   F. Massage reddened areas to improve blood return and assist with healing.

6. Which instruction would the nurse give the assistive personnel (AP) about how to perform skin care on a client at risk for pressure injury because of immobility and incontinence?
    A. Use an antibiotic soap and rinse with hot water to remove all soap residue.
    B. Scrub vigorously to ensure that all dried feces are removed.
    C. After cleaning, apply a light layer of powder or talc directly on the perineum.
    D. Clean the skin and moisturize with dimethazone, zinc oxide, lanolin, or petrolatum.

7. How will the nurse document assessment findings on a client's coccyx region that is reddened, is intact, and does not blanch when pressure is applied?
    A. Stage 1 pressure injury
    B. Stage 2 pressure injury
    C. Stage 3 pressure injury
    D. Unstageable pressure injury

8. What would the nurse be sure to do before documenting a client's pressure injury changes with a series of photographs?
    A. Close the door and turn on the overhead light.
    B. Pull the bedside curtains for client privacy.
    C. Obtain informed consent from the client.
    D. Consult with the primary health care provider.

9. Which clients with pressure injuries would the nurse assess as at **high** risk for development of infection? **Select all that apply.**
    A. Client with rotator cuff injury awaiting surgery
    B. Older client with a low white blood cell (WBC) count
    C. Client with type 1 diabetes mellitus
    D. Older client with high cholesterol who walks a mile every day
    E. Client with chronic obstructive pulmonary disease (COPD) on steroids
    F. Older client with large abdominal incision who needs help with repositioning

10. Which finding indicating infection in a client would the nurse report to the health care provider **immediately**?
    A. Progressive decrease in injury size and depth
    B. Presence of granulation and re-epithelialization
    C. Beefy red color that grows and fills in the wound
    D. Changes in the quantity, color, or odor of exudate

11. How does the nurse determine which dressing is **best** for a client with a stage 3 pressure injury over the left trochanter area that has a thick exudate?
    A. Select a dressing that helps remove debris by mechanical débridement.
    B. Obtain a prescription to consult with the certified wound care specialist.
    C. Expect the primary health care provider to prescribe a drug for topical débridement.
    D. Obtain a prescription for the type of dressing from primary health care provider.

12. What would the nurse direct the home assistive personnel (AP) to do for an older client who wants to avoid dry skin?
    A. Assist with a complete bath or shower only every other day (wash face, axillae, perineum, and any soiled areas with soap daily).
    B. Generously apply oil and leave it on for 20 minutes; then bathe the client, especially the genital and axillary areas.
    C. Use an antimicrobial skin soap and wash the client carefully; then apply alcohol-based astringent, especially to the legs and arms.
    D. Use hot water with a deodorant soap; then gently pat the client dry and apply oil and cream to the skin.

13. Which intervention would the nurse use to reduce shearing force for an obese client who is on bedrest for the next 3 days?
    A. Place the client in a high Fowler's position.
    B. Instruct the client to use arms and legs to push when moving in bed.
    C. Place the client in a side-lying position at a 30-degree tilt.
    D. Assist the client to get up three to four times daily to a recliner chair.

14. Which finding, when assessing a client's wound for signs of healing or infection, indicates to the nurse that healing is progressing as expected?
    A. Wound surface is excessively moist with a deep reddish-purple color
    B. Area appears pale pink, progressing to a spongy texture with a beefy red color
    C. Eschar starts to lift and separate from the tissue beneath, which appears dry and pale
    D. Tissue is soft and more yellow with substantially increased exudates

15. Which conditions will the nurse consider to be contributing factors for a client with chronic pressure injuries? **Select all that apply.**
    A. Malnutrition
    B. Peripheral vascular disease
    C. Incontinence
    D. Immobility
    E. Pressure relief mattresses
    F. Prolonged bedrest

16. When would the nurse expect to culture a client's pressure injury wound?
    A. Routinely every other day with a sterile culture swab
    B. When there is any exudate from the wound
    C. When clinical or systemic signs of infection are present
    D. When the pressure injury wound first becomes apparent

17. Which client would the nurse monitor carefully when continuous negative-pressure wound therapy (NPWT) is used to facilitate healing?
    A. Client with diabetes mellitus
    B. Client receiving anticoagulation
    C. Client with severe pain
    D. Client hypertension

18. Which expected outcomes are appropriate for a client with a pressure injury? **Select all that apply.**
    A. Client will rate pain at an acceptable level
    B. Client will remain free from local or systemic infections
    C. Client will re-establish skin tissue integrity and restore skin barrier function
    D. Client will verbalize that wound is smaller
    E. Client's wound will show granulation and decrease in size
    F. Client will consume a diet rich in carbohydrates

19. Which **priority** nursing interventions focus on increasing client comfort and preventing skin injury when the client has pruritus? **Select all that apply.**
    A. Administering prescribed antihistamines or topical drugs
    B. Keeping client's fingernails trimmed short
    C. Instructing assistive personnel (AP) to trim toenails
    D. Applying mittens or gloves to client's hands at night
    E. Maintaining daily fluid intake of 3000 mL unless contraindicated
    F. After bathing, patting skin dry rather than rubbing

20. What would the nurse suspect when a client is admitted with a rash of white or red edematous papules or plaques that developed after the client ate seafood?
    A. Urticaria
    B. Pruritus
    C. Eczema
    D. Psoriasis

21. Which question would the nurse ask a client, who has nonspecific eczematous dermatitis, to determine if avoidance therapy is an appropriate intervention?
    A. "Have you noticed a change in the appearance of a mole?"
    B. "Have you used any new soaps, detergents, or personal care products?"
    C. "Does anyone residing in your household have a similar skin problem?"
    D. "Do you have a history of surgery for removal of skin growths?"

22. Which **essential** teaching would the nurse provide for a client who is prescribed diphenhydramine to treat urticaria (hives)?
    A. Warm environments and warm showers will accelerate metabolism and recovery.
    B. Use an emollient cream or lotion after bathing to reduce the itching.
    C. Avoid alcohol consumption, which can potentiate the sedative effects of this drug.
    D. Use an antibacterial soap when bathing and apply topical antibiotic cream after.

23. Which characteristics would the nurse expect to assess for a client with plaque psoriasis? **Select all that apply.**
    A. Raised, red patches covered with silvery white scales
    B. White pustules surrounded by reddened skin
    C. Affected areas usually include scalp, knees, elbows, lower back
    D. Usually starts after a streptococcal infection
    E. May be itchy, painful, or bleeding
    F. Affected areas usually include hands and feet

24. Which **essential** teaching would the nurse provide for a younger female client with psoriasis who is prescribed tazarotene?
    A. This drug can reduce the effectiveness of hormone-based contraceptives.
    B. Tazarotene should be applied to each lesion for only a short period of time.
    C. This drug can help relieve chronic psoriasis but may cause acne.
    D. Tazarotene can cause birth defects even when applied topically.

25. In addition to topical drugs for psoriasis, which therapies would the nurse teach a client to reduce symptoms? **Select all that apply.**
    A. Ultraviolet (UV) irradiation
    B. Oral antibiotics
    C. Photochemotherapy with psoralen
    D. Surgical excision
    E. Excimer lasers
    F. Systemic therapy

26. Which actions would the nurse teach a client and family to use to stop the spread of methicillin-resistant *Staphylococcus aureus* (MRSA)? **Select all that apply.**
    A. Wash your hands with soap and warm water before and after touching the infected area or handling the bandages.
    B. Shower (rather than bathe) daily, using an antibacterial soap.
    C. Sleep in a separate bed from others until the infection is cleared.
    D. Do not share clothing, washcloths, towels, athletic equipment, shavers or razors, or any other personal items.
    E. Avoid close contact with others, including participation in contact sports, until the infection has cleared.
    F. Wash all soiled clothing and linens with hot water and laundry detergent. Dry clothing either in a hot dryer or outside on a clothesline in the sun.

27. For which client would the nurse notify the primary health care provider when a Zostavax vaccine for shingles is prescribed?
    A. Client with diabetes
    B. Client with immunosuppression
    C. Client with Raynaud's disease
    D. Client with hypertension

28. Which information would the nurse teach a client about treatment of pediculosis pubis?
    A. Pubic lice are found only in the genital region of the body.
    B. Abstain from sexual intercourse with any infected person.
    C. Treatment of this condition involves shaving genital hair.
    D. Over-the-counter lindane is a topical drug used to kill the lice.

29. Which condition would the nurse suspect when observing linear ridges on the inner aspects of the wrists and the client reports intense itching especially at night?
    A. Dermatitis
    B. Body lice
    C. Scabies
    D. Head lice

30. Which is the nurse's **best** response when a client diagnosed with bedbug bites states he or she is embarrassed, showers every day, and lives in a clean environment?
    A. "Have you been travelling or staying in a hotel?"
    B. "No need for embarrassment, these things happen."
    C. "Showering will not kill bedbugs."
    D. "Have you seen bedbugs on your clothing?"

31. What type of healing does the nurse assess when a client's surgical wound edges are approximated, closed with sutures, and there is no inflammation?
    A. Healing by third intention
    B. Healing by granulation
    C. Healing by first intention
    D. Healing by second intention

32. How long would the nurse expect a client's partial-thickness wound to heal by epithelialization?
    A. 24 hours
    B. 48 hours
    C. 2 to 3 days
    D. 5 to 7 days

33. What **priority** complication would the nurse suspect when assessing a client with an electrical burn that has an entrance wound on the right shoulder and an exit wound through the left side ribs?
    A. Kidney failure
    B. Cardiac dysrhythmias
    C. Gastrointestinal ileus
    D. Fractured ribs

34. Which assessment findings would the emergency department (ED) nurse expect when a client has a smoke-related inhalation injury? **Select all that apply.**
    A. Soot around the nose or mouth
    B. Singed nasal hairs
    C. Hoarseness of speech
    D. Shortness of breath
    E. Cherry red skin
    F. Cough

35. What is the **priority** focus of prehospital care for a client with a chemical injury burn?
    A. Decontamination
    B. Fluid balance
    C. Airway control
    D. Preventing infection

36. Which teaching strategies would the nurse include when instructing clients about how to prevent burn injuries? **Select all that apply.**
    A. Hot water heaters should be set below 150°F (65.5°C).
    B. Never add a flammable substance to an open flame.
    C. Use sunscreen and protective clothes to avoid sunburn.
    D. Avoid smoking when drinking alcohol or taking drugs that induce sleep.
    E. When space heaters are used, keep flammable objects away from them.
    F. If using home oxygen, do not smoke in the room where oxygen is in use.

37. What would be the nurse's **best** action when a client with a burn injury develops a brassy cough, increased difficulty swallowing, and progressive hoarseness?
    A. Place the client on continuous pulse oximetry.
    B. Instruct the AP to check vital signs every 30 minutes.
    C. Activate the Rapid Response Team.
    D. Establish a second IV access.

38. Which is the **best** action for the nurse to take prior to changing the dressing of a client with a burn injury?
    A. Allow the client to rest and nap for an hour.
    B. Give pain medication 30 minutes prior to dressing change.
    C. Instruct the AP to give the client a complete bath.
    D. Leave the wound open to air for 30 minutes.

39. Which are priorities of care when providing care for a client with a burn injury during the emergent phase? **Select all that apply.**
    A. Securing the airway
    B. Maintaining nutrition status
    C. Supporting circulation and perfusion
    D. Maintaining body temperature
    E. Keeping client comfortable with analgesics
    F. Psychosocial adjustment

40. Which factors increase the risk of complications from a burn injury in an older adult client? **Select all that apply.**
    A. Slower healing time
    B. Thinner skin
    C. Increased inflammatory response
    D. Increased pulmonary compliance
    E. Medical conditions such as diabetes
    F. Increased immune response

41. Which client does the nurse consider to be at **highest** risk for development of skin cancer?
    A. Dark-skinned male who works as a lab technician
    B. Light-skinned female who works as a lifeguard every summer
    C. Older adult who enjoys gardening and wears a large hat
    D. Younger adult who works as a home health assistant

42. Which preventive strategies for skin cancer would the nurse teach to clients and families? **Select all that apply.**
    A. Avoiding sun exposure between 11 a.m. and 3 p.m.
    B. Wearing a hat, opaque clothing, and sunglasses when you are in the sun
    C. Using tanning beds no more than 30 minutes twice a week
    D. Taking pictures of lesions and comparing them month by month
    E. Keeping a "body map" of your skin spots, scars, and lesions
    F. Using sunscreens if your sun exposure will be more than an hour

43. What would the help-line nurse advise a client who states that a skin lesion's color has changed, its size has increased, and its border is irregular?
    A. "Contact your primary health care provider immediately."
    B. "Continue to monitor the changes and take pictures to show your primary health care provider."
    C. "You should go to the nearest emergency department and have the lesion evaluated."
    D. "It may not be anything to worry about, but make an appointment within the next month."

44. Which finding when the nurse assesses a nevus on a client's back would be of concern and warrant further investigation?
    A. Regular and well-defined borders
    B. Uniform dark brown color
    C. Rough surface
    D. Report of itching and bleeding

45. Which client is most likely to be a candidate for Mohs surgery?
    A. Client with squamous cell carcinoma on the nose
    B. Client with joint contractures from burn injuries to the elbows
    C. Client with infected pressure injury in deep tissues over the coccyx
    D. Client with the need to have excessive breast tissue removed

46. What is the **priority** action for the nurse and other interprofessional team members when caring for a client with Stevens-Johnson syndrome?
    A. Treat the subjective symptoms of pain and itching.
    B. Closely observe for signs of renal failure.
    C. Protect against localized skin infection.
    D. Identify the offending drug and discontinue it.

Chapter 23 Answer Key

1. C
   A pressure injury (PI) is a loss of tissue integrity. It is caused when the skin and underlying soft tissue are compressed between a bony prominence and an external surface. This results in reduced tissue perfusion and gas exchange, which eventually leads to cell death. Most frequently these injuries are found on the sacrum, hips, and heels.

2. A, C, D, E
   Factors that increase the risk for development of pressure injuries include lack of mobility, exposure of skin to excessive moisture (e.g., urinary or fecal incontinence), malnourishment, and aging skin. Clients with cognitive decline or impairment are at risk if they are unable to fully participate in care. Individuals with peripheral vascular disease and/or diabetes mellitus are at risk, as they may experience impaired sensory perception as well as delayed wound healing. The client who is ambulatory with occasional urinary incontinence is not at increased risk, nor is the confused client who can use the bathroom with assistance as long as they receive the care necessary to use the bathroom and keep their skin clean and dry.

3. B
   Malnutrition increases the risk for skin breakdown and delayed wound healing. The nurse collaborates with the registered dietitian nutritionist (RDN) to help the client eat a well-balanced diet, especially emphasizing protein.

4. A
   If the nurse suspects that tunneling is present ("hidden" wounds that extend from the primary wound into surrounding tissues), he or she uses a cotton-tipped applicator to probe gently for a much larger tunnel or pocket of necrotic tissue beneath the opening, estimates the size and location of any tunneled areas, and documents the findings.

5. A, B, D, E
   See Best Practice for Patient Safety & Quality Care (QSEN) Prevents Pressure Injuries in your text book. All of the responses except two are appropriate interventions. Donut-shaped pillows are not used because these can damage capillary beds and increase tissue necrosis. Reddened areas are not massaged because this increases the risk for skin breakdown.

6. D
   The skin is cleaned as soon as possible after soiling occurs and at routine intervals, and is then moisturized with dimethazone, zinc oxide, lanolin, or petrolatum. Incontinence products are changedd frequently and the skin is inspected at least every 2 hours, especially under these products.
   Skin is washed, not scrubbed, with clean, warm water and mild soap, using only the amount of pressure needed to clean. Skin is patted dry, not rubbed.

7. A

Stage 1 pressure injuries are non-blanchable erythema of intact skin. Characteristics include: intact skin with localized area of non-blanchable erythema (may appear differently in skin with darker pigmentation); may be preceded by changes in sensation, temperature or firmness; and color changes are **not** purple or maroon. See Key Features of Pressure Injuries in your text.

8. C

Serial photographs of the wound are very helpful in documenting changes in wound appearance and progress toward healing. Policies on photographic documentation vary between agencies but require informed consent from the client or durable power of attorney if the client is unable to provide consent.

9. B, C, E, F

Clients with diabetes are slow to heal and the longer the incision is open the greater the risk for infection. Low WBC count leaves the client unable to fight infection. Steroid therapy interferes with the actions of the immune system. The client with the large abdominal incision is at risk because of difficulty with healing. The client awaiting surgery and the client with high cholesterol who walks daily are **not** at increased risk for infection from a pressure injury.

10. D

In the presence of a pressure injury, the following changes are reported to the primary health care provider: sudden deterioration of the ulcer, with an increase in the size or depth of the lesion; changes in the color or texture of the granulation tissue; and changes in the quantity, color, or odor of exudate.

11. B

Specific dressings, because there are so many and recommendations are so specialized based on the individual client's needs, are often recommended by the wound nurse. The unit nurse will collaborate closely with this member of the interprofessional team to determine the most appropriate dressing.

12. A

To assist an older adult in prevention of dry skin, the nurse would teach the AP to help the client take a complete bath or shower **every other day** (wash face, axillae, perineum, and any soiled areas with soap daily), using tepid water. See Patient and Family Education: Preparing for Self-Management — Prevention of Dry Skin in your text for additional interventions to prevent dry skin.

13. C

Shearing forces are generated when the skin itself is stationary and the tissues below the skin (e.g., fat, muscle) shift or move. The movement of the deeper tissue layers reduces the blood supply to the skin, leading to skin hypoxia, anoxia, ischemia, inflammation, and necrosis. To reduce pressure, the head of the bed is NOT elevated above 30 degrees to prevent shearing. When a client is positioned on his or her side, the position is kept at a 30-degree tilt (avoiding 90-degree positions).

14. B

Granulation tissue is a sign of healing tissue. It may be pale pink (early granulation) to beefy red; healthy tissue is moist and slightly spongy. Eschar is an indicator of necrotic tissue, increased exudate often indicates infection, and deep red, maroon, or purple indicates a suspected deep-tissue injury.

15. A, B, C, D, F

Contributing factors for chronic pressure injuries include: prolonged bedrest and/or immobility; incontinence; diabetes mellitus and/or peripheral vascular disease; malnutrition; and decreased sensory perception or cognitive problems. A pressure relieving mattress would help prevent pressure injuries.

16. C

Wound culturing is not routinely performed, unless there is lack of healing and signs of persistent infection are present. If performed, a tissue culture is done. Clinical indicators of infection (e.g., cellulitis, exudate changes, increase in injury size or depth) and systemic signs of bacteremia (e.g., fever, elevated white blood cell [WBC] count) are used to diagnose an infection.

17. B
The nurse would recognize that continuous negative-pressure wound therapy (NPWT) is used with caution with clients on anticoagulant therapy because NPWT increases the risk for bleeding at the application site. He or she would respond by consulting with members of the interprofessional team, such as the primary health care provider and wound care nurse, to ensure that anticoagulant status was appropriately monitored.

18. B, C, E
The expected outcomes for a client with a pressure injury include that the client will: experience progress toward wound healing by second intention as evidenced by granulation, epithelialization, contraction, and reduction or resolution of wound size; re-establish skin tissue integrity and restore skin barrier function; and remain free from local or systemic infections.

19. A, B, D, E, F
All of these interventions are appropriate except that a podiatrist should trim the client's toenails, not an AP or a family member.

20. A
Urticaria (hives) is a rash of white or red edematous papules or plaques of various sizes. This problem is usually caused by exposure to allergens, which releases histamine into the skin. Blood vessel dilation and plasma protein leakage lead to formation of lesions or wheals.

21. B
Avoidance therapy is used to reverse the reaction and clear the rash when the initiating cause is known. For example, if a new soap for hand-washing causes contact dermatitis of the hands, the client is taught to avoid that substance.

22. C
Antihistamines provide some relief from itching but may not keep the client totally comfortable. The sedative effects of these drugs may be better tolerated if most of the daily dose is taken near bedtime. The client is taught about possible side effects like drowsiness, and reminded to avoid driving, use of machinery, concurrent use of alcohol or other drugs, and making decisions that require clarity of thought.

23. A, C, E
Plaque psoriasis is the most common form of psoriasis. It is described as: raised, red patches covered with silvery white scales; usually found on scalp, knees, elbows, lower back; and may be itchy, painful, or bleeding. White pustules surrounded by reddened skin occurs with pustular psoriasis which usually occurs on hands and feet. Guttate psoriasis usually occurs after a streptococcal infection.

24. D
Tazarotene is a teratogenic substance (e.g., can cause birth defects). Women who are pregnant, or who plan to become pregnant, are instructed to avoid use of this drug, and to use effective contraception even if pregnancy is desired while using this drug. Corticosteroids provide anti-inflammatory effects. Anthralin is a hydrocarbon with action similar to tar which can help relieve chronic psoriasis. It should be applied to each lesion for a short period of time.

25. A, C, E, F
Ultraviolet (UV) irradiation has been shown to be beneficial in controlling psoriatic lesions. Photochemotherapy can be given by administration of psoralen, a photosensitizer, taken either orally or within a bath, followed by ultraviolet A (UVA) radiation. Excimer lasers emit UVB light and can be used for localized lesion treatment. Whether administered in a continuous or pulsed exposure, this modality allows for better focus on the lesions and reduces exposure to the surrounding normal skin. Oral systemic agents are often prescribed for clients with more than 5% body surface area affected by psoriasis (e.g., methotrexate, folic acid, and systemic retinoids). Oral antibiotics and surgical excision are **not** interventions of choice for this problem.

26. A, B, C, D, E, F

Preventing skin infection, especially bacterial and fungal infections, involves avoiding the offending organism and practicing good hygiene to remove the organism before infection can occur. Handwashing and not sharing personal items with others are the best ways to avoid contact with these organisms, including MRSA. In your text, see Patient and Family Education: Preparing for Self-Management: Preventing the Spread of MRSA for a list of strategies to teach clients and family members to prevent infection spread to other body areas and to other people.

27. B

Zostavax (zoster vaccine live) should not be given to clients with severe immunosuppression, those who are taking drugs that reduce immunity, individuals who are undergoing radiation or chemotherapy, or those with cancer affecting the bone marrow or lymphatic system.

28. B

Pediculosis pubis causes intense itching of the vulvar or perirectal region. Pubic lice can be contracted from infested bed linens or during sexual intercourse with an infected individual, so it is essential to avoid infected individuals. Although these lice are usually found in the genital region, they can also infest the axillae, the eyelashes, and the chest. The treatment of pediculosis involves using chemicals to kill the parasites (e.g., topical sprays, creams, and shampoos). Topical agents include permethrin cream or malathion lotion. Oral agents such as ivermectin may also be used. Over-the-counter lindane, a topical drug, has been used in the past as a pediculocide. It is no longer recommended as the first line of treatment for pediculosis because of possible neurologic adverse effects.

29. C

Scabies is a contagious skin infection caused by mite infestations. It is transmitted by close contact with an infested person or infested bedding. Curved or linear ridges in the skin are characteristic of scabies. The itching is very in-tense, and clients often report that it becomes unbearable at night. The webs of the fingers and on the inner aspects of the wrists are where the linear ridges are most commonly found.

30. A

Bedbug infestations are increasingly common as a result of travel and resistance to pesticides. Clients are taught to: examine hotel rooms and sleeping quarters, especially in crevices of box springs; place luggage on a rack away from the bed when traveling; place used/worn clothing into a sealed plastic bag when traveling; and carefully examine used items from garage sales before bringing them home. Bedbugs often live in mattresses and fabric upholstery, and in cracks and crevices of furniture. The most common mode of infestation is carrying the bug home from an infested environment such as a hotel room. Options B, C, and D do not respond to the client's concerns.

31. C

A wound without tissue loss, such as a clean laceration or a surgical incision, can be closed with sutures, staples, or adhesives. The wound edges are brought together with the skin layers lined up in correct anatomic position (approximated) and held in place until healing is complete. This type of wound represents healing by first intention, in which the closed wound eliminates dead space and shortens the phases of tissue repair.

32. D

Partial-thickness wounds are superficial with minimal loss of tissue integrity from damage to the epidermis and upper dermal layers. These wounds heal by re-epithelialization, the production of new skin cells by undamaged epidermal cells in the basal layer of the dermis, which also lines the hair follicles and sweat glands. In a healthy adult, healing of a partial-thickness wound takes about 5 to 7 days.

33. B

An electrical injury occurs when an electrical current enters the body. Tissue injury occurs when electrical energy converts to heat energy as it travels through the body. Once the current penetrates the skin causing the entry wound, it flows through the body damaging tissues in its path until leaving the body at the exit wound. The path of this client's electrical injury flows across the chest through the myocardium causing damage to the heart, which can lead to dysrhythmias.

34. A, B, C, D, F
With a suspected inhalation injury, the nurse would assess the mouth, throat, and nose for signs of soot. He or she would also listen for coughing, shortness of breath, or hoarseness of the voice which may indicate smoke inhalation. Cherry red skin is a sign of carbon monoxide poisoning, not inhalation injury.

35. A
Acids and alkalines are the most common chemical substances that can inflict burns. Decontamination is the focus for prehospital emergency responders. Contaminated clothing is removed and chemicals in powder form are brushed off.

36. B, C, D, E, F
All of the options presented are appropriate teaching points for prevention of burn injuries except A. Water heaters should be set below 120°F (49°C).

37. C
The nurse would monitor a client's respiratory efforts closely to recognize possible airway involvement. For a burn client in the resuscitation phase who is hoarse, has a brassy cough, drools, has difficulty swallowing, or produces an audible breath sound on exhalation, the nurse responds by immediately positioning the client upright, applying oxygen, and notifying the Rapid Response Team.

38. B
Because dressing changes can be uncomfortable, giving pain medication at least 30 minutes ahead of time can make the procedure less painful and more comfortable.

39. A, C, D, E
The priorities of care during the emergent phase include (1) securing the airway, (2) supporting circulation and perfusion, (3) maintaining body temperature, (4) keeping the client comfortable with analgesics, and (5) providing emotional support.

40. A, B, E
Thinner skin increases the depth of injury even when the exposure to the cause of injury is of shorter duration. Slower healing time leads to longer time with open areas, which results in a greater risk for infection. Pre-existing conditions such as diabetes can lead to slower healing time. Decreased (not increased) inflammatory and immune responses would increase risk for complications. Increased pulmonary compliance would not affect an older adult's risk for complications with burn injuries. See Patient-Centered Care: Older Adult Considerations
Age-Related Changes Increasing Complications from Burn Injury in your text.

41. B
Overexposure to sunlight is the major cause of skin cancer. Because sun damage is an age-related skin finding, screening for suspicious lesions is an important part of physical assessment.

42. A, B, D, E
All options are appropriate except C and F. Tanning bed should be completely avoided, and whenever a client's skin will be exposed to sunlight, a sunscreen should be used.

43. A
It is essential that the client contact the primary health care provider if any of these findings are noted: a change in the color of a lesion, especially if it darkens or shows evidence of spreading; a change in the size of a lesion, especially rapid growth; a change in the shape of a lesion, such as a sharp border becoming irregular or a flat lesion becoming raised; redness or swelling of the skin around a lesion; a change in sensation,

especially itching or increased tenderness of a lesion; or a change in the character of a lesion, such as oozing, crusting, bleeding, or scaling.

44. D

Melanomas are pigmented cancers arising in the melanin-producing epidermal cells. Most often they start as the benign growth of a nevus (mole). Normal nevi have regular, well-defined borders and are uniform in color, ranging from light colors to dark brown. The lesion's surface may be rough or smooth. Those with irregular or spreading borders, and/or multiple colors, are abnormal. Other suspicious features include sudden changes in lesion size and reports of itching or bleeding.

45. A

Mohs surgery is a specialized form of excision usually for basal and squamous cell carcinomas when they occur on the face, nose, or other areas of thin skin that may affect the cosmetic outcome.

46. D

Stevens-Johnson syndrome (SJS) and toxic epidermal necrolysis (TEN) are life-threatening cutaneous reactions most commonly triggered by drugs. Drugs most commonly associated with SJS/TEN include allopurinol, carbamazepine, lamotrigine, phenobarbital, phenytoin, and sulfasalazine. The response will continue and worsen if exposure to the drug continues.

24 CHAPTER

Assessment of the Respiratory System

1. Which description of respiratory physiologic features is correct?
   A. The elastic tissues of the tracheobronchial tree are the major structures responsible for gas exchange.
   B. The epiglottis closes during speech to divert air movement into and through the vocal cords to produce sound.
   C. Any problem with the right lung interferes with gas exchange and perfusion to a greater degree than a problem in the left lung.
   D. The left lung is responsible for approximately 60% of gas exchange and the right lung is responsible for 60% of pulmonary perfusion.

2. What is the **priority** or **most relevant** medical-surgical concept for the nurse when performing an assessment of a client's respiratory system?
   A. Perfusion
   B. Gas exchange
   C. Acid-base balance
   D. Cellular regulation

3. Which client conditions does the nurse recognize as most likely to cause a "left shift" of the oxyhemoglobin dissociation curve? **Select all that apply**.
   A. Alkalosis
   B. Increased body temperature
   C. Reduced blood and tissue pH
   D. Increased metabolic demands
   E. Reduced blood and tissue levels of oxygen
   F. Reduced blood and tissue levels of diphosphoglycerate (DPG)

4. Which assessment findings are **most important** for the nurse to determine when assessing a client with dyspnea? **Select all that apply.**
   A. Onset of or when the client first noticed dyspnea
   B. Results of most recent pulmonary function test
   C. Conditions that relieve the dyspnea sensation
   D. Whether or not dyspnea interferes with ADLs
   E. Inspection of the external nose and its symmetry
   F. Whether stridor is present with dyspnea

5. The nurse assessing a client's respiratory status finds fremitus has increased from the assessment performed yesterday. For which possible respiratory problem will the nurse assess further?
   A. Pneumothorax
   B. Pneumonia
   C. Pleural effusion
   D. Emphysema

6. Which factor does the nurse teach clients as the **most common** cause of chronic respiratory problems and physical limitations?
   A. Annual chest x-ray exposure to ionizing radiation
   B. Age-related decreased strength of respiratory muscles
   C. Failure to receive influenza and pneumonia vaccinations
   D. Smoking cigarettes or chronic exposure to cigarette smoke

7. Which question will the nurse ask **first** when a client reports a persistent, nagging cough?
   A. "Have you been running a fever?"
   B. "Do you have pain when coughing?"
   C. "How long has your cough been present?"
   D. "Do you have a family history of lung cancer?"

8. How will the nurse document the pack-year smoking history for a client who reports smoking a pack of cigarettes a day for 10 years, quitting for 4 years, and then smoking 2 packs a day for the last 25 years?
   A. 30 years
   B. 35 years
   C. 45 years
   D. 60 years

9. Which statements made by a client indicate to the nurse the need for additional education regarding smoking-related health risks? **Select all that apply**.
   A. "I have heard that cigarette smoking can cause both lung problems and heart problems."
   B. "I don't worry about lung problems because, unlike my wife, I don't smoke daily."
   C. "I worry about lung diseases because I borrow cigarettes when I'm out with friends."
   D. "I use a hookah when I smoke, but I'm trying to quit because I know it's not good for me."
   E. "I don't worry about lung problems because no one in my family has ever had lung cancer."
   F. "I am trying to get my college-age daughter to 'vape' rather than smoke because it is safer than cigarettes."

10. Which statements indicate to the nurse that a client has a strong addiction to cigarette smoking. **Select all that apply**.
    A. "I smoke a cigarette when I wake up before I make coffee."
    B. "To reduce my children's exposure, I only smoke outdoors."
    C. "I used to just 'bum' cigarettes but now I buy a pack daily for myself."
    D. "I only watch movies on television rather than at a theater because I can smoke at home."
    E. "Last night I woke up at 2:00 a.m. and 5:00 a.m. to smoke two cigarettes each time."
    F. "Last year when I had pneumonia, I didn't smoke for 2 weeks but started again when I was well."

11. Which respiratory changes does the nurse expect to find in an 82-year-old client who has no indicators of respiratory disease? **Select all that apply**.
    A. Exhalation is twice as long as inhalation
    B. Wheezing on arising every morning
    C. Decreased force of cough
    D. Increased anteroposterior diameter
    E. Shortness of breath at rest
    F. Softer voice

12. Which precaution to **prevent harm** is **most important** for the nurse to teach a client who is newly prescribed to take varenicline?
    A. Avoid crowds and people who are ill because your immunity is reduced while on this drug.
    B. Immediately report any change in thought process or suicide ideation because this drug can alter behavior.
    C. Be sure to remain in an upright position for an hour after taking the drug to avoid esophageal reflux and ulceration.
    D. Do not smoke cigarettes or use nicotine in any form while on this drug because the risk for heart attack or stroke is increased.

13. What type of assessment information does the nurse expect to gather when asking a client who has a respiratory problem whether the symptoms are worse at work or at home?
    A. Exposure to respiratory infections
    B. Presence of inherited predisposition
    C. Possible particulate matter exposure
    D. Possible continuation of a childhood respiratory problem

14. When the SpO_2 of a client with very dark skin reads 91%, which additional assessments will the nurse perform to determine the client's gas exchange adequacy? **Select all that apply**.
    A. Examine the color of oral mucosa.
    B. Ask the client to rate his or her dyspnea.
    C. Reapply the pulse oximeter to the earlobe.
    D. Use capnography to assess end-tidal CO_2 levels.
    E. Examine the color of the sclera closest to the iris.
    F. Compare the temperature of the right foot to that of the left.

15. How will the nurse document the respiratory assessment findings on auscultation that are heard as squeaky, musical continuous sounds when the client inhales and exhales?
    A. Fine crackles
    B. Coarse crackles
    C. Wheezes
    D. Rhonchi

16. Which findings noted during assessment of a client who reports a respiratory problem will the nurse document as abnormal? **Select all that apply**.
    A. Moveable trachea
    B. Use of pursed-lip breathing
    C. Intercostal space two finger-breadths wide
    D. Flat percussive sound in the upper center chest
    E. No breath sounds heard below the diaphragm
    F. Rough scratching sounds over the right lower lobe

17. With which client will the nurse expect to find a "barrel chest" on respiratory assessment?
    A. 22-year-old with mild, intermittent asthma
    B. 28-year-old with cystic fibrosis
    C. 55-year-old with chronic emphysema
    D. 60-year-old with bilateral pneumonia

18. Which arterial blood gas (ABG) values from an 86-year-old client does the nurse consider to be normal?
    A. pH 7.32, PaO_2 94 mm Hg, $PaCO_2$ 42 mm Hg
    B. pH 7.35, PaO_2 90 mm Hg, $PaCO_2$ 52 mm Hg
    C. pH 7.45, PaO_2 88 mm Hg, $PaCO_2$ 48 mm Hg
    D. pH 7.47, PaO_2 98 mm Hg, $PaCO_2$ 30 mm Hg

19. How will the nurse categorize a client's level of dyspnea who reports no shortness of breath (SOB) at rest, fair to moderate SOB with activity, some SOB while dressing, and has to stop to catch his breath when going up a flight of stairs?
    A. Class II
    B. Class III
    C. Class IV
    D. Class V

20. Which client assessment finding does the nurse recognize as an **immediate** gas exchange and perfusion problem?
    A. Pursed-lip breathing
    B. Clubbed fingers
    C. Barrel chest
    D. Cyanosis

21. What is the nurse's **best** response to a client who says he is afraid to have pulmonary function testing (PFTs) because it may reveal that he has lung cancer?
    A. "This test can establish whether lung cancer is present at a very early stage when the disease is more curable."
    B. "Because this test is noninvasive, it is less likely to cause you pain or increase your risk for infection."
    C. "These tests only determine whether your breathing is normal and cannot diagnose lung cancer."
    D. "There is nothing to fear because a local anesthetic is used."

22. Which are the nurse's priority actions when caring for a client who has labored, shallow respirations and a respiratory rate of 32 breaths/min with a pulse oximetry reading of 85%? **Select all that apply**.
    A. Notify the respiratory therapist to give the client a breathing treatment.
    B. Start oxygen using a nasal cannula at a rate of 2 L/min.
    C. Assess other indicators of adequate gas exchange.
    D. Obtain an order for a stat arterial blood gas (ABG).
    E. Assist with coughing and deep-breathing exercises.
    F. Place the client in an upright position.

23. Which client descriptions of sputum production alert the nurse to the possibility of a current respiratory problem? **Select all that apply**.
    A. Totals about 2 ounces daily
    B. Is streaked with mucous
    C. Is clear and thin
    D. Is frothy and pink
    E. Has a foul odor
    F. Is colorless

24. Which end-tidal carbon dioxide level in a client being monitored with capnography after anesthesia indicates to the nurse a possible **early** problem affecting gas exchange?
    A. 28 mm Hg
    B. 40 mm Hg
    C. 58 mm Hg
    D. 80 mm Hg

25. What is the **priority action to prevent harm** for a nurse to take before allowing a client who had a flexible bronchoscopy 2 hours ago to drink or eat?
    A. Assessing pulse oximetry to be sure oxygen saturation has returned to normal
    B. Measuring the client's end-tidal carbon dioxide level
    C. Asking whether the client has any nausea
    D. Checking for return of the gag reflex

26. Which assessment findings on a client who had a bronchoscopy using the local anesthetic benzocaine spray along with light sedation are most important to report to the health care provider who performed the procedure? **Select all that apply**.
    A. Oxygen saturation is 60% and does not increase with supplemental oxygen.
    B. Twenty minutes after the procedure, the client remains drowsy.
    C. Client coughed on first being awake but is no longer coughing.
    D. The client reports having a sore throat.
    E. Oral mucous membranes are cyanotic.
    F. Sputum is grossly bloody.

27. Which client will the nurse assess **most often** for the possibility of a postprocedure pneumothorax?
    A. Pulmonary function testing
    B. Flexible bronchoscopy
    C. Laryngoscopy
    D. Thoracentesis

Chapter 24 Answer Key

1. C
   The right lung is larger and has more diffusing surface and more blood vessels than does the left lung. All lung functions (gas exchange and perfusion) are greater in the right lung, which means that problems in the right lung more severely affect (reduce) gas exchange than do similar problems in the left lung. Surfactant reduces surface tension rather than increases it. Gas exchange does not occur within the tracheobronchial tree because the tissues are too thick for adequate diffusion of gas in either direction.

2. B
    Although all four concepts are associated with the respiratory system, the main function of the respiratory system is gas exchange. The other three concepts are dependent on gas exchange for proper activity.

3. A, F
    The oxyhemoglobin dissociation curve is shifted to the left when conditions are present that reduce overall oxygen needs. This left shift makes it harder for oxygen to dissociate from the hemoglobin molecule. Such conditions are those associated with slower or lower metabolism and oxygen need. These include less DPG, and alkalosis (fewer hydrogen ions). Reduced pH, increased metabolic demand, increased body temperature, and hypoxia are all associated with increased oxygen need and a right shift in the oxyhemoglobin dissociation curve.

4. A, C, D, F
    Dyspnea, especially if it is new onset, is a sensitive indicator of the possible presence of life-threatening respiratory problems. Dyspnea is subjective and determining onset, relieving factors, interference with ADLs, and presence of stridor should be elicited from the client to help assess severity and determine the level of intervention needed. Pulmonary functioning and inspection of the external nose are objective data.

5. B
    Fremitus is a vibration that can be felt on the chest wall when the client speaks. It is decreased if the transmission of sound waves from the larynx to the chest wall is slowed, such as when the pleural space is filled with air (pneumothorax) or fluid (such as with a pleural effusion) or when the bronchus is obstructed. Fremitus is increased with pneumonia and lung abscesses because the increased density of the chest enhances transmission of the vibrations.

6. D
    Although age-related decreased muscle strength can increase the work of breathing and not having up-to-date immunizations increases the

risk for respiratory infection, exposure to cigarette smoke (directly or indirectly as secondhand smoke) is the single most common factor causing chronic respiratory problems and physical limitations. Ionizing radiation exposure is an uncommon source of respiratory injury and chronic respiratory problems.

7. C
    A cough is a common symptom with a variety of respiratory problems and some cardiac problems, and must be thoroughly assessed. The first cough assessment questions should be to determine the extent and duration of when it occurs.

8. D
    Pack-years are calculated by multiplying the number of packs smoked per day by the number of years of smoking at that rate. One pack per day X 10 years = 10 pack-years, plus 2 packs per day X 25 years = 50 years. Total is 50 plus 10 for 60 pack-years.

9. B, E, F
    Anyone who lives with a smoker has passive exposure to smoke and has a greater risk for lung problems than those who never experience exposure to cigarette smoke. Passive smoking contributes to health problems, especially when chronic exposure occurs in small, confined spaces. Lung cancer is an environmentally acquired malignancy. Current evidence does not associate any genetic mutation with an increased risk for lung cancer. New evidence from the Centers for Disease Control and Prevention indicate that vaping as a form of nicotine delivery is at least as problematic for lung disease as cigarette smoking is. Statements B, E, and F are recognized by the nurse as gaps in the client's knowledge of the health risk. The other three statements indicate the client is aware of health risks.

10. A, D, E
    Indicators of strong nicotine dependence includes the need to wake up in the middle of the night to smoke, to find it difficult not to smoke

in places where smoking is prohibited (such as movie theaters), having a cigarette within the first 5 to 10 minutes after waking up, and smoking during illness.

11. A, C. D, F

A respiratory cycle consists of one inhalation followed by one exhalation. The normal respiratory cycle has an exhalation period that is twice as long as inhalation. Vocal cords slacken with age and the voice becomes softer. All muscles of inhalation weaken and lose strength with age, making coughs less forceful. With normal aging, the anteroposterior diameter enlarges. (It is much more exaggerated in obstructive respiratory disorders). Wheezing on arising is not normal at any age. Although older adults may develop some shortness of breath on exertion or exercise, shortness of breath at rest is not a normal age-related finding.

12. B

This drug has psychotropic properties and can increase feelings of self-harm or suicide ideation. It does not contain nicotine and can be used at the same time as nicotine to gradually reduce the urge to smoke. Varenicline does not induce esophageal irritation or ulcers nor does it reduce immunity.

13. C

In using the I-PREPARE model to determine whether a respiratory problem is possibly caused by particulate matter exposure (PME), the nurse investigates all aspects of a client's work history for exposure to industrial dusts, fumes, or chemicals. Occupations with higher risk for exposures include bakers, coal miners, stone masons, cotton handlers, woodworkers, welders, potters, plastic and rubber manufacturers, printers, farm workers, those working in grain elevators or flour mills, and steel foundry workers. A key indicator of PME is when breathing difficulties are less severe when away from the work environment. Answers to this question do not determine whether the problem is inherited, a continuation of a childhood disorder, or infectious in nature.

14. A, D

The color of the oral mucous membranes is related to blood oxygenation rather than skin pigmentation and can be used to determine whether the client has any degree of cyanosis. Measurement of capnography for end-tidal CO_2 levels is a very sensitive indicator of gas exchange adequacy. If this measure is normal, gas exchange is adequate even when pulse oximetry is low. Dyspnea is a subjective sensation and does not accurately indicate adequacy of gas exchange. The earlobe is also pigmented and moving the sensor to the earlobe is not likely to result in an accurate result. The color of the sclera is not related to blood flow and oxygenation. This area is the one used to assess for jaundice, not gas exchange. Foot temperature is not used to assess gas exchange adequacy.

15. C

Squeaky, musical continuous sounds heard when the client inhales and exhales are abnormal (adventitious) and described as wheezes. Fine crackles are heard as popping, discontinuous high-pitched sounds at the end of inhalation. Coarse crackles are a rattling sound. Rhonchi are heard as low-pitched continuous snoring sounds.

16. B, C, F

The trachea should be midline and slightly moveable. Pursed-lip breathing is abnormal and generally used only in clients who have obstructive disease with air trapping. The space between the ribs (intercostal space) should be only one finger-breadth wide. A flat percussive sound is expected in the upper center chest because the sternum is located there. No breath sounds are heard below the diaphragm because the lungs are located above the diaphragm. Rough scratching sounds heard over the right lower lobe are an abnormal sound known as a pleural friction rub.

17. C

A barrel chest occurs when air trapping and increased residual volume is severe and long-standing, such as in chronic emphysema. Neither pneumonia nor cystic fibrosis cause air trapping. Although asthma can result in air trapping, this does not happen with mild disease occurring intermittently. Although the anteroposterior chest diameter does increase somewhat as a result of normal aging, it does not increase to the point that it is equal to or greater than the lateral chest diameter.

18. A

Adults over 60 years of age usually have a slightly lower than normal pH and slightly lower PaO_2 levels (slightly acidotic). $PaCO_2$ levels are not affected by increasing age alone. Normal arterial pH is 7.35-7.45.

19. B

Clients with class III dyspnea report that shortness of breath commonly occurs during usual activities such as showering or dressing, but the patient can manage without assistance from others (although the client may consider asking for help because self-care is too time-consuming). Dyspnea is not present at rest and client can walk for more than a city block at own pace but cannot keep up with others of own age. Usually clients must stop to catch their breath partway up a flight of stairs.

20. D

Finger clubbing and a barrel chest take many months to years of inadequate gas exchange to develop. Pursed-lip breathing is a learned behavior to compensate for loss of elastic recoil. Only cyanosis reflects an immediate decrease in gas exchange and/or perfusion.

21. C

PFTs are noninvasive, which makes them painless and without risk for infection; however, they cannot diagnose lung cancer. The fear of a lung cancer diagnosis is this client's concern, not fear of pain or discomfort.

22. B, C, F

The client is demonstrating difficulty breathing and ineffective gas exchange with hypoxemia. Placing the client in an upright position may improve respiratory effectiveness. Oxygen therapy is an appropriate immediate action to prevent harm. Pulse oximetry is usually a good indicator of gas exchange; however, the equipment may be faulty or the probe incorrectly placed. Therefore, assessing other indicators of adequate gas exchange is an appropriate early action. None of the other actions will have an immediate effect on gas exchange,

23. B, D, E

Sputum is continually produced in all clients. The sputum of a client with no respiratory problem is thin, clear, colorless, has no odor, and is less than 90 mL daily. Excessive pink, frothy sputum is common with pulmonary edema. Bacterial pneumonia often produces rust-colored sputum, and a lung abscess may cause foul-smelling sputum. Clients with chronic bronchitis, especially smokers, have thicker sputum with mucous.

24. C

The normal value of the partial pressure of end-tidal carbon dioxide ranges between 20 and 40 mm Hg. Thus options A and B are within the normal range. 58 mm Hg indicates a relatively early problem with effective gas exchange. Option D represents a severe or late problem with gas exchange.

25. D

A flexible bronchoscopy is often performed using light sedation or local anesthesia, both of which can reduce the gag reflex. When the gag reflex is reduced or not intact, the risk for aspiration increases. Oxygen saturation and end-tidal carbon dioxide levels do not determine whether the client's gag reflex has returned. Although nausea should be ruled out, the priority action to prevent harm is ascertaining the presence of an intact gag reflex.

26. A, E, F

The cyanosis and low oxygen saturation that does not improve with supplemental oxygen are very serious and could indicate methemoglobinemia associated with the use of benzocaine spray, which requires immediate intervention to prevent death. Grossly bloody sputum is not a normal expectation after the procedure and could herald hemorrhage. Most clients have a sore throat after bronchoscopy and remain somewhat drowsy for an hour or more after sedation. Neither of these responses are caused for alarm, nor is a reduction in coughing.

27. D

A pneumothorax (collapsed lung) is most common after invasive procedures that allow air into the intrapleural space, such as with a thoracentesis that involves having a needle penetrate through the chest wall into the pleural space. Pulmonary function testing is noninvasive; a flexible bronchoscopy does not penetrate the chest wall, and a laryngoscopy does not enter the lungs.

25 CHAPTER

Concepts of Care for Patients Requiring Oxygen Therapy or Tracheostomy

1. Which statements about oxygen therapy are true? **Select all that apply**.
   A. When oxygen therapy is successful, hypercarbia is cured.
   B. Oxygen therapy must be monitored to prevent explosions.
   C. The oxygen provided during oxygen therapy is considered a drug.
   D. Nurses must know the purposes and expected outcomes for each client prescribed oxygen therapy.
   E. Because oxygen is a normal component of atmospheric air, its use as therapy is completely safe.
   F. When oxygen therapy increases the client's oxygen saturation to 99%, hypoxia and hypoxemia are cured.

2. What is the nurse's **best** response to a client who asks whether he can use a computer in the same room while using oxygen therapy?
   A. "Yes, as long as the cord is not frayed and has a three-pronged plug."
   B. "Yes, but only in battery mode to prevent the possibility of sparks."
   C. "No, overheating of the unit could cause the oxygen to explode."
   D. "No, only approved medical electronic equipment can be used during oxygen therapy."

3. In what situations will the nurse consider oxygen therapy as possibly beneficial for a client? **Select all that apply**.
   A. Anemia
   B. Hypoxia
   C. Hypothermia
   D. Hypertension
   E. Pneumonia
   F. Venous insufficiency

4. Which manifestations in a client receiving oxygen therapy at 60% for more than 24 hours alerts the nurse to the possibility of oxygen toxicity?
   A. Oxygen saturation greater than 100%
   B. Decreased rate and depth of respiration
   C. Wheezing on inhalation and exhalation
   D. Discomfort or pain under the sternum

5. Which condition does the nurse suspect when noting that a client who is receiving 40% oxygen therapy now has new onset of crackles and decreased breath sounds on auscultation?
   A. Alveolar drying
   B. Arterial hypoxemia
   C. Chronic hypercarbia
   D. Absorptive atelectasis

6. What is the **priority** action for the nurse to take to **prevent harm** when caring for a client who is receiving oxygen at 5 L/min by nasal cannula?
   A. Switch to a mask delivery system.
   B. Humidify the oxygen with sterile water.
   C. Add extension tubing for client mobility.
   D. Check to ensure the delivery equipment is plugged into a grounded outlet.

7. Which parameters will the nurse monitor to ensure that a client's gas exchange response to oxygen therapy is adequate? **Select all that apply**.
   A. Level of consciousness
   B. Respiratory pattern
   C. Oxygen flow rate
   D. Pulse oximetry
   E. Respiratory rate
   F. Blood pressure

8. Which action does the nurse caring for a client receiving humidified oxygen take to **prevent harm** from potential infection?
   A. Never draining fluid from the water trap back into the nebulizer
   B. Administering the prescribed antibiotic for a current infection
   C. Always wearing gloves when changing the oxygen tubing
   D. Not allowing live or cut flowers into the client's room

9. With which client prescribed to receive oxygen therapy does the nurse suggest using a face tent rather than a nasal cannula?
   A. Client with severe sleep apnea
   B. Client with facial trauma
   C. Client who is confused
   D. An unconscious client

10. Which actions are **most important** for a nurse to take to **prevent harm** when caring for a client who is receiving oxygen therapy with a nasal cannula? **Select all that apply**.
    A. Making sure that the prongs on the nasal cannula are properly positioned in the nares
    B. Applying a water-soluble gel to the nares as needed
    C. Adjusting the flow rate between 1 and 8 L/min based on the client's report of dyspnea
    D. Removing the cannula during meals
    E. Checking the client's skin under the cannula and behind the ears
    F. Maintaining a flow rate below 20%

11. Which **priority** action does the nurse perform to **prevent harm** for a client receiving oxygen therapy through a nonrebreather mask?
    A. Preventing the reservoir bag from inflating to more than one-half full
    B. Ensuring that valves and flaps are patent, functional, and not stuck
    C. Switching to partial rebreather mask for more precise FiO_2
    D. Ensuring that the flow rate does not exceed 6 L/min

12. Which clients could benefit from the use of noninvasive positive-pressure ventilation (NPPV)? **Select all that apply**.
    A. 22-year-old with an acute asthma attack
    B. 36-year-old with sleep apnea
    C. 40-year old with acute pneumothorax
    D. 50-year-old with cardiopulmonary arrest
    E. 64-year-old with acute exacerbation of COPD
    F. 72-year-old with cardiogenic pulmonary edema

13. For which activity does the nurse teach the client who is receiving oxygen by a transtracheal oxygen (TTO) delivery system to switch to a nasal cannula oxygen delivery system?
    A. Eating a meal
    B. Sleeping at night
    C. Cleaning the catheter
    D. Performing mouth care

14. Which factors does the home health nurse identify as safety hazards in the home of a client requiring home oxygen therapy? **Select all that apply**.
    A. Three-pronged outlets in every room
    B. Bottle of wine in the kitchen area
    C. Candles on the mantelpiece
    D. Pack of cigarettes on the coffee table
    E. Electric heater with a frayed cord in the bathroom
    F. Computer with a three-pronged plug

15. What information will the nurse explain to the family of a client who has been prescribed to receive transtracheal oxygen (TTO) therapy? **Select all that apply**.
    A. Cures sleep apnea
    B. Prevents nitrogen toxicity
    C. Delivers oxygen directly into the lungs
    D. Less likely to cause pressure injury to the skin
    E. Used with mechanical ventilation
    F. Provides high humidity with oxygen delivery

16. What is the nurse's **best first** action when a client's heart rate changes from 78 beats/min to 48 beats/min during nasotracheal suctioning?
    A. Immediately stop suctioning.
    B. Gently pinch the client's cheek
    C. Administer oxygen by mask at 2 L/min
    D. Document the change as the only action

17. Which instructions must the nurse provide to an assistive personnel (AP) prior to feeding a client who is at risk for aspiration? **Select all that apply**.
    A. Position the client in the most upright position possible.
    B. Provide adequate time; do not "hurry" the client.
    C. Provide sips of water through a straw between bites of food to help with swallowing.
    D. Encourage the client to "tuck" his or her chin down and move the forehead forward while swallowing.
    E. If the client coughs, stop the feeding until he or she indicates that the airway has been cleared.
    F. Allow the client to indicate when he or she is ready for the next bite.

18. With which clients does the nurse anticipate probable placement of a **temporary tracheostomy**? **Select all that apply.**
    A. 28-year-old who became quadriplegic from a C-2 spinal transection
    B. 36-year-old with permanent brain damage after a traumatic brain injury
    C. 45-year-old with facial and oral cavity burns
    D. 56-year-old with stage IV lung cancer
    E. 69-year-old unable to wean from a ventilator
    F. 72-year-old with an acute airway obstruction caused by epiglottitis

19. How will the nurse determine whether a postoperative client has subcutaneous emphysema following the creation of a tracheostomy?
    A. Checking the volume of the pilot balloon
    B. Listening for airflow through the tube
    C. Palpating for air under the skin
    D. Assessing oxygen saturation

20. What is the **most appropriate** action for the nurse to take to prevent accidental decannulation of client's tracheostomy tube?
    A. Obtaining an order for continuous upper extremity restraints
    B. Securing the tube in place using twill ties or commercial fasteners
    C. Allowing at least 2 inches of space between the ties and the client's neck
    D. Instructing the client to hold the tube in place with a tissue while coughing

21. Which **necessary** equipment does the nurse ensure is kept at the bedside of a client with a newly created tracheostomy? **Select all that apply.**
    A. Oxygen
    B. Resuscitation bag
    C. Pair of wire cutters
    D. Oxygen tubing
    E. Suction equipment
    F. Tracheostomy tray with tube and obturator

22. Which complication of a tracheostomy does the nurse suspect in a client who has difficulty breathing, noisy respirations, difficulty inserting a suction catheter, and thick, dry secretions?
    A. Accidental decannulation
    B. Aspiration pneumonia
    C. Pneumothorax
    D. Tube obstruction

23. What is the nurse's best **first** action when a client who is 4 days postoperative with a tracheostomy suddenly sneezes during tracheostomy care and the tube falls out onto the bed linens?
    A. Ventilate the client with 100% oxygen and notify the Rapid Response Team.
    B. Quickly and gently replace the tube with a clean cannula kept at the bedside.
    C. Clean and rinse the tube with sterile solution and gently replace it.
    D. Apply oxygen with a facemask and prepare the client for surgery.

24. Which action will the nurse take to **prevent harm** from tracheomalacia in a client who has a newly created tracheostomy?
    A. Maintaining the tracheal cuff pressure between 14 and 20 mm Hg
    B. Wrapping gauze around the tube to prevent bleeding at the site
    C. Performing suctioning only when the client requests this action
    D. Changing the dressing whenever it becomes moist

25. With which clients who have tracheostomies will the nurse remain extra vigilant for possible tracheal tissue injury? **Select all that apply.**
    A. 26-year-old who is 6 months pregnant
    B. 30-year-old who also has seasonal asthma
    C. 42-year-old taking corticosteroids daily for a chronic inflammatory condition
    D. 50-year-old on hormone replacement therapy for menopause
    E. 61-year-old with chronic alcoholism and malnutrition
    F. 78-year-old who also has early-stage prostate cancer

26. What is the reason that the nurse performing tracheal suctioning on a client applies continuous suction only during catheter withdrawal?
    A. To promote adequate oxygenation during the procedure
    B. To prevent dropping of secretions into the trachea
    C. To assist the client in effective coughing efforts
    D. To ensure the catheter does not go beyond the carina

27. Which actions reflect proper techniques for the nurse to use when performing deep suctioning on a client with a tracheostomy or endotracheal tube? **Select all that apply.**
    A. Preoxygenate the client for at least 30 seconds before suctioning.
    B. Instruct the client that he or she is going to be suctioned.
    C. Quickly insert the suction catheter until resistance is met.
    D. Suction the client for at least 30 seconds to ensure effective secretion removal.
    E. Repeat suctioning for four to five total suction passes.
    F. Apply intermittent suction while withdrawing the suction catheter.

28. Which activities are **most** important for the nurse to teach a client with a temporary tracheostomy to **avoid** until cleared by the surgeon? **Select all that apply.**
    A. Swimming
    B. Driving a car
    C. Riding a bicycle
    D. Paddleboarding
    E. Engaging in sexual intercourse
    F. Participating in airplane travel

29. Which precaution is **most important** for the nurse to take to **prevent harm** when caring for a client who is breathing on his own and has a fenestrated tracheostomy tube with a cuff?
    A. Keeping the cuff inflated to prevent secretions from entering the lung
    B. Providing mouth care with sterile solutions at least every 4 to 6 hours
    C. Deflating the cuff before capping the tube with the decannulation cap
    D. Ensuring that a manual resuscitation bag accompanies the client whenever he or she is out of the room

30. With which interprofessional team members does the nurse expect to collaborate in preparing a client and family for home care with a permanent tracheostomy without oxygen therapy? **Select all that apply**.
    A. Discharge planner
    B. Pharmacologist
    C. Registered dietitian nutritionist
    D. Respiratory therapist
    E. Social worker
    F. Wound care specialist

Chapter 25 Answer Key

1. C, D
   Oxygen is both an atmospheric gas and a drug. Nurses must be knowledgeable about oxygen hazards before starting oxygen therapy and understand the rationale and the expected outcome of oxygen therapy for each client prescribed to receive oxygen. Although oxygen therapy can improve a client's oxygen saturation, it does not cure the underlying cause of hypoxia or hypoxemia. Also, hypercarbia is an increase in the client's arterial blood level of carbon dioxide, which has many causes. Oxygen therapy does not cure hypercarbia. The presence of oxygen supports combustion but this gas does not explode. Although oxygen therapy has many benefits, if used at too high a delivery rate or for an extended period of time, oxygen toxicity can occur and cause serious injury.

2. A
   A computer is safe to use in rooms where oxygen is in use if it is grounded (has three prongs) and is plugged into grounded outlets to prevent fires from electrical arcing sparks. Frayed cords are not used because they can spark and ignite a flame. Batteries are just as likely to spark as electrical cords. Oxygen does not explode even when equipment is overheated.

3. A, B, E
   Oxygen therapy is usually beneficial with any acute or chronic respiratory problem that interferes with gas exchange. It is also useful in some nonpulmonary conditions such as anemia, cardiac problems, and sepsis. It does not have a beneficial effect on hypertension and cannot improve venous insufficiency.

4. D
   Oxygen toxicity damages the alveolar membrane, stimulating the formation of a hyaline membrane and impairing gas exchange. Clients become increasingly more dyspneic and hypoxic. Initial manifestations include dyspnea, nonproductive cough, chest pain beneath the sternum, and GI upset. Oxygen saturation falls, not increases. Breathing becomes more rapid with the sensation of dyspnea. Wheezing represents airway obstruction, not damage to the alveolar membrane.

5. D
   Nitrogen composes 79% of room air and maintains patent airways and inflated alveoli. When high oxygen levels are delivered, nitrogen is diluted, oxygen diffuses from the alveoli into the blood, and the alveoli collapse. Collapsed alveoli cause absorptive atelectasis, which is detected as crackles and decreased breath sounds on auscultation. Dry alveoli would not create crackles. Hypercarbia and hypoxemia may increase respiratory rate but neither problem affects breath sounds.

6. B

Oxygen therapy can dry out mucous membranes. When the prescribed oxygen flow rate is higher than 4 L/min, the delivery system is humidified to prevent harm with loss of tissue integrity. A nasal cannula can be used to deliver oxygen at a rate of 5 L/min. Extension tubing can increase the client's risk for falls and does not prevent harm from oxygen delivery. Hospital oxygen delivery equipment is not electrified.

7. A, B, D, E

The parameters that would change based on adequacy of gas exchange include level of consciousness (decreases when gas exchange is poor), respiratory pattern (requires increased effort and exertion with poor gas exchange), pulse oximetry (decreases with poor gas exchange), and respiratory rate (increases with poor gas exchange). The oxygen flow rate is not a client indicator of gas exchange. Blood pressure is not directly affected by changes in gas exchange.

8. A

Condensation often forms in the tubing and can be a source of infection with bacteria or fungus. The nurse removes condensation as it collects by disconnecting the tubing and emptying the water without allowing any water to drain back into the nebulizer system or tubing. Gloves are not needed to change tubing. Live or cut flowers do not represent an infection risk unless the client is very immunosuppressed. Administering antibiotics for a current infection does not prevent a potential infection.

9. B

A face tent puts minimal pressure on facial tissues and allows greater humidification. Facial trauma is one criterion for its use. A confused client is more likely to try and remove a face tent or mask than a nasal cannula. Sleep apnea is not helped by oxygen therapy delivered either with a nasal cannula or a face tent. There is no increased benefit in using a face tent versus a nasal cannula for oxygen delivery to an unconscious client.

10. A, B, E

If the nasal cannula is not properly positioned in the nares, oxygen therapy is ineffective, which could cause the client harm.

The presence of a nasal cannula can irritate the nares and cause harm with loss of skin integrity. Lubricating the nares and assessing the skin under the cannula and behind the ears helps prevent skin breakdown.

The flow rate is not adjusted based on the sensation of dyspnea, which is subjective and often does not reflect gas exchange effectiveness or oxygen saturation.

The presence of a cannula does not interfere with eating and removing the cannula during meals may cause harm by increasing hypoxemia.

The flow rate by nasal cannula can be increased above 20% without causing harm.

11. B

The nonrebreather mask has a one-way valve between the mask and the reservoir and has two flaps over the exhalation ports. The valve allows the patient to draw all needed oxygen from the reservoir bag, and the flaps prevent room air from entering through the exhalation ports. During exhalation, air leaves through these exhalation ports while the one-way valve prevents exhaled air from re-entering the reservoir bag. If the flaps or valve should fail, the patient would inhale room air and exhale CO_2 with each breath, which decreases oxygen delivery and cause hypoxemia. The flow rate must be kept between 10 and 15 L/min for the nonrebreather mask to be effective. A partial rebreather mask would be less precise.

12. A, B, E, F

Noninvasive positive-pressure ventilation (NPPV) uses positive pressure to keep alveoli open and improve gas exchange without the dangers of intubation for clients with dyspnea, hypercarbia, acute exacerbations of chronic obstructive pulmonary disease (COPD), cardiogenic pulmonary edema, acute asthma attacks, and sleep apnea. A client in cardiac arrest would need intubation. An acute pneumothorax would not be helped with NPPV.

13. C

A transtracheal oxygen (TTO) delivery system involves passing a catheter into the trachea through a small incision with the client under local anesthesia, delivering oxygen directly to the lungs. Thus, the mouth is not involved and this delivery is not disrupted by eating, drinking, or performing oral care. If the catheter is properly attached to the client, it is no more likely to become dislodged during sleep than is a nasal cannula. To maintain adequate gas exchange and oxygenation, the client should receive supplemental oxygen through a nasal cannula delivery system whenever the transtracheal catheter is not in place for any reason, such as when cleaning it.

14. C, D, E

Items that should not be present in the same room in which oxygen is in use include anything with an open flame (candles, cigarettes) and frayed electrical wires. The three-pronged outlets and plugs are grounded and not a safety hazard with oxygen therapy. Drinking wine (in moderation) either by the client or family members is not a safety hazard with oxygen therapy.

15. C, D

Transtracheal oxygen (TTO) is a long-term method of delivering oxygen directly into the lungs with the use of a small, flexible catheter in the trachea through a small incision. TTO reduces loss of tissue integrity from nasal prongs and is less visible.

TTO does not cure sleep apnea and is not used for assisting in any type of pressure or mechanical ventilation.

Nitrogen toxicity is not a real problem with oxygen therapy.

The typical TTO set-up may not be associated with humidification.

16. A

The change in heart rate is a serious response to suctioning. The client is experiencing vagal stimulation and bradycardia from the presence of the suction catheter in the tracheopharyngeal area. Such stimulation can lead to severe hypotension, heart block, and asystole. Administering oxygen would be a good second action, but the first action is to stop the activity causing the problem. The client's response is not related to a lack of being alert.

17. A, B, D, E, F

Options A, B, D, E, and F are recommended to prevent aspiration as described in the Best Practice for Patient Safety & Quality Care: Preventing Aspiration While Swallowing box. Water and thin liquids are avoided during meals, especially delivered through a straw, because they are difficult for the client to control and may slide into the trachea when the epiglottis is open.

18. C, F

Temporary tracheostomies are performed when conditions that are expected to resolve endanger the airway. Such conditions include facial and oral cavity burns and epiglottitis. A C-2 spinal cord transection resulting in quadriplegia is unlikely to resolve and neither will the permanent brain damage. A client with difficulty breathing as a result of stage IV lung cancer would not be a candidate unless a specific temporary condition requiring tracheostomy were also present. Clients who are unable to wean from a ventilator are among the most common people who have a permanent tracheostomy.

19. C

Subcutaneous emphysema occurs when there is an opening or tear in the trachea and air escapes into the fresh tissue planes of the neck. This condition is identified by inspecting for puffiness in the skin and palpating for air under the skin, felt as a crackling sensation when pressing on the skin around the new tracheostomy. Subcutaneous emphysema cannot be determined by changes in oxygen saturation, changes in airflow through the tube, or by knowing the volume of the pilot balloon around the cuff.

20. B

Keeping the tube in place with twill ties or commercial tube holders that allow only the space of one finger between the client's neck and the ties helps prevent accidental decannulation. Two inches of space is very loose and does not keep the tube secure. The tube should be secured well enough that the client does not need to hold it in place when coughing or moving. Restraints are not an acceptable means of preventing decannulation.

21. A, B, D, E, F

For safety in case of accidental decannulation within the first 72 hours after creation of a tracheostomy, necessary bedside equipment includes a tracheostomy insertion tray with a tube of the same type (including an obturator) and size (or one size smaller). Until the tube is reinserted, the client will need to be ventilated manually with a manual resuscitation bag and facemask connected to oxygen. Wire cutters are not needed because a tracheostomy is not wired in place.

22. D

Indicators of tube obstruction include difficulty breathing; noisy respirations; difficulty inserting a suction catheter; thick, dry secretions; and high peak pressures (if a mechanical ventilator is used). Indications of accidental decannulation are obvious with no cannula in the tracheostomy and greatly decreased oxygen saturation. The major indications of a pneumothorax include absence of breath sounds on the affected side and tracheal deviation away from the affected side. Indications of aspiration pneumonia include reduced breath sounds on the affected side with no other particular signs or symptoms.

23. B

If decannulation occurs after 72 hours, the nurse at the bedside may be able to secure the airway by extending the patient's neck and opening the tissues of the stoma with a curved Kelly clamp and then, insert the fresh and clean tube with obturator inserted into the tracheostomy site. If the nurse is unsuccessful at this

attempt, the Rapid Response Team is initiated quickly. The nurse does not use the previous tracheostomy tube and obturator.

24. A

Although most actions listed are correct to perform on a client with a tracheostomy, only maintaining the cuff pressure between 14 and 20 mm Hg helps prevent tracheomalacia. Wrapping gauze around the tube can prevent site bleeding and changing moist dressings helps prevent both infection and skin breakdown. A major indicator of the need for suctioning is the client's request that it be performed; however, while this action does help prevent trauma that could result in intermittent rubbing of the tube against tracheal tissues, only maintaining a lower cuff pressure results in continuous protection against tracheal trauma and potential tracheomalacia.

25. C, E, F

Clients at high risk for tracheal tissue injury with a tracheostomy include those who are malnourished, dehydrated, hypoxic, older, or receiving corticosteroids. Pregnancy, seasonal asthma, and menopausal hormone replacement therapy are not factors known to increase the risk for tissue injury.

26. B

Although the process of suctioning of a client with a tracheostomy occurs on only an intermittent basis (unlike gastric suctioning that often is a continuous process), the application of suction during the process only occurs during catheter withdrawal and is continuous during the withdrawal to prevent the suctioned secretions from falling out of the catheter and back into the client's airway. Oxygenation is never adequate during suctioning, which is why the entire process is limited to a maximum of 15 seconds. Suctioning often stimulates coughing but that is not the reason why continuous suctioning occurs only during withdrawal. Only measuring the length of the suction tube and not inserting it too deeply prevents the catheter from going beyond the carina.

27. A, B, C

As described in the Best Practice for Patient Safety & Quality Care: Suctioning the Artificial Airway box, correct suctioning techniques include instructing the client about suctioning, preoxygenating the client, and quickly inserting the suction catheter until resistance is met. To prevent hypoxemia, pain, and tissue injury, suctioning lasts 10 to 15 seconds per catheter insertion and is repeated for no more than three passes. Suction is only applied during catheter withdrawal and is continuous during withdrawal to prevent the suctioned secretions from falling out of the catheter and back into the client's airway.

28. A, D

It is important for the client to avoid getting water or particulate matter into the trachea through the tracheostomy, which eliminates swimming and paddleboarding because of the risk for immersing the tracheostomy in water. All other activities in this list are acceptable for a client with a tracheostomy to perform.

29. C

A fenestrated tube has openings that permit air to flow through it or around it into the natural airway so the patient can cough and speak when the inner cannula is not in place and the plug or stopper is locked in place. If the stopper is in place with the tube cuff inflated and the fenestrated tube is capped, the client has no airway. Mouth care for a client with a tracheostomy does not need to be performed using sterile solutions. Although having a manual resuscitation bag accompany the client is a reasonable action, the most important action for safety with a fenestrated tube is always ensuring the cuff is deflated before capping the tube.

30. A, C, D, E

Care for the patient requiring long-term or permanent tracheostomy is best when a team approach is used. In addition to the nurse, interprofessional team members most commonly include the primary health care provider, respiratory therapist, registered dietitian nutritionist, discharge planner, and social worker. A pharmacologist is generally not involved. A wound care specialist is only involved when the incision is not healing properly and is not an expected member of the interprofessional team under normal circumstances.

26 CHAPTER

Concepts of Care for Patients with Noninfectious Upper Respiratory Problems

1. Which structures are the most critical to keep patent for effective gas exchange? **Select all that apply**.
   A. Nose
   B. Larynx
   C. Trachea
   D. Oropharynx
   E. Laryngopharynx
   F. Maxillary sinuses

2. With which client will the nurse remain **most** alert for development of airway obstruction from a mucoid impaction?
   A. 34-year-old client with a head injury who is comatose
   B. 44-year-old client with jaws wired together after facial trauma
   C. 64-year-old client with Alzheimer disease who wanders from room to room
   D. 74-year-old client who has had an endotracheal tube in place for the past 4 days

3. What is the **priority action** for a nurse to take to **prevent harm** when a client who is talking and laughing while eating begins to choke on a piece of meat?
   A. Initiate chest compressions.
   B. Perform abdominal thrusts (Heimlich maneuver).
   C. Deliver several sharp blows between the scapulae.
   D. Attempt to remove the obstruction with oral suction.

4. Which type of respiratory support does the nurse prepare for a client with severe angioedema and tongue swelling from exposure to seafood who has stridor and an oxygen saturation of 70%?
   A. Nasal BiPAP
   B. Tracheotomy
   C. Cricothyroidotomy
   D. Endotracheal intubation

5. Which statements about obstructive sleep apnea (OSA) are true? **Select all that apply**.
   A. A main feature is hypopnea
   B. Results from chronic sinusitis
   C. Associated with frequent nightmares
   D. Most commonly diagnosed by flexible bronchoscopy
   E. Causes fragmented nighttime sleep and daytime drowsiness
   F. Is most common in people who have longer than average neck length

6. With which client does the nurse anticipate possible complications from obstructive sleep apnea (OSA) following abdominal surgery?
   A. 28-year-old who is 80 lb (36.4 kg) overweight and has a short neck
   B. 48-year-old who has type 1 diabetes and chronic sinusitis
   C. 58-year-old who has had gastroesophageal reflux disease for 10 years
   D. 78-year-old who wears upper and lower dentures and has asthma

7. Which subjective symptoms will the nurse expect a client with obstructive sleep apnea to report or describe? **Select all that apply**.
   A. Excessive daytime sleepiness
   B. Loss of taste sensation
   C. Excessive production of sputum
   D. Decreased ability to concentrate
   E. Irritability
   F. Heavy snoring

8. Which actions will the nurse suggest to a client to help improve **mild** obstructive sleep apnea (OSA)? **Select all that apply**.
   A. Sleeping on the side rather than in a supine position
   B. Using continuous positive airway pressure (CPAP) every night
   C. Losing weight to come within 10% of his or her ideal weight
   D. Using an oral position-fixing device to prevent tongue subluxation
   E. Consulting with an oral surgeon about removal of wisdom teeth
   F. Taking an over-the-counter sleep aid to achieve a deeper sleep

9. For which possible long-term health changes will the nurse assess a client who has moderate to severe obstructive sleep apnea (OSA)? **Select all that apply**.
   A. Anemia
   B. Chronic obstructive pulmonary disease
   C. Decreased cognition
   D. Diabetes mellitus
   E. Resistant hypertension
   F. Stroke

10. With which clients will the nurse be alert for an increased risk of obstructive sleep apnea OSA? **Select all that apply**.
    A. 26-year-old woman who had tonsils and adenoids removed as a child
    B. 35-year-old man who is a marathon runner
    C. 48-year-old woman who has a short neck and a small chin
    D. 56-year-old man who smokes two packs of cigarettes daily
    E. 65-year-old man who is malnourished and has chronic obstructive pulmonary disease (COPD)
    F. 80-year-old woman who is cognitively impaired from Alzheimer disease

11. Which precaution related to noninvasive positive pressure ventilation (NPPV) by continuous positive airway pressure (CPAP) is **most important** for the nurse to teach a client with obstructive sleep apnea (OSA) who is being managed by CPAP?
    A. Use the CPAP machine only for the first 2 hours of sleep.
    B. Avoid using the CPAP equipment when you have a respiratory infection.
    C. Ensure the mask or nasal pillows fits tightly over your nose and/or mouth.
    D. Ensure that there are no open flames (fireplace or candles) in the room when CPAP is in use.

12. What is the **best first** action for the nurse to take to prevent harm for a client 12 hours after a modified uvulopalatopharyngoplasty (modUPPP) who now has stridor and excessive drooling along with an increasing end-tidal carbon dioxide level?
    A. Use a soft catheter to suction the oral cavity.
    B. Reposition the client to his or her right side.
    C. Apply an ice collar to the client's neck.
    D. Call the Rapid Response Team.

13. Which discharge precautions will the nurse teach a client and family after extensive surgery for obstructive sleep apnea (OSA)? **Select all that apply**.
    A. Avoid aspirin or aspirin-containing products.
    B. Drink cool liquids and eat soft foods for a week or two.
    C. Use a firm toothbrush and floss four times daily to prevent infection.
    D. Try to go as long as possible between dosage of pain medication to reduce the risk for addiction.
    E. Examine your mouth and throat daily for any thick drainage and pus or a beefy red color.
    F. Go to the nearest emergency department if you see any amount of blood in your saliva or mucous.

14. What is the nurse's **best** response when a client who is 2 days postoperative from a modified uvulopalatopharyngoplasty (modUPPP) states disappointment at still snoring?
    A. I will report this complication to your surgeon immediately.
    B. Snoring for a few weeks after surgery is normal because of tissue swelling.
    C. Just because you are snoring doesn't mean your obstructive sleep apnea still exists.
    D. You may need a prescription for antibiotics because snoring after this surgery is an indication of infection.

15. Which action will the nurse perform **first** for a client with an active nosebleed (epistaxis)?
    A. Have the client sit upright with the head forward.
    B. Apply direct lateral pressure to the nose.
    C. Apply ice to the back of the client's neck.
    D. Insert nasal packing.

16. Which precaution is **most important** for the nurse to teach a client, who is a secretary, and just had nasal tubes removed after a posterior nasal bleed?
    A. Avoid NSAIDs for at least 1 week.
    B. Wait 4 weeks before returning to work.
    C. If bleeding recurs, call 911 immediately.
    D. Do not blow your nose for at least a month.

17. What is the **priority action** for a nurse to take to **prevent harm** when caring for a client with fresh packing in place for a posterior nosebleed?
    A. Assessing the airway
    B. Preventing dehydration
    C. Ensuring adequate humidification
    D. Monitoring for potential infection

18. Which interventions are **most appropriate** for the nurse to teach a client with a nasal fracture to reduce bleeding from the injury? **Select all that apply.**
    A. "Avoid blowing or picking the nose."
    B. "Drink at least 2000 mL of fluid daily."
    C. "Take the antibiotics for as long as they are prescribed."
    D. "Take in only liquids and eat no solid food for at least a week."
    E. "Change the drip (moustache) dressing as soon as it becomes wet."
    F. "Use acetaminophen for pain rather than aspirin or other NSAIDS."

19. Which complication of nasal fracture does the nurse suspect when a client's clear nasal secretions react positively when tested for glucose?
    A. Jaw fracture
    B. Facial fracture
    C. Vertebral fracture
    D. Skull fracture

20. What is the nurse's best **first** action when a postoperative client with a rhinoplasty repeatedly swallows?
    A. Ask the client if a sore throat is present.
    B. Examine the throat for bleeding.
    C. Provide ice chips to reduce pain.
    D. Notify the surgeon.

21. Which instructions will the nurse give to a client after rhinoplasty to **prevent harm** from bleeding? **Select all that apply**.
    A. Limit or avoid straining during bowel movements (e.g., Valsalva maneuver).
    B. Do not sniff upwards or blow your nose.
    C. Sneeze with your mouth closed for a few days after packing is removed.
    D. Cough forcefully twice daily to keep your airways clear.
    E. Avoid aspirin-containing products or NSAIDs.
    F. Use a humidifier to prevent mucosal drying.

22. Which procedure will the nurse prepare to assist with for a client who arrives in the emergency department with a severe crush injury to the face with blood gurgling from the mouth and nose and obvious respiratory distress?
    A. Tracheotomy
    B. Needle thoracotomy
    C. Nasal airway insertion
    D. Endotracheal tube insertion

23. Which discharge care issues are a **priority** for the nurse to teach a client with facial trauma who has undergone surgical intervention to wire the jaw shut? **Select all that apply**.
    A. Oral care
    B. Position restrictions
    C. Use of wire cutters
    D. Oxygen therapy
    E. Aspiration prevention
    F. Dental liquid diet

24. Which assessment finding on a client with significant and obvious facial trauma after being struck repeatedly in the face does the nurse recognize as a **priority** for immediate action?
    A. Asymmetry of the mandible
    B. Swollen lips and missing teeth
    C. Pain upon palpation over the nasal bridge
    D. Restlessness with high-pitched respirations

25. Which assessment finding indicates to the nurse that a client who sustained laryngeal trauma and is being treated with humidified oxygen that further action is needed urgently?
    A. Respiratory rate 24 breaths/min, Pao_2 90-100 mm Hg, no difficulty with communication
    B. Pulse oximetry 96%, anxious, fatigued, blood in sputum, abdominal breathing
    C. Confused and disoriented, difficulty producing sounds, pulse oximetry 80%
    D. Anxious, respiratory rate 30 breaths/min, talking rapidly about the accident, warm to touch

26. Which client symptom suggests the possibility of sinus cancer to the nurse?
    A. Blurred vision
    B. Intermittent nasal obstruction
    C. Long-term bloody nasal discharge
    D. Reduction of nasal mucous production

27. How will the nurse determine whether a client who suffered severe laryngeal trauma has subcutaneous emphysema?
    A. Using a stethoscope to assess for adventitious lung sounds
    B. Listening for stridor or a change in voice quality
    C. Palpating for air under the skin
    D. Assessing oxygen saturation

28. Which changes does the nurse teach adults to be aware of as warning signs of head and neck cancer? **Select all that apply**.
    A. Weight gain
    B. Lump in mouth, neck, or throat
    C. Change in fit of dentures
    D. Difficulty swallowing
    E. Intermittent bilateral ear pain
    F. Numbness in the mouth, lips, or face

29. What is the nurse's **best** response when a 62-year-old client whose brother was just diagnosed with head and neck cancer asks what he could do to reduce his risk for also developing this cancer?
    A. "Because head and neck cancer has a strong hereditary component, participating in screening twice yearly is critical for you."
    B. "Always wear sunscreen with a 50% or greater protection factor whenever you are outdoors."
    C. "Avoid shouting and singing to prevent stress to your vocal cords and larynx."
    D. "Stop smoking and drink alcohol only in moderation."

30. With which members of the interprofessional team will the nurse **most commonly** collaborate in providing comprehensive care to clients with head and neck cancer and their families? **Select all that apply**.
    A. Clergy
    B. Pharmacologist
    C. Physical therapist
    D. Registered dietitian nutritionist
    E. Respiratory therapist
    F. Speech-language pathologist

31. How will the nurse document the pack-year smoking history for a client who reports smoking three packs of cigarettes daily for 5 years, two packs daily for 10 years, and 1 pack daily for 3 years?
    A. 38 pack-years
    B. 48 pack-years
    C. 58 pack-years
    D. 68 pack-years

32. For which side effects will the nurse prepare the client who is to receive 6 weeks of external beam radiation therapy for throat cancer? **Select all that apply**.
    A. Dry mouth
    B. Taste changes
    C. Scalp alopecia
    D. Bowel changes
    E. Increased fatigue
    F. Dry, red, and peeling skin
    G. Difficulty swallowing
    H. Numbness and tingling in fingers and toes

33. Which action will the nurse recommend for the client who suffers from chronic xerostomia induced by radiation treatment for head and neck cancer?
    A. Eat six smaller meals instead of three larger ones daily.
    B. Wash the area carefully twice a day with soap and water.
    C. Try using a moisturizing mouth spray.
    D. Avoid carbonated beverages.

34. Which client will the nurse educate about relevant lifestyle modifications to decrease the risk for head and neck cancer?
    A. 64-year-old woman previously treated for breast cancer
    B. 57-year-old man with chronic alcoholism
    C. 34-year-old man who snorts cocaine
    D. 28-year-old woman with diabetes

35. Which care issue will the nurse consider to be the highest **priority to prevent harm** when caring for a client after a supraglottic laryngectomy for head and neck cancer?
    A. Preventing aspiration
    B. Preventing wound infection
    C. Maintaining communication
    D. Maintaining adequate nutrition

36. What is the **priority action** for the nurse to take **first to prevent harm** for a client whose tissue flap over the carotid artery after head and neck surgery is spurting bright red blood?
    A. Take the client's blood pressure.
    B. Call the Rapid Response Team.
    C. Apply immediate, direct pressure to the site.
    D. Apply a bulky sterile dressing and secure the airway.

37. Which assessment finding does the nurse expect for a client who has had a neck dissection with removal of muscle tissue, lymph nodes, and the 11th cranial nerve?
    A. Loss of sensation for taste and smell discrimination
    B. Shoulder drop with limitation of movement
    C. Asymmetrical eye movements and decreased visual acuity
    D. Facial swelling with discoloration and bruising around the eyes

38. Which side effect will the nurse teach a client with head and neck cancer who is taking the biotherapy cetuximab to expect?
    A. Hemorrhagic cystitis
    B. Persistent severe nausea and vomiting
    C. Exercise intolerance and increased fatigue
    D. Development of rash and dry peeling skin

Chapter 26 Answer Key

1. B, C, D
   The larynx, trachea, and oropharynx are structures that lead directly to the lungs and must remain patent for gas exchange. The laryngopharynx lies behind the trachea and leads to the esophagus. The nose and maxillary sinuses warm and filter air inspired through the nares; however, gas exchange can be adequate even if these structures were completely blocked.

2. A
   A mucoid impaction, also known as inspissated secretions, is a condition in which thickly crusted oral and nasopharyngeal secretions build up in the oropharynx leading to a partial or complete airway obstruction and potential asphyxiation. This condition is caused by poor oral hygiene and is most likely to occur in those who have an altered mental status and level of consciousness, are dehydrated, are unable to communicate, are unable to cough effectively, or are at risk for aspiration. The comatose client is most at risk. The client with Alzheimer disease is less at risk because of being ambulatory. Although the client who is intubated may be at risk for impacted secretions, the endotracheal tube prevents asphyxiation. The client whose jaws are wired together is less at risk because of age and has no other cognitive or physical disability.

3. D
   If possible, the obstruction is removed manually or by oral suction. Abdominal thrust maneuver is performed when a known airway obstruction exists and manual removal is not possible. Cardiac compressions are not sufficient to force an airway obstruction out of the airway. Initiating the Rapid Response Team is appropriate if the abdominal thrusts are not effective at removing the obstruction.

4. C
   Stridor is a sound made from a laryngeal obstruction, not just an oral obstruction. The fact that her oxygen saturation is so low indicates that this is a critical emergency and that her airway is going to become completely obstructed very soon. Nasal BiPAP is not at all helpful here and it is unlikely that endotracheal intubation would be successful with this much edema. A tracheotomy would work but takes more time. Also, because this is a temporary condition that should respond well to anaphylaxis therapy, cricothyroidotomy is the best choice and this is what the nurse should have prepared for the Rapid Response Team.

5. A, C, E
OSA usually occurs with sleep time hypopnea (lower than normal respiratory rate and depth insufficient for effective gas exchange). The sleep pattern in OSA is fragmented and prevents the deep sleep needed for best physiologic restoration, leading to chronic excessive daytime sleepiness. The associated hypoxia triggers frequent nightmares. It is common in people who have shorter necks and retracted jaws. Chronic sinusitis is not a cause of OSA. OSA is not diagnosed by any one blood test or imaging method, but by an overnight sleep study using polysomnography. The most definitive assessment to determine the presence of OSA is an overnight sleep study known as **polysomnography** in which the client is directly observed during a full sleep time while wearing a variety of monitoring equipment to evaluate depth of sleep, type of sleep, respiratory effort, oxygen saturation, carbon dioxide exhalation, and muscle movement.

6. A
The two biggest risk factors for OSA are obesity and a short neck. It is an anatomical problem, not a disease-related one. Diabetes is not related to OSA, especially type 1, which is not associated with obesity. GERD can damage the larynx over time but does not cause the tongue to subluxate, which is what obstructs the airway. Dentures alone (whether in or out) do not contribute to the ongoing problem of OSA.

7. A, D, E, F
Adult clients with OSA usually have chronic excessive daytime sleepiness, an inability to concentrate, morning headache, and irritability and are reported by family members as being heavy snorers. This problem does not increase sputum production and does not change the sensation of taste.

8. A, C, D
Recommended interventions and actions to improve mild OSA include avoidance of the supine position for sleep, reducing obesity, and the use of position-fixing devices that reduce obstruction by supporting the lower jaw or

preventing subluxation of the tongue from slipping backward during sleep. CPAP is recommended for moderate OSA. The presence of wisdom teeth does not increase the risk for or severity of obstructive sleep apnea. Taking sleep-inducing medication, either prescribed or over-the-counter, does not prevent sleep apnea and may make the condition worse.

9. C, D, E, F
Chronic OSA is associated with cardiovascular changes, especially hypertension that may not respond as expected to prescribed drug therapy. Additional long-term effects of chronic OSA include increased risk for stroke, cognitive deficits, weight gain, diabetes, and cardiovascular disease. Anemia is not caused by OSA. Although COPD may be worsened by OSA, it is not caused by OSA.

10. C, D,
Anatomic features such as a short neck and small chin increase the risk for development of OSA. Cigarette smoking also increases the risk.
An athletic lifestyle (associated with normal weight and good muscle tone) reduces the risk for OSA.
Younger age, female gender, and removal of adenoids and tonsils reduce the risk for OSA.
COPD and malnutrition do not increase the risk for OSA.
Cognitive impairment alone does not increase the risk.

11. C
The effectiveness of CPAP for holding the airway open is dependent on maintaining a tight seal over the orifice(s). For OSA, CPAP uses room air and there are no restrictions for using it in a room with open flames.

12. D
The client is displaying multiple indications of airway narrowing or partial obstruction (e.g., increased respiratory effort, presence of stridor or crowing, drooling or an inability to swallow oral secretions, reduction in the size of the oropharynx, decreasing oxygen saturation, rising end-tidal carbon dioxide level). The Rapid

Response Team is needed to initiate interventions to prevent a partial obstruction from becoming a complete obstruction. None of the other actions will open the airway or prevent obstruction.

13. A, B, E

There is a continued risk for bleeding after this surgery because of mouth movements and eating. Avoiding aspirin, aspirin-containing products, and NSAIDs helps reduce this risk. Swallowing is difficult and the tissues are easily traumatized. Drinking cool liquids and eating soft foods make swallowing easier. The mouth and throat are not sterile environments and infection risk remains after surgery until all tissues have healed. The client is taught to examine the mouth and throat for indications of infection, such as purulent drainage or a change in mucous membrane color from pink to beefy red.

Toothbrushing and flossing are avoided for several weeks to prevent tissue trauma.

This surgery is painful because of the high number of pain receptors in the mouth. Clients are taught to take prescribed pain medication around the clock on a schedule to avoid excessive pain.

Blood mixed in with saliva or mucous is expected and not a cause for concern. Heavy bleeding and the presence of large clots are a cause for concern.

14. B

Surgery in the mouth and throat usually causes swelling because of the highly vascular nature of the tissue. This swelling may allow snoring to continue for a few weeks until all swelling is gone. Snoring is not a complication and is not an indication of infection. Option C is not incorrect but not likely to allay the client's concern.

15. A

Placing the client in an upright position with the head forward reduces the risk for blood entering the throat and being aspirated. Applying lateral pressure is done after positioning the client. Applying ice to the back of the neck does not stop or slow epistaxis. Usually insertion of packing is done by a primary health care provider. Also, even if performed by a nurse, it is not done before proper positioning.

16. C

The most important of all these precautions is to get emergency treatment as soon as any rebleeding occurs. The tissue is fragile and could rebleed easily and excessively. It is important for the client to avoid the issues that could lead to bleeding, such as nose-blowing and the use of NSAIDs, but it is more important to stop the bleeding as soon as possible. Because this client's occupation is sedentary (being a secretary), he or she could return to work within a day or two as long as the usual precaution regarding heavy lifting is observed.

17. A

While all actions are appropriate, the priority is airway assessment. Posterior nasal packing can slip and cause airway obstruction.

18. A, F

Blowing or picking the nose can further damage the mucosa and lead to bleeding. Aspirin and other NSAIDs increase the risk for bleeding, acetaminophen does not. Clients can eat soft and solid foods as soon as they feel like it. Taking antibiotics for as long as prescribed and drinking plenty of fluids are healthy actions, but do not decrease the risk for bleeding. Changing the drip dressing does not apply pressure to the area and does not decrease bleeding risk.

19. D

Clear fluid draining from one or both nares after a simple nasal fracture that tests positive for glucose is cerebral spinal fluid (CSF) and indicates a serious injury (e.g., skull fracture). None of the other complications are indicated by a leakage of CSF.

20. B

Assessing how often the patient swallows after nasal surgery is a priority because repeated swallowing may indicate posterior nasal bleeding.

21. A, B, E, F
To prevent bleeding, the client is instructed to avoid forceful coughing or straining during a bowel movement, not to sniff upward or blow the nose, and not to sneeze with the mouth closed for the first few days after the packing is removed. Avoiding aspirin and other NSAIDs also helps to prevent bleeding, as does humidifying the environment.

22. A
The client's airway is at risk with the profuse blood flow through the nose and mouth and an emergency tracheotomy is needed. Even insertion of an endotracheal tube is dangerous because it is unlikely the emergency health care provider will be able to visualize the vocal cords and epiglottis. An injury to the face does not cause a pneumothorax. Thus, a thoracotomy would be of no benefit. Nasal airway insertion is not attempted with a crush injury to the face and would not protect the client's airway.

23. A, C, E, F
With jaw wiring, the client cannot open his or her mouth, making oral care and nutrition more challenging, especially because this fixation often remains in place for 6 to 10 weeks. A dental liquid diet is needed and meticulous oral care with an irrigating device is required to prevent infection and dental decay. Because the client cannot open his or her jaws and eject vomit, if vomiting occurs the wires must be cut to prevent aspiration. Neither position restrictions nor oxygen therapy are required as part of home care after this procedure.

24. D
Although all assessment findings are abnormal and will require eventual intervention, the finding of restlessness with high-pitched sounds on respiration indicates ineffective gas exchange and must be addressed first and quickly.

25. C
The findings listed in option C indicate hypoxemia and inadequate gas exchange while receiving oxygen. These changes are associated with inadequate gas exchange and must be addressed urgently.

26. C
The onset of sinus cancer is slow, and symptoms resemble sinusitis. These include persistent nasal obstruction, drainage, bloody discharge, and pain that persists after treatment of sinusitis.

27. C
Subcutaneous emphysema occurs when there is an opening or tear in the trachea and air escapes into the fresh tissue planes of the neck. This condition is identified by inspecting for puffiness in the skin and palpating for air under the skin, felt as a crackling sensation when pressing on the skin around the injured area. Subcutaneous emphysema cannot be determined by changes in oxygen saturation, changes in voice quality, or the presence of adventitious lung sounds.

28. B, C, D, F
The warning signs of head and neck cancer include: pain; lump in the mouth, throat, or neck; difficulty swallowing; color changes in the mouth or tongue to red, white, gray, dark brown, or black; oral lesion or sore that does not heal in 2 weeks; persistent or unexplained oral bleeding, numbness of the mouth, lips, or face; change in the fit of dentures; burning sensation when drinking citrus juices or hot liquids; persistent, unilateral (not intermittent or bilateral) ear pain; hoarseness or change in voice quality; persistent or recurrent sore throat, shortness of breath; and anorexia and weight loss (not weight gain).

29. D
No hereditary component has been identified to increase the risk for head and neck cancer. Although many head and neck cancers are squamous cell, which is a type of skin cancer, these cancers develop inside the oropharyngeal area and are not associated with external skin cancers on the head or the neck. Vocal cord abuse is associated with some types of head and

neck cancer; however, the two most important risk factors for head and neck cancer are tobacco and alcohol use, especially in combination. Other risk factors include chronic laryngitis, exposure to chemicals, dust, poor oral hygiene, long-term or severe gastroesophageal reflux disease, and oral infection with the human papillomavirus. Of all the cancer prevention activities this client could perform, smoking cessation and reduction of alcohol intake (or elimination of alcohol intake) are the most effective.

30. D, E, F
The three health care professionals who work with the nursing staff, patient, and family closely after surgery are the respiratory therapist, registered dietitian nutritionist, and speech-language pathologist. In addition, a psychiatric mental health professional is often involved in supporting the client and family while they learn to deal with appearance changes, lifestyle changes, and the possibility of disease progression. For some clients, members of the clergy are requested as part of the team. Pharmacologists and physical therapists are less involved in providing care to these clients and their families.

31. A
Pack-years are calculated by multiplying the number of packs smoked per day by the number of years of smoking at that rate. Three packs per day × 5 years = 15 pack-years, two packs per day × 10 years = 20 pack-years, plus 1 pack per day × 3 years = 3 pack-years. Total is 15, plus 20, plus 3 for 38 pack-years.

32. A, B, E, F, G
Radiation therapy is local therapy and most effects on normal tissues are those in the radiation path, which, in this case, is the skin and deeper throat tissues. Generalized side effects from radiation therapy include taste changes and intense fatigue over time, although the exact mechanisms responsible for these effects are not clear. Scalp alopecia will not occur from external beam radiation to the throat. Dry

mouth and difficulty swallowing are likely to occur because the salivary glands and esophagus are in the radiation path. The fingers and toes are not in the radiation path and will not be affected.

33. C
Xerostomia is a dry mouth that may be permanent after radiation therapy that includes the mouth and throat. Moisturizing sprays, increased water intake, and humidification can help ease the discomfort. Changing the volume of food eaten does not reduce the dry mouth. The mouth is not washed with soap and water. If the oral mucous membranes are intact, there is no need to avoid carbonated beverages.

34. B
The two primary lifestyle choices that greatly increase the risk for development of head and neck cancer are cigarette smoking and alcohol consumption, particularly three or more ounces of alcohol daily. These are modifiable risk factors. Previous treatment for breast cancer does not increase the risk and is not modifiable, neither is diabetes. Although cocaine use is modifiable, it is not a known cause of head and neck cancer.

35. A
All care issues listed are important. The one with the highest priority for the client after a supraglottic laryngectomy is preventing aspiration because of the altered swallow mechanism caused by the surgery. Aspiration can occur quickly and result in pneumonia, weight loss, and prolonged hospitalization. This client is still able to speak although the voice quality will have changed.

36. C
Bright red blood spurting from the flap indicates carotid artery rupture, which is an emergency. To prevent harm from stroke or death, the nurse will first immediately place constant pressure over the site and maintain direct manual, continuous pressure on the carotid artery. The nurse has another person call the Rapid

Response Team or surgeon and starts immediately transporting the client to the operating room for carotid resection.

37. B

The 11th cranial nerve is the accessory nerve which controls the motor function of the sternocleidomastoid and trapezius muscles. During a neck dissection, this nerve is damaged on one side and results in poor function of those innervated muscles on that side. Neck dissection does not affect visual, taste, or smell function, nor does it result in bruising around the eyes.

38. D

Cetuximab is a biotherapy (targeted therapy) that is an epidermal growth factor receptor inhibitor (EGFRI). Although it is a targeted therapy, this drug blocks EGFRs in normal tissues as well as those in the tumor. As a result, severe skin reactions are common and difficult for the patient.

27 CHAPTER

Concepts of Care for Patients with Noninfectious Lower Respiratory Problems

1. Which characteristics are most commonly associated with asthma? **Select all that apply**.
   A. Airway hyperresponsiveness
   B. Narrowed airway lumen
   C. Chronic bronchitis
   D. Dilated alveoli
   E. Excessive inflammation
   F. Leukocyte activation
   G. Reversible airway obstruction
   H. Bronchiolar smooth muscle constriction

2. Which client with asthma does the nurse consider to have the **highest risk** for a fatal outcome of an acute attack?
   A. 24-year-old with exercise-induced wheezing
   B. 45-year-old recovering from pneumonia
   C. 58-year-old who has type 2 diabetes mellitus
   D. 76-year-old with hypertension

3. How will the nurse categorize the level of asthma control for a client who reports usually waking at night with wheezing at least three times weekly and needing to use the prescribed reliever inhaler to stop the episodes?
   A. Controlled
   B. Partly controlled
   C. Minimally controlled
   D. Uncontrolled

4. Which symptom in a client having an acute asthma episode indicates to the nurse that the attack is becoming more severe?
   A. Loud wheezing is heard on inhalation as well as exhalation.
   B. The end-tidal carbon dioxide level is decreasing.
   C. The respiratory cycle is becoming shorter.
   D. The client's heart rate is decreasing.

5. Which arterial blood gas (ABG) value indicates to the nurse that a client with asthma demonstrating increased respiratory effort is in the early phase of the attack?
   A. $Paco_2$ of 60 mm Hg
   B. $Paco_2$ of 30 mm Hg
   C. pH of 7.40
   D. Pao_2 of 86 mm Hg

6. Which assessment findings does the nurse expect to see in a client having an acute asthma attack? **Select all that apply**.
   A. Audible wheezing
   B. Breathlessness while speaking
   C. Clubbing of the fingers
   D. Cyanosis of the nail beds
   E. Use of pursed-lip respirations
   F. Sternal retractions

7. Which key elements will the nurse teach or reinforce to a client for self-management with a personal asthma action plan? **Select all that apply**.
   A. A schedule for prescribed daily controller drug(s) and directions for prescribed reliever drug
   B. Daily assessment of symptom severity with a peak flow meter
   C. Client-specific daily asthma control assessment questions
   D. Directions for adjusting the daily controller drug schedule
   E. Emergency actions to take when asthma is not responding to controller and reliever drugs
   F. When to contact the primary health care provider (in addition to regularly scheduled visits)

8. Which statement(s) regarding drug therapy for asthma is(are) true? **Select all that apply**.
   A. A nursing priority for clients prescribed interleukin-5 antagonists is teaching them the correct subcutaneous technique for self-injection.
   B. Increases in a client's forced expiratory volume in the first second (FEV_1) is a positive indicator for asthma diagnosis.
   C. Inhaled anti-inflammatory drugs are always used for asthma control and never for acute asthma rescue.
   D. Reliever drugs are delivered by inhaler and controller drugs are taken orally.
   E. Metered dose inhalers are most effective with the use of a spacer.
   F. Oxygen is considered a type of asthma control drug.
   G. Daily magnesium sulfate prevents asthma attacks.

9. Which parameter indicates to the nurse that the medication administered to the client 5 minutes ago for an acute asthma attack is effective?
   A. SpO_2 decreased from 85% to 78%.
   B. Peak expiratory flow increased from 50% to 70%.
   C. The obvious use of accessory muscles during inhalation.
   D. Active bubbling in the humidifier chamber of the oxygen delivery system.

10. Which asthma drugs or drug categories have the **primary purpose** of asthma relief (rescue) rather than asthma control? **Select all that apply**.
    A. Anti-inflammatories
    B. Cholinergic antagonists
    C. Immunoglobulin E (IgE) antagonists
    D. Interleukin antagonists
    E. Long-acting beta agonists
    F. Short-acting beta agonists

11. Which suggestions will the nurse make to a client with asthma who is a runner to **prevent** an exercise-induced attack? **Select all that apply**.
    A. Use your reliever inhaler before starting your run.
    B. Dress in extra clothing during cold weather.
    C. Run on an indoor track during cold weather.
    D. Use pursed-lip breathing during the run.
    E. Exercise early in the morning before the day becomes too warm.
    F. Avoid eating eat solid foods before starting your run.

12. Which factors or conditions that increase the risk for development of chronic obstructive pulmonary disease (COPD) will the nurse include in preparing client education materials? **Select all that apply**.
    A. Alpha$_1$-antitrypsin (AAT) deficiency
    B. Chronic exposure to inhalation irritants
    C. Cigarette smoking
    D. History of asthma
    E. Mutations in the *CFTR* gene
    F. Pulmonary protease deficiency

13. Which arterial blood gas (ABG) value in a client with COPD does the nurse interpret as hypercarbia?
    A. pH = 7.19
    B. HCO_3^- = 33 mEq/L
    C. $Paco_2$ = 72 mm Hg
    D. Pao_2 = 92 mm Hg

14. Which common features of chronic obstructive pulmonary disease COPD does the nurse recognize as increasing a client's risk for respiratory infection? **Select all that apply**.
    A. Acidosis
    B. Ineffective cough
    C. Poor ciliary function
    D. Inadequate nutrition
    E. Excessive thick mucus
    F. Right-sided heart failure

15. Which symptom in a client with chronic obstructive pulmonary disease (COPD) does the nurse associate directly with chronic hypoxemia?
    A. Finger clubbing
    B. Barrel chest
    C. Pursed-lip breathing
    D. Increased mucous production

16. Which signs or symptoms in a client with long-standing chronic obstructive pulmonary disease (COPD) indicate to the nurse the possibility of cor pulmonale? **Select all that apply**.
    A. Dependent edema
    B. Distended neck veins
    C. Systemic high blood pressure
    D. Hypoxemia and acidosis
    E. Paralysis of airway cilia
    F. Swollen liver

17. Which nonpulmonary change in a client with chronic obstructive pulmonary disease (COPD) indicates to the nurse that the disorder may becoming more serious?
    A. Abdominal muscles contract on exhalation
    B. Increased urinary output at night
    C. Morning sputum production
    D. Weight loss of 11 lb (5 kg)

18. What is the nurse's **best** response to a client with chronic obstructive pulmonary disease (COPD) who is prescribed an inhaled long-acting beta$_2$ agonist and asks why the drug can't be taken as a pill?
    A. "Drugs taken by inhaler work more slowly and remain in the system longer."
    B. "Drugs taken by inhaler have no side effects and are less expensive."
    C. "Drugs taken by mouth are more expensive because they must be sterile."
    D. "Drugs taken by mouth have systemic side effects and are harder to control."

19. What is the nurse's **best** response to a client with chronic obstructive pulmonary disease (COPD) who states that there is no reason to quit cigarette smoking now that the disease has already been diagnosed?
    A. If you stop smoking now, the damage to your lungs can be reversed.
    B. Smoking cessation can slow the rate of your disease progression.
    C. You are correct, nothing will change the course of the disease now.
    D. You can serve as a role model to others by quitting smoking.

20. After collaboration with the registered dietitian nutritionist, the nurse expects to reinforce which nutritional changes to the client with chronic obstructive pulmonary disease (COPD)? **Select all that apply**.
    A. Increasing protein intake
    B. Avoiding dry or crumbly food
    C. Eating all fruit and vegetables raw
    D. Eating six smaller meals instead of three larger ones daily
    E. Drinking as much fluid as possible during meals to reduce coughing
    F. Greatly increasing the percentage of carbohydrates consumed daily

21. Which statement by a client with chronic obstructive pulmonary disease (COPD) indicates to the nurse a need for additional teaching about the disorder?
    A. "I have to be careful because I am susceptible to respiratory infections."
    B. "If the disease becomes more severe, I might develop serious heart failure."
    C. "My COPD is serious, but it can be reversed if I follow my treatment plan."
    D. "The lack of oxygen could cause my heart to beat in an irregular pattern."

22. With which client who has chronic obstructive pulmonary disease (COPD) does the nurse suspect that chronic bronchitis is more of a problem than emphysema?
    A. 52-year-old with an alpha$_1$-antitrypsin (AAT) deficiency
    B. 60-year-old with a 60 pack-year cigarette smoking history
    C. 66-year-old with chronic hypoxia, Paco$_2$ of 40 mm Hg, and cyanosis
    D. 70-year-old with Paco$_2$ of 65 mm Hg, dependent edema, and Spo$_2$ of 93%

23. What is the nurse's **best first** action to **prevent harm** for a client with chronic obstructive pulmonary disease (COPD) who is 1 day postoperative and now has an SpO$_2$ of 83%?
    A. Apply oxygen.
    B. Raise the head of the bed.
    C. Recheck the SpO$_2$ on a different body area.
    D. Instruct the client to use the incentive spirometer immediately.

24. Using the GOLD classification system, how will the nurse categorize the severity of respiratory impairment for a client with chronic obstructive pulmonary disease (COPD) whose FEV$_1$ now consistently measures 60% of the predicted value for the client's age?
    A. Mild
    B. Moderate
    C. Severe
    D. Very severe

25. The nurse will recognize which differences in common drug therapy for a client who has chronic obstructive pulmonary disease (COPD) from that prescribed for clients with asthma? **Select all that apply**.
    A. Addition of mucolytics
    B. Absence of reliever drugs
    C. Daily use of nebulizer delivery
    D. Addition of cholinergic antagonists
    E. Controllers in combinations of three drugs
    F. Increased use of immunoglobulin E (IgE) antagonists

26. With clients from which racial or ethnic group will the nurse make sure to ask about family members with cystic fibrosis when performing a pulmonary assessment?
    A. Asian Americans
    B. African Americans
    C. European Americans
    D. Hispanic or Latino Americans

27. Which assessment findings will the nurse expect to find in a 32-year-old client who was diagnosed with cystic fibrosis (CF) at age 6 months? **Select all that apply**.
    A. Arterial blood gases with a higher than normal pH
    B. History of frequent respiratory infections
    C. Cough and sputum production
    D. Chest muscle weakness
    E. Decreased exercise tolerance
    F. Barrel-shaped chest

28. Which laboratory test will the nurse expect to be ordered as **most appropriate** for an adult client who has persistent pulmonary symptoms to determine whether cystic fibrosis (CF) is the cause?
    A. Sweat chloride level
    B. Alpha$_1$-antitrypsin (AAT) levels
    C. Arterial blood gas (ABG) analysis
    D. Genetic analysis of the *CFTR* gene

29. Which precaution is **most important** for the nurse to teach a client who has cystic fibrosis?
    A. Report a weight change of 2 pounds to your health care provider immediately.
    B. Use supplemental oxygen whenever your oxygen saturation is less than 95%.
    C. Eat six small meals each day instead of only three larger ones.
    D. Avoid crowds and people who are ill.

30. Which activities will the nurse indicate are safe to perform without causing lung problems for a client with cystic fibrosis (CF) who had a bilateral lung transplant 6 months ago? **Select all that apply**.
    A. Bowling
    B. Hiking
    C. Playing chess with a friend with asthma
    D. Riding a bicycle
    E. Sledding
    F. Swimming

31. Which client with a respiratory problem having a sudden onset of extreme shortness of breath causes the nurse to suspect primary pulmonary arterial hypertension (PAH) as a possible cause of the problem?
    A. 27-year-old woman whose mother died of PAH
    B. 55-year-old man with a 70 pack-year smoking history
    C. 65-year-old woman with chronic obstructive pulmonary disease (COPD)
    D. 70-year-old man who had a pneumonectomy 1 year ago for lung cancer

32. Which subjective assessment findings will the nurse expect in a client who has just been diagnosed with early-stage pulmonary arterial hypertension (PAH)?
    A. Difficulty concentrating and anorexia
    B. Dyspnea and fatigue
    C. Cyanosis and finger clubbing
    D. Hypotension and headache

33. What are the **critical priority actions** for the nurse to take to **prevent harm** when caring for a client with pulmonary artery hypertension who is receiving an infusion of a prostacyclin through a small portable IV pump? **Select all that apply**.
    A. Ensuring the infusion is never interrupted
    B. Monitoring arterial blood gas values (ABGs)
    C. Assessing for new-onset angina-like chest pain
    D. Teaching the client about anticoagulation therapy
    E. Avoiding the use of the pump line for delivery of other drugs
    F. Using strict aseptic technique when changing drug cassettes and site dressings

34. Which instructions are **most important** for the nurse to teach a female client with pulmonary artery hypertension (PAH) who is prescribed an oral endothelin-receptor antagonist therapy at home? **Select all that apply**.
    A. Report any yellowing of the skin or whites of the eyes to your pulmonologist immediately.
    B. If you are sexually active, be sure to use two reliable methods of contraception.
    C. Get up slowly from a lying or sitting position.
    D. Do not break, chew, or crush the drug tablet.
    E. Take the drug with a full glass of water.
    F. Avoid drinking alcoholic beverages.

35. Which drugs or drug classes will the nurse expect to be prescribed to slow disease progression for a client who has early-stage idiopathic pulmonary fibrosis? **Select all that apply**.
    A. Antibiotics
    B. Bronchodilators
    C. Corticosteroids
    D. Morphine
    E. Nintedanib
    F. Pirfenidone

36. Which assessment findings will the nurse associate with the possibility of lung cancer? **Select all that apply**.
    A. Dyspnea
    B. Persistent cough
    C. Abdominal pain
    D. Change in voice quality
    E. Use of accessory muscles
    F. Dark yellow-colored sputum

37. For which side effects of therapy will the nurse prepare a client who is about to begin external beam radiation for lung cancer?
    A. Constipation
    B. Scalp alopecia
    C. Chest skin redness and peeling
    D. Persistent abdominal pain and vomiting

38. Which new-onset problem in a client diagnosed with advanced lung cancer indicates to the nurse probable metastasis?
    A. Anorexia
    B. Bone pain
    C. Insomnia
    D. Dyspnea

39. Which action will the nurse perform to promote comfort for a client with dyspnea from advanced lung cancer?
    A. Providing supplemental oxygen via cannula or mask
    B. Providing nonopioid pain medication when the client requests it
    C. Encouraging coughing, deep-breathing, and independent ambulation
    D. Placing the client in a supine position with a pillow under the knees and legs

40. What is the nurse's **best** action to **prevent harm** when caring for a client with a chest tube in place that has drained 110 mL during the past hour?
    A. Gently "milk" the tubing using a hand-over-hand technique.
    B. Reposition the client to the operative side.
    C. Check the chest tube system for leaks.
    D. Notify the surgeon immediately.

41. The chest tube of a client who is 12 hours postoperative from a lobectomy separates from the drainage system. What is the nurse's best **first** action?
    A. Immediately call the surgeon or Rapid Response Team.
    B. Notify respiratory therapy to set up a new drainage system.
    C. Cover the insertion site with a sterile occlusive dressing and tape down on three sides.
    D. Place the end of the disconnected tube into a container of sterile water positioned below the chest.

42. Which observation of a client's chest tube setup indicates to the nurse a leak is present in the system?
    A. Cessation of fluctuation in the water-seal chamber
    B. Increase of bubbling in the suction chamber
    C. Continuous bubbling in the water-seal chamber
    D. Decreased drainage in the collection chamber

43. Which problem has the **highest priority** for the nurse to help the wife of a client with late-stage small cell lung cancer to provide symptom management in the home?
    A. Continuing weight loss
    B. Constipation
    C. Severe pain
    D. Fatigue

Chapter 27 Answer Key

1. A, B, E, F, G, H

   Asthma is a chronic disease in which reversible airway obstruction occurs intermittently, reducing airflow. Airway obstruction occurs by excessive inflammation and airway tissue sensitivity (hyperresponsiveness) with bronchoconstriction. Lumens are narrowed by inflammation and constriction of bronchiolar smooth muscle. Inflammation begins with leukocyte activation, especially of the eosinophils and the neutrophils. Airway hyperresponsiveness and constriction of bronchial smooth muscle narrow the tubular structure of the airways.

   Asthma is an airway disease and the alveoli are not directly affected. Infectious or inflammatory chronic bronchitis is not a feature or characteristic of asthma.

2. D

   Although asthma can be fatal at any age, asthma-related deaths are highest in adults aged over 65 years. Lung and airway changes as a part of the aging process make breathing problems more serious in the older adult. Also, older adults have a decreased sensitivity of beta-adrenergic receptors, which then no longer respond as quickly or as strongly to agonists and beta-adrenergic drugs, which are often used as rescue therapy during an acute asthma attack.

3. D

   The client meets the criteria for uncontrolled asthma, which are that any of these symptoms occur three or more times per week:

   Daytime symptoms of wheezing, dyspnea, coughing

   Waking from night sleep with symptoms of wheezing, dyspnea, coughing

   Reliever (rescue) drug needed more than twice weekly

4. A

   Respiratory effort is needed for inhalation to overcome the elastic recoil of the lungs, whereas exhalation is a largely passive event not requiring muscle effort. Thus, when airflow is impaired, wheezing is heard first on exhalation.

   As the impairment becomes worse, the client has audible or even loud wheezing on inhalation as well as exhalation. With narrowed airways, air movement out and in is impeded and the actual respiratory cycle becomes longer. As the effectiveness of ventilation decreases, gas exchange decreases and carbon dioxide levels in exhaled air increases. Heart rate increases rather than decreases whenever gas exchange is impaired.

5. B

   ABG levels show the effectiveness of gas exchange. Early in the attack, the arterial carbon dioxide level ($PaCO_2$) may be decreased as the client increases the breathing rate and depth. Later in an asthma episode, $PaCO_2$ rises indicating carbon dioxide retention. The pH is in the normal range and the PaO_2 is low, which usually occurs later in the attack as respiratory effort becomes less effective.

6. A, B, D, F

   Common symptoms during an asthma attack are an audible wheeze and increased respiratory rate making the client breathless and unable to speak more than a few words between breaths. If hypoxemia is present, cyanosis of the nail beds and oral mucous membranes may be present. Clients may need to use accessory muscles to help breathe during an attack, which is seen as muscle retraction at the sternum.

   Clubbing of the fingers occurs only with disorders that are associated with chronic, continuous hypoxia, not an intermittent problem of asthma. Clients who have COPD use pursed-lip respirations, which are slow and deep, and those having an acute asthma attack do not use this form of respiration.

7. A, C, D, E, F

   All the above-listed elements are key parts of a personal asthma action plan except for option B. At one time, clients were instructed to assess their asthma severity at least daily with a peak flow meter. However, this process is now only recommended for those clients whose asthma is not well controlled.

8. C, E

Inhaled anti-inflammatory drugs help prevent asthma attacks from occurring but their actions are too slow to help stop an actual attack.

Without a spacer, drug doses delivered by metered dose are more likely to stick to oral mucus membranes or to be exhaled through the nose instead of reaching the lower airways, which are the sites of action.

Although some interleukin-5 antagonists are injected subcutaneously, the drug is associated with a relatively high risk for inducing anaphylaxis and must be administered by a health care professional in a setting prepared to handle emergency management of anaphylaxis.

Narrowing of the airways during an asthma attack causes a decrease in forced expiratory volume in the first second (FEV_1), not an increase.

Both asthma reliever and control drugs may be delivered by inhaler.

Oxygen is a drug but its use does not prevent or control an asthma attack, it only supports gas exchange during an attack.

Magnesium sulfate may be used during status asthmaticus but is not a controller drug. Its use in status asthmaticus is controversial.

9. B

Peak flow measures the effectiveness of expiratory efforts. An increased peak flow rate indicates less obstruction and greater movement of air with expiratory effort. Decreased SpO_2 would indicate a worsening of the condition, not effectiveness of the therapy. The use of accessory muscles indicates that the work of breathing has increased. The active bubbling in the humidification chamber is not related to the client's respiratory effort or the drug therapy's effectiveness.

10. F

Only short-acting beta$_2$ agonists work rapidly enough to cause bronchodilation to be effective as asthma reliever or rescue drugs. The others have a much slower onset of action. Although cholinergic antagonists are sometimes used as a reliever drug, this is not their primary purpose.

11. A, C

Use of a reliever inhaler before exercise begins can help prevent an asthma attack by inducing or increasing bronchodilation.

Exercising in cold, dry air is an airway irritant that usually exacerbates exercise-induced asthma. Changing the environment during cold weather by running on an indoor track can help prevent an attack.

Dressing warmly does not affect the temperature of the inhaled air or reduce exercise-induced asthma as a trigger.

Using pursed-lip breathing does not contribute to bronchodilation.

Exercising before the day becomes too warm is a good idea for other reasons, but does not help prevent exercise-induced asthma.

Although eating solid food before running may cause discomfort during the run, it does not trigger exercise-induced asthma.

12. A, B, C, D

Well known factors or conditions associated with development of COPD include cigarette smoking, chronic exposure to inhalation irritants, and AAT deficiency. A newer identified factor is asthma. The incidence of COPD is reported to be 12 times greater among adults with asthma than among adults without asthma.

Mutations in the *CFTR* gene cause cystic fibrosis, not COPD. One of the pathologic mechanisms for the injury to elastic tissues leading to emphysema is an excess of pulmonary proteases.

13. C

All of the ABG values are abnormal. Hypercapnia is an elevated arterial carbon dioxide level (also known as hypercarbia). The pH is low, indicating acidosis; however, it does not indicate that hypercapnia is the cause. The bicarbonate level is elevated but only indicates that the acidosis is chronic, not that hypercapnia is present. The carbon dioxide is very high, indicating hypercapnia (normal is 35 to 45 mm Hg). The oxygen level is low, indicating hypoxemia but not hypercapnia.

14. B, C, D, E

A major factor that increases the risk for respiratory infection in a client with COPD is the presence of excessive thick mucus. It is a fertile medium for the growth of microorganisms. Thus, any problem that reduces the client's ability to cough up the mucus increases the risk, such as an ineffective cough and poor ciliary function. Clients with inadequate nutrition have weaker muscles, which also reduce coughing effectiveness.

Acidosis does not directly increase the risk for respiratory infection. Right-sided heart failure results in systemic edema, which has little if any effect on risk for infection. (Left-sided failure would cause pulmonary edema and increase infection risk.)

15. A

Chronic hypoxemia from any pathologic condition (pulmonary or cardiovascular) causes finger clubbing. Barrel chest is caused by air trapping. Pursed-lip breathing is a change in breathing pattern taught to clients with COPD to prevent both airway and alveolar collapse. Increased mucous production is a result of the presence of airway inflammation and chronic bronchitis, not hypoxemia.

16. A, B, F

Cor pulmonale is right-sided heart failure that develops as a result of the right ventricle overworking to pump blood into the lungs that have a high vascular pressure from long-term COPD. Blood backs up into the venous vascular system, causing dependent edema, distended neck veins (even when the client is in the upright position), nausea and other GI problems, and a swollen and tender liver. Systemic blood pressure is actually low because not as much blood is getting to the left side of the heart, which is responsible for mean arterial pressure.

Hypoxemia and acidosis to some degree are present in all clients with COPD, not just those who have cor pulmonale. Paralysis of cilia is common in anyone who smokes cigarettes and is not a specific sign or symptom of cor pulmonale.

17. D

Unplanned weight loss is likely when COPD severity increases because the work of breathing increases metabolic needs. In addition, increasing dyspnea and mucus production often result in poor food intake and inadequate nutrition, which also contribute to weight loss.

18. D

When used as prescribed, inhaler drugs go more to the site where the intended responses are needed (the airways) and less drug is absorbed systemically. Thus, inhaled drugs have fewer side effects (but still have side effects). Oral drugs always have systemic side effects.

19. B

Nothing reverses the existing lung damage of COPD; however, reducing or eliminating the exposure to cigarette smoke can reduce the severity of the symptoms (especially the cough and mucous production) and slow the progression of the disorder.

20. A, B, D

The client with COPD often has nausea, early satiety, poor appetite, and meal-related dyspnea. The work of breathing raises total calorie and protein needs, which can lead to protein-calorie malnutrition. Although all food groups are important, recommendations include increasing proteins and relying less on carbohydrates. To avoid early satiety, clients are instructed to avoid drinking liquids with meals and to eat smaller meals more frequently. Dry or crumbly food is avoided because these foods increase coughing, which may make the client too fatigued to eat. Food that requires a lot of chewing also may make the client too fatigued to eat. Fruits and vegetables that are cooked and require less chewing are recommended.

21. C

The tissue damage to the pulmonary system caused by COPD is not reversible; however, progression may be delayed when a client is adherent to the prescribed treatment plan. Complications of COPD include increased susceptibility to respiratory infection, hypoxia-induced cardiac dysrhythmias, and heart failure.

22. C
Clients with COPD whose pathology is chronic bronchitis rather than emphysema do not retain CO_2 because the alveoli are not affected and have no difficulty eliminating this gas. The bronchitis narrows the upper airways reducing oxygenation leading to chronic hypoxia and hypoxemia, resulting in a cyanotic appearance. Cigarette smoking and an AAT deficiency are associated with development of emphysema and CO_2 retention.

23. A
All actions are appropriate for the nurse to take to help this client. The SpO_2 of 83% indicates hypoxemia and this must be corrected first with supplemental oxygen. Ideally, a client with COPD does not have an SpO_2 of less than 88%. It is possible that the pulse oximeter is not working properly or is incorrectly positioned providing a falsely low SpO_2 but applying oxygen to improve gas exchange is the priority before checking the accuracy of the reading.

24. B
The GOLD classification identifies a consistent FEV_1 between 50% to 79% of predicted in a client with COPD as moderate severity. Mild severity has an FEV_1 equal to or greater than 80%, severe between 30% to 49%, and very severe less than 30% of predicted.

25. A, C, E
All drugs commonly used for asthma control and relief are also used for COPD. An additional drug category for COPD management is the mucolytics, some of which are delivered by nebulizer daily. The focus for COPD management is on long-term control therapy with longer-acting drugs in two- and three-drug combinations. These are not recommended (and some are contraindicated) for asthma management.

Although cholinergic antagonists are used more commonly for COPD, they are also prescribed for asthma control. IgE antagonists are not prescribed for COPD because disease symptoms are not caused by allergens.

26. C
CF is most common among whites, especially European Americans from northern Europe, and about 4% (1 in 29) are carriers.

27. B, C, E, F
Pulmonary symptoms are usually the most obvious problems caused by CF and are progressive. Respiratory infections are frequent or chronic with exacerbations. Clients usually have chest congestion, limited exercise tolerance, cough, sputum production, use of accessory muscles, and decreased pulmonary function (especially forced vital capacity [FVC] and forced expiratory volume in the first second of exhalation [FEV_1]). Chest x-rays show infiltrate and an increased anteroposterior diameter leading to a barrel chest.

Clients with long-standing CF do not have chest muscle weakness because of the constant increased respiratory effort needed to breathe. A higher than normal ABG pH indicates alkalosis, not the acidosis most commonly present in these clients.

28. A
The defect in the *CFTR* gene that causes CF results in a high concentration of chloride ions being present in the affected client's sweat. It is a quick, noninvasive, and inexpensive way to determine whether or not the client has any form of CF. Genetic analysis of the *CFTR* gene to determine the exact mutation is performed later after the diagnosis is made to assess which therapy may be beneficial. Alpha$_1$-antitrypsin (AAT) levels are normal in CF. ABGs are nonspecific and only indicate gas exchange adequacy or inadequacy (and whether the problem is chronic or acute), not CF.

29. D
The most common cause of death for a client with cystic fibrosis is respiratory failure from a respiratory infection. Avoiding infection in this population is critical for survival. While many

clients who have CF are underweight and need to maintain good nutrition, changes in weight and food intake patterns are not as critical as avoiding infection. Supplemental oxygen use is based on client manifestations. Its use is not as critical as avoiding infection.

30. A, B, C, D, E, F
After healing from lung transplantation surgery, there are no activity restrictions related to the new lungs.

31. A
Although rare, primary PAH has a genetic component and is more common among women than men. Smoking does not contribute to the development of primary PAH but may play more of a role in secondary PAH. As COPD progresses, it does increase pulmonary vascular pressures but this is a type of secondary PAH, not primary. Lung removal does not cause primary PAH in the remaining lung.

32. B
The most common early symptoms are dyspnea and fatigue in an otherwise healthy adult. At this time, gas exchange and oxygenation remain adequate as a result of increased respiratory rate. Cyanosis occurs later and finger clubbing takes months of hypoxemia to develop. Pulmonary vessels are constricted as are systemic vessels, leading to hypertension.

33. A, E, F
The effectiveness of parenteral prostacyclin therapy for PAH depends on continuous infusion and interrupting the therapy even for a few minutes can have adverse effects. The line is dedicated to the use of the prostacyclin administration only to prevent disruption of therapy or the dilution of the drug concentration. A major cause of death in clients receiving this therapy is sepsis because the continuous IV infusion allows direct access of microorganisms to the blood stream. Strict asepsis is needed to prevent this potentially fatal complication.
Monitoring ABGs, although important, is not a critical priority.

The client is likely to go home on anticoagulant therapy but at this time, teaching is not the priority.
Prostacyclin induces vasodilation and does not cause angina-like symptoms.

34. A, B, C, D, E, F
Although the oral endothelin-receptor antagonist drugs are beneficial to clients with PAH, they are dangerous drugs with many side effects, including liver toxicity (so clients must avoid alcohol consumption and assess daily for indications of jaundice), postural hypotension, and inducing birth defects. These drugs are not to be crushed, chewed, or broken, and must be taken with a full glass of water.

35. C, E, F
Pulmonary fibrosis is an example of excessive wound healing. Once lung injury occurs, inflammation begins tissue repair and continues beyond normal healing time, causing fibrosis and scarring, which thicken alveolar tissues and make gas exchange difficult. Drug therapy for slowing disease progression includes anti-inflammatory/immunosuppressants (corticosteroids) and drugs that inhibit fibrous growth (nintedanib, pirfenidone). Antibiotics and morphine are prescribed as needed during the course of the disease but do not slow disease progression. Because the disorder affects the lung tissue and not the airways, bronchodilators are not part of therapy for idiopathic pulmonary fibrosis.

36. A, B, D, E
Common symptoms of lung cancer include hoarseness, cough, sputum production, hemoptysis, shortness of breath, labored breathing, and reduced endurance. Abdominal pain is not associated with lung cancer. Although increased sputum production occurs, it is frequently blood-tinged. Dark yellow sputum is associated with respiratory infections, especially viral pneumonia.

37. C
Radiation therapy is local and only the tissues in the path of the radiation beam are affected

directly, in this case the chest. The skin of the chest will develop irritation, redness, peeling, and loss of chest hair. Scalp hair is unaffected. The abdomen is not in the radiation path, thus constipation is not an expected side effect of the therapy and neither are abdominal pain and persistent vomiting.

38. B
A common site for metastasis of lung cancer is the bone, which increases the pressure in the bone and causes pain. Anorexia and weight loss are common with advanced lung cancer as a result of increasing shortness of breath and the energy needed for the increased work of breathing. Dyspnea occurs as a result of the primary tumor in the lungs or airways and not metastasis.

39. A
Only providing supplemental oxygen can reduce dyspnea. Nonopioids do not relieve dyspnea although opioids may. Coughing, deep-breathing, and independent ambulation may all make dyspnea worse as will being in a supine position.

40. D
Chest tube drainage of more than 70 mL/hr at any time after surgery is excessive and may

indicate internal bleeding. This finding is reported immediately to the surgeon.

41. D
This soon after surgery an open chest drainage tube can have air suck through it back into the client's chest and collapse the lung. This is an emergency. Although the surgeon or Rapid Response Team should be called, the nurse first prevents the situation from becoming worse by sealing the tube with water. Because the chest tube is still in place in the client, using an occlusive dressing will not help prevent a lung collapse. Setting up a new drainage system can wait until after the tube is secured.

42. C
Bubbling of the water in the water-seal chamber indicates air drainage from the client whenever he or she exhales, coughs, or sneezes. Continuous or excessive bubbling in the water-seal chamber indicates an air leak.

43. C
Although all the listed problems are important, effective pain management is the most important issue for this client an3d family.

28
CHAPTER

Concepts of Care for Patients with Infectious Respiratory Problems

1. Which information will the nurse include when providing community education on prevention of seasonal influenza? **Select all that apply**.
   A. Adults older than 65 years should get the Prevnar-13 vaccination yearly.
   B. All adults younger than 49 years should receive a quadrivalent immunization annually.
   C. Sneeze into a disposable tissue or into your sleeve instead of your hand.
   D. Avoid large crowds during spring and summer to limit the chance for getting the flu.
   E. Wash your hands frequently and after blowing your nose, coughing, or sneezing.
   F. Call your provider for an antiviral prescription within 3 days of getting symptoms.

2. What action by the assisted living facility nurse is **most appropriate** to prevent influenza spread when a resident client tests positive for influenza A?
   A. Prepare to administer antibiotics.
   B. Have the resident eat meals in his or her room.
   C. Provide oseltamivir to the staff.
   D. Arrange a follow-up chest x-ray in 2 weeks.

3. What is the nurse's **best response** when a 65-year-old client with no health problems states that he had a flu shot last year and asks if it is necessary to have it again this year?
   A. "No, because once you get a flu shot, it lasts for several years and is effective against many different viruses."
   B. "Yes, because the immunity against the virus wears off, increasing your chances of getting the flu."
   C. "Yes, because the vaccine guards against a few specific viruses and reduces your chances of acquiring flu and is only effective for 1 year."
   D. "No, flu shots are only for high-risk clients and you are not considered to be at high risk."

4. For which client does the nurse recommend vaccination with the influenza "super vaccine"?
   A. 19-year-old living in a college dormitory
   B. 36-year-old who has type 1 diabetes mellitus
   C. 50-year-old who just underwent aortic valve replacement
   D. 75-year old community-dwelling client after hip replacement surgery

5. For which serious complications of the infection will the nurse caring for a client who has seasonal influenza continuously monitor? **Select all that apply**.
   A. Chronic obstructive pulmonary disease (COPD)
   B. Fever
   C. Hypertension
   D. Pneumonia
   E. Renal failure
   F. Sepsis

6. In the event of a new pandemic influenza outbreak, such as COVID-19, what is the nurse's primary role?
   A. Immediately report new cases to the Centers for Disease Control and Prevention (CDC).
   B. Administer oxygen, standard antibiotics, and supportive therapies to clients.
   C. Prevent the spread of infection to other employees and clients.
   D. Ensure all unit staff have annual influenza vaccination.

7. Which information does the community health nurse include when preparing an information packet about a potential pandemic influenza outbreak? **Select all that apply**.
   A. In the event of an outbreak, do not eat any cooked or uncooked meat from exotic animals.
   B. Have on hand a minimum of 2 weeks' supply of food, water, and routine prescription drugs.
   C. Listen to public health announcements and early warning signs for disease outbreaks.
   D. Avoid traveling to areas where there has been a suspected outbreak of disease.
   E. Obtain a supply of antiviral drugs such as oseltamivir.
   F. In the event of an outbreak, avoid going to public areas such as churches or schools.

8. The nurse is caring for a client who just returned from an extended trip overseas. The client has severe headache, muscle aches, fever, fatigue, sore throat and cough with acute respiratory distress. Which nursing action is appropriate? **Select all that apply**.
   A. Ask the client about exposure to anyone who was ill.
   B. Use only gown and gloves when entering this client's room.
   C. Prepare to administer isoniazid when the first dose is available.
   D. Explain that visitors will not be allowed into the care unit.
   E. Obtain arterial blood gases and monitor oxygen status.
   F. Obtain sputum cultures for acid-fast bacilli.

9. Which actions help the nurse caring for a client with a pandemic influenza such as COVID-19 to prevent contracting the virus? **Select all that apply**.
   A. Wearing eye protection during suctioning
   B. Keeping the door of the client's room closed
   C. Changing the water in the oxygen nebulizer daily
   D. Checking results of the client's sputum cultures daily
   E. Washing hands after removing gowns, gloves, and masks
   F. Using a powered air-purifying respirator (PAPR) when in the client's room

10. Which clients will the nurse recognize to be at risk for developing pneumonia? **Select all that apply**.
    A. 72-year-old with chronic confusion
    B. 66-year-old with influenza
    C. 55-year-old with atrial fibrillation who is taking an oral anticoagulant
    D. 40-year-old being mechanically ventilated and is orally colonized with Gram-negative bacteria
    E. 35-year-old with hyperthyroid disease
    F. 28-year-old who is extremely malnourished

11. Which laboratory result for a client with pneumonia will the cause the nurse to **collaborate quickly** with the primary health care provider?
    A. White blood cell (WBC) count of 14,526/mm^3
    B. Pao$_2$ 68 mm Hg
    C. Paco$_2$ 48 mm Hg
    D. Fasting blood glucose 146 mg/dL

12. Which assessment finding on a client with pneumonia who is receiving IV antibiotics and oxygen by nasal cannula indicates to the nurse that initial goals for this client have been met?
    A. Client is alert and oriented to person, place, and time.
    B. Blood pressure is within normal limits and client's baseline.
    C. Skin behind the ears demonstrates no redness or irritation.
    D. Urine output has been >30 mL/hr per foley catheter.

13. Which factor will the nurse recognize as increasing a client's risk for developing community-acquired pneumonia (CAP)?
    A. Obtaining an influenza vaccination in November rather than September
    B. Having received a pneumococcal vaccination
    C. Using tobacco and alcohol often and regularly
    D. Living alone and preparing own meals

14. Which client assessment findings alert the nurse to the possibility of uncomplicated community-acquired pneumonia (CAP)? **Select all that apply**.
    A. Abdominal pain
    B. Back pain
    C. Chest discomfort
    D. Dyspnea
    E. Increased sputum production
    F. Fever

15. Which **priority** action will the nurse take to help prevent the complication of pneumonia for a client who is postoperative from extensive abdominal surgery?
    A. Monitoring chest x-rays and WBC counts for early signs of infection
    B. Monitoring lung sounds every shift and encouraging fluids
    C. Teaching coughing, deep-breathing exercises, and use of incentive spirometry
    D. Encouraging hand hygiene among all caregivers, clients, and visitors

16. Which specific signs and symptoms does the nurse expect to see in an 80-year-old client admitted with bacterial pneumonia? **Select all that apply**.
    A. Confusion
    B. Decreased oxygen saturation
    C. Productive cough
    D. Weakness and fatigue
    E. Elevated white blood cell (WBC) count
    F. Fever

17. Which chest x-ray finding will the nurse expect to see for a client suspected to have pneumonia?
    A. Patchy areas of increased density
    B. "Ground-glass" appearance of the lung
    C. Mediastinal widening
    D. Large hyperinflated airways

18. For which client with pneumonia and hypoxemia will the nurse **avoid** the use of oxygen therapy? **Select all that apply**.
    A. 28-year-old with community-acquired pneumonia
    B. 38-year-old with fractured ribs
    C. 48-year-old with type 2 diabetes mellitus
    D. 58-year-old client with metastatic breast cancer
    E. 68-year-old with chronic obstructive pulmonary disease
    F. 78-year-old with acute confusion

19. Which additional client condition(s) or factor(s) will the nurse recognize as increasing the risk for ventilator-associated pneumonia (VAP)? **Select all that apply**.
    A. History of alcohol use and cigarette smoking
    B. Presence of feeding tube
    C. Unplanned weight loss
    D. IV therapy with normal saline
    E. Tooth loss and mouth sores
    F. Bacterial colonization of the airway

20. Which changes in signs and symptoms in a client with bacterial pneumonia does the nurse report to the primary health care provider as indicators of possible empyema? **Select all that apply**.
    A. Increased production of thick yellow sputum
    B. Reduced chest wall motion on one side
    C. Decreased breath sounds
    D. Flat percussion
    E. Persistent fever
    F. Wheezing

21. Which clients will the nurse recognize as at higher risk for having active tuberculosis (TB) in North America? **Select all that apply**.
    A. 22-year-old college student sharing a room in a dormitory
    B. 28-year-old man with HIV-III (AIDS)
    C. 48-year-old homemaker who volunteers at a soup kitchen
    D. 55-year-old homeless man with alcoholism who stays weekly in a shelter
    E. 60-year-old migrant farm worker from Mexico
    F. 68-year-old man incarcerated for 20 years

22. Which assessment findings for a community-dwelling client who reports "not feeling well" for about 2 months indicate to the nurse the possibility of active tuberculosis (TB)? **Select all that apply**.
    A. Fatigue
    B. Weight gain
    C. Night sweats
    D. Back soreness
    E. Persistent cough
    F. Low-grade fever
    G. Shortness of breath
    H. Blood-streaked sputum

23. Which assessment finding for a client who received the subcutaneous Mantoux skin test 72 hours ago will the nurse interpret as a positive test result for tuberculosis (TB)?
    A. Test area is red, warm, and blistered.
    B. A flat, erythematous skin rash is present at the test site.
    C. Induration/hardened area measures 5 mm or greater.
    D. Induration/hardened area measures 10 mm or greater.

24. What is the **best** explanation a nurse will provide to a client whose skin test result for tuberculosis (TB) is positive?
    A. "There is active disease, but you are not yet infectious to others."
    B. "There is active disease, and you need to start drug therapy immediately."
    C. "You have been infected, but this does not mean active disease is present."
    D. "A repeat skin test is necessary because the test could give a false-positive result."

25. Which action will the nurse take to prevent infection when a 95-year-old nursing home resident has a productive cough, fever, chills, and a history of night sweats but the client's Mantoux test for tuberculosis (TB) is negative?
    A. Use Standard Precautions alone because the client does not have TB.
    B. Use Airborne Precautions because the client is at high risk for TB.
    C. Use Airborne Precautions until a chest x-ray shows the client not to have active TB.
    D. Use Standard Precautions alone because the client is taking penicillin therapy for another respiratory infection.

26. Which drugs and side effects will the nurse plan to teach a client with active non–drug-resistant tuberculosis (TB) who is being discharged on first-line therapy? **Select all that apply**.
    A. Rifampin; contact lenses can become stained orange
    B. Isoniazid; report yellowing of the skin or darkened urine
    C. Pyrazinamide; maintain a fluid restriction of 1200 mL/day
    D. Ethambutol; report any changes in vision
    E. Amoxicillin; take this drug with food or milk

27. Which action to **prevent harm** is **most important** for a nurse to include when teaching a client with tuberculosis (TB) about the prescribed first-line drug therapy?
    A. "Wear a mask for the first 8 weeks on therapy at home and when away from home."
    B. "Do not drink alcohol in any quantity while taking these drugs."
    C. "Avoid grapefruit and grapefruit juice while taking these drugs."
    D. "Restrict fluid intake to 2 quarts of liquid a day."

28. Which client factors does the nurse consider a reason for implementation of a directly observed therapy (DOT) for antimicrobial therapy for tuberculosis (TB)? **Select all that apply**.
    A. Client is homeless.
    B. Client is often confused.
    C. TB is multidrug resistant.
    D. Client has gained 11 lb (5 kg) in 8 weeks.
    E. The main prescribed drug is bedaquiline.
    F. Symptoms have decreased after 4 weeks of therapy.

29. What does the nurse suggest when the client prescribed first-line therapy for tuberculosis develops nausea from the drugs?
    A. "Stop taking the drugs."
    B. "Try taking the drugs at bedtime."
    C. "Take the drugs on an empty stomach."
    D. "Take the drugs individually throughout the day."

30. What is the nurse's **best** response when the family of a client who has been receiving first-line therapy for tuberculosis (TB) for 8 weeks and has shown clinical improvement asks if the client is still infectious?
    A. "He or she will remain infectious until the entire treatment period is completed."
    B. "The ability to spread the infection remains as long as his or her skin test remains positive."
    C. "Although he or she is no longer infectious, treatment may need to continue for at least 18 more weeks."
    D. "His or her sputum will likely always remain infectious although treatment is not needed after the cough has resolved."

31. What recommendations does the nurse make to the client who has rhinosinusitis? **Select all that apply**.
    A. Get plenty of rest, at least 8-10 hours per day.
    B. Keep fluid intake between 1000 and 1200 mL/day.
    C. Use a humidifier to help relieve congestion.
    D. Use nasal saline irrigation to safely relieve symptoms.
    E. Try sleeping with the head of your bed flat for better drainage.
    F. Limit exposure to any allergic causes.

32. Which side effects of first-generation antihistamines to treat sinusitis does the nurse caution the family of an older client to observe for? **Select all that apply**.
    A. Insomnia
    B. Hypotension
    C. Confusion
    D. Dry mouth
    E. Constipation
    F. Increased urine output

33. For which symptom does the nurse teach the client who is going home with a peritonsillar abscess to go to the emergency department immediately?
    A. Persistent cough
    B. Sore throat
    C. Nausea and vomiting
    D. Stridor or excessive drooling

34. Which additional assessment finding in a client who has a severe sore throat with pain that radiates behind the ear and difficulty swallowing supports the nurse's suspicion that the client may have a peritonsillar abscess?
    A. Deviated uvula
    B. Bad breath
    C. Coated tongue
    D. Beefy red mucous membranes

35. Which question is **most important** to ask a client who may have an **endemic** respiratory infection with fever, cough, headache, muscle aches, chest pain, and night sweats, and tests negative to the common forms of influenza? **Select all that apply**.
    A. Do you have any known allergies?
    B. What medications do you take daily?
    C. Do you have a chronic illness of any kind?
    D. Where have you traveled in the past 2 to 4 weeks?
    E. Have you ever been ill with these symptoms before?
    F. What type of heating system do you have in your home?

Chapter 28 Answer Key

1. B, C, E

   Option A is incorrect because Prevnar-13 is a pneumonia vaccine (not for influenza) and is only given once.

   Option B is correct because this is the injectable form of the influenza vaccine that is recommended for adults aged 50 and younger to receive as an immunization yearly.

   Option C is correct because this technique is the one recommended by the CDC to limit infection spread.

   Option D is incorrect because influenza season in North America is in the fall and winter.

   Option E is correct because this action can limit infection spread.

   Option F is incorrect because these drugs are effective only if taken within 24 to 48 hours after symptoms begin.

2. B

   Unless this client develops complications, he or she is most likely going to be managed at the assisted living facility. Influenza is highly contagious. Keeping the client in his or her room rather than going to the dining room and eating with other residents will help prevent infection spread. Antibiotics are not used for influenza. The staff should not, at this time, require oseltamivir unless they have symptoms of influenza. This is not a pandemic influenza and oseltamivir is not used for prophylaxis in this situation. Unless the client develops signs and symptoms of pneumonia, an x-ray is not indicated.

3. C

   Seasonal influenza can be prevented or its severity reduced when adults receive an annual influenza vaccination containing antigens to the three to four specific viral strains that are most likely to cause illness during that year's influenza season. There are many influenza viruses and their specific prevalences change each year. Thus, annual influenza vaccination is needed.

4. D

For adults aged over 65 years, a new formulation is available, known as a "senior flu shot," which is a higher dose, quadrivalent vaccine designed for more effective protection for adults with age-related reduced immunity.

5. D, F

The two most common complications of seasonal influenza are pneumonia and sepsis.

Influenza is not a risk factor for development of chronic obstructive pulmonary disease.

Fever is a symptom of influenza, not a complication.

Hypertension is not associated with influenza.

Renal failure can accompany sepsis but is not associated with seasonal influenza although it is associated with MERS.

6. C

The primary nursing role is helping to contain the outbreak by preventing spread of the infection to employees, other clients, and visitors. The facility's administrators have the responsibility to report the infection. Antibiotics do not combat influenza. Annual influenza vaccinations are not effective against new pandemic influenzas and the nurse can only recommend annual vaccination to co-workers not ensure compliance.

7. B, C, D, F

When a pandemic influenza appears in a community, it is announced at large and containment actions are instituted. Containment recommendations include staying home and avoiding public areas for at least 2 weeks. Thus, people should have a 2-week supply of food, water, and their usual prescription drugs in order to stay home and avoid coming into contact with infected individuals.

Influenza in pandemic form is a respiratory illness that spreads through person-to-person contact and not through the intestinal tract.

Unless a person has influenza symptoms or lives with a person who actually has influenza, antiviral drugs are not prescribed.

8. A, D, E

A is correct. This client has recently traveled overseas and may have been exposed to COVID-19. It is critical to determine whether the client has been in contact with anyone who has symptoms of COVID-19.

B is not correct. Although Contact Precautions should be used, Airborne Precautions must also be instituted.

C is not correct. Isoniazid is used only for tuberculosis. The sudden and rapid onset of this client's respiratory distress is not consistent with tuberculosis.

D is correct because Covid-19 is highly contagious and strict containment is required.

E is correct because any client with acute respiratory distress can have progression to complete respiratory failure. Arterial blood gas results help determine the adequacy of gas exchange and the need for oxygen therapy and/or mechanical ventilation.

F is incorrect. This test is only for tuberculosis. The sudden and rapid onset of this client's respiratory distress is not consistent with tuberculosis.

9. A, E, F

Wearing eye protection while suctioning the client protects the nurse from contact with infected droplets. Using PAPR protects the nurse from inhalation exposure to the virus. Washing hands after removing gowns, gloves, masks, and eyewear protects the nurse from direct contact with the virus.

Keeping the door of the client's room closed is a good action to take but does not protect the nurse in the room with the client. Changing the water in the nebulizer protects the client, not the nurse. Testing for pandemic influenza viruses is not performed by sputum culture.

10. A, B, D, F

Clients with chronic confusion are at higher risk for pneumonia because of reduced ability to know when to take precautions to avoid infection. This client's risk is also increased because of age-related reduced immunity and may have a higher risk for aspiration pneumonia.

Influenza is a very common cause of pneumonia.

Mechanical ventilation greatly increases the risk for ventilator-associated pneumonia as the lower respiratory system is more open with by-passing of some anatomy safe-guards, the mouth may be colonized with organisms that can translocate to the lungs, and oral secretions can be aspirated into the lungs.

Anyone who is severely malnourished has an increased risk for infectious pneumonia because of reduced immunity.

Neither atrial fibrillation nor anticoagulant therapy increases pneumonia risk.

Hyperthyroidism has no direct on risk for any type of pneumonia.

11. B

Although all values are abnormal ($Paco_2$ is only slightly elevated), they are expected findings in clients with pneumonia or any other severe infection. The very low Pao_2 level indicates severe hypoxemia and great risk for death without immediate intervention.

12. A

One of the first signs and symptoms of pneumonia in an older adult is acute confusion as a result of impaired gas exchange. A client with pneumonia who is alert and oriented to person, place, and time is responding well to appropriate therapy for the disorder. The blood pressure is not an indicator of effective management of pneumonia and neither is urine output. The skin behind the client's ears being intact is important and desirable, but not an outcome indicator for pneumonia management.

13. C

Chronic tobacco use (especially cigarette smoking) is associated with an increased risk for community-acquired pneumonia by reducing immunity within the pulmonary system. It also increases the inflammatory response with more secretions that provide a nutrient environment for microorganisms. Chronic alcohol consumption also reduces general immunity and may lead to malnutrition, another pneumonia risk factor. Although being immunized against influenza later in the fall, protection against influenza should be sufficient within 3 weeks. Receiving a pneumococcal vaccination reduces pneumonia risk. Living alone and preparing his or own meals does not increase a person's risk for infection or pneumonia.

14. C, D, E, F

Common uncomplicated community-acquired pneumonia signs and symptoms include chest pain or discomfort, myalgia, headache, chills, fever, cough, tachycardia, dyspnea, tachypnea, hemoptysis, and sputum production. Abdominal pain is not associated with pneumonia. Back pain is only present when pneumonia is complicated by pleural inflammation.

15. C

All actions listed are helpful for pneumonia prevention. However, the most common cause of pneumonia after abdominal surgery is decreased mobility causing atelectasis and pulmonary fluid stasis. This noninfectious type of pneumonia can be prevented by having the postoperative client cough, turn, move about as much as possible, and perform deep-breathing exercises, such as the use of incentive spirometry.

16. A, B, D

The older adult with pneumonia has weakness, fatigue, lethargy, confusion, and poor appetite. Fever and an elevated WBC count are often absent initially because of the older client's reduced immune and inflammatory responses (the WBC count may not be elevated until the infection is severe). The older client often does not cough with pneumonia, but hypoxemia is often present.

17. A

The classic chest x-ray findings for a client with pneumonia is patchy areas of increased density in the involved lung areas. A "ground-glass" appearance is associated with acute respiratory distress syndrome. Mediastinal widening is associated with inhalation anthrax. Large, hyperinflated lungs occur with chronic obstructive pulmonary disease.

18. None of the above
All clients with pneumonia who have hypoxemia require oxygen therapy, even the client who has chronic obstructive pulmonary disease.

19. B, E, F
A feeding tube prevents full closure of the epiglottis making aspiration into the airway easier when an endotracheal tube is also in place. Colonization of any part of the airway with bacteria allows direct translocation into the lower respiratory tract and lungs. The presence of tooth loss and mouth sores adds additional loss of barrier function and increases microorganism presence in the oral cavity, a major cause of VAP.

    Although alcohol use and cigarette smoking increase the risk for infectious pneumonia, they do not generally increase the risk for VAP. Weight loss alone does not increase the risk for VAP.

20. B, C, D, E
Pulmonary empyema is a collection of pus in the pleural space (not in the lungs) most commonly caused by pneumonia or another pulmonary infection. Its manifestations include reduced chest wall motion, reduced or absent or fremitus, flat percussion, and decreased breath sounds. The client has either a persistent fever despite antibiotic therapy or recurrence of fever. Although empyema fluid is thick, purulent, and foul-smelling, the client cannot cough it up because it is in the pleural space and not in the lungs. Wheezing does not occur because the fluid is not in the airways.

21. B, D, E, F
Many people are exposed to the TB organism and do not develop active disease if they are otherwise healthy and immunocompetent. The college student living in a dormitory and the homemaker working in a soup kitchen are not at high risk. The man with HIV-III is severely immunocompromised despite his age, as is the client who is homeless and suffers from alcoholism. Poor immigrants from less affluent countries, such as Mexico, and those who live in crowded areas such as long-term care facilities, prisons, homeless shelters, and mental

health facilities, are at high risk for developing active TB.

22. A, C, E, F, G, H
Indications of TB include persistent cough, unintended weight loss, anorexia, night sweats, hemoptysis, shortness of breath, low-grade fever, and chills. Back soreness is not a common symptom of TB.

23. D
An area of induration (localized swelling with hardness of soft tissue), not just redness, measuring 10 mm or greater, indicates exposure to and possible active infection with TB.

24. C
A positive reaction to a TB indicates exposure to TB or the presence of inactive (dormant) disease, not active disease. Additional testing is needed to rule out or confirm active TB.

25. C
When clients are very old or have severe immunodeficiency, their Mantoux skin tests may be negative even when active TB is present because their reduced immunity may result in too few immune system cells and cell products to mount an immune response to the test (anergy). Therefore, Airborne Precautions are used in addition to Standard Precautions with any older client who presents with clinical indications of TB until other tests also rule it out.

26. A, B, D
Amoxicillin is not prescribed for TB. Pyrazinamide, although prescribed for TB, calls for an increase in fluids, not fluid restriction. Rifampin, isoniazid, and ethambutol are first-line drugs for TB therapy and have side effects. The side effects listed with these drugs are appropriate to teach the client.

27. B
All the first-line drugs for TB are liver toxic and can cause liver damage. Drinking alcohol compounds this damage and should be ingested only in small quantities, if at all. Fluids are to be increased, not decreased. Clients do not need to wear masks in their own homes because family

members and anyone else living in the home have already been heavily exposed to the bacillus. Grapefruit does not affect the absorption or metabolism of these drugs.

28. A, B, C, E
Successful treatment of TB requires that prescribed antitubercular drugs be taken daily, exactly as prescribed, for as long as they are prescribed. Adherence is more difficult for anyone who is homeless or confused. When the disease is drug-resistant, adherence is even more important to prevent the client's death from disease progression. Bedaquiline is prescribed only for multidrug-resistant TB and has life-threatening serious side effects. For this reason, DOT therapy is recommended for bedaquiline.
Weight gain and reduced symptoms are signs that therapy is effective, indicating that the client is adhering to the therapy regimen.

29. B
It is critically important to continue taking these drugs. Often, taking the drugs at bedtime prevents the client from being aware of nausea. Taking the drugs on an empty stomach would enhance their absorption and generally increase the likelihood of nausea. Taking the drugs throughout the day could prolong the sensation of nausea.

30. C
Generally, clients who have shown clinical improvement after 8 weeks of therapy are no longer infectious but must continue the prescribed therapy for at least 18 more weeks. Once the infection has been eradicated, the sputum is no longer infectious. The skin test remains positive after successful treatment of TB and is not an indication of infectious status.

31. A, C, D, F
Rhinosinusitis is often managed at home. In addition to decongestants and any needed antimicrobials, recommendations include supportive therapy such as humidification, nasal irrigation, getting plenty of rest, increasing fluid intake, and sleeping with the head of the bed elevated. Regardless of the cause of

rhinosinusitis, discomfort increases when exposures to allergens occur.

32. A, C, D, E
First-generation antihistamines may not be appropriate drugs for older adults because these clients often have reduced drug clearance resulting in higher risk for confusion and anticholinergic effects such as dry mouth, constipation, difficulty sleeping, and hypertension. The anticholinergic effects can also include urinary retention.

33. D
Stridor and/or drooling indicate at least a partial airway obstruction. The client needs immediate care to prevent the partial obstruction from becoming a complete obstruction, leading to death. Persistent cough, sore throat, and nausea and vomiting are not life-threatening.

34. A
A major indication of a peritonsillar abscess is a collection of pus behind the tonsil causing swelling on one side of the throat that pushes the uvula toward the unaffected side. Bad breath and a coated tongue can occur with any sore throat. Beefy red mucous membranes occur with any oral infection.

35. B, C, D
An endemic respiratory infection is one in which the causative organism is much more common within a geographic location. Adults living in these areas have often developed some immunity to the organism over time and usually only develop the infection if they come into contact with large numbers of the organism or have a severely reduced immune response. Those who do not live in the region may have no immunity to it and become ill after traveling in the area and becoming exposed. Important questions related to a potential endemic respiratory infection include history of recent travel (and the exact location visited), whether the client is taking a drug that reduces immunity, and whether he or she has a chronic illness that would either reduce immunity or increase susceptibility. Questions pertaining to allergies, the type of heating system used, and whether or not the client has ever had these symptoms before are less important.

29
CHAPTER

Critical Care of Patients with Respiratory Emergencies

1. Which factors or conditions are major risk factors for venous thromboembolism (VTE) leading to pulmonary embolism (PE)? **Select all that apply**.
   A. Obesity
   B. Pregnancy
   C. Malnutrition
   D. Cigarette smoking
   E. Prolonged immobility
   F. Use of anticoagulants
   G. Central venous catheters
   H. Chronic obstructive pulmonary disease (COPD)

2. Which client will the nurse assess **most frequently** for a venous thromboembolism (VTE) to **prevent harm** from a pulmonary embolism (PE)?
   A. 75-year old with left heart failure
   B. 65-year-old with breast cancer
   C. 55-year-old after a total knee replacement
   D. 44-year-old with type 2 diabetes mellitus

3. Which additional assessment findings support the nurse's suspicion that the client who reports a sudden onset of shortness of breath may have a pulmonary embolism (PE)? **Select all that apply?**
   A. SpO_2 85%
   B. Hoarseness
   C. Diaphoresis
   D. Hypertension
   E. Crushing chest pain radiating to the jaw
   F. Crackles in a lower lung lobe

4. In addition to arterial blood gas levels, for which diagnostic test will the nurse prepare a client who is suspected to have a pulmonary embolism (PE)?
   A. Computed tomography pulmonary angiography
   B. Carbon monoxide diffusion capacity
   C. Pneumoencephalogram
   D. 12-lead ECG

5. Which action will the nurse instruct an assistive personnel (AP) to **avoid performing** on a client after abdominal surgery to **prevent harm** from a pulmonary embolism?
   A. Encouraging fluid intake
   B. Massaging the client's calves
   C. Ambulating the client in the hall
   D. Changing the client's position every 2 hours

6. Which actions are **most appropriate** for the nurse to take *immediately* when a client has indications of a pulmonary embolism (PE)? **Select all that apply**.
   A. Apply oxygen.
   B. Reassure the client.
   C. Increase the IV flow rate.
   D. Elevate the head of the bed.
   E. Initiate the Rapid Response Team.
   F. Instruct the client to not cross his or her legs.

7. What changes in care orders does the nurse anticipate in response to reporting to the primary health care provider that a client who has been receiving heparin IV for the past 3 days may have received twice the prescribed dose? **Select all that apply**.
   A. Activated partial thromboplastin time (aPTT)
   B. International normalized ratio (INR)
   C. Arterial blood gas (ABG) values
   D. Protamine sulfate
   E. Prothrombin time
   F. Vitamin K

8. Which change in a client's laboratory values does the nurse interpret as being consistent with the presence of a pulmonary embolism (PE)?
   A. pH 7.36
   B. Elevated D-dimer
   C. Low levels of factor V Leiden
   D. Decreased leukocyte count

9. In addition to the pulmonary health care provider, with which members of the interprofessional team does the nurse expect to collaborate to achieve the desired outcomes of care for a client hospitalized with a large pulmonary embolism? **Select all that apply**.
   A. Occupational therapist
   B. Pastoral care workers
   C. Physical therapist
   D. Registered dietitian nutritionist
   E. Respiratory therapist
   F. Social worker

10. Which symptoms indicate to the nurse that the management of a client with a pulmonary embolism (PE) is **not effective**? **Select all that apply**.
    A. Partial thromboplastin time (PTT) is 2.0 times normal
    B. ECG shows increasing dysrhythmias
    C. Client has stopped sweating
    D. Neck veins are distended
    E. Sacral edema is present
    F. Pulse oximetry is 88%

11. The nurse anticipates a prescription for which drug when the client with a pulmonary embolism being managed with IV crystalloids remains hypotensive with a low cardiac output?
    A. Alteplase
    B. Warfarin
    C. Morphine
    D. Dobutamine

12. Which client information indicates to the nurse that management of a pulmonary embolism (PE) is effective? **Select all that apply**.
    A. Pulse oximetry of 95%
    B. Arterial blood gas, pH of 7.28
    C. Client's desire to go home
    D. Absence of pallor or cyanosis
    E. Mental status at client's baseline
    F. Palpable peripheral pulses

13. Which precaution is a **priority** for the nurse to teach a client as part of discharge instructions after a pulmonary embolism (PE) to **prevent harm**?
    A. Report excessive bleeding immediately.
    B. Take your pulse and temperature twice daily.
    C. Drink at least 3 L of water or other fluids daily.
    D. Avoid crowds, small children, and people who are ill.

14. By which critical arterial blood gas (ABG) values will the nurse interpret as meeting the classification for acute respiratory failure? **Select all that apply**.
    A. $Paco_2$ 39 mm Hg
    B. $Paco_2$ 62 mm Hg
    C. Pao_2 78 mm Hg
    D. Pao_2 55 mm Hg
    E. pH value of < 7.3
    F. Sao_2 80%

15. Which client processes does the nurse understand contribute to or cause pure ventilatory failure? **Select all that apply**.
    A. Hematologic disease
    B. Loss of lung elastic tissue
    C. Weak diaphragm contraction
    D. Stiffness of the chest wall
    E. Infectious diseases such as pneumonia
    F. Defect in the respiratory control center of the brain

16. Which action is most important for the nurse to perform **first** for a client suspected of having acute respiratory failure?
    A. Initiating an IV
    B. Applying oxygen
    C. Calling the Rapid Response Team
    D. Asking the client about a history of respiratory disorders

17. Which conditions or changes are responsible for the problems associated with acute respiratory distress syndrome (ARDS)? **Select all that apply**.
    A. Increased lung fluid
    B. Systemic inflammatory response
    C. Dried out and flaky pulmonary epithelium
    D. Decreased lung volume
    E. Refractory hypoxemia
    F. Excessive surfactant production

18. Which client will the nurse consider to be at greatest risk for acute respiratory distress syndrome (ARDS)?
    A. 22-year-old who received 10 units of blood after a motor vehicle accident
    B. 24-year-old with asthma who has not taken prescribed asthma medications for 2 weeks
    C. 62-year-old with chronic obstructive pulmonary disease who has pneumonia
    D. 78-year-old with chronic heart failure and pulmonary edema

19. Which assessment will the nurse perform **first** when a client at risk for acute respiratory distress syndrome (ARDS) becomes cyanotic and diaphoretic?
    A. Compare current ECG tracing with baseline measurement.
    B. Measure the blood pressure in both arms.
    C. Auscultate breath sounds bilaterally.
    D. Measure pulse oximetry.

20. Which phase of acute respiratory syndrome (ARDS) case management does the nurse identify for a client who has been intubated for 6 days and has progressive hypoxemia that responds poorly to high levels of oxygen?
    A. Resolution phase
    B. Recovery phase
    C. Exudative phase
    D. Fibrosing alveolitis phase

21. Which action does the nurse take **first** when a client who is intubated and being mechanically ventilated has an oxygen saturation of 89%, a heart rate of 120 beats/min, is increasingly agitated and restless, and has lung sounds that are diminished on one side?
    A. Notify the provider and prepare for re-intubation or repositioning the tube.
    B. Document the findings and request a prescription for a sedative.
    C. Call respiratory therapy to obtain a set of arterial blood gases.
    D. Reposition the tube and call radiology for a stat chest x-ray.

22. What is the nurse's **best** action on finding that the cuff pressure of the client's endotracheal tube is 25 cm water?
    A. Move the endotracheal tube to the other side of the mouth.
    B. Remove 10 cm water pressure of air from the cuff.
    C. Add 10 cm water pressure of air to the cuff.
    D. Document the finding as the only action.

23. Which assessment finding in a client with an endotracheal tube most strongly indicates to the nurse that the tube remains correctly in the trachea and is not in the esophagus?
    A. Stomach contents cannot be aspirated.
    B. Oxygen saturation is greater than 50%.
    C. End-tidal carbon dioxide level is 38 mm Hg.
    D. No air is heard in the stomach when auscultated with a stethoscope.

24. Which information is **most relevant** for the nurse to document after a client has been successfully intubated by the health care provider? **Select all that apply.**
    A. Level of the tube
    B. IV fluid infusion rate
    C. Presence (or absence) of dysrhythmias
    D. Presence of bilateral and equal breath sounds
    E. Changes in vital signs during the procedure
    F. Placement verification by end-tidal carbon dioxide levels

25. For which problems will the nurse specifically assess when the high-pressure alarm of a client's mechanical ventilator sounds? **Select all that apply.**
    A. Mucus plug
    B. Bronchospasm
    C. Client coughing
    D. Air leak in tube cuff
    E. Client fighting the ventilator
    F. Ventilator tubing disconnected

26. Which clients will the nurse expect to **most likely** need to be intubated and mechanically ventilated? **Select all that apply.**
    A. 25-year-old with burns who has severe swelling of oral mucosa
    B. 38-year-old with copious secretions and ineffective cough
    C. 45-year-old with SpO_2 of 93% on a high-flow oxygen face mask
    D. 56-year-old with pneumonia, increasing fatigue, and shallow respirations
    E. 62-year-old with COPD who is able to cough and has an SpO_2 of 90%
    F. 72-year-old with moderate heart failure and orthopnea

27. Which action will the nurse take **first** to **prevent harm** for a client being mechanically ventilated who is biting and chewing at the endotracheal tube (ET)?
    A. Request an order for soft wrist restraints.
    B. Immediately suction the client's mouth.
    C. Administer a paralyzing agent.
    D. Insert an oral airway.

28. What are the characteristics of a mechanical ventilator that is pressure-cycled? **Select all that apply.**
    A. Its main function is to provide positive pressure only during expiration to keep lungs partially inflated.
    B. Air is forced into the lungs during inhalation until a preset pressure is reached.
    C. The client's own inspiratory efforts control the volume provided.
    D. It usually requires either a tracheostomy or endotracheal tube.
    E. A safety feature is that a client cannot be hyperventilated.
    F. Tidal volumes and inspiratory times are varied.

29. Which action will the nurse perform **first** when performing a check of the ventilator equipment after determining the client's gas exchange status?
    A. Turning off the alarms during the system check
    B. Checking the cuff pressure on the endotracheal tube
    C. Comparing the actual settings with the prescribed settings
    D. Draining the condensation from the ventilator trap tubing

30. Which action does the nurse take to **prevent harm** through loss of tracheal tissue integrity in a client with an endotracheal tube (ET) who is being mechanically ventilated?
    A. Inserting an oral airway
    B. Providing meticulous oral care every 8 hours
    C. Deflating the cuff for 15 minutes every 2 hours
    D. Maintaining cuff inflation pressure less than 30 cm H_2O

31. Which actions are **most important** for the nurse to perform to prevent a mechanically ventilated client from developing ventilator-associated pneumonia (VAP)? **Select all that apply**.
    A. Preventing aspiration
    B. Performing oral care every at least 12 hours
    C. Suctioning every 1-2 hours around the clock
    D. Turning and repositioning client every 2 hours
    E. Preventing pressure ulcers around the mouth
    F. Keeping the HOB elevated at least 30 degrees

32. Which assessment finding for a client who is receiving mechanical ventilation in synchronized intermittent mandatory ventilation (SIMV) mode indicates to the nurse probable readiness to be weaned?
    A. Fever from a respiratory infection has resolved.
    B. Client is alert and oriented to place and person.
    C. Client receives 1-2 mechanical ventilator breaths/min.
    D. Arterial blood gas values are maintained within normal limits.

33. Which assessment finding does the nurse expect for a client who was extubated 2 hours ago?
    A. Restlessness
    B. Hoarseness
    C. Dyspnea
    D. Stridor

34. Which conditions indicate to the nurse that a client being mechanically ventilated needs to be suctioned? **Select all that apply**.
    A. Presence of ronchi when listening to breath sounds
    B. Presence of moisture in the ventilator tubing
    C. Audible secretions in the endotracheal tube
    D. Low-pressure alarm sounds
    E. Increased peak inspiratory pressure (PIP)
    F. Tubing becomes disconnected from the ventilator

35. Which assessment is **most important** for the nurse to perform for a client with chest trauma who is at high risk for a pulmonary contusion?
    A. Observing for chest movements
    B. Aulscultating for breath sounds
    C. Listening for hyperresonance
    D. Observing for deviation

36. Which intervention will the nurse expect to be prescribed for a client who has a simple fracture of three ribs on the right side after a fall?
    A. Cricothyroidotomy
    B. Mechanical ventilation
    C. Tight bandage around chest
    D. Pain control for adequate breathing

37. Which assessment findings indicate to the nurse that a client with a flail chest may require mechanical ventilation?
    A. Constant pain and anxiety
    B. Hypoxemia and hypercarbia
    C. Paradoxical chest movements
    D. Tachycardia and hypertension

38. For which client does the nurse expect interventions to include an open thoracotomy?
    A. 28-year-old with a hemothorax and a 1500 mL blood loss from the chest tube
    B. 45-year-old with a tension pneumothorax and tracheal deviation toward the unaffected side
    C. 60-year-old with a simple pneumothorax and hyperresonance on the affected side
    D. 70-year-old with a simple fracture of four ribs on the left side and mild heart failure

Chapter 29 Answer Key

1. A, B, D, E, G
    Major conditions and factors that increase the risk for VTE leading to PE are prolonged immobility, central venous catheters, major surgery (especially abdominal or lower limb), pregnancy, obesity, advancing age, general and genetic conditions that increase blood clotting, history of previous thromboembolism, smoking, estrogen therapy, heart failure, stroke, cancer (particularly lung or prostate), and trauma. Anticoagulant therapy decreases the risk for VTE and increases the risk for uncontrolled bleeding. Malnutrition is more likely to decrease the formation of clotting factors, decreasing the risk for VTE. COPD does not directly increase the risk for clot formation.

2. C
    VTEs leading to PE most often form in a vein in the legs or the pelvis, especially after total joint replacement surgery. The surgery disrupts some venous blood flow and most clients are less mobile for days after the surgery, which also increases the risk. Left heart failure may increase the risk for stroke, but not PE. Any client with cancer forms clots more easily but not to the same degree that knee replacement surgery does. Diabetes mellitus does not increase clotting risk.

3. A, C, F
    Common assessment findings for PE include sudden onset of stabbing chest pain, apprehension, restlessness, feeling of impending doom, cough, hemoptysis, diaphoresis, increased respiratory rate, hypotension, crackles in the affected lung areas, pleural friction rub, tachycardia, S_3 or S_4 heart sound, low-grade fever, petechiae over chest and axillae, and decreased arterial oxygen saturation.
    The lungs are affected, not the trachea or the vocal cords so there is no change in voice quality. Crushing chest pain that radiates to the jaw is associated with myocardial infarction, not PE.

4. A
    Computed tomography pulmonary angiography (CT-PA) is most commonly used for diagnosis of PE and may also diagnose other pulmonary abnormalities causing the client's symptoms. Carbon monoxide diffusion capacity is part of pulmonary function testing but cannot help diagnose a PE. A pneumoencephalogram is a brain test, not a pulmonary test. A 12-lead ECG may show changes related to hypoxia but has no specific diagnostic value for PE.

5. B
    Massaging the calves could cause an existing venous thrombus in the lower legs (most common place of formation) to break up and form emboli that could travel to the lungs. Increasing fluid intake, ambulation, and changing positions frequently reduces the risk for clot formation.

6. A, B, D, E
    The client with a PE is hypoxic and has difficulty breathing. Applying oxygen and elevating the head of the bed can help ease respiratory difficulty. PE is a serious emergency and the Rapid Response Team is initiated to begin appropriate diagnostic and management efforts as quickly as possible. The client is usually apprehensive or frightened. Reassuring him or her and staying with the client is also a priority.
    Increasing the IV flow rate does not improve pulmonary gas exchange. Although avoiding the action of crossing the legs can help prevent a clot, this action does not do anything to make a difference for an already formed clot that has moved into the lung.

7. A, D
    The client has been receiving an excessive dose of heparin. The aPTT will help assess this client's degree of bleeding risk. Depending on the results of this test, the client may need a heparin antidote, which is protamine sulfate.
    ABGs, INR, and prothrombin time do not indicate the effects of heparin. Vitamin K is an antidote for warfarin but has no effect on heparin levels.

8. B
    The D-dimer level rises with fibrinolysis, making it consistent with a PE. However, other diagnostic testing is still needed to determine

whether a PE has occurred. A pH of 7.36 is normal. Factor V Leiden, is a mutated form of factor V. Its value is absent unless a client has the genetic mutation. High levels of factor V Leiden are associated with PE and other types of excessive clotting. The leukocyte count is either unchanged or higher with a PE if inflammation also is present.

9. A, B, C, D, E, F
All of the health care workers listed above are essential parts of the interprofessional team caring for a client with PE. Respiratory therapists assist with prescribed oxygen therapy and delivery needs. Physical therapists can help the client maintain muscle conditioning. Occupational therapists provide information and home set-up suggestions to help clients conserve energy when endurance is affected. Registered dietitian nutritionists assess clients' caloric and protein needs and plan personalized interventions to meet these needs. Pastoral care workers and clergy may help clients who experience spiritual distress with this life-altering condition. Social workers together with home care nurses determine which types of home modifications and durable supplies would be most helpful in maintaining functional ability for self-management of ADLs.

10. B, D, E, F
Indications of a worsening PE include increasing dyspnea, dysrhythmias, distended neck veins, pedal or sacral edema, increasing crackles or other abnormal lung sounds, and cyanosis of the lips, conjunctiva, oral mucosa, and nail beds. The distended neck veins and sacral edema are associated with increasing pulmonary pressures from an extending PE that cause right-sided heart failure and systemic edema. Dysrhythmias and low pulse oximetry are indicators of hypoxemia from decreased pulmonary gas exchange.

The desired therapeutic PTT for anticoagulation therapy of a client with PE is 1.5 to 2.5 times the normal. Stopping sweating is not associated with a PE.

11. D
Dobutamine is an inotropic agent that increases myocardial contractility and can help increase

cardiac output and raise blood pressure. Alteplase is a fibrinolytic agent that can help dissolve a PE but has no direct effect on cardiac output or hypotension. Warfarin is an oral anticoagulant that has no direct effect on either cardiac output or hypotension. Morphine is an opioid pain medication that can lower blood pressure further.

12. A, D, E, F
A pulse oximetry reading of 95%, absence of cyanosis or pallor, a return of the client's mental status to baseline, and palpable peripheral pulses all indicate adequate perfusion and gas exchange (the desired outcomes of PE management). The client's desire to go home could occur even when he or she is still dangerously hypoxemic. An arterial blood gas of 7.28 means the client is acidotic and is not a positive indicator of PE therapy effectiveness.

13. A
The client with a PE is discharged from the hospital when hypoxemia and hemodynamic instability have resolved and adequate anticoagulation has been achieved. However nearly all clients are on anticoagulation therapy for some time at home and remain at high risk for excessive bleeding. Drinking plenty of fluids and assessing pulse and temperature are important but do not have the same priority as bleeding. A PE does not drastically increase the client's risk for acquiring an infection spread by person-to-person contact.

14. B, D, E, F
The critical ABG values that define or classify a respiratory problem as acute respiratory failure are a partial pressure of arterial oxygen (Pao_2) of less than 60 mm Hg (hypoxemic/oxygenation failure), or a partial pressure of arterial carbon dioxide ($Paco_2$) of more than 45 mm Hg occurring with acidemia (pH < 7.35), and arterial oxygen saturation (Sao_2) less than 90%. A $Paco_2$ of 39 mm Hg is a normal ABG finding, not a critical value. Although a Pao_2 of 78 mm Hg is abnormally low, it is still above 60 and does not meet the criteria.

15. B, C, D, F
Ventilatory failure is a problem in which air movement or ventilation is inadequate and blood flow (perfusion) is normal. It occurs when the chest pressure does not change enough to permit air movement into and out of the lungs. Common problems leading to pure ventilatory failure include a physical problem of the lungs or chest wall, a defect in the respiratory control center in the brain, or poor function of the respiratory muscles (especially the diaphragm). Hematologic disease usually causes oxygen failure with an inadequate amount of red blood cells and/or hemoglobin. Pneumonia impairs perfusion and gas exchange rather than ventilation, resulting in oxygen failure rather than ventilatory failure.

16. B
Oxygen therapy is appropriate for any client with acute hypoxemia caused by acute respiratory failure and is started first (while another person is calling the Rapid Response Team). Even if the hypoxemia is not caused by acute respiratory failure it is still the best first action.

17. A, B, D, E
The syndrome of ARDS that occurs after lung injury involves a variety of pathologic consequences that impair gas exchange. These changes start with a local inflammatory response in the lung membranes with movement of fluid from the pulmonary capillaries into the lungs, increasing lung fluid and decreasing the area of the membrane available for gas exchange. Injury and inflammation of the type II pneumocytes decrease surfactant production and make lung volumes decrease at the same time that lung fluid increases. The inflammation persists and becomes systemic, which also increases the fluid (containing more protein) in the lungs with capillary dilation. Blood moves through the lungs but is poorly oxygenated causing hypoxemia that does not improve when oxygen is administered (refractory hypoxemia).

18. A
Extensive trauma alone can cause an excessive release of intracellular enzymes that can damage lung cells and lead to ARDS. The 10 units of blood indicate severe trauma. In addition, with massive transfusions there is redistribution of large volumes of blood into the pulmonary circulation, which increases pulmonary capillary hydrostatic pressure contributing to movement of fluid into lung tissue causing noncardiac pulmonary edema. Plasma proteins from this edema start inflammatory processes in the lung tissues leading to ARDS.

19. D
In early ARDS, hypoxemia may be the only abnormal assessment finding and can be life threatening. Changes in breath sounds usually occur later in ARDS. Blood pressure changes and ECG changes are not specific for ARDS.

20. D
In the fibrosing alveolitis phase, increased lung injury leads to pulmonary hypertension and fibrosis. The body attempts to repair the damage, and increasing lung involvement reduces gas exchange and oxygenation even when higher levels of oxygen are supplied. The exudative stage occurs within the first 24 to 48 hours of the syndrome. Both the resolution and recovery stage show decreasing or absent hypoxemia.

21. A
With the decreased oxygen saturation and decreased breath sounds on one side, the endotracheal tube is incorrectly positioned into one bronchus. For effective gas exchange, the tube must be repositioned, which is a performed by the primary health care provider, not the nurse.

22. D
The cuff pressure should be maintained between 20 and 30 cm of water for effectiveness without causing trauma. Thus 25 cm is normal and air does not need to be added or removed from the cuff. The only action needed is to document the assessment finding. Moving the endotracheal tube to the opposite side of the mouth is not an action that addresses cuff pressure although it can help prevent mouth trauma.

23. C

The end-tidal carbon dioxide level is within the normal range. If the endotracheal tube were in the esophagus or stomach rather than the trachea, it would be very low or undetectable. The lack of aspiration of stomach contents is not conclusive for correct placement and neither is the fact that air cannot be heard in the stomach. Oxygen saturation should always be greater than 50% and should be much higher if the tube is correctly placed.

24. A, C, D, E, F

Documentation of the level of the tube is relevant to help health care providers know if there is a change in its position. Dysrhythmias can occur during and shortly after intubation as a result of hypoxia. Assessment and documentation of the presence of bilateral and equal breath sounds is critical to note because it demonstrates that the intubation process was correct and successful. Documenting the client's responses during intubation helps identify possible problems resulting from the intubation. Verification of correct tube placement is critical to know because if tube placement is incorrect, the procedure will need to be repeated. The rate of the IV fluid infusion can be documented but is not relevant to the procedure of intubation.

25. A, B, C, E

Common causes of alarms indicating high pressure include: presence of increased airway secretions or mucous plugs, client coughing or gaging, client fighting or "bucking" the ventilator, anything that decreases airway size (i.e., bronchospasms), presence of a pneumothorax, displacement of the endotracheal tube further into the tracheobronchial tree, and external obstruction of the tubing.

An air leak in the tube cuff or disconnection of the ventilator tubing results in low pressure, not high pressure.

26. A, B, D

The client with burns and swelling of the oral mucosa also probably has injury to the pharynx and larynx that will cause a partial or complete airway obstruction. Any client with copious secretions and an ineffective cough is at risk for obstruction and impaired ventilation. The client with pneumonia has decreased gas exchange and must increase ventilatory effort to maintain oxygenation. As his or her respirations become more shallow and fatigue increases, mechanical ventilation is needed for support.

The client on a high-flow oxygen mask who is maintaining an SpO_2 of 93% and the client with COPD who is maintaining it at 90% do not meet criteria for mechanical ventilation (at this time). The client with heart failure and orthopnea would not be helped by mechanical ventilation.

27. D

The ET must be kept stable to ensure it remains properly placed. Biting or chewing on the tube can destabilize it. A simple way to prevent this is by inserting an oral airway. Chewing and biting the ET is not an indication of the need for suctioning. Use of a paralyzing agent or requesting an order for restraints is a more drastic measure and neither step is taken as the first action.

28. B, D, F

With pressure-cycled ventilators, the machine pushes or forces air into the lungs for inhalation until a preset airway pressure is reached. This type of ventilation is generally considered invasive and usually requires either a tracheostomy tube or an endotracheal tube for function. The tidal volumes and inspiratory times vary because neither volume nor time are responsible for inhibiting the inhalation, only pressure.

It is not controlled in any way by the client's respiratory efforts and does not have the main function of providing positive pressure during exhalation only. Any type of ventilator can cause hyperventilation if the settings are not appropriate for the client.

29. C

The nurse always assesses the client before the assessing the ventilator. The first action to prevent harm and ensure adequate gas exchange is to compare the current or actual ventilator settings with those prescribed by the pulmonary health care provider. When settings are not correct for the client's condition, under ventilation or over ventilation can occur. Both problems can cause complications. The next action is to check the cuff pressure on the endotracheal or tracheostomy tube. Draining the condensation is important but is not the priority first action. Ventilator alarms are **NOT** turned off.

30. D
An overinflated cuff can cause tissue injury and necrosis of the tracheal tissue. Although cuff pressure must be adequate to prevent leaks, it is critical to keep the pressure no higher than 30 cm H_2O. Meticulous oral care can help maintain tissue integrity of oral mucous membranes but does not help tracheal tissue integrity. Deflating the cuff reduces the effectiveness of the endotracheal tube for adequate ventilation and increases the risk that it may dislodge. Inserting an oral airway can help reduce the risk for some complications but does not help prevent injury to the trachea.

31. A, B, D, E, F
Implementation of the recommended ventilator bundle to prevent VAP includes:
Keeping the head of the bed elevated at least 30 degrees
Performing oral care per agency policy (usually brushing teeth at least every 12 hours and antimicrobial rinse)
Oral pressure injury prophylaxis
Preventing aspiration
Pulmonary hygiene (i.e., chest physiotherapy, postural drainage, and turning and positioning)
Suctioning is not performed on a scheduled basis, but only when there are indications that it is needed.

32. C
SIMV allows spontaneous breathing at the client's own rate and tidal volume between the ventilator breaths. The number of mechanical breaths (SIMV breaths) is gradually decreased (e.g., from 12 to 2) as the client resumes spontaneous breathing. When the client requires only 1 to 2 SIMV breaths/min, he or she is considered ready for weaning and removal from the ventilator.

33. B
A normal and expected assessment finding soon after intubation is hoarseness from irritation by the endotracheal tube against the vocal cords and other soft tissues. Restlessness, dyspnea, and stridor are not an expected finding after extubation and their presence is associated with impaired ventilation and gas exchange, which are indications for reintubation.

34. A, C, E
The most common indicator of the need for suctioning is the presence of coarse crackles (rhonchi) over the trachea. Other indicators or conditions requiring suctioning include excessive secretions, increased peak airway (inspiratory) pressure (PIP), and decreased breath sounds.

35. B
Clients with a pulmonary contusion often first present with decreased breath sounds or crackles and wheezes over the affected area. Later symptoms include bruising over the injury, dry cough, tachycardia, tachypnea, and dullness to percussion. Paradoxical chest movement occurs with a flail chest. Percussive hyperresonance and tracheal deviation are indications of a pneumothorax, not a pulmonary contusion.

36. D
The client with a simple fracture of three ribs will be in pain and may try to avoid deep breathing to prevent movement of the damaged ribs. Pain control measures are needed to ensure the client continues to breathe deeply and frequently enough to prevent stasis pneumonia. Cricothyroidotomy is performed when emergency tracheotomy is needed. Mechanical ventilation is not needed to manage simple rib fracture. Tight bandaging around the chest is avoided to prevent compromising the client's ability to breathe sufficiently.

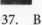

37. B

Mechanical ventilation is needed for a client with a flail chest if respiratory failure occurs, as evidenced by severe hypoxemia and hypercarbia. Constant pain and anxiety are expected and managed but not with mechanical ventilation. Paradoxical chest movement is a flail chest and not alone an indication for mechanical ventilation.

38. A

An open thoracotomy is needed when there is initial blood loss of 1000 mL from the chest or persistent bleeding at the rate of 150 to 200 mL/hr over 3 to 4 hours. Open thoracotomy is not required for simple rib fractures, simple pneumothorax, or a tension pneumothorax.

30

CHAPTER

Assessment of the Cardiovascular System

1. Which statement **best** defines the cardiovascular concept of preload?
   A. Amount of resistance the ventricles must overcome to eject blood through the semilunar valves and into the peripheral blood vessels
   B. Degree of myocardial fiber stretch at the end of diastole and just before the heart contracts
   C. The volume of blood ejected each minute by the heart
   D. Force of blood exerted against the vessel walls

2. Which statements about the structure of the heart are accurate? **Select all that apply.**
   A. The heart normally pumps about 5 L of blood per minute.
   B. A muscular wall called the septum separates only the ventricles of the heart.
   C. The pericardium is a covering that protects the heart.
   D. The left ventricle pumps deoxygenated blood to the lungs.
   E. The right ventricle pumps blood into the aorta and systemic arterial system.
   F. Coronary artery blood flow occurs primarily during diastole.

3. What is the **lowest** mean arterial pressure (MAP) necessary to perfuse the major organs of the body?
   A. 90 to 100 mm Hg
   B. 80 to 90 mm Hg
   C. 70 to 80 mm Hg
   D. 60 to 70 mm Hg

4. What would the nurse calculate the cardiac output to be when the client's heart rate is 68 beats/min and the stroke volume is 50 mL?
   A. 3400 L/min
   B. 4000 L/min
   C. 4400 L/min
   D. 4800 L/min

5. What is the client's pulse pressure when the nurse finds that his or her blood pressure is 148/86 mm Hg?
   A. 48 mm Hg
   B. 56 mm Hg
   C. 62 mm Hg
   D. 86 mm Hg

6. Which statements about blood pressure are accurate? **Select all that apply.**
   A. The right ventricle of the heart generates the greatest amount of blood pressure.
   B. Diastolic blood pressure is primarily determined by the amount of peripheral vasoconstriction.
   C. Systolic blood pressure is the amount of pressure or force generated by the left ventricle to distribute blood into the aorta with each contraction of the heart.
   D. Diastolic pressure is the highest pressure generated during contraction of the ventricles.
   E. To maintain adequate blood flow through the coronary arteries, mean arterial pressure (MAP) must be at least 90 mm Hg.
   F. Paradoxical blood pressure is an exaggerated decrease in systolic pressure by more than 10 mm Hg during the inspiratory phase of the respiratory cycle.

7. What possible causes would the nurse consider when assessing a client and finding a hyperkinetic pulse? **Select all that apply.**
   A. Sepsis
   B. Sedentary lifestyle
   C. Pain
   D. Fever
   E. Anxiety
   F. Thyrotoxicosis

8. For which pathophysiological conditions can a normal healthy heart adapt to maintain perfusion to the body tissues?
   A. Menses and gastroesophageal reflux disease
   B. Stress and infection
   C. Kidney stones and peripheral vascular disease
   D. Bleeding and shortness of breath

9. Before administering which class of drugs would the nurse always check the client's heart rate?
   A. Beta blockers
   B. Diuretics
   C. Anticoagulants
   D. Nonsteroidal anti-inflammatories

10. What is the nurse's **first** action when the health care provider prescribes orthostatic blood pressure checks for a client?
    A. Wait for 1 minute before auscultating blood pressure while the client is sitting.
    B. Instruct the client to sit on the side of the bed before checking blood pressure.
    C. Measure the blood pressure after the client has been supine for 3 minutes.
    D. Tell the client to change positions rapidly between blood pressure checks.

11. Which mechanisms regulate and mediate blood pressure? **Select all that apply.**
    A. Kidneys
    B. Gastrointestinal system
    C. Autonomic nervous system
    D. Respiratory system
    E. Endocrine system
    F. Carbon dioxide elimination

12. When a client is hypovolemic, which tissue reacts and sends fewer impulses to the CNS?
    A. Baroreceptors
    B. Central chemoreceptors
    C. Stretch receptors
    D. Kidney receptors

13. Which cardiovascular assessment changes would the nurse expect in an older client? **Select all that apply.**
    A. Presence of murmurs
    B. Atrial dysrhythmias
    C. Fewer premature ventricular contractions
    D. Very short QT interval on ECG
    E. Increased dizziness
    F. Positive orthostatic blood pressure

14. Which assessment factors for a 62-year-old client would the nurse recognize as modifiable risk factors for heart disease? **Select all that apply.**
    A. History of smoking
    B. Age
    C. Obesity
    D. Ethnic background
    E. Sedentary lifestyle
    F. Gender

15. Which questions would the nurse ask to assess a client's nicotine dependence? **Select all that apply.**
    A. "What brand of cigarettes do you smoke?"
    B. "Do you smoke even when you are ill?"
    C. "How soon after you wake up in the morning do you smoke?"
    D. "What happened the last time you tried to quit smoking?"
    E. "Do you wake up in the middle of the night to smoke?"
    F. "Do you find it difficult not to smoke in places where smoking is prohibited?"

16. Which statement by a client to the nurse indicates an understanding of cigarette usage related to cardiovascular risks?
    A. "I don't smoke as much as I used to and I'm down to half a pack a day."
    B. "I need to be completely cigarette free for at least 3 years."
    C. "I started smoking a few years ago but I plan to quit in a year or two."
    D. "I smoke to relax like when I go out with friends or when I drink."

17. What is the **priority** medical-surgical concept when the nurse is assessing a client with cardiovascular disease (CVD)?
    A. Acid-base balance
    B. Fluid and electrolyte balance
    C. Gas exchange
    D. Perfusion

18. Which exercise regimen would the nurse teach an older adult is best to meet guidelines for physical fitness to promote heart health?
    A. Golfing for 4 hours once a week
    B. Brisk walk for 20 to 30 minutes each day
    C. Bike ride for 6 hours every Saturday
    D. Running for 15 minutes twice a week

19. Which American Heart Association guidelines would the nurse teach a client to fight obesity and improve cardiovascular health? **Select all that apply.**
    A. Don't consume more calories than you can use in a day.
    B. Consume foods that contain vitamins, minerals, and fiber.
    C. Choose foods that are healthy and low in calories.
    D. Avoid gas-producing vegetables such as cabbage or broccoli.
    E. Eat vegetables, fruit and whole-grain foods.
    F. For calcium, choose whole milk dairy products.

20. Which triad of symptoms would the nurse assess for in a woman at risk for cardiovascular disease? **Select all that apply.**
    A. Severe chest pain
    B. Feeling of abdominal fullness
    C. Chronic fatigue despite adequate rest
    D. Extremity pain
    E. Dyspnea or inability to catch her breath
    F. Intermittent claudication

21. Which statement about the peripheral vascular system is accurate?
    A. The velocity of blood flow depends on the diameter of the blood vessel lumen.
    B. The parasympathetic nervous system has the largest effect on blood flow to organs.
    C. Veins have valves that direct blood flow to the heart and prevent backflow.
    D. Blood flow decreases and blood tends to clot as the viscosity decreases.

22. What does the nurse suspect when assessing a client at risk for CVD who states, "my right foot turns very dark red when I sit too long and when I put my foot up, it turns pale?"
    A. Central cyanosis
    B. Arterial insufficiency
    C. Peripheral cyanosis
    D. Venous insufficiency

23. How many cigarette pack-years has this client smoked: Smoked half a pack a day for 6 years?
    A. ½ pack-year
    B. 1 pack-year
    C. 2 pack-years
    D. 3 pack-years

24. When the nurse assesses a client in the clinic for a physical examination and finds decreased skin temperature, what does this **most** likely indicate?
    A. Renal failure
    B. Arterial insufficiency
    C. Anemia
    D. Central cyanosis

25. What is the correct technique for the nurse to use to check a client's lower extremities using the ankle-brachial index?
    A. Blood pressure in the legs is measured with the client supine; then the client stands for 5 minutes and blood pressure is measured in the arms.
    B. A blood pressure cuff is applied to the lower extremities and the systolic pressure is measured by Doppler ultrasound at both the dorsalis pedis and posterior tibial pulses.
    C. The dorsalis pedis and posterior tibial pulses are manually palpated and compared bilaterally for strength and equality and compared to a standard index.
    D. A blood pressure cuff is applied to the lower extremities to observe for an exaggerated decrease in systolic pressure of more than 10 mm Hg during inspiration.

26. What is the best technique for assessing a client's right lower leg for arterial insufficiency?
    A. Palpate the peripheral arteries using a head-to-toe approach with side-to side comparison.
    B. Check all pulse points in the right leg in dependent and supine positions.
    C. Palpate the major arteries including the femoral, and observe for pallor.
    D. Use a Doppler to find the dorsalis pedis and posterior tibial pulses in the right leg.

27. What common assessment finding would the nurse expect to find in an older adult with cardiovascular disease?
    A. Lower leg swelling
    B. Pericardial friction rub
    C. S_4 heart sound
    D. Change in point of maximal impulse (PMI) location

28. Which client has an abnormal heart sound?
    A. S_3 in a 54-year-old
    B. S_1 in a 45-year-old
    C. S_2 in a 38-year-old
    D. S_3 in a 25-year-old

29. What does the nurse suspect when a client who had a bruit on assessment during the previous 2 days does not have a bruit on assessment today?
    A. The prescribed antiplatelet therapy is working.
    B. The problem has resolved spontaneously.
    C. The previous findings may have been an anomaly.
    D. The occlusion of the blood vessel is now 90%.

30. Which techniques would the medical/surgical nurse use when inspecting a client's precordium? **Select all that apply.**
    A. Look at the chest from the side, at a right angle, and downward over areas of the precordium where vibrations are visible.
    B. Note any movement over the aortic, pulmonic, and tricuspid areas.
    C. Use percussion over the heart area to determine its size.
    D. Observe for the location of the point of maximal impulse (PMI) and note any shift.
    E. Palpate the areas over the aortic, pulmonic, and tricuspid valves.
    F. Listen to the heart sounds in a systematic order.

31. What is the nurse's **best** action when auscultating S_1 for a client is difficult?
    A. Ask the assistive personnel (AP) to do a 12-lead electrocardiogram (ECG).
    B. Auscultate with the bell of the stethoscope instead of the diaphragm.
    C. Have the client lean forward or roll to his or her left side.
    D. Instruct the client to take deep breaths and hold them for 5 seconds.

32. Which may be causes of a client's pericardial friction rub? **Select all that apply.**
    A. Myocardial infarction
    B. Pulmonary edema
    C. Cardiac tamponade
    D. Infection
    E. Inflammation
    F. Thoracotomy

33. Which is the most common and normal response by a client to a cardiovascular illness?
    A. Denial
    B. Fear
    C. Loss of control
    D. Depression

34. Which assessment data would the nurse expect for a client diagnosed with angina? **Select all that apply.**
    A. Pain relieved at rest
    B. Sudden onset of pain
    C. Intermittent pain relieved by sitting upright
    D. Substernal pain that may spread across chest, back, and arms
    E. Sharp, stabbing pain that is moderate to severe
    F. Pain that usually lasts less than 15 minutes

35. Which questions would the nurse ask a client when a client is admitted reporting chest pain? **Select all that apply.**
    A. "How do you feel about the chest pain?"
    B. "How long does the pain last and how often does it occur?"
    C. "Where does the pain occur and what does it feel like?"
    D. "Have you had other symptoms that occur with the chest pain and what are they?"
    E. "What activities were you doing when the pain occurred?"
    F. "Is this episode of chest pain different from other episodes you have had?"

36. What does the nurse suspect when a client states "I get short of breath whenever I lie down for several hours?"
    A. Dyspnea on exertion
    B. Orthopnea
    C. Paroxysmal nocturnal dyspnea
    D. Fatigue

37. Which actions by an older adult are likely to cause the experience of syncope? **Select all that apply.**
    A. Walking briskly for 20 minutes
    B. Turning the head
    C. Laughing
    D. Performing a Valsalva maneuver
    E. Rapidly swallowing fluids
    F. Shrugging the shoulders

38. What is the priority problem when a nurse assesses a client with CVD and notes skin that is pale, cool, and moist?
    A. Skin integrity
    B. Abnormal body temperature
    C. Peripheral neurovascular dysfunction
    D. Decreased perfusion

39. What is the **best** advice the nurse would give to a client with moderate-to-severe cramping sensation in their legs or buttocks associated with an activity such as walking?
    A. "Elevating the affected extremity may help relieve the pain."
    B. "Resting or lowering the affected extremity can relieve the pain."
    C. "Placing a nitroglycerine tablet under your tongue may relieve the pain."
    D. "Losing some weight can take pressure off the extremity and relieve the pain."

40. Which information from a client's medical history causes the nurse to check for abnormalities of the heart valves?
    A. Staphylococcal infections of the skin
    B. Yeast infections of the vagina
    C. Fungal infections on the toe nails
    D. Streptococcal infections of the throat

41. Which client serum lipid tests suggest an increased risk for cardiovascular disease (CVD)? **Select all that apply.**
    A. HDL 65 mg/dL
    B. LDL 170 mg/dL
    C. Triglycerides 185 mg/dL
    D. Total cholesterol 175 mg/dL
    E. VLDL 39 mg/dL
    F. Total cholesterol 250 mg/dL

42. Which laboratory value test elevation does the nurse consider **most** significant in the diagnosis of a client's myocardial infarction (MI)?
    A. Troponin T and I
    B. Myoglobin
    C. Highly sensitive C-reactive protein
    D. Creatinine kinase MB

43. What action does the nurse plan to take prior to a cardiac catheterization when a client states he or she has an allergy to seafood and iodine-containing dyes?
    A. Inform the cardiologist because the test must be delayed for a week.
    B. Prepare to administer anticoagulation therapy before the test.
    C. Administer an antihistamine and / or a steroid before the test.
    D. Instruct the client that the test will be conducted using noncontrast dye.

44. Which statements about intravascular ultrasonography (IVUS) are accurate? **Select all that apply.**
    A. A flexible catheter with a miniature transducer is introduced at the distal tip to view the coronary arteries.
    B. Injection of a contrast dye through a catheter permits viewing the coronary arteries.
    C. The catheter has a transducer which emits sound waves that reflect off the plaque and the arterial wall to create an image of the blood vessel.
    D. The catheter is advanced through either the inferior or the superior vena cava and is guided by fluoroscopy.
    E. IVUS can be used in vessels as small as 2 mm to assess the nature of plaques or vessel condition following an intervention.
    F. The cardiologist advances the catheter against the blood flow from the femoral, brachial, or radial artery up the aorta, across the aortic valve, and into the left ventricle.

45. Which action does the nurse perform to prevent kidney toxicity when caring for a client after cardiac catheterization?
    A. Assess pedal pulses every 15 minutes.
    B. Provide intravenous and oral fluids for 12 to 24 hours.
    C. Check the catheterization site every hour for 8 hours.
    D. Keep the catheterized extremity straight for 6 hours.

46. Which instructions would the nurse give the LVN/LPN monitoring a client after cardiac catheterization by radial artery approach? **Select all that apply.**
    A. Monitor the client's vital signs every 15 minutes for 1 hour.
    B. Assess the insertion site for bloody drainage or hematoma.
    C. Keep the client in bed for at least 6 hours.
    D. Assess peripheral pulses and skin temperature and color with every vital sign check.
    E. Monitor intake and output.
    F. Provide oral fluids for adequate contrast excretion.

47. Which tests will the nurse teach a client are routinely done for follow-up monitoring when the client is discharged with a prescription for warfarin?
    A. Complete blood count and platelet count
    B. Partial thromboplastin time (PTT) and serum potassium
    C. Prothrombin time (PT) and international normalized ratio (INR)
    D. Serum and urine electrolyte studies

48. Which instruction would the nurse give a client who is to have an exercise electrocardiography test?
    A. "Someone must drive you home because of sedative effects of the medications."
    B. "Wear comfortable loose-fitting clothes and supportive, rubber-soled shoes."
    C. "Avoid smoking or drinking alcohol for at least a week before the test."
    D. "Do not eat or drink anything after midnight."

49. Which parameter indicates to the nurse that a client's exercise electrocardiogram (ECG) should be stopped?
    A. Increase in heart rate
    B. Increase in blood pressure
    C. ECG shows P waves before every QRS complex
    D. ECG shows ST-segment depression

50. Which medications will the nurse expect the cardiologist to put on hold before an exercise stress test?
    A. Acetaminophen and bronchodilator
    B. Atenolol and diltiazem
    C. Vitamins and iron
    D. Colace and aspirin

51. Which statement best describes the functional capability of a client who is categorized as New York Heart Association Class II?
    A. Ordinary physical activity results in fatigue, palpitations, dyspnea, and anginal pain.
    B. Ordinary physical activity does not cause undue fatigue, palpitation, dyspnea, or anginal pain.
    C. Less than ordinary physical activity causes fatigue, palpitation, dyspnea, or anginal pain.
    D. If any physical activity is undertaken, discomfort is increased.

Chapter 30 Answer Key

1. B
   The stretch imposed on the muscle fibers results from the volume contained within the ventricle at the end of diastole. Preload is determined by the amount of blood returning to the heart from both the venous system (right heart) and the pulmonary system (left heart) (left ventricular end-diastolic [LVED] volume). Option A describes the concept of afterload. Option C describes the concept of cardiac output and Option D is the definition of blood pressure.

2. A, C, F
   Options A, C, and F are accurate. The septum separates the atria and the ventricles. The right ventricle pumps deoxygenated blood to the pulmonary artery and lungs, while the left ventricle pumps blood to the aorta and the systemic arterial system.

3. D
   A MAP between 60 and 70 mm Hg is necessary to maintain perfusion of major body organs, such as the kidneys and brain.
   While all of these MAPs will maintain perfusion to the major organs, this question asks for the **lowest** MAP necessary to maintain major organ perfusion and therefore option D is the best response.

4. A
   Cardiac output (CO), is the amount of blood pumped from the left ventricle each minute. CO depends on the relationship between heart rate (HR) and stroke volume (SV); it is the product of these two variables: CO = SV × HR i.e., 50 × 68 = 3400 mL/min.

5. C
   The difference between the systolic and diastolic values is referred to as pulse pressure. 148 − 86 = 62 mm Hg.

6. B, C, F
   The left ventricle generates the greatest amount of blood pressure. To maintain adequate blood flow through the coronary arteries, MAP must be at least 60 mm Hg. Systolic pressure is the highest pressure during contraction of the ventricles. Options B, C, and F are accurate.

7. A, C, D, E, F
   A hyperkinetic pulse is a large, "bounding" pulse caused by an increased ejection of blood. It occurs in clients with a high cardiac output (e.g., with exercise [not sedentary], sepsis, or thyrotoxicosis) and in those with increased sympathetic system activity (e.g., with pain, fever, or anxiety).

8. B

The healthy heart can adapt to various pathophysiologic conditions (e.g., stress, infections, hemorrhage) to maintain perfusion to the various body tissues.

9. A

An increase in circulating catecholamines (e.g., epinephrine and norepinephrine) usually causes an increase in HR and contractility. Many cardiovascular drugs, particularly beta blockers, block this sympathetic (fight or flight) pattern by decreasing the HR. The nurse would check to be sure that the heart rate was not too slow before administering a beta blocker.

10. C

Postural (orthostatic) hypotension occurs when the BP is not adequately maintained while moving from a lying to a sitting or standing position. It is defined as a decrease of more than 20 mm Hg of the systolic pressure or more than 10 mm Hg of the diastolic pressure and a 10% to 20% increase in heart rate. To detect orthostatic changes in BP, first measure the BP when the client is supine. After remaining supine for at least 3 minutes, the client changes position to sitting or standing. Normally systolic pressure drops slightly or remains unchanged as the client rises, whereas diastolic pressure rises slightly. After the position change, wait for at least 1 minute before auscultating BP and counting the radial pulse. The cuff should remain in the proper position on the client's arm. Observe and record any signs or symptoms of dizziness. If the client cannot tolerate the position change, return him or her to the previous position of comfort.

11. A, C, E

The three mechanisms that regulate and mediate blood pressure: the autonomic nervous system (ANS), which excites or inhibits sympathetic nervous system activity in response to impulses from chemoreceptors and baroreceptors; the kidneys, which sense a change in blood flow and activate the renin-angiotensin-aldosterone mechanism; and the endocrine system, which releases various hormones (e.g., catecholamine, kinins, serotonin, histamine) to stimulate the sympathetic nervous system at the tissue level.

12. C

Stretch receptors in the vena cava and the right atrium are sensitive to pressure or volume changes. When a client is hypovolemic, stretch receptors in the blood vessels sense a reduced volume or pressure and send fewer impulses to the CNS. This reaction stimulates the sympathetic nervous system to increase the heart rate and constrict the peripheral blood vessels. Impulses from these baroreceptors inhibit the vasomotor center which results in a drop in BP. Central chemoreceptors in the respiratory center of the brain are also stimulated by hypercapnia (an increase in partial pressure of arterial carbon dioxide [$Paco_2$]) and acidosis. The kidneys retain sodium and water so BP tends to rise because of fluid retention and activation of the renin-angiotensin-aldosterone mechanism.

13. A, B, E, F

Calcification of heart valves can cause murmurs. Pacemaker cells decrease in number which can lead to atrial dysrhythmias and increased (not fewer) premature ventricular contractions. The size of the left ventricle increases which can lead to widened QRS complexes and longer (not shorter) QT intervals. Baroreceptors become less sensitive which can lead to positive orthostatic blood pressure and dizziness as well as fainting.

14. A, C, E

Modifiable risk factors are personal lifestyle habits, including cigarette smoking, physical inactivity, obesity, and psychological variables. Nonmodifiable (uncontrollable) risk factors include the client's age, gender, ethnic origin, and a family history of cardiovascular disease.

15. B, C, E, F

Determine nicotine dependence by asking questions such as: How soon after you wake up in the morning do you smoke?; Do you wake up in the middle of the night to smoke?; Do you find it difficult not to smoke in places where smoking is prohibited?; and Do you smoke even when you are ill?

16. B

Three to four years after a client has stopped smoking, his or her CVD risk appears to be similar to that of a person who has never smoked. The client is still smoking in the other responses and is still at risk for CVD.

17. D

The priority concept when assessing for cardiovascular disease is perfusion. The interrelated concept for this chapter is fluid and electrolyte balance. Gas exchange and acid-base balance are more pertinent to respiratory and renal illnesses.

18. B

In the United States the recommended exercise guidelines are: 150 minutes of moderate exercise or 75 minutes of vigorous exercise per week (or a combination of the two) plus completing muscle-strengthening exercises at least 2 days per week. Regular physical activity (not just once a week) promotes cardiovascular fitness and produces beneficial changes in blood pressure and levels of blood lipids and clotting factors.

19. A, B, C, E

The American Heart Association provides guidelines to combat obesity and improve cardiac health, including ingesting more nutrient-rich foods that have vitamins, minerals, fiber, and other nutrients but are low in calories. To get the necessary nutrients, teach clients to choose foods such as vegetables, fruits, unrefined whole-grain products, and fat-free (not whole milk) dairy products most often. Also teach clients to not eat more calories than they can burn every day. Vegetables such as cabbage and broccoli are good sources of nutrients.

20. B, C, E

Some clients, especially women, do not experience pain in the chest but, instead, feel discomfort or indigestion. Women often present with a "triad" of symptoms. In addition to indigestion or a feeling of abdominal fullness, chronic fatigue despite adequate rest and feelings of an "inability to catch my breath" (dyspnea) are also common in heart disease.

21. C

Veins in the superficial and deep venous systems (except the smallest and the largest veins) have valves that direct blood flow back to the heart and prevent backflow. Skeletal muscles in the extremities provide a force that helps push the venous blood forward. Veins have the ability to accommodate large shifts in volume with minimal changes in venous pressure.

22. B

Rubor (dusky redness) that replaces pallor in a dependent foot suggests arterial insufficiency. Central cyanosis involves decreased oxygenation of the arterial blood in the lungs and appears as a bluish tinge of the conjunctivae and the mucous membranes of the mouth and tongue. Peripheral cyanosis occurs when blood flow to the peripheral vessels is decreased by peripheral vasoconstriction. Venous insufficiency is a result of prolonged venous hypertension that stretches and damages the valves which can lead to backup of blood, edema, and decreased tissue perfusion.

23. D

Pack-years are the number of packs of cigarettes per day multiplied by the number of years the client has smoked. ½ x 6 = 3 pack-years.

24. B

Decreased blood flow results in decreased skin temperature. It is lowered in several clinical conditions, including heart failure, peripheral vascular disease, and shock. It can be assessed for symmetry by touching different areas of the body with the dorsal (back) surface of the hand or fingers.

25. B

The ankle-brachial index (ABI) can be used to assess the vascular status of the lower extremities. A BP cuff is applied to the lower extremity just above the malleolus. The systolic pressure is measured by Doppler ultrasound at both the dorsalis pedis and posterior tibial pulses. The higher of these two pressures is then divided by the higher of the two brachial pulses to obtain the ABI. Normal values for the ABI are 1.00 or higher because BP in the legs is usually higher than BP in the arms.

26. A

Assessment of arterial pulses provides information about vascular integrity and circulation. For clients with suspected or actual vascular disease, major peripheral pulses should be assessed for presence or absence, amplitude, contour, rhythm, rate, and equality. Palpate the peripheral arteries in a head-to-toe approach with a side-to-side comparison.

27. C

This question asks for a finding related to aging. An atrial gallop (S_4) may be heard in clients with hypertension, anemia, ventricular hypertrophy, MI, aortic or pulmonic stenosis, and pulmonary emboli. It may also be heard with advancing age because of a stiffened ventricle. Edema, friction rubs, and PMI changes occur with CVD but are not just age related.

28. A

An S_3 gallop in clients older than 35 years is considered abnormal and represents a decrease in left ventricular compliance. It can be detected as an early sign of heart failure or as a ventricular septal defect. An S_3 heart sound is most likely to be a normal finding in those younger than 35 years. S_1 and S_2 are both normal heart sounds.

29. D

Bruits are swishing sounds that may occur from turbulent blood flow in narrowed or atherosclerotic arteries. Assess for the absence or presence of bruits by placing the bell of the stethoscope on the neck over the carotid artery while the client holds his or her breath. Normally there are no sounds if the artery has uninterrupted blood flow. A bruit may develop when the internal diameter of the vessel is narrowed by 50% or more, but this does not indicate the severity of disease in the arteries. Once the vessel is blocked 90% or greater, the bruit often cannot be heard.

30. A, B, D

Inspect the chest from the side, at a right angle, and downward over areas of the precordium where vibrations are visible. Cardiac motion is of low amplitude, and sometimes the inward movements are more easily detected by the naked eye. Note any prominent pulses. Movement over the aortic, pulmonic, and tricuspid areas is abnormal. Pulses in the mitral area (the apex of the heart) are considered normal and are referred to as the apical impulse, or the point of maximal impulse (PMI). The PMI should be located at the left fifth intercostal space (ICS) in the midclavicular line. If it appears in more than one ICS and has shifted lateral to the midclavicular line, the client may have left ventricular hypertrophy. Palpation and percussion are usually not performed by medical/surgical nurses. Listening to the heart sounds would be part of auscultation assessment.

31. C

When there is difficulty hearing heart sounds, have the client lean forward or roll to his or her left side. These actions move the heart closer to the chest wall and can facilitate hearing the heart sounds more clearly.

32. A, C, D, E, F

A pericardial friction rub originates from the pericardial sac and occurs with the movements of the heart during the cardiac cycle. They are usually transient and are a sign of inflammation, infection, or infiltration. They may be heard in clients with pericarditis resulting from MI, cardiac tamponade, or post-thoracotomy. Pulmonary edema is not a cause of a pericardial friction rub.

33. A

A common and normal response is denial, which is a defense mechanism that enables the client to cope with threatening circumstances. He or she may deny the current cardiovascular condition, may state that it was present but is now absent, or may be excessively cheerful. Denial becomes maladaptive when the client is noncompliant or does not adhere to the interdisciplinary plan of care.

34. A, B, D, F

Angina pain is usually sudden in onset, in response to exertion, emotion, or extremes in temperature. It is usually located on the left side of chest without radiation but can be substernal and may spread across the chest and the back and/or down the arms. It usually lasts less than 15 minutes and is relieved with rest, nitrate administration, or oxygen therapy. See Table 30.1 in the text.

35. B, C, D, E, F

If pain is present, ask whether it is different from any other episodes of pain. Ask the client to describe which activities he or she was doing when it first occurred, such as sleeping, arguing, or running (precipitating factors). If possible, the client should point to the area where the chest pain occurred (location) and describe if and how the pain radiated (spread). In addition, ask how the pain feels and whether it is sharp, dull, or crushing (quality of pain). To understand the severity of the pain, ask the client to grade it from 0 to 10, with 10 indicating severe pain (intensity). He or she may also report other signs and symptoms that occur at the same time (associated symptoms), such as dyspnea, diaphoresis (excessive sweating), nausea, and vomiting. Other factors that need to be addressed are those that may have made the chest pain worse (aggravating factors) or less intense (relieving factors). Asking how the client feels about the pain should be part of the psychosocial assessment.

36. C.

Paroxysmal nocturnal dyspnea (PND) develops after the client has been lying down for several hours. In this position, blood from the lower extremities is redistributed to the venous system, which increases venous return to the heart. A diseased heart cannot compensate for the increased volume and is ineffective in pumping the additional fluid into the circulatory system. Pulmonary congestion results, and the client awakens abruptly, often with a feeling of suffocation and panic. He or she sits upright and dangles the legs over the side of the bed to relieve the dyspnea. This sensation may last for 20 minutes. Dyspnea associated with activity is dyspnea on exertion. Orthopnea is dyspnea whenever a client lies flat and

may require three to four pillows for sleep. Fatigue is a feeling of tiredness as a result of activity.

37. B, D, F

Syncope in an older adult may result from hypersensitivity of the carotid sinus bodies in the carotid arteries. Pressure applied to these arteries while turning the head, shrugging the shoulders, or performing a Valsalva maneuver (bearing down during defecation) may stimulate a vagal response and syncope. Walking, laughing, or swallowing fluids does not usually cause syncope in older adults.

38. D

Decreased perfusion is manifested as cool, pale, and moist skin. If there is normal blood flow or adequate perfusion to a given area in light-colored skin, it appears pink, perhaps rosy, and is warm.

39. B

Clients who report a moderate-to-severe cramping sensation in their legs or buttocks associated with an activity such as walking have intermittent claudication related to decreased arterial tissue perfusion. Resting or lowering the affected extremity to decrease tissue demands or to enhance arterial blood flow usually relieves claudication pain. Leg pain that results from prolonged standing or sitting is related to venous insufficiency from either incompetent valves or venous obstruction. Elevating the extremity may relieve this pain. Nitroglycerine is given to relieve angina. Weight loss will not relieve the pain of intermittent claudication.

40. D

Ask clients about recurrent tonsillitis, streptococcal infections, and rheumatic fever because these conditions may lead to valvular abnormalities of the heart.

41. B, C, E, F

See Laboratory Profile Cardiovascular Assessment Box in text. This box lists the normal results and states which lipid results increase the risk for CVD. The desired ranges for lipids are:

Total cholesterol less than 200 mg/dL; Triglycerides between 40 and 160 mg/dL for men and between 35 and 135 mg/dL for women; HDL more than 45 mg/dL for men; more than 55 mg/dL for women ("good" cholesterol); and LDL less than 130 mg/dL; VLDL is 7-32 mg/dL or 0.18-0.83 mmol/L (SI units). A fasting blood sample for the measurement of serum cholesterol levels is preferable to a nonfasting sample.

42. A
Troponin is a myocardial muscle protein released into the bloodstream with injury to myocardial muscle. Troponins T and I are not found in healthy clients, so any rise in values indicates cardiac necrosis or acute MI. Before the development of highly sensitive troponin levels, providers relied on creatinine kinase (CK), its isoenzyme (CK-MB), and myoglobin to assist with diagnosis of acute myocardial infarction. Highly sensitive C-reactive protein (hsCRP) has been the most studied marker of inflammation.

43. C
Before the procedure, question the client about any history of allergy to iodine-based contrast agents. An antihistamine or steroid may be given to a client with a positive history or to prevent a reaction. The test does not need to be delayed and contrast dye is necessary to see any coronary artery blockages. Anticoagulants would not be given because that would cause bleeding.

44. A, C, E
Options A, C, and E are accurate about the intravascular ultrasonography (IVUS) procedure. Options B, D, and F are descriptions related to the usual cardiac catheterization procedure.

45. B
Contrast-induced renal dysfunction can result from vasoconstriction and the direct toxic effect of the contrast agent on the renal tubules. Hydration pre- and post-study helps eliminate or minimize contrast-induced renal toxicity.

46. A, B, D, E, F
All options except C are correct for safe recovery of the client after a cardiac catheterization. Keeping the client in bed for more than 2 hours is not necessary when the radial approach is used for the test.

47. C
Prothrombin time (PT) and international normalized ratio (INR) are used when initiating and maintaining therapy with oral anticoagulants, such as sodium warfarin. They measure the activity of prothrombin, fibrinogen, and factors V, VII, and X. INR is the most reliable way to monitor anticoagulant status in warfarin therapy. The therapeutic ranges vary significantly based on the reason for the anticoagulation and the client's history. The normal INR is 0.8-1.1. An INR range of 2.0-3.0 is generally an effective therapeutic range for people taking warfarin.

48. B
Clients are advised to wear comfortable, loose clothing and rubber-soled, supportive shoes. Instruct the client to get plenty of rest the night before the procedure. He or she may have a light meal 2 hours before the test but should avoid smoking or drinking alcohol or caffeine-containing beverages on the day of the test. Usually cardiovascular drugs such as beta blockers or calcium channel blockers are withheld on the day of the test to allow the heart rate to increase during the stress portion of the test. Sedation drugs are not given with this test.

49. D
Increases in heart rate and blood pressure are expected. P waves before each QRS complex is a normal finding. The client exercises until one of these findings occurs: a predetermined HR is reached and maintained; signs and symptoms such as chest pain, fatigue, extreme dyspnea, vertigo, hypotension, and ventricular dysrhythmias appear; or significant ST-segment depression or T-wave inversion occurs.

50. B

Usually cardiovascular drugs such as beta blockers (e.g., atenolol) or calcium channel blockers (e.g., cardizem) are withheld on the day of the test to allow the heart rate to increase during the stress portion of the test. The drugs listed in options A, C, and D do not generally affect heart rate.

51. A

With regard to physical activity, the New York Heart Association Functional Classification of Cardiovascular Disability describes the four classes as follows: Class I, ordinary physical activity does not cause undue fatigue, palpitation, dyspnea, or anginal pain; Class II, ordinary physical activity results in fatigue, palpitation, dyspnea, or anginal pain; Class III, less than ordinary physical activity causes fatigue, palpitation, dyspnea, or anginal pain; and Class IV, if any physical activity is undertaken, discomfort is increased.

31
CHAPTER

Concepts of Care for Patients with Dysrhythmias

1. Which **priority** concept does the nurse focus on when a client is diagnosed with a dysrhythmia?
   A. Clotting
   B. Fluid and electrolyte balance
   C. Perfusion
   D. Acid-base balance

2. Which normal heart rates does the nurse expect to be initiated by the primary pacemaker of the heart (SA Node) in clients when the heart rate is regular? **Select all that apply.**
   A. 55 beats/min
   B. 62 beats/min
   C. 74 beats/min
   D. 86 beats/min
   E. 98 beats/min
   F. 110 beats/min

3. Which waveform does the nurse recognize as atrial depolarization when a client is placed on a cardiac monitor?
   A. P wave
   B. PR segment
   C. QRS complex
   D. T wave

4. How would the nurse **best** interpret the electrocardiogram (ECG) of a younger athletic client which shows sinus bradycardia with a rate of 54 beats/min?
   A. It is the body's attempt to compensate for a decreased stroke volume by decreasing heart rate.
   B. The sinus bradycardia provides an adequate stroke volume that is associated with cardiac conditioning.
   C. The client has a rapid filling rate that lengthens diastolic filling time and leads to decreased cardiac output.
   D. This is a common finding in healthy adults of all ages and would be considered a normal finding.

5. To determine if a client has a pulse deficit, what procedure would the nurse follow?
   A. Assess the apical and radial pulses for a full minute and calculate the difference.
   B. Check the client's blood pressure and subtract the diastolic from the systolic pressure.
   C. Take the client's pulse rate while supine, then in a standing position.
   D. Assess the radial pulse for a minute, have the client rest, then check the radial pulse again.

6. Which ECG waveforms and intervals are the normal measurements or positions? **Select all that apply.**
   A. PR interval 0.12-0.20 second
   B. QRS complex 0.06-0.10 second
   C. PR segment isoelectric line
   D. QT interval less than half of the R to R interval
   E. U wave follows T wave if present
   F. TP segment one block above isoelectric line

7. Which definition **best** describes the electro-physiologic property called automaticity of myocardial pacemaker cells?
   A. The ability of atrial and ventricular muscle cells to shorten their fiber length in response to electrical stimulation, causing sufficient pressure to push blood forward through the heart
   B. The ability to send an electrical stimulus from cell membrane to cell membrane
   C. The ability of nonpacemaker heart cells to respond to an electrical impulse that begins in pacemaker cells
   D. The ability of cardiac cells to generate an electrical impulse spontaneously and repetitively

8. To best perform a 12-lead ECG on a client, how does the nurse place the leads on the client?
   A. Four leads are placed on the limbs and four are placed on the chest.
   B. The negative electrode is placed on the left arm and the positive electrode is placed on the right leg.
   C. Four leads are placed on the limbs and six are placed on the chest.
   D. The negative electrode is placed on the right arm and the positive electrode is placed on the left leg.

9. Where will the nurse place the leads on a client for a five-lead continuous monitoring system? **Select all that apply.**
   A. Right arm electrode just below the right clavicle
   B. Left arm electrode just below the left clavicle
   C. Right leg electrode on the highest palpable rib, on the right midclavicular line
   D. Left leg electrode on the lowest palpable rib, on the left midclavicular line
   E. Fifth electrode placed to obtain one of the six chest leads
   F. Left arm electrode just above the left clavicle

10. Which condition is indicated when the nurse notes ST segment elevation or one to two small blocks on a client's ECG?
    A. Ventricular irritability
    B. Subarachnoid hemorrhage
    C. Myocardial injury or ischemia
    D. Malfunction of the SA node

11. Which serum electrolyte would the nurse check after noting tall and peaked T waves on a client's ECG?
    A. Sodium
    B. Potassium
    C. Magnesium
    D. Chloride

12. Which actions are responsibilities of the monitor technician? **Select all that apply.**
    A. Report client rhythm and significant changes to the nurse.
    B. Notify the health care provider of any pertinent changes.
    C. Print routine ECG strips for each monitored client.
    D. Apply battery-operated transmitter leads to clients.
    E. Watch the bank of cardiac monitors on a client care unit.
    F. Interpret rhythm strips for each monitored client.

13. Which would be the **best** method for the nurse to confirm a report from the monitor technician about a change in a monitored client's heart rate?
    A. Count QRS complexes in a 6-second strip and multiply by 10.
    B. Analyze the ECG rhythm strip using an ECG caliper.
    C. Assess the client's heart rate directly by checking the apical pulse.
    D. Request that the monitor technician run an ECG strip for a minute.

14. What is the **first** step when the nurse analyzes a client's ECG rhythm strip?
    A. Analyze the P waves
    B. Determine the heart rate
    C. Measure the QRS complex
    D. Assess for ST-segment elevation

15. Which questions would the nurse use to assess a client's P wave on an ECG rhythm strip? **Select all that apply.**
    A. Do all P waves look similar?
    B. Are P waves present?
    C. Does one P wave follow each QRS complex?
    D. Are P waves occurring regularly?
    E. Are the P waves greater than 0.20 second?
    F. Are P waves smooth, rounded, and upright?

16. Which criteria support the nurse's assessment that a client's ECG rhythm strip shows a normal sinus rhythm (NSR)?
    A. PR interval is 0.24 second.
    B. Atrial and ventricular rates are 58 beats/min.
    C. Atrial and ventricular rates are regular.
    D. P waves are present before every QRS complex.
    E. QRS duration is consistent at 0.08 second.
    F. Atrial and ventricular rates are 82 beats/min.

17. What is the **priority** action for the nurse when the monitor technician states that a client's telemetry monitor shows a rhythm that appears as a wandering or fuzzy baseline?
    A. Check to see if the client has a do-not-resuscitate order.
    B. Assess the client to differentiate artifact from an actual lethal rhythm.
    C. Immediately obtain a 12-lead ECG to assess the actual rhythm.
    D. Ask the assistive personnel (AP) to take a set of vital signs on the client.

18. Which actions would the nurse take when the monitor technician states that a client's telemetry ECG signal transmission is not very clear? **Select all that apply.**
    A. Ensure that the gel on each electrode is moist and fresh.
    B. Clean the skin and clip hairs if necessary.
    C. Abrade the skin by rubbing briskly with a rough washcloth.
    D. Make sure that the skin is free of lotion or any other substance.
    E. Clean the skin with povidone-iodine before applying electrodes.
    F. Check to be sure that electrodes are not placed over scar tissue.

19. Which conditions would the nurse suspect when a client's telemetry ECG rhythm strip shows ST elevation of 1.5 mm (1.5 small blocks)? **Select all that apply.**
    A. Pericarditis
    B. Hypokalemia
    C. Myocardial infarction
    D. Ventricular hypertrophy
    E. Endocarditis
    F. Hyperkalemia

20. What does the nurse determine is the client's heart rate when assessing a 6-second telemetry ECG strip with five QRS complexes?
    A. 30 beats/min, bradycardia
    B. 40 beats/min, bradycardia
    C. 50 beats/min, bradycardia
    D. 60 beats/min, normal

21. Which signs and symptoms would the nurse expect to assess in a client with sinus tachycardia? **Select all that apply.**
    A. Fatigue
    B. Shortness of breath
    C. Decreased oxygen saturation
    D. Decreased blood pressure
    E. Anginal pain
    F. Widened QRS complexes

22. What does the nurse suspect when assessing a client's telemetry ECG strip and noting a wide distorted QRS complex of 0.14 second followed by a P wave?
    A. Delayed time of the impulse through the ventricles
    B. Problem with speed set on the ECG telemetry monitor
    C. Wide but normal complex with no cause for concern
    D. Premature ventricular complex followed by atrial contraction

23. Which causes would the nurse recognize as leading to increased atrial irritability and premature atrial contractions (PACs) in a client's myocardium? **Select all that apply.**
    A. Caffeine intake
    B. Anxiety
    C. Syncope
    D. Stress in life
    E. Infection
    F. Pulmonary hypotension

24. Which dysrhythmia does the nurse consider life threatening because it causes the ventricles to quiver and results in the absence of cardiac output for a client?
    A. Asystole
    B. Ventricular tachycardia
    C. Atrial fibrillation
    D. Ventricular fibrillation

25. Which nursing actions have **priority** when a client with acute supraventricular tachycardia (SVT) is to be administered adenosine by the health care provider? **Select all that apply.**
    A. Have injectable beta-blocker drugs at the bedside.
    B. Give the drug slowly over 1-2 minutes.
    C. Ensure that emergency equipment is at the bedside.
    D. Follow the drug injection with a normal saline bolus.
    E. Monitor the client for bradycardia, nausea, and vomiting.
    F. Prepare for synchronized cardioversion after giving the adenosine.

26. Which risk factors for atrial fibrillation would the nurse monitor for in client? **Select all that apply.**
    A. Peripheral vascular disease
    B. Hypertension
    C. Chronic obstructive pulmonary disease
    D. Diabetes mellitus
    E. Excessive alcohol intake
    F. Mitral valve disease

27. When a client has been in atrial fibrillation for 3 days and is scheduled for an elective cardioversion, what **priority** teaching does the nurse provide to the client?
    A. Consume potassium-rich food sources such as bananas.
    B. Report muscle tremors or weakness to the health care provider.
    C. Get up slowly when getting out of bed or a chair.
    D. Watch for any sign of bleeding and report this to your health care provider.

28. Which actions are essential nursing care for a client **immediately** after elective cardioversion? **Select all that apply.**
    A. Administer oxygen.
    B. Assess vital signs and level of consciousness.
    C. Provide sips of water or ice chips.
    D. Monitor for dysrhythmias.
    E. Maintain an open airway.
    F. Document the results of the cardioversion.

29. Which client assessment takes **priority** when the nurse begins his or her shift?
    A. Client with chronic atrial fibrillation and ventricular rate of 72 beats/min
    B. Client with sinus tachycardia and occasional premature atrial contractions (PACs)
    C. Client with paroxysmal supraventricular tachycardia (PSVT) that terminated
    D. Client with atrial fibrillation and sustained rapid ventricular response

30. How does the nurse interpret a client's telemetry ECG strip that shows four successive premature ventricular contractions (PVCs)?
    A. The monitor is showing two PVC couplets in a row.
    B. This rhythm is ventricular asystole as seen in a dying heart.
    C. The client had an episode of nonsustained ventricular tachycardia (NSVT).
    D. The nurse must check the client for loose leads and artifact.

31. Which procedure would the nurse provide teaching about to a client who has chronic atrial fibrillation and is at increased risk for a stroke, but is not a candidate for anticoagulation?
    A. Radiofrequency catheter ablation (RCA)
    B. Left atrial appendage (LAA) occlusion
    C. Biventricular pacing
    D. Surgical maze procedure

32. After calling for help, when the nurse finds a client in his or her room without a pulse, apneic and unconscious, which action should be taken **next**?
    A. Begin cardiac compressions.
    B. Establish IV access.
    C. Give supplemental oxygen.
    D. Defibrillate the client.

33. Which drug does the nurse prepare to administer to a client diagnosed with the dysrhythmia torsades de pointes?
    A. Calcium chloride
    B. Epinephrine
    C. Magnesium sulfate
    D. Adenosine

34. When would the telemetry unit nurse use temporary transcutaneous pacing for a client? **Select all that apply.**
    A. Only when a client's ECG shows a bradydysrhythmia and the client is asymptomatic
    B. When a client's ECG strip shows atrial fibrillation with a rapid ventricular response
    C. Only as a temporary emergency measure until invasive pacing method can be started
    D. When a client is experiencing syncope, dizziness and fainting
    E. Only until the client's heart rhythm returns to normal
    F. When invasive pacing is not immediately available

35. Which ECG strip pattern is evidence to the nurse that a client's temporary transvenous pacemaker has successfully depolarized the ventricles?
    A. A pacer spike followed by a QRS complex
    B. Two spikes followed by a QRS complex
    C. A pacer spike before and after the QRS complex
    D. No pacer spike but regular QRS complexes

36. Which statements about permanent pacemakers are accurate? **Select all that apply.**
    A. Permanent pacemakers are powered by lithium batteries that last over 20 years.
    B. Permanent pacemakers are available as pacemaker/defibrillator devices.
    C. Biventricular pacemakers allow synchronized depolarization of the ventricles.
    D. Permanent pacemakers are used to treat disorders such as complete heart block.
    E. A client with a new pacemaker should avoid lifting his or her arm over the head for at least 6 months.
    F. The pulse generator for a permanent pacemaker is usually implanted in the left subclavian area.

37. Which are nursing responsibilities for the care of a client with a newly implanted permanent pacemaker? **Select all that apply.**
    A. Assess the implantation site for bleeding, swelling, redness, tenderness, or infection.
    B. Administer short-acting sedatives as needed and prescribed.
    C. Monitor the ECG rhythm strip to ensure that the pacemaker is working correctly.
    D. Observe for overstimulation of the chest wall, which might cause pneumothorax.
    E. Assess that the implantation site dressing is clean and dry.
    F. Teach the client about initial activity restrictions.

38. Which important teaching points would the nurse discuss with a client who receives a new permanent pacemaker? **Select all that apply.**
    A. Report any pulse rate that is lower than the rate set on the pacemaker.
    B. Avoid sources of strong electromagnetic fields such as magnets.
    C. If the surgical incision is near the shoulder, be sure to perform daily range of motion.
    D. Carry a pacemaker identification card and wear a medical alert bracelet.
    E. Avoid tight clothing to prevent pressure over the pacemaker generator.
    F. It is safe to go through airport security because the pacemaker will not set off the alarms.

39. Which safety precaution **must** be taken before defibrillating a client with ventricular fibrillation (VF)?
    A. Make sure that the defibrillator is set on the synchronous mode.
    B. Be sure to hyperventilate the client before the defibrillation.
    C. Command all health care team members to stand clear of the client's bed.
    D. Disconnect the monitor leads to prevent electrical shocks to the client.

40. For which cardiac dysrhythmia(s) would an automatic external defibrillator (AED) instruct the nurse to immediately defibrillate an unconscious client at an outpatient clinic? **Select all that apply.**
    A. Paroxysmal supraventricular tachycardia
    B. Pulseless electrical activity
    C. Ventricular fibrillation
    D. Pulseless ventricular tachycardia
    E. Nonsustained ventricular tachycardia
    F. Atrial fibrillation with rapid ventricular response

41. What effect does the nurse expect a Class IV drug to have on a client's cardiac conduction system?
    A. Slow the flow of calcium into the cell during depolarization to depress automaticity
    B. Stabilize membranes to decrease myocardial contractility
    C. Decrease heart rate and conduction velocity
    D. Lengthen the absolute refractory period and prolong repolarization

42. Which descriptions are characteristics of Class III antidysrhythmic drugs? **Select all that apply.**
    A. Increase force of contraction
    B. Lengthen absolute refractory period
    C. Include hypertension as a side effect for some drugs
    D. Include bradycardia as a side effect for some drugs
    E. Prolong QT interval
    F. Prolong repolarization

43. Which beta-blocker drug approved for treating dysrhythmias is also a Class III antidysrhythmic drug?
    A. Sotalol
    B. Esmolol
    C. Propranolol
    D. Acebutolol

44.   Interpret the following rhythm strip

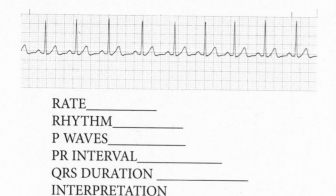

    RATE_____
    RHYTHM_____
    P WAVES_____
    PR INTERVAL_____
    QRS DURATION _____
    INTERPRETATION_____

45.   Interpret the following rhythm strip

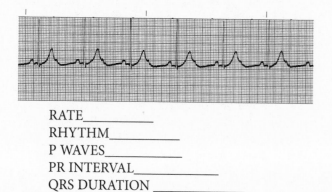

    RATE_____
    RHYTHM_____
    P WAVES_____
    PR INTERVAL_____
    QRS DURATION _____
    INTERPRETATION_____

46.   Interpret the following rhythm strip

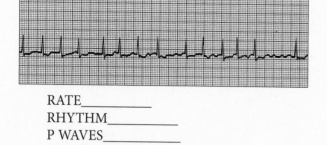

    RATE_____
    RHYTHM_____
    P WAVES_____
    PR INTERVAL_____
    QRS DURATION _____
    INTERPRETATION_____

47.   Interpret the following rhythm strip

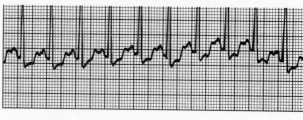

    RATE_____
    RHYTHM_____
    P WAVES_____
    PR INTERVAL_____
    QRS DURATION _____
    INTERPRETATION_____

48.   Interpret the following rhythm strip

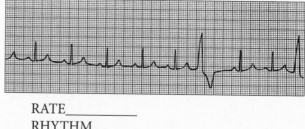

    RATE_____
    RHYTHM_____
    P WAVES_____
    PR INTERVAL_____
    QRS DURATION _____
    INTERPRETATION_____

49.   Interpret the following rhythm strip

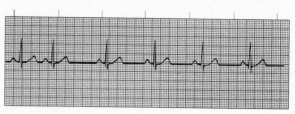

    RATE_____
    RHYTHM_____
    P WAVES_____
    PR INTERVAL_____
    QRS DURATION _____
    INTERPRETATION_____

50. Interpret the following rhythm strip

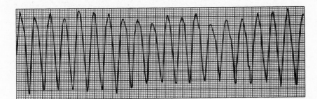

RATE_____
RHYTHM_____
P WAVES_____
PR INTERVAL_____
QRS DURATION _____
INTERPRETATION_____

51. Interpret the following rhythm strip

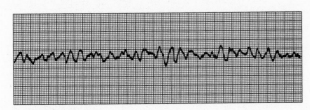

RATE_____
RHYTHM_____
P WAVES_____
PR INTERVAL_____
QRS DURATION _____
INTERPRETATION_____

52. Interpret the following rhythm strip

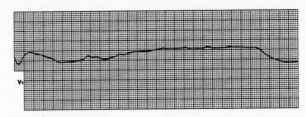

RATE_____
RHYTHM_____
P WAVES_____
PR INTERVAL_____
QRS DURATION _____
INTERPRETATION_____

Chapter 31 Answer Key

1. C
    Perfusion is the priority concept for the client with dysrhythmias. It occurs when there is adequate arterial blood flow through the peripheral tissues (peripheral perfusion) and blood that is pumped by the heart to oxygenate major body organs (central perfusion). Perfusion is a normal physiologic process of the body; without adequate perfusion, cell death can occur. When a client has a dysrhythmia, often perfusion is inadequate. Clotting and fluid and electrolyte balance are interrelated concepts for dysrhythmias. Acid-base imbalance may be a result of inadequate perfusion.

2. B, C, D, E
    The SA node is the heart's primary pacemaker. It can spontaneously and rhythmically generate electrical impulses at a rate of 60 to 100 beats/min and therefore has the greatest degree of automaticity (pacing function). Heart rates less than 60 beats/min are bradycardias and heart rates greater than 100 beats/min are tachycardias.

3. A

Impulses from the sinus node move directly through atrial muscle and lead to atrial depolarization, which is reflected in a P wave on the electrocardiogram (ECG). Atrial muscle contraction should follow. The PR segment reflects impulses slowing down or being delayed in the AV node before proceeding to the ventricles. QRS complexes reflect ventricular depolarization and T waves reflect ventricular repolarization.

4. B

Well-conditioned athletes with bradycardia have a hypereffective heart in which the strong heart muscle provides an adequate stroke volume and a low heart rate to achieve a normal cardiac output. This is not a common finding in adults of all ages, but an indicator of dysrhythmia in older adults. Decreasing heart rate in most adults results in decreased cardiac output.

5. A

Pulse deficit is the difference between the apical and peripheral (e.g., radial) pulses. If the apical pulse differs from the radial pulse rate, a pulse deficit exists and indicates that the heart is not pumping adequately to achieve optimal perfusion to the body. The difference between systolic and diastolic pressures is the pulse pressure. When a client's blood pressure and pulse are taken first lying down and then sitting or standing, that is orthostatic vital signs.

6. A, B, C, D, E

All of these statements are correct except F. The TP segment should return to and be located on the isoelectric line.

7. D

The electrophysiologic properties of specialized myocardial cells regulate heart rate and rhythm and possess unique properties: automaticity, excitability, conductivity, and contractility. Automaticity (pacing function) is the ability of cardiac cells to generate an electrical impulse spontaneously and repetitively. Excitability is the ability of nonpacemaker heart cells to respond to an electrical impulse that begins in pacemaker cells. Conductivity is the ability to send an electrical stimulus from cell membrane to cell membrane. Contractility is the ability of atrial and ventricular muscle cells to shorten their fiber length in response to electrical stimulation, causing sufficient pressure to push blood forward through the heart.

8. C

The 12-lead ECG provides 12 views of the electrical activity of the heart. There are six unipolar (or V) *chest leads,* determined by the placement of the chest electrode. The four limb electrodes are placed on the extremities which provide the 12 views. Positioning of the electrodes is crucial in obtaining an accurate ECG. Comparisons of ECGs taken at different times will be valid only when electrode placement is accurate and identical at each test. In many cases, a surgical marker is used to assure consistent placement of the leads.

9. A, B, D, E

If the monitoring system provides five electrode cables, place the electrodes as follows: right arm electrode just below the right clavicle; left arm electrode just below the left clavicle; right leg electrode on the lowest palpable rib, on the right midclavicular line; left leg electrode on the lowest palpable rib, on the left midclavicular line; and fifth electrode placed to obtain one of the six chest leads.

10. C

The normal ST segment begins at the isoelectric line. ST elevation or depression is significant if displacement is 1 mm (one small box) or more above or below the line and is seen in two or more leads. ST elevation may indicate problems such as myocardial infarction, pericarditis, and hyperkalemia. ST depression is associated with hypokalemia, myocardial infarction, or ventricular hypertrophy.

11. B

T waves may become tall and peaked; inverted (negative); or flat as a result of myocardial ischemia, potassium or calcium imbalances, medications, or autonomic nervous system effects.

12. A, C, E, F

Most acute care facilities have monitor technicians who are specially educated in ECG monitoring and rhythm interpretation. Their responsibilities include: watching a bank of monitors on a unit; printing ECG rhythm strips routinely and as needed; interpreting rhythms; and reporting the client's rhythm and significant changes to the nurse. The nurse would be responsible for notifying the cardiac health care provider (HCP) of changes, and the nurse or a qualified AP would apply the leads to a monitored client.

13. C

The best and most direct method of checking the client for a change in heart rate is to assess the apical pulse for a full minute. All of the other responses are indirect methods and do not include assessing the client which is the most important action in this situation.

14. B

Analysis of an ECG rhythm strip requires a systematic approach using an eight-step method. The first step is to determine the heart rate. This is commonly accomplished by use of the 6-second strip method. Normal heart rate is 60-100 per minute. Less than 60 is bradycardia and more than 100 is tachycardia. Analyzing P waves is the 3rd step; measuring the QRS duration is 5th; and measuring the PR interval is the 4th step.

15. A, B, D, F

Ask these five questions when analyzing P waves: Are P waves present?; Are the P waves occurring regularly?; Is there one P wave for each QRS complex?; Are the P waves smooth, rounded, and upright in appearance; or are they inverted?; and Do all P waves look similar?

16. C, D, E, F

Normal sinus rhythm (NSR) is the rhythm originating from the sinoatrial (SA) node (dominant pacemaker) that meets these ECG criteria: Rate: atrial and ventricular rates of 60 to 100 beats/min; Rhythm: atrial and ventricular rhythms regular; P waves: present, consistent configuration, one P wave before each QRS complex; PR interval: 0.12 to 0.20 second and constant; and QRS duration: 0.06 to 0.10 second and constant.

17. B

Artifact is interference seen on the monitor or rhythm strip, which may look like a wandering or fuzzy baseline. It can be caused by client movement, loose or defective electrodes, improper grounding, or faulty ECG equipment such as broken wires or cables. Some artifacts can mimic lethal dysrhythmias such as ventricular tachycardia (with toothbrushing) or ventricular fibrillation (with tapping on the electrode). Assess the client to differentiate artifact from actual lethal rhythms! Do not rely only on the ECG monitor.

18. A, B, D, F

The clarity of continuous ECG monitor recordings is affected by skin preparation and electrode quality. To ensure the best signal transmission and decrease skin impedance, clean the skin and clip hairs if needed. Make sure that the area for electrode placement is dry. The gel on each electrode must be moist and fresh. Attach the electrode to the lead cable and then to the contact site. The contact site should be free of any lotion, tincture, or other substance that increases skin impedance. Electrodes cannot be placed on irritated skin or over scar tissue.

19. A, C, F

ST elevation may indicate problems such as myocardial infarction, pericarditis, and hyperkalemia. ST depression is associated with hypokalemia, myocardial infarction, or ventricular hypertrophy. Endocarditis is an infection of the endocardium and usually affects the heart valves.

20. C

The most common method is to count the number of QRS complexes in 6 seconds and multiply that number by 10 to calculate the rate for a full minute. This client has five QRS complexes in a 6-second strip. So, 5 times 10 equals 50 beats/min, which is a bradycardia.

21. A, B, C, D, E
For clients with sinus tachycardia, assess for fatigue, weakness, shortness of breath, orthopnea, decreased oxygen saturation, increased pulse rate, and decreased blood pressure. Also assess for restlessness and anxiety from decreased cerebral perfusion and for decreased urine output from impaired renal perfusion. The client may also have anginal pain and palpitations. The ECG pattern may show T-wave inversion or ST-segment elevation or depression (not wide QRS complexes) in response to myocardial ischemia.

22. D
Premature ventricular complexes (PVCs), also called premature ventricular contractions, result from increased irritability of ventricular cells and are seen as early ventricular complexes followed by a pause. They appear as widened QRS complexes and sometimes the P waves follow the QRS complexes. They may be all the same shape (unifocal) or different shapes (multifocal). PVCs are common and increase with age.

23. A, B, D, E
The causes of atrial irritability that can lead to PACs include: stress; fatigue; anxiety; inflammation; infection; intake of caffeine, nicotine, or alcohol; and drugs such as epinephrine, sympathomimetics, amphetamines, digoxin, or anesthetic agents. PACs may also result from myocardial ischemia, hypermetabolic states, electrolyte imbalance, or atrial stretch.

24. D
Ventricular fibrillation (VF) is a cardiac dysrhythmia that results from electrical chaos in the ventricles; impulses from many irritable foci fire in a totally disorganized manner so that ventricular contraction cannot occur; there is no cardiac output or pulse and therefore no cerebral, myocardial, or systemic perfusion. This rhythm is rapidly fatal if not successfully terminated within 3 to 5 minutes. Ventricular tachycardia and asystole are also life-threatening dysrhythmias. With atrial fibrillation there is loss of the atrial contribution to cardiac output, but the ventricles are usually still putting out adequate cardiac output.

25. C, D, E
Adenosine is used to terminate the acute episode and is given rapidly (over several seconds) followed by a normal saline bolus. Side effects of adenosine include significant bradycardia with pauses, nausea, and vomiting. Beta blockers would not be given because they would cause increased bradycardia. The purpose of the drug is to terminate the dysrhythmia so cardioversion is not necessary.

26. B, D, E, F
Risk factors for atrial fibrillation include hypertension (HTN), previous ischemic stroke, transient ischemic attack (TIA) or other thromboembolic event, coronary heart disease, diabetes mellitus, heart failure, obesity, hyperthyroidism, chronic kidney disease, excessive alcohol use, and mitral valve disease. This dysrhythmia also increases with age.

27. D
When the onset of AF is greater than 48 hours, the client must take anticoagulants for at least 3 weeks (or until the INR is 2 to 3) before the elective cardioversion to prevent clots from moving from the heart to the brain or lungs. Teaching the client to monitor for bleeding and reporting this to the primary health care provider (HCP) are essential when a client is prescribed an anticoagulant drug.

28. A, B, D, E, F
Nursing care after cardioversion includes: maintaining a patent airway; administering oxygen; assessing vital signs and the level of consciousness; administering antidysrhythmic drug therapy, as prescribed; monitoring for dysrhythmias; assessing for chest burns from electrodes; providing emotional support; and documenting the results of cardioversion. Sips of water and ice chips would not be provided until the client's gag reflex returned.

29. D

The nurse would want to assess all four clients. However, the client with atrial fibrillation with sustained rapid ventricular response is at highest risk for decreased cardiac output and development of symptoms. Therefore this client would need to be assessed first.

30. C

Three or more successive PVCs in a row are usually called nonsustained ventricular tachycardia (NSVT). Two PVCs in a row make a couplet. Artifact appears as a fuzzy or wandering baseline. Ventricular asystole is generally described as a flat line although P waves may still be seen.

31. B

For clients who are at high risk for stroke and who are not candidates for anticoagulation, the left atrial appendage (LAA) occlusion device may be an option. The LAA is the most common site of blood clot development leading to the risk of stroke. Inserted percutaneously via the femoral vein, a device to occlude the LAA is delivered via a transseptal puncture. Radiofrequency catheter ablation (RCA) is an invasive procedure that may be used to destroy an irritable focus in atrial or ventricular conduction. Biventricular pacing is used with clients who have heart failure and conduction disorders. The surgical maze procedure is an open-chest surgical technique performed with coronary artery bypass grafting (CABG).

32. A

The desired outcomes of collaborative care are to resolve VF promptly and convert it to an organized rhythm. Therefore, the priority is to defibrillate the client immediately according to ACLS protocol. If a defibrillator is not readily available, as would likely be the case in a client's room, high-quality CPR must be initiated and continued until the defibrillator arrives.

33. C

Magnesium is used to treat the life-threatening ventricular tachycardia called torsades de pointes. Often a client with this dysrhythmia is hypomagnesemic which causes increased ventricular irritability. Adenosine treats PSVT; epinephrine increases atrial irritability and heart rate; and calcium chloride is used in cardiac resuscitation, arrhythmias, hypermagnesemia, calcium channel blocker overdose, and beta-blocker overdose.

34. C, E, F

Transcutaneous pacing is used as an emergency measure to provide demand ventricular pacing in a profoundly bradycardic or asystolic client until invasive pacing can be used or the client's heart rate returns to normal. This method of pacing is painful and may require administration of pain and sedative medications for the client to tolerate the therapy. Transcutaneous pacing is used only as a temporary measure to maintain heart rate and perfusion until a more permanent method of pacing is used.

35. A

When a pacing stimulus is delivered to the heart, a spike (or pacemaker artifact) is seen on the monitor or ECG strip. When the pacer spike is followed by a QRS complex, this pattern indicates ventricular depolarization and is referred to as capture (the pacemaker successfully depolarized the ventricles).

36. B, C, D, F

The average life of lithium batteries that power permanent pacemakers is 10 years. A biventricular pacemaker may be used to coordinate contractions between the right and left ventricles. The electrophysiologist implants the pulse generator in a surgically made subcutaneous pocket at the shoulder in the right or left subclavicular area, which may create a visible bulge. Permanent pacemaker insertion is performed to treat conduction disorders that are not temporary, including complete heart block. Combination pacemaker/defibrillator devices are available. If the surgical incision is near either shoulder, advise the client to avoid lifting the arm over the head or lifting more than 10 lb for the next

4 weeks because this could dislodge the pacemaker wire.

37. A, C, E, F

After the procedure, monitor the ECG rhythm to check that the pacemaker is working correctly. Assess the implantation site for bleeding, swelling, redness, tenderness, and infection. The dressing over the site should remain clean and dry. The client should be afebrile and have stable vital signs. The electrophysiologist prescribes initial activity restrictions, which are then gradually increased. Observe for muscle contractions over the diaphragm that are synchronous with the heart rate. Pneumothorax is usually not a complication of pacemaker implantation. Sedative drugs are often given to clients receiving transcutaneous pacing but not for permanent pacemaker insertion.

38. A, B, D, E

The client would inform airport personnel of the pacemaker before passing through a metal detector and show them the pacemaker identification card. The metal in your pacemaker will trigger the alarm in the metal detector device. Instruct the client to avoid lifting the arm over the head or lifting more than 10 lb for the next 4 weeks because this could dislodge the pacemaker wire. Teach the client to report any pulse rate lower than that set on the pacemaker. Tell clients to avoid sources of strong electromagnetic fields, such as magnets and telecommunications transmitters. Carry a pacemaker identification card provided by the manufacturer and wear a medical alert bracelet at all times.

39. C

Before defibrillation, loudly and clearly command all personnel to clear contact with the client and the bed and check to see they are clear before the shock is delivered. This safety measure prevents health care team members from receiving a shock when the client is defibrillated. Synchronous mode is used for cardioversion. Disconnection of the monitor leads would prevent assessing the effectiveness of the defibrillation shock. Hyperventilation of the client will not keep the health care team safe.

40. C, D

Defibrillation shocks are recommended by AEDs only for ventricular fibrillation and pulseless ventricular tachycardia.

41. A

Class IV antidysrhythmics slow the flow of calcium into the cell during depolarization, thereby depressing the automaticity of the sinoatrial (SA) and atrioventricular (AV) nodes, decreasing the heart rate, and prolonging the AV nodal refractory period and conduction. Calcium channel blockers, such as verapamil hydrochloride and diltiazem hydrochloride, are Class IV drugs. They are used to treat supraventricular tachycardia (SVT) and atrial fibrillation (AF) to slow the ventricular response.

42. B, D, F

Class III antidysrhythmics lengthen the absolute refractory period and prolong repolarization and the action potential duration of ischemic cells. Class III drugs include amiodarone and ibutilide and are used to treat or prevent ventricular premature beats, VT, and VF. Bradycardia is a side effect with sotalol and amiodarone. Hypertension is not a side effect of these drugs.

43. A

Sotalol hydrochloride is an antidysrhythmic agent with both noncardioselective beta-adrenergic blocking effects (Class II) and action potential duration prolongation properties (Class III). It is an oral agent that may be used for the treatment of documented ventricular dysrhythmias such as VT that are life threatening.

44. RATE 80 beats/min; RHYTHM Regular; P WAVES one for each QRS; PR Interval 0.16 second; QRS DURATION 0.10 second; INTERPRETATION Normal sinus rhythm

45. RATE Variable about 130 beats/min; RHYTHM Irregularly irregular; P WAVES None, fibrillatory waves; PR Interval none; QRS duration 0.08 second; INTERPRETATION Atrial fibrillation with rapid ventricular response

46. RATE 50 beats/min; RHYTHM Regular; P WAVES one for each QRS; PR INTERVAL 0.20 second; QRS DURATION 0.08 second; INTERPRETATION Sinus bradycardia

47. RATE 150 beats/mmin; RHYTHM Regular; P WAVES one for each QRS; PR INTERVAL 0.12 second; QRS DURATION 0.04 second; INTERPRETATION Sinus tachycardia

48. RATE About 80 beats/min RHYTHM Regular except one premature complex; P WAVES one per QRS except early wide complex; PR INTERVAL 0.20 second; QRS DURATION 0.04 second; INTERPRETATION Sinus rhythm with a premature ventricular complex (PVC)

49. RATE 60 beats/min; RHYTHM Regular except one premature complex; P WAVES one before each QRS complex; PR INTERVAL 0.20 second; QRS DURATION 0.08 second; INTERPRETATION Sinus rhythm with one premature atrial contraction (PAC)

50. RATE About 200 beats/min; RHYTHM Regular with wide QRS complexes; P WAVES none; PR INTERVAL None; QRS DURATION wide 0.28 second; INTERPRETATION Ventricular tachycardia

51. RATE Cannot be determined; RHYTHM Chaotic; P WAVES None; PR INTERVAL None; QRS DURATION None; INTERPRETATION Ventricular fibrillation (life threatening)

52. RATE None; RHYTHM None; P WAVES None; PR INTERVAL None; QRS DURATION None; IITERPRETATION Ventricular asystole

32
CHAPTER

Concepts of Care for Patients with Cardiac Problems

1. What is the **priority** concept for a client who has heart failure?
   A. Gas exchange
   B. Perfusion
   C. Comfort
   D. Infection

2. When a client develops heart failure, what **initial** compensatory mechanism of the heart does the nurse expect to occur that will maintain cardiac output (CO)?
   A. Parasympathetic stimulation
   B. Ventricular hypertrophy
   C. Sympathetic stimulation
   D. Renin-angiotensin activation system

3. What does the nurse suspect when assessment of a client with HF reveals pulses that alternate in strength?
   A. Pulsus alternans
   B. Pulsus paradoxus
   C. Orthostatic hypotension
   D. Angina

4. When would the nurse expect the release of B-type natriuretic peptide (BNP) for a client with heart failure?
   A. When the client has an enlarged liver
   B. When a client's ejection fraction is lower than normal
   C. When a client develops ventricular hypertrophy
   D. When a client has fluid overload

5. When a client admits that he or she sometimes has trouble catching his or her breath, which question would the nurse ask to obtain more information about the client's symptoms?
   A. "Do you have a history of any medical problems like high blood pressure?"
   B. "What did your health care provider tell you about your diagnosis?"
   C. "What was your most strenuous activity during the past week?"
   D. "How do you feel about being told that you have heart failure?"

6. What assessment findings would the nurse expect to find in a client with right heart failure? **Select all that apply.**
   A. Weight loss
   B. Dependent edema
   C. Neck vein distention
   D. Angina
   E. Hepatomegaly
   F. Weak peripheral pulses

7. What **early** sign of left ventricular failure is a client most likely to report to the nurse?
   A. Nocturnal coughing
   B. Swollen legs
   C. Weight gain
   D. Nocturia

8. Based on the etiology and main cause of heart failure, the nurse knows that which client has the **greatest** need for health promotion measures to prevent heart failure?
   A. Client with asthma
   B. Client with renal insufficiency
   C. Client with hypertension
   D. Client with Parkinson disease

9. Which assessment findings would the nurse expect to find in a client with left heart failure? **Select all that apply.**
   A. Wheezes or crackles
   B. Jugular vein distention
   C. S_3 heart sound
   D. Paroxysmal nocturnal dyspnea
   E. Ascites
   F. Oliguria during the day

10. Which statement by a client with a history of hypertension and heart problems would cause the nurse to suspect development of heart failure?
    A. "I've had a fever frequently."
    B. "I noticed a very fine red rash on my chest."
    C. "I get a pain in my shoulder when I cough."
    D. "I've had to remove all of my rings for the past month."

11. What is the **most** reliable method of monitoring for fluid gain or loss in a client with heart failure?
    A. Check for pitting edema in dependent body parts.
    B. Auscultate the lungs for worsening crackles or wheezes.
    C. Weigh the client daily at the same time and using the same scale.
    D. Assess the client's skin turgor and condition of mucous membranes.

12. Which major self-management categories will the nurse include when teaching a client, newly diagnosed with heart failure, who is about to be discharged? **Select all that apply.**
    A. Symptoms, what to do when they get worse
    B. Medications
    C. Activity
    D. Heart transplants
    E. Weight
    F. Diet

13. When the client asks the nurse about the **best** method of diagnosing heart failure, what teaching would the nurse provide?
    A. Radionuclide studies
    B. Echocardiography
    C. Multigated acquisition (MUGA) scan
    D. Pulmonary artery catheter

14. Which **early** symptoms indicate to the nurse that a client's HF is getting worse and pulmonary edema is developing? **Select all that apply.**
    A. Crackles in the lung bases
    B. Frothy, blood-tinged sputum
    C. Dyspnea at rest
    D. Cyanosis
    E. Disorientation
    F. Level of crackles rises higher in the lungs

15. Which interventions would the nurse expect to include in the care of a client with pulmonary edema caused by HF? **Select all that apply.**
    A. Sodium restriction
    B. Fluid restriction
    C. Administration of potassium supplement
    D. Position client in semi-Fowler or high-Fowler
    E. Weekly weight monitoring
    F. Administration of loop diuretics

16. Which instruction would the nurse give the assistive personnel (AP) who is helping a client with HF and excessive aldosterone secretion?
    A. Restrict the client's fluids to 2 L/day and keep accurate intake and output.
    B. Severely restrict fluids to 500 mL of fluid plus the client's urine output from the past 24 hours.
    C. Give the client as much water as he or she wants to prevent dehydration.
    D. Frequently offer the client ice chips and moistened mouth swabs and limit fluids to 1 L/day.

17. What are the **priority** nursing actions related to caring for an older adult client with HF who is prescribed digoxin? **Select all that apply.**
    A. Monitor the ECG strip for early signs of toxicity such as bradycardia.
    B. Auscultate the apical pulse heart rate and rhythm for a full minute before administering the drug.
    C. Observe for signs of toxicity, which are often nonspecific such as anorexia, fatigue, and blurred vision.
    D. Report any changes in heart rate or rhythm to the health care provider.
    E. Monitor serum digoxin and potassium levels.
    F. Check the health care provider's prescription for parameters to hold the drug.

18. To improve gas exchange, how much supplemental oxygen would the nurse provide a client with HF?
    A. 2 L/min by nasal canula
    B. 100% by nonrebreather mask
    C. Within the range prescribed by the HCP to keep saturation at 90% or more
    D. 50% by endotracheal tube and mechanical ventilator

19. Which are **potential** benefits of a client receiving the drug digoxin?
    A. Reduced heart rate
    B. Increased contractility
    C. Venous vasodilation
    D. Slowed conduction through the AV node
    E. Inhibition of sympathetic activity with enhanced parasympathetic activity
    F. Enhanced renal excretion of sodium and water

20. When a client has an ejection fraction of less than 30%, about which potential treatment does the nurse prepare to educate the client?
    A. Heart transplant
    B. Implantable cardioverter/defibrillator
    C. Ventricular reconstructive procedure
    D. Implanted mechanical pump

21. When a client with heart failure walks 200 feet down the hall and develops a feeling of heaviness in the legs, how does the nurse interpret this finding?
    A. The client is building endurance.
    B. The activity is appropriate.
    C. The client could walk farther.
    D. The activity is too stressful.

22. What is the **priority** intervention when a client comes to the emergency department (ED) with extreme anxiety, tachycardia, struggling for air, and a moist cough productive of frothy and blood-tinged sputum?
    A. Prepare for endotracheal intubation and mechanical ventilation.
    B. Administer high-flow oxygen therapy by face mask.
    C. Prepare for continuous positive airway pressure ventilation.
    D. Apply a pulse oximeter and a cardiac monitor.

23. Which drugs would the nurse prepare to administer to a client with HF who has developed pulmonary edema? **Select all that apply.**
    A. Nitroglycerin sublingual
    B. Lorazepam IV
    C. Oxygen at 1 L/min nasal canula
    D. Furosemide IV
    E. Metoprolol IV
    F. Nitroglycerin IV

24. Which key points would the nurse include when teaching a client about signs and symptoms of return or worsening of heart failure, that must be reported to the primary health care provider? **Select all that apply.**
    A. Cold symptoms (e.g., cough) lasting more than 3 to 5 days
    B. Rapid weight loss of 3 lb in a week
    C. Excessive awakening at night to urinate
    D. Increase in exercise tolerance lasting 2 to 3 days
    E. Development of dyspnea or angina at rest or worsening angina
    F. Increased swelling in feet, ankles, or hands

25. Which statement by a client with heart failure indicates to the nurse the need for additional teaching?
    A. "If my heart feels like it's racing, I should call my health care provider."
    B. "I must weigh myself once a week and watch for signs of fluid retention."
    C. "I'll need periods of rest and activity and I should avoid activity after meals."
    D. "I'll need to consider and plan my activities for the day, and rest as needed."

26. Which findings would the nurse expect in a client with mitral valve stenosis? **Select all that apply.**
    A. A client with mild mitral valve stenosis will likely be asymptomatic.
    B. Classic signs include dyspnea, angina, and syncope.
    C. Rumbling apical diastolic murmur
    D. Syncope on exertion
    E. Sinus tachycardia
    F. Right-sided heart failure with jugular (neck) vein distention

27. For which finding in a client with mitral valve stenosis would the nurse **immediately** notify the primary health care provider because of the potential for decompensation?
    A. Slow, bounding peripheral pulses associated with bradycardia
    B. An increase and decrease in pulse rate that follows inspiration and expiration
    C. An irregular heart rhythm and ECG strip that indicate atrial fibrillation
    D. An increase in pulse rate and blood pressure after exertion

28. Which are the characteristics that the nurse would expect when a client is diagnosed with mitral valve prolapse (MVP)? **Select all that apply.**
    A. Valve leaflets enlarge and bulge up into the left atrium during systole.
    B. Hepatomegaly is a late sign.
    C. Most clients are asymptomatic and this abnormality is benign.
    D. Many clients have normal heart rates and blood pressures.
    E. Older adults have increased risk for mitral valve prolapse.
    F. A midsystolic click and late systolic murmur is best heard at the apex of the heart.

29. Which signs and symptoms would the nurse expect to assess when a client is diagnosed with aortic stenosis? **Select all that apply.**
    A. Dyspnea on exertion
    B. Atypical chest pain
    C. Angina
    D. Hemoptysis
    E. Harsh, systolic crescendo-decrescendo murmur
    F. Orthopnea

30. Which **urgent** intervention is required when the nurse reviews the results of diagnostic testing for a client with aortic stenosis and discovers that the surface area of the valve is less than 1 cm?
    A. Surgical aortic heart valve replacement
    B. Aortic valvuloplasty in the cardiac catheterization laboratory
    C. Physical therapy to create an individualized exercise program
    D. Therapy with drugs that will increase myocardial contractility

31. Which type of heart valvular disease does the nurse suspect when a client's assessment reveals pitting edema?
    A. Aortic valve stenosis and regurgitation
    B. Mitral valve stenosis and regurgitation
    C. Mitral valve prolapse
    D. Tricuspid valve prolapse

32. Which client with valvular heart disease would benefit from the nonsurgical invasive procedure balloon valvuloplasty?
    A. Older adult who needs a valve replacement
    B. Middle-aged adult whose open-heart surgery failed
    C. Young adult with a genetic valve defect
    D. Older adult who is not a surgical candidate

33. Which **essential** medications would the nurse provide teaching about postoperatively for a client who received a prosthetic valve replacement?
    A. Immunosuppressants
    B. Antibiotics
    C. Anticoagulants
    D. Diuretics

34. Which **priority** information would the nurse be sure to provide for a client who is scheduled for mitral valve replacement with a xenograft valve?
    A. "You will need an individualized exercise program to develop collateral circulation."
    B. "Your xenograft valve will need to be replaced in about 7 to 10 years."
    C. "You must take and record your temperature daily and watch for signs of rejection."
    D. "You will require frequent laboratory tests to monitor your coagulation status."

35. Which topics would the nurse be sure to cover when providing discharge instructions for a client with prosthetic valve surgery? **Select all that apply.**
    A. Avoid heavy lifting for 3 to 6 weeks.
    B. Report dyspnea, syncope, dizziness, edema, and palpitations to your health care provider.
    C. Use an electric razor to avoid skin cuts.
    D. Increase your consumption of foods that are high in vitamin K.
    E. Notify your health provider for any bleeding or excessive bruising.
    F. Watch for and report any fever or drainage and redness at the surgical site.

36. Which complication is a client at **most** risk for when the nurse notes that excessive fluid was seen in the pericardial cavity on echocardiogram?
    A. Cardiac tamponade
    B. Pericardial friction rub
    C. Systemic emboli
    D. Splinter hemorrhages

37. Which assessment findings would cause the nurse to suspect cardiac tamponade in a client? **Select all that apply.**
    A. Neck vein distention
    B. Paradoxical pulse
    C. Hypertension
    D. Muffled heart sounds
    E. Tachycardia
    F. Petechiae

38. Which clients are at **greatest** risk for development of infective endocarditis? **Select all that apply.**
    A. Clients after myocardial infarction
    B. Clients who are IV drug users
    C. Clients with poor dental health
    D. Clients with opioid addictions
    E. Clients with systemic alterations in immunity
    F. Clients postoperative after valve replacement

39. Which findings does the nurse expect when assessing a client with infective endocarditis? **Select all that apply.**
    A. Grating pain that is aggravated by breathing
    B. Osler nodes on palms of hands and soles of feet
    C. Splinter hemorrhages
    D. Janeway lesions on the hands and feet
    E. Anorexia and weight loss
    F. Pericardial friction rub

40. Which treatment **best** applies to the care of a client newly diagnosed with infective endocarditis?
    A. Long-term anticoagulant therapy with IV heparin followed by oral warfarin
    B. Hospitalization for initial IV antibiotics, followed by continued IV antibiotics at home
    C. Complete bedrest for the duration of the treatment with subcutaneous enoxaparin
    D. Administration of IV penicillin, followed by oral penicillin for 6 to 10 weeks

41. Which **priority** teaching would the nurse provide to a client with infective endocarditis who is scheduled for an invasive dental procedure?
    A. "Be sure to use your nitroglycerin whenever you experience chest pain."
    B. "Remind your health care provider to provide you with a prescription for prophylactic antibiotics."
    C. "Get up slowly after taking each dose of your antihypertensive medication."
    D. "Your health care provider will instruct you to have blood drawn to check your anticoagulation status."

42. What does the nurse suspect when a client describes substernal pain that radiates to the left shoulder, is grating, and worsens with inspiration and coughing?
    A. Chronic constrictive pericarditis
    B. Cardiac tamponade
    C. Hypertrophic cardiomyopathy
    D. Acute pericarditis

43. What is the **best** method for the nurse to use when auscultating a client's pericardial friction rub with a stethoscope?
    A. Place the bell just below the left clavicle.
    B. Place the diaphragm at the apex of the heart.
    C. Place the diaphragm at the left lower sternal border.
    D. Place the bell at several points while the client holds his or her breath.

44. Which signs or symptoms would the nurse expect when assessing a client with chronic constrictive pericarditis? **Select all that apply.**
    A. Exertional fatigue and dyspnea
    B. Dependent edema
    C. Crackles and wheezes
    D. Hepatic engorgement
    E. Pink, frothy sputum
    F. Decreased appetite

45. What does the nurse instruct a client with pericarditis to do to make him or her will feel more comfortable?
    A. Lie down and bend the legs at the knees.
    B. Sit in a semi-Fowler position with pillows under each arm.
    C. Sit up and lean forward.
    D. Lie on the side in a fetal position.

46. Which are proposed criteria for diagnosis of a client with acute pericarditis? **Select all that apply.**
    A. Chest pain that lasts longer than 3 months
    B. Pericardial chest pain
    C. Presence of a pericardial friction rub
    D. New ST elevation in all ECG leads or PR-segment depression
    E. New or worsening pericardial effusion
    F. Hepatic engorgement

47. What is the **definitive** treatment for chronic constrictive pericarditis?
    A. Pericardiocentesis
    B. Surgical removal of the pericardium
    C. Placement of a pericardial drain
    D. Creation of a pericardial window

48. Which are potential causes of dilated cardiomyopathy? **Select all that apply.**
    A. Alcohol abuse
    B. Sedentary lifestyle
    C. Cigarette smoking
    D. Infection
    E. Chemotherapy
    F. Poor nutrition

49. Which type of cardiomyopathy may present with sudden death as the first symptom?
    A. Dilated
    B. Arrhythmogenic right ventricular
    C. Restrictive
    D. Hypertrophic

50. Which criteria are appropriate for a client with dilated cardiomyopathy to become a candidate for heart transplant surgery? **Select all that apply.**
    A. Life expectancy greater than 2 years
    B. Age generally less than 65 years
    C. New York Heart Association Class III or IV

D. Normal or only slightly increased pulmonary vascular resistance
E. Consumes less than five to six beers per day
F. Absence of active infection

51. Which assessment findings would suggest to the nurse that a client who received a heart transplant was experiencing organ rejection? **Select all that apply.**
    A. Shortness of breath
    B. Hypotension
    C. Abdominal pain
    D. Decreased activity tolerance
    E. Fluid gain (edema, increased weight)
    F. Atrial fibrillation or flutter

Chapter 32 Answer Key

1. B
   The priority concept for a client with heart failure (HF) is perfusion. Interrelated concepts include gas exchange and comfort.

2. C
   In heart failure (HF), stimulation of the sympathetic nervous system (e.g., increasing catecholamines) as a result of tissue hypoxia represents the most immediate compensatory mechanism. This results in an immediate increase in cardiac output. Later compensatory mechanisms include activation of renin-angiotensin system and myocardial hypertrophy.

3. A
   Pulsus alternans is a type of pulse in which a weak pulse alternates with a strong pulse despite a regular heart rhythm; seen in clients with severely depressed cardiac function such as heart failure. Pulsus paradoxus is an exaggerated decrease in systolic blood pressure by more than 10 mm Hg during the inspiratory phase of the respiratory cycle (normal is 3 to 10 mm Hg); indicative of cardiac tamponade, constrictive pericarditis, and pulmonary hypertension. Angina is chest pain. Orthostatic hypotension occurs when there is a systolic blood pressure decrease of at least 20 mm Hg or a diastolic blood pressure decrease of at least 10 mm Hg

within 3 minutes of a client moving from a lying to a sitting or standing position.

4. D
   B-type natriuretic peptide (BNP) is a peptide produced and released by the ventricles when the client has fluid overload as a result of heart failure. BNP levels increase with age and are generally higher in healthy women than in healthy men.

5. C
   Assess activity tolerance by asking whether the client can perform normal ADLs or climb flights of stairs without fatigue or dyspnea. Many clients with heart failure (HF) experience weakness or fatigue with activity or have a feeling of heaviness in their arms or legs. Ask about their ability to perform simultaneous arm and leg work (e.g., walking while carrying a bag of groceries). Such activity may place an unacceptable demand on the failing heart. To gather more data, ask the client to identify his or her most strenuous activity in the past week.

6. B, C, E
   Assessment findings of right ventricular failure are related to systemic congestion. They include: jugular (neck vein) distention; enlarged liver and spleen; anorexia and nausea; dependent

edema (legs and sacrum); distended abdomen; swollen hands and fingers; polyuria at night; weight gain; and increased blood pressure (from excess volume) or decreased blood pressure (from failure).

7. A
The client in early HF describes a cough that is irritating, nocturnal (at night), and usually nonproductive. As HF becomes very severe, he or she may begin expectorating frothy, pink-tinged sputum, a sign of life-threatening pulmonary edema.

8. C
Heart failure (HF) is caused by systemic hypertension in most cases. Some clients experiencing myocardial infarction (MI, "heart attack") also develop HF. The next most common cause is structural heart changes, such as valvular dysfunction, particularly pulmonic or aortic stenosis, which leads to pressure or volume overload on the heart.

9. A, C, D, F
Signs and symptoms of left heart failure are related to decreased cardiac output (CO) and pulmonary congestion. Those associated with decreased CO include: fatigue; weakness; oliguria during the day (nocturia at night); angina; confusion, restlessness; dizziness; tachycardia, palpitations; pallor; weak peripheral pulses; and cool extremities. Those related to pulmonary congestion include: hacking cough, worse at night; dyspnea/breathlessness; crackles or wheezes in lungs; frothy, pink-tinged sputum; tachypnea; and; S_3/S_4 summation gallop.

10. D
Clients may notice that their shoes fit more tightly, or their shoes or socks may leave indentations on their swollen feet. They may have removed their rings because of swelling in their fingers and hands.

11. C
Edema is an extremely unreliable sign of HF. Be sure that accurate daily weights are taken to document fluid retention. Assessing weight at the same time of the morning using the same scale is important. Weight is the most reliable indicator of fluid gain and loss! Ask about weight gain. An adult may retain 4 to 7 liters of fluid (10 to 15 lb [4.5 to 6.8 kg]) before pitting edema occurs. Increasing crackles or wheezes can indicate that the client's HF is getting worse but does not indicate weight. Skin turgor and mucous membranes indicate fluid balance but not weight in a client.

12. A, B, C, E, F
One standard and frequently used self-management plan is called **MAWDS**. The major teaching areas for this plan include:
   Medications: Take medications as prescribed and do not run out; know the purpose and side effects of each drug; and avoid NSAIDs to prevent sodium and fluid retention.
   Activity: Stay as active as possible but don't overdo it; know your limits; and be able to carry on a conversation while exercising.
   Weight: Weigh each day at the same time on the same scale to monitor for fluid retention.
   Diet: Limit daily sodium intake to 2 to 3 g as prescribed; limit daily fluid intake to 2 liters.
   Symptoms: Note any new or worsening symptoms and notify the health care provider immediately.

13. B
Echocardiography is considered the best tool in diagnosing heart failure. Radionuclide studies (thallium imaging or technetium pyrophosphate scanning) can also indicate the presence and some causes of HF. Multigated acquisition (MUGA) scans, also called multigated blood pool scans, provide information about left ventricular ejection fraction and velocity, which are typically low in clients with HF. Placement of a pulmonary artery catheter is done in an

intensive care unit. This catheter can provide direct measures of pressures in the heart and cardiac output.

14. A, C, E

    Assess for and report early symptoms, such as crackles in the lung bases, dyspnea at rest, disorientation, and confusion, especially in older clients. Later, the level of the fluid progresses from the bases to higher levels in the lungs as the condition worsens. The client in acute pulmonary edema is typically extremely anxious, tachycardic, and struggling for air. As pulmonary edema becomes more severe, he or she may have a moist cough productive of frothy, blood-tinged sputum; and his or her skin may be cold, clammy, or cyanotic.

15. A, D, F

    Reducing sodium and water retention will decrease the workload of the heart. The primary health care provider may restrict sodium intake in an attempt to decrease fluid retention. Weigh the client daily. Remember that 1 kg of weight gain or loss equals 1 liter of retained or lost fluid. The same scale should be used every morning before breakfast for the most accurate assessment of weight. Loop diuretics such as furosemide, torsemide, and bumetanide are most effective for treating fluid volume overload. If the client has dyspnea, place in a high-Fowler position with pillows under each arm to maximize chest expansion and improve gas exchange. Potassium supplements may be needed for potassium replacement, but it does not improve pulmonary edema.

16. A

    Clients with excessive aldosterone secretion may experience thirst and drink 3 to 5 liters of fluid each day. As a result, their fluid intake may need to be limited to a more normal 2 L/day. Supervise assistive personnel (AP) to ensure that they limit the prescribed intake and accurately record intake and output.

17. A, B, C, D, E, F

    All of these responses are appropriate to the care of an older adult with heart failure who has been prescribed digoxin. Often the cardiac

health care provider will have the nurses hold a client's digoxin dose if the heart rate is less than 50 to 60 beats/min.

18. C

    Provide the necessary amount of supplemental oxygen within a range prescribed by the cardiac health care provider to maintain oxygen saturation at 90% or greater.

19. A, B, D, E

    The potential benefits of digoxin include: increased contractility; reduced heart rate (HR); slowing of conduction through the atrioventricular node; and inhibition of sympathetic activity while enhancing parasympathetic activity. Diuretics (especially loop and thiazide) enhance excretion of water and sodium. Nitrates are venous vasodilators.

20. B

    Because these clients are at high risk for sudden cardiac death, clients with an ejection fraction of less than 30% are considered candidates for an implantable cardioverter/defibrillator (ICD).

21. D

    Many clients with heart failure (HF) experience weakness or fatigue with activity or have a feeling of heaviness in their arms or legs while walking for a distance. Such activity may place an unacceptable demand on the failing heart.

22. B

    The **priority** nursing action is to administer oxygen therapy at 5 to 12 L/min by simple face-mask or at 6 to 10 L/min by nonrebreathing mask with reservoir (which may deliver up to 100% oxygen) to promote gas exchange and perfusion. In addition, if the client is not hypotensive, place him or her in a sitting (high-Fowler) position with the legs down to decrease venous return to the heart. Apply a pulse oximeter and titrate the oxygen flow to keep the client's oxygen saturation above 90%. If supplemental oxygen does not resolve the client's respiratory distress, collaborate with the respiratory therapist and cardiac health care provider for more aggressive therapy, such as continuous positive airway pressure (CPAP) or bi-level positive airway pressure (BiPAP) ventilation. Intubation and mechanical ventilation may be needed for some clients.

23. A, D, F
If the client's systolic blood pressure is above 100, administer sublingual nitroglycerin (NTG) as prescribed to decrease afterload and preload every 5 minutes for three doses while establishing IV access for additional drug therapy. IV nitroglycerin may also be administered. Give furosemide (a rapid-acting loop diuretic) IV push (IVP) over 1 to 2 minutes to **avoid** ototoxicity. IV morphine sulfate may be prescribed, 1 to 2 mg at a time, to reduce venous return (preload), decrease anxiety, and reduce the work of breathing; however there is discussion about the benefits of using this drug for HF. Oxygen should be given high-flow with a face mask, not at 1 L/minute. Oral beta blockers are often prescribed for clients with heart failure and continued after discharge. IV lorazepam is used for sedation.

24. A, C, E, F
Teach the client and caregiver to immediately report to the primary health care provider the occurrence of *any* of these symptoms, which could indicate worsening or recurrent heart failure: rapid weight gain (3 lb in a week or 1 to 2 lb overnight); decrease in exercise tolerance lasting 2 to 3 days; cold symptoms (cough) lasting more than 3 to 5 days; excessive awakening at night to urinate; development of dyspnea or angina at rest or worsening angina; and increased swelling in the feet, ankles, or hands.

25. B
The client is taught to weigh himself or herself every day (not once a week). The other statements indicate that the client has an appropriate understanding of the treatment regimen for heart failure.

26. A, B, C, F
Key features of mitral valve stenosis include fatigue; dyspnea of exertion; orthopnea; paroxysmal nocturnal dyspnea; hemoptysis; hepatomegaly; neck vein distention; pitting edema, atrial fibrillation; and rumbling apical diastolic murmur. Syncope on exertion occurs with aortic stenosis and sinus tachycardia with aortic regurgitation.

27. C
Because the development of atrial fibrillation in a client with mitral valve stenosis indicates that the client may decompensate, the health care provider should be notified immediately of changes to the heart rhythm. Increase and decrease in pulse rate that varies with inspiration and expiration is characteristic of sinus arrythmia. An increase in heart rate and blood pressure is common for most clients. Bounding arterial pulses are associated with aortic regurgitation.

28. A, C, D, F
With MVP, the valvular leaflets enlarge and prolapse (bulge) upward into the left atrium during systole. This abnormality is usually benign. However, it may progress to pronounced mitral regurgitation in some clients. A normal heart rate and BP are usually found on physical examination. A midsystolic click and a late systolic murmur may be heard at the apex of the heart. MVP often begins in younger adults and has a familial tendency. Hepatomegaly occurs with mitral stenosis, not MVP.

29. A, C, E, F
Signs and symptoms of aortic stenosis include dyspnea on exertion; angina; syncope on exertion; fatigue, orthopnea, paroxysmal nocturnal dyspnea; and harsh, systolic crescendo-decrescendo murmur. Atypical chest pain is characteristic of mitral valve prolapse and hemoptysis occurs with mitral stenosis.

30. A
As stenosis worsens, cardiac output becomes fixed and cannot increase to meet the demands of the body during exertion and symptoms develop. Eventually the left ventricle fails, blood backs up in the left atrium, and the pulmonary

system becomes congested. Right-sided HF can occur late in the disease. When a client has aortic stenosis and the surface area of the valve becomes 1 cm or less, surgery is indicated on an urgent basis!

31. B

Pitting edema is characteristic of mitral valve stenosis and regurgitation. Left heart failure eventually leads to signs of right heart failure with signs of peripheral volume overload such as hepatomegaly and pitting edema.

32. D

Balloon valvuloplasty, an invasive nonsurgical procedure, is possible for stenotic mitral and aortic valves; however, careful selection of clients is needed. It may be the initial treatment of choice for people with noncalcified, mobile mitral valves. Clients selected for aortic valvuloplasty are usually older and are at high risk for surgical complications. The benefits of this procedure for aortic stenosis tend to be short lived, rarely lasting longer than 6 months. Aortic valvuloplasty may be beneficial as a bridge to either surgical or percutaneous aortic valve replacement.

33. C

When a client has a mechanical valve, lifelong anticoagulant therapy with warfarin is required. Teach the client that the international normalized ratio (INR) will need to be monitored frequently. The therapeutic goal for clients with mechanical heart valves is 3.0 to 4.0

34. B

Biologic valve replacements may be xenograft (from other species), such as a porcine valve (from a pig) or a bovine valve (from a cow). Because tissue valves are associated with little risk for clot formation, long-term anticoagulation is not indicated. Xenografts are not as durable as prosthetic valves and usually must be replaced every 7 to 10 years.

35. B, C, E, F

A client receiving a prosthetic valve will be taking anticoagulants for the rest of his or her life. Teach nutritional considerations (if taking warfarin) and the prevention of bleeding. For example, the client is taught to avoid foods high in vitamin K, especially dark green leafy vegetables, and to use an electric razor to avoid skin cuts. Also teach him or her to report any bleeding or excessive bruising to the primary health care provider. Reinforce how to care for the sternal incision and instruct him or her to watch for and report any fever, drainage, or redness at the site. Most clients return to normal activity after 6 weeks, but should avoid heavy physical activity involving their upper extremities for 3 to 6 **months** to allow the incision to heal. Teach the client to report any changes in cardiovascular status, such as dyspnea, syncope, dizziness, edema, and palpitations.

36. A

Cardiac tamponade is compression of the myocardium by fluid that has accumulated around the heart. This compresses the atria and the ventricles, prevents them from filling adequately, and reduces cardiac output.

37. A, B, D, E

Findings of cardiac tamponade include: jugular venous (neck vein) distention; paradoxical pulse, also known as pulsus paradoxus; tachycardia; muffled heart sounds; and hypotension (not hypertension).

38. B, C, D, E, F

Infective endocarditis occurs primarily in clients with injection drug use (IDU), and who have had valve replacements, have experienced systemic alterations in immunity, or have structural cardiac defects. It is not associated with myocardial infarction or cardiac dysrhythmias. Possible ports of entry for infecting organisms include: the oral cavity (especially if dental procedures have been performed); skin rashes, lesions, or abscesses; infections (cutaneous, genitourinary, GI, systemic); and surgery or invasive procedures, including IV line placement. These clients are also at risk for infective endocarditis.

39. B, C, D, E
Manifestation of infective endocarditis include: fever associated with chills, night sweats, malaise, and fatigue; anorexia and weight loss; cardiac murmur (newly developed or change in existing); development of heart failure; evidence of systemic embolization; petechiae; splinter hemorrhages; Osler nodes (on palms of hands and soles of feet); Janeway lesions (flat, reddened maculae on hands and feet); Roth spots (hemorrhagic lesions that appear as round or oval spots on the retina); and positive blood cultures.

40. B
Antimicrobials are the main treatment for infective endocarditis, with the choice of drug depending on the specific organism involved. Because vegetations surround and protect the offending microorganism, an appropriate drug must be given in a sufficiently high dose to ensure its destruction. Antimicrobials are usually given IV, with the course of treatment lasting 4 to 6 weeks. For most bacterial cases, the ideal antibiotic is one of the penicillins or cephalosporins. Clients may be hospitalized for several days to institute IV therapy and then are discharged for continued IV therapy at home.

41. B
Clients with infective endocarditis must be taught to request a prescription for prophylactic antibiotics whenever any invasive dental or oral procedure is scheduled. This includes clients with a previous history of endocarditis and cardiac transplant or valve recipients.

42. D
A client with acute pericarditis would experience substernal precordial pain that radiates to the left side of the neck, the shoulder, or the back. The pain is classically grating and oppressive and is aggravated by breathing (mainly on inspiration), coughing, and swallowing. The pain is worse when the client is in the supine position and may be relieved by sitting up and leaning forward.

43. C
A pericardial friction rub may be heard with the diaphragm of the stethoscope positioned at the left lower sternal border. This scratchy, high-pitched sound is produced when the inflamed, roughened pericardial layers create friction as their surfaces rub together.

44. A, B, D
Clients with chronic constrictive pericarditis (lasting longer than 3 months) have signs of right-sided HF, including elevated systemic venous pressure with jugular distention, hepatic engorgement, and dependent edema. Exertional fatigue and dyspnea are common.

45. C
The pain is worse when a client with acute pericarditis is in the supine position and may be relieved by sitting up and leaning forward.

46. B, C, D, E
The proposed diagnostic criteria for acute pericarditis are presence of two of the following: pericardial chest pain; presence of pericardial rub; new ST elevation in all ECG leads or PR-segment depression; and new or worsening pericardial effusion.

47. B
The definitive treatment for chronic constrictive pericarditis is surgical excision of the pericardium (pericardiectomy). Pericardiocentesis, placement of a drain, or creation of a pericardial window are all interventions for clients with acute pericarditis.

48. A, D, E, F
Causes of dilated cardiomyopathy may include alcohol abuse, chemotherapy, infection, inflammation, and poor nutrition.

49. D
Sudden death may be the first symptom of hypertrophic cardiomyopathy (HCM), although the primary symptoms of HCM are exertional dyspnea, angina, and syncope. The chest pain is

atypical in that it usually occurs at rest, is prolonged, has no relation to exertion, and is not relieved by the administration of nitrates. A high incidence of ventricular dysrhythmias is also associated with HCM.

50. B, C, D, F

    Candidate selection criteria for heart transplantation include: life expectancy less than 1 year; age generally less than 65 years; New York Heart Association (NYHA) Class III or IV; normal or only slightly increased pulmonary vascular resistance; absence of active infection; stable psychosocial status; and no evidence of current drug or alcohol misuse.

51. A, B, D, E, F

    Signs and symptoms of heart transplant rejection include: shortness of breath; fatigue; fluid gain (edema, increased weight); abdominal bloating; new bradycardia; hypotension; atrial fibrillation or flutter; decreased activity tolerance; and decreased ejection fraction (late sign).

33 CHAPTER

Concepts of Care for Patients with Vascular Problems

1. What are the **priority** nursing care concepts for clients with vascular problems?
   A. Perfusion and fluid balance
   B. Clotting and immunity
   C. Inflammation and perfusion
   D. Perfusion and clotting

2. Which factors would the nurse note as increasing the risk for atherosclerosis with an older African-American client? **Select all that apply.**
   A. 20-year history of type 2 diabetes
   B. Nutrition includes three to four diet sodas per day
   C. Sedentary lifestyle
   D. 25 pounds overweight
   E. Father with history of colon cancer
   F. Grandmother died after heart attack

3. What is the nurse's **best** response when a client asks about the difference between arteriosclerosis and atherosclerosis?
   A. Arteriosclerosis is the sudden blockage of an artery while atherosclerosis is formation of plaque in arteries.
   B. Atherosclerosis is forming plaques in arteries but arteriosclerosis is thickening of arterial walls associated with aging.
   C. Arteriosclerosis is hardening of arterial walls while atherosclerosis involves permanent localized dilation of arteries
   D. Atherosclerosis is thickening of arterial walls but arteriosclerosis is clot formation usually in the deep veins.

4. Which control systems play an important role in maintaining a client's blood pressure? **Select all that apply.**
   A. The arterial baroreceptor system
   B. Elevated lipid levels
   C. Regulation of body fluid volume
   D. Dietary saturated fats and sodium
   E. Vascular autoregulation
   F. The renin-angiotensin-aldosterone system

5. Which lifestyle changes would the nurse teach a client to help control hypertension? **Select all that apply.**
   A. Weight reduction if overweight or obese.
   B. Implement a healthy diet such as the DASH diet.
   C. Decrease smoking and nicotine use.
   D. Use relaxation techniques to decrease stress.
   E. Restrict sodium by not adding salt at the table.
   F. Increase activity by use of a structured exercise program.

6. When the nurse performs blood pressure screenings, which clients would be referred for further evaluation? **Select all that apply.**
   A. Diabetic client with blood pressure 118/76 mm Hg
   B. Client with heart disease and blood pressure 148/90 mm Hg
   C. Renal failure client with blood pressure of 180/90 mm Hg
   D. Client with no known health problems and blood pressure of 106/70 mm Hg
   E. Client with muscle cramping taking a statin drug with blood pressure 124/82 mm Hg
   F. COPD client with blood pressure 158/88 mm Hg

7. How does the nurse **best** interpret a client's low-density lipoprotein cholesterol (LDL-C) value which is greater than 190 mg/dL and does not respond to dietary intervention?
   A. The client should have total cholesterol and LDL-C testing repeated during the next routine examination.
   B. The client should be instructed to exercise 6 to 7 days per week to help bring the LDL-C level over time.
   C. The client should be evaluated for secondary causes of hyperlipidemia and treated with statin therapy because of the high LDL-C level.
   D. The client should be followed every 6 months routinely to check lipid profiles and detect trends in the values.

8. Which drug would the nurse expect the primary health care provider to prescribe for a client to **decrease** blood pressure, decrease triglycerides, increase high-density lipoprotein cholesterol (HDL-C), and lower low-density lipoprotein cholesterol (LDL-C)?
   A. Advicor
   B. Caduet
   C. Vytorin
   D. Ezetimibe

9. Which instructions would the nurse give a client for following dietary recommendations of the American College of Cardiology (ACC) and the American Heart Association (AHA)? **Select all that apply.**
   A. Consume a dietary pattern that emphasizes intake of lean protein.
   B. Consume low-fat dairy products, poultry, and fish.
   C. Lower sodium intake to no more than 2400 mg/day.
   D. Engage in aerobic physical activity six to seven times a week.
   E. Limit intake of sweets and red meats.
   F. Eat legumes, tropical vegetable oils (e.g., canola oil), and nuts.

10. What **priority** teaching would the nurse provide for a client who will be discharged with a prescription for atorvastatin?
    A. "Take over-the-counter ranitidine when you experience nausea or vomiting."
    B. "Go to the emergency department if you experience a nagging, nonproductive cough."
    C. "You can use acetaminophen if the drug causes mild to moderate headaches."
    D. "Immediately report any muscle cramping to your primary health care provider."

11. Which techniques would the nurse use when performing an initial cardiovascular assessment on a middle-aged client? **Select all that apply.**
    A. Check blood pressure on the dominant arm.
    B. Palpate all of the major pulse sites.
    C. Auscultate bruits in the radial and brachial arteries.
    D. Palpate and compare temperature differences in the lower extremities.
    E. Check the client for orthostatic hypotension.
    F. Perform bilateral but separate palpation on the carotid arteries.

12. What is the nurse's **best** explanation to a client for use of **low**-dose niacin to decrease LDL-C and very-low-density lipoprotein (VLDL) cholesterol levels?
    A. It will prevent muscle myopathies.
    B. It works well to prevent elevated blood pressure.
    C. It helps reduce side effects of flushing and feeling too warm.
    D. It will help prevent the undesirable side effect of hypokalemia.

13. Which piece of equipment would the nurse recommend for a client to manage hypertension at home?
    A. Blood pressure monitoring device
    B. Stationary exercise bicycle
    C. Blood glucose monitoring device
    D. Kitchen food scale

14. Which condition would the nurse suspect when a client has these findings (BP 200/130 mm Hg; sudden headache, blurred vision, and dyspnea)?
    A. Sustained hypertension
    B. Primary hypertension
    C. Secondary hypertension
    D. Malignant hypertension

15. What drug would the nurse expect to be prescribed for a client with hypertension and for whom lifestyle modifications have failed to control blood pressure?
    A. Thiazide diuretic
    B. Calcium channel blocker
    C. Angiotensin-converting enzyme inhibitor
    D. Beta blocker

16. What frequency of drug dosage therapy would the nurse advocate for an older client with hypertension who lives alone and is able to manage his or her self-care?
    A. Four times a day
    B. Three times a day
    C. Twice a day
    D. Once a day

17. For which client would the nurse question the prescription of hydrochlorothiazide?
    A. Client with asthma
    B. Client with hypokalemia
    C. Client with hyperkalemia
    D. Client with chronic airway limitation

18. What would be the nurse's **best** action when a client reports dizziness when changing position from sitting to standing and a sudden dry cough after starting a prescription of captopril?
    A. Instruct the client to change positions slowly and take an over-the-counter cough syrup.
    B. Tell the client to take the drug at bedtime and use over-the-counter throat lozenges.
    C. Notify the primary health care provider immediately about these side effects.
    D. Teach the client to increase fluid intake to at least 3 L/day.

19. Which action increases the effectiveness of angiotensin II receptor blockers (ARBs) and angiotensin-converting enzyme inhibitors (ACEIs) in controlling hypertension for African-American clients?
    A. The ARB or ACEI is given with a diuretic, beta blocker, or a calcium channel blocker.
    B. A much higher dose of ARB or ACEI is prescribed for an African-American client.
    C. The ARB or ACEI is combined with rigorous lifestyle modifications.
    D. Clients take the ARB or ACEI around the clock on an individualized schedule.

20. Which nursing interventions promote a client's compliance with antihypertensive therapy? **Select all that apply.**
    A. Provide oral and written instructions related to all prescribed medications.
    B. Give the client a list of resources for finding additional information on prescribed drugs.
    C. Stress that suddenly stopping beta blockers can cause angina or heart attack.
    D. Suggest that the client have a home scale for weight monitoring.
    E. Advocate for medications that are taken three times a day for better BP control.
    F. Teach clients to report unpleasant side effects to the primary health care provider.

21. Which assessment findings indicate to the nurse that a client has stage III peripheral arterial disease (PAD)? **Select all that apply.**
    A. Pain is described as numbness, burning, toothache-type pain.
    B. Muscle pain, cramping, or burning occurs with exercise and is relieved with rest.
    C. Pain is relieved by placing the extremity in a dependent position.
    D. Ulcers and blackened tissue occur on the toes, forefoot, and heel.
    E. Pain usually occurs in the distal part of the extremity (toes, arch, forefoot, or heel).
    F. Pain while resting commonly awakens the client at night.

22. What would the nurse suspect when assessing a client's lower extremities and finding decreased pedal pulses, skin that is cool to touch, loss of hair, and thickened toenails?
    A. Peripheral venous disease
    B. Raynaud's syndrome
    C. Deep vein thrombosis
    D. Peripheral arterial disease

23. Which relatively **new** therapy would be tried for clients with familial hypercholesterolemia or for those who are unable to reduce LDLs with existing therapies?
    A. PCSK9 inhibitors
    B. Nicotinic acid
    C. Lovaza (omega-3 ethyl esters)
    D. Combination drugs (e.g., Caduet)

24. Which features would the nurse recognize as indicating that a client had a venous ulcer? **Select all that apply.**
    A. No claudication or rest pain
    B. Ulcer located in the ankle area
    C. Brown pigmentation
    D. Very little granulation tissue present
    E. Ulcer bed is pink
    F. Pulses are present

25. Which clients are at **increased** risk for peripheral arterial disease (PAD)? **Select all that apply.**
    A. Client with anemia
    B. Client with hypertension
    C. Client with diabetes mellitus
    D. Client who smokes cigarettes
    E. Client who is African American
    F. Client who is extremely thin

26. Which symptom causes **most** clients to seek medical attention for peripheral arterial disease (PAD)?
    A. Pain at rest
    B. Rubor in the extremity
    C. Muscle atrophy
    D. Intermittent claudication

27. What symptom would the nurse expect on assessment of a client with inflow peripheral arterial disease?
    A. Frequent episodes of rest pain
    B. Burning or cramping in the calves, ankles, feet, or toes after walking
    C. Waking often at night for pain relieved by hanging feet off the bed
    D. Discomfort in the lower back, buttocks, or thighs after walking

28. What is the nurse's **best** response when a client with peripheral arterial disease asks why he or she should exercise when walking causes pain?
    A. "This type of therapy is free and you can do it by yourself to improve the muscle tone in your legs."
    B. "The cramping will eventually stop if you continue the exercise routine. When you have too much pain, just rest a little while."
    C. "Exercise can improve blood flow to your legs because small blood vessels will compensate for the blood vessels that are blocked off."
    D. "Exercise is a nonsurgical, noninvasive technique used to increase arterial blood flow to your affected leg."

29. What would the nurse teach a client with peripheral arterial disease about positioning and position changes?
    A. Change positions slowly when getting out of bed.
    B. Sleep with legs elevated above the heart if legs are swollen.
    C. Avoid crossing legs at all times.
    D. Sit upright in a chair if legs are not swollen.

30. Which information would the nurse be sure to include when teaching a client with peripheral arterial disease about methods to promote vasodilation? **Select all that apply.**
    A. Maintain a warm environment at home.
    B. Wear socks or insulated shoes at all times.
    C. Prevent cold exposure to the affected limb.
    D. Apply direct heat to the involved limb with a heating pad.
    E. Completely abstain from smoking or chewing tobacco.
    F. Avoid emotional stress and excessive caffeine.

31. Which drugs are useful in promoting circulation for clients with **chronic** peripheral arterial disease? **Select all that apply.**
    A. Aspirin
    B. Ezetimibe
    C. Pentoxifylline
    D. Clopidogrel
    E. Cilostazol
    F. Propranolol

32. Which statements about percutaneous vascular interventions are accurate? **Select all that apply.**
    A. One or more arteries are dilated with a balloon catheter to open the vessel(s).
    B. Stents are often placed to ensure adequate blood flow.
    C. Placement of stents results in a longer hospitalization.
    D. Some clients are occlusion free for 3 to 5 years.
    E. Clients who are candidates must have occlusions or stenoses that are accessible to the catheter.
    F. A percutaneous vascular intervention is considered to be a minor surgical procedure.

33. What nursing actions are included in the routine postprocedural care for a client after percutaneous vascular intervention? **Select all that apply.**
    A. Observe for bleeding at the puncture site.
    B. Perform frequent distal pulse checks on both limbs.
    C. Provide supplemental oxygen at 5 L per nasal cannula.
    D. Administer antiplatelet therapy as prescribed.
    E. Monitor for signs of shock.
    F. Check vital signs frequently as ordered.

34. During which timeframe is it **most** important for the nurse to monitor a client for graft occlusion after receiving revascularization with graft placement?
    A. First 2 hours
    B. First 24 hours
    C. Days 1 and 2 postoperative
    D. During the first week

35. Which method would the postanesthesia care unit (PACU) nurse use to assess the patency of the graft after a client's arterial revascularization with graft placement?
    A. Gently palpate the site every 15 minutes for the first hour and assess for warmth, redness, and swelling.
    B. Ask the client if there is any pain or loss of sensation anywhere in the extremity.
    C. Check the dorsalis pedis and post tibial pulses for the first hour, then every 2 hours.
    D. Check the affected extremity, comparing it to the unaffected, for changes in color, temperature, and pulse intensity every 15 minutes for the first hour, then hourly.

36. What would the nurse expect to find in the history of a client admitted with acute arterial occlusion?
    A. History of chronic venous stasis disease treated with debridement
    B. Acute myocardial infarction or atrial fibrillation within the previous weeks
    C. Episode of blunt trauma that occurred several months ago
    D. Family history of coronary artery disease

37. What would be the **priority** nursing action when a client experiences increasing pain, swelling, and tenseness after thrombectomy?
    A. Elevate the affected extremity and apply ice packs.
    B. Prepare to initiate systemic thrombolytic therapy.
    C. Report these symptoms to the health care provider immediately.
    D. Administer the prescribed pain medication as soon as possible.

38. Which statements are accurate about a client's true aneurysm? **Select all that apply.**
    A. The aneurysm may be described as fusiform or saccular.
    B. An aneurysm is formed when blood accumulates in the wall of an artery.
    C. The aneurysm creates a permanent dilation of an artery.
    D. A true aneurysm can occur as a result of trauma to the arterial walls.
    E. A congenitally weakened arterial wall may result in an aneurysm.
    F. The aneurysm section of the arterial wall is enlarged to at least twice its normal diameter.

39. What is the nurse's **best** interpretation when reviewing a client's abdominal CT scan and noting that there is an outpouched segment coming off the abdominal aorta?
    A. Dissecting aneurysm
    B. Saccular aneurysm
    C. Fusiform aneurysm
    D. False aneurysm

40. Which location would the nurse expect to be the most common for a client to form an aneurysm?
    A. Femoral artery
    B. Radial artery
    C. Thoracic aorta
    D. Abdominal aorta

41. What would the nurse assess for when a client is suspected of having an abdominal aortic aneurysm? **Select all that apply.**
    A. Chest pain and shortness of breath
    B. Abdominal, flank, or back pain
    C. Gnawing pain unaffected by movement
    D. Pulsation in the upper abdomen
    E. Auscultation of a bruit in the upper abdomen
    F. Palpation of a mass in the upper abdomen

42. Which diagnostic tests would the health care provider prescribe to confirm a diagnosis of abdominal aortic aneurysm (AAA) suspected in a client? **Select all that apply.**
    A. Chest x-ray
    B. Ultrasound
    C. Electrocardiogram
    D. Magnetic resonance imaging
    E. Computed tomography scan
    F. Cardiac catheterization

43. What is the **best** nonsurgical intervention for a client with a 3-cm abdominal aortic aneurysm to decrease the risk of rupture?
    A. Bedrest with bathroom privileges until the aneurysm shrinks
    B. Maintenance of normal blood pressure and avoidance of hypertension
    C. Heparin followed by warfarin therapy to prevent clotting
    D. Intraarterial thrombolytic therapy to dissolve any existing clots

44. Which symptoms would indicate to the nurse that a client's aneurysm had ruptured? **Select all that apply.**
    A. Hypotension
    B. Diaphoresis
    C. Decreased level of consciousness
    D. Loss of pulses distal to rupture
    E. Bradypnea
    F. Scant urine output

45. Which are complications that the nurse would monitor for after a client receives an endovascular stent graft for emergent repair of an abdominal aortic aneurysm? **Select all that apply.**
    A. Bleeding
    B. Misplacement of stent graft
    C. Dissecting aneurysm
    D. Peripheral embolization
    E. Endoleak
    F. Aneurysm rupture

46. Which activity would the nurse advise during the recovery period for a client returning home after AAA repair?
    A. Climbing a flight of stairs
    B. Driving a car
    C. Playing golf
    D. Gradually increased walking

47. What is the nurse's **priority** action when a client with AAA suddenly exhibits decreased level of consciousness, blood pressure 82/48 mm Hg, irregular apical pulse, and perfuse diaphoresis?
    A. Alert the Rapid Response Team.
    B. Establish IV access.
    C. Place the client on a cardiac monitor.
    D. Auscultate for bruit and palpate for a mass.

48. Which findings would the nurse expect to assess when a client presents with a thoracic aortic aneurysm? **Select all that apply.**
    A. Tachycardia
    B. Hoarseness
    C. Shortness of breath
    D. Paralytic ileus
    E. Difficulty swallowing
    F. Visible mass above the suprasternal notch

49. Which drug would the nurse prepare to administer when a client enters the emergency department with chest pain described as a "tearing" sensation, diaphoresis, blood pressure of 200/130 mm Hg, weak pulses, and a sense of apprehension?
    A. Oral beta blocker such as atenolol
    B. Calcium channel blocker such as amlodipine
    C. IV beta blocker such as esmolol
    D. Antianginal drug such as nitroglycerin

50. What does the nurse suspect when assessing a client on bedrest and finding that he or she has a left calf that is swollen, warm to touch, reddened, and moderately painful?
    A. Raynaud's syndrome
    B. Cellulitis
    C. Arterial occlusion
    D. Deep vein thrombosis

51. Which nonsurgical management techniques would the nurse expect when caring for a client with DVT? **Select all that apply.**
    A. Gradual increase in ambulation as tolerated by the client
    B. Elevation of legs when in bed or sitting in a chair
    C. Knee- or thigh-high compression stockings
    D. Massage to ease the client's calf pain
    E. Anticoagulant drugs as prescribed
    F. Complete bedrest for up to 4 weeks

52. For prevention of DVT, which drug would the nurse expect the health care provider to prescribe?
    A. Thrombolytic therapy
    B. IV unfractionated heparin
    C. Novel oral anticoagulants (NOACs)
    D. Subcutaneous low–molecular-weight heparin (LMWH)

53. What is the recommended therapeutic range for the international normalized ratio (INR) for a client receiving warfarin sodium to prevent DVT and decrease the risk for stroke?
    A. 2.0-2.5
    B. 1.5-2.0
    C. 1.0-1.5
    D. 0.5-1.0

54. Which are characteristics a nurse would expect in clients with Raynaud's disease? **Select all that apply.**
    A. Occurs more often in young women
    B. Claudication in feet and lower extremities is present
    C. Clients experience cold intolerance
    D. Occurs only in upper extremities
    E. Causes red-white-blue skin color changes on exposure to cold or stress
    F. Occurs often in smokers especially young men

55. What is the **most** important teaching point for the nurse to emphasize with a client who has Buerger's disease?
    A. Decrease intake of fats and reduce cholesterol to reverse the disease process.
    B. Limit exposure to extreme warm temperatures because of vasodilation.
    C. Cease cigarette smoking and all exposure to tobacco to arrest the disease process.
    D. Perform exercises of fingers and toes at least twice a day to slow the disease process.

56. What is the nurse's **best** advice for a client, who is an avid golfer, but has been recently diagnosed with thoracic outlet syndrome?
    A. Check your blood pressure in both arms daily.
    B. Rest whenever shortness of breath occurs.
    C. Avoid walking for long distances.
    D. Don't elevate your arms above your head.

57. Which drug would the nurse expect to administer to a client with Raynaud's or Buerger's disease?
    A. Captopril
    B. Nifedipine
    C. Warfarin
    D. Atorvastatin

58. What is the **priority** action for the nurse when a client is to have unfractionated heparin (UFH) discontinued and to start receiving subcutaneous low–molecular-weight heparin (LMWH)?
    A. Discontinue the UFH at least 30 minutes before giving the first LMWH injection.
    B. Check the aPTT and INR laboratory results before giving the first LMWH injection.
    C. Assess the client's IV site and convert it to a saline lock before starting LMWH.
    D. Instruct the client about the need for frequent laboratory test to ensure the LMWH is working.

59. What are the purposes for a client with a venous stasis ulcer to be prescribed the topical drug Accuzyme? **Select all that apply.**
    A. Improve circulation
    B. Promote healing
    C. Eliminate infection
    D. Chemically debride the ulcer
    E. Eliminate necrotic tissue
    F. Prevent stasis

60. Which statements pertaining to the use of an Unna boot for a client are accurate? **Select all that apply.**
    A. It is used to heal peripheral arterial ulcers.
    B. It is constructed from gauze and zinc oxide.
    C. It promotes venous return and prevents stasis.
    D. It is changed by the health care provider every 3 to 4 days.
    E. It forms a sterile environment for the ulcer.
    F. The client is instructed to report any increase in pain.

61. Which are conservative management measures for a client's varicose veins? **Select all that apply.**
    A. Graduated compression stockings (GCSs)
    B. Surgical ligation and removal of veins
    C. Exercise to increase venous return
    D. Sclerotherapy
    E. Elevating the extremities
    F. Endovenous ablation

62. Which essential teaching would the nurse provide for a client being discharged with chronic venous insufficiency? **Select all that apply.**
    A. Elevate your legs at least 20 minutes four to five times a day.
    B. Avoid crossing legs at all times.
    C. Wear compression stocking at night during sleep.
    D. Avoid standing still for any length of time.
    E. Keep legs and feet positioned below the heart for better perfusion.
    F. Avoid tight restrictive pants, girdles, or garters.

Chapter 33 Answer Key

1. D
   The priority care concepts for clients with vascular problems are perfusion and clotting. Inflammation is an interrelated concept for these clients.

2. A, C, D, F
   Risk factors for atherosclerosis include: low HDL-C, high LDL-C, increased triglycerides, genetic predisposition, diabetes mellitus, obesity, hypertension, sedentary lifestyle, smoking, stress, African American or Hispanic ethnicity, older adult, and diet high in saturated and *trans* fats, cholesterol, sodium, and sugar.

3. B
   Arteriosclerosis is a thickening, or hardening, of the arterial wall which is often associated with aging. Atherosclerosis is a type of arteriosclerosis that involves the formation of plaque within the arterial wall and is the leading contributor to coronary artery and cerebrovascular disease. A sudden blockage is an acute arterial occlusion. Permanent dilation of arteries occurs with an aneurysm. Clot formation in the deep veins is a deep vein thrombosis (DVT).

4. A, C, E, F
   Stabilizing mechanisms exist in the body to exert overall regulation of systemic arterial pressure and to prevent circulatory collapse. Four control systems play a major role in maintaining blood pressure: the arterial baroreceptor system, regulation of body fluid volume, the renin-angiotensin-aldosterone system, and vascular autoregulation. Some elevated lipid levels contribute to development of atherosclerosis and arterial disease. A diet high in saturated fats and sodium is a risk factor for development of atherosclerosis.

5. A, B, D, F
   The nurse would teach all clients about lifestyle changes to help control hypertension including: restrict dietary sodium according to ACC/AHA guidelines (not adding table salt is often not enough); reduce weight if overweight or obese; implement a heart-healthy diet, such as the DASH diet; increase physical activity with a structured exercise program; abstain or decrease alcohol consumption (no more than one drink a day for women and two drinks a day for men); stop smoking and tobacco use; and use relaxation techniques to reduce stress.

6. B, C, E, F
    The client with heart disease has stage 1 hypertension. The client with renal failure has very high blood pressure and stage 2 hypertension. The client taking the statin drug should be referred for a change in drug therapy because muscle cramps are a side effect of these drugs and this indicates that the client is not tolerating the statin. The client with COPD also has stage 2 hypertension (See Table 33.1). The diabetic client and the client with no known health problems both have normal blood pressure readings.

7. C
    Increased low-density lipoprotein cholesterol (LDL-C) ("bad" cholesterol) levels and low high-density lipoprotein cholesterol (HDL-C) ("good" cholesterol) indicate that a person is at an increased risk for atherosclerosis. For clients with elevated total cholesterol and LDL-C levels that do not respond adequately to dietary intervention, the primary health care provider prescribes a cholesterol-lowering agent, most likely a 3-hydroxy-3-methylglutaryl coenzyme A (HMG-CoA) reductase inhibitors or "statin" (e.g., lovastatin, simvastatin, atorvastatin), which would successfully reduce total cholesterol in most clients when used for an extended period.

8. B
    Amlodipine and atorvastatin are combined as Caduet to decrease blood pressure while decreasing triglycerides (TGs), increasing HDL-C, and lowering LDL-C. Vytorin (ezetimibe and simvastatin) is a combination of a selective inhibitor of intestinal cholesterol and statin used to treat elevated cholesterol. Ezetimibe is in a class of medications called cholesterol-lowering medications. It works by preventing the absorption of cholesterol in the intestine. Advicor is a combination of niacin XR and lovastatin used to lower cholesterol and triglyceride (fat) levels in the blood.

9. B, C, E, F
    The ACC and AHA publish dietary recommendations for lowering LDL-C levels. These recommendations are based on the best current evidence from randomized controlled trials and include: consume a dietary pattern that emphasizes intake of vegetables, fruits, and whole grains; consume low-fat dairy products, poultry (without the skin), fish, legumes, nontropical (e.g., canola) vegetable oils, and nuts; limit intake of sweets, sugar-sweetened beverages, and red meats; aim for a dietary pattern that includes 5% to 6% of calories from saturated fat; and limit *trans* fats.

10. D
    Statins reduce cholesterol synthesis in the liver and increase clearance of LDL-C from the blood. Therefore, they are contraindicated in clients with active liver disease or during pregnancy because they can cause muscle myopathies and marked decreases in liver function. Statins also have the potential for interactions with other drugs, such as warfarin, cyclosporine, and selected antibiotics. They are discontinued if the client has muscle cramping or elevated liver enzyme levels.

11. B, C, D, E, F
    Because of the high incidence of hypertension in clients with atherosclerosis, assess the blood pressure in **both** arms. Palpate pulses at all the major sites on the body and note any differences. Palpate each carotid artery **separately** to prevent blocking blood flow to the brain! Also feel for temperature differences in the lower extremities and check capillary filling. Prolonged capillary filling (>3 seconds in young to middle-aged adults; >5 seconds in older adults) generally indicates poor circulation. Many clients with vascular disease have a bruit in the larger arteries, which can be heard with a stethoscope or Doppler probe. A bruit is a turbulent, swishing sound, which can be soft or loud in pitch. It is heard as a result of blood trying to pass through a narrowed artery. A bruit is considered abnormal, but it does not indicate the severity of disease. Bruits often occur in the carotid, aortic, femoral, and popliteal arteries. Orthostatic hypotension is checked

because it is a frequent side effect of antihypertensive drugs.

12. C
Low doses of niacin are recommended because many clients experience flushing and a very warm feeling all over with higher doses. Higher doses can also result in an elevation of hepatic enzymes. In statin-intolerant clients, niacin can be useful to help lower LDL cholesterol levels in combination with other drugs.

13. A
The nurse would teach the client to obtain an ambulatory BP monitoring (ABPM) device for use at home so the pressure can be checked daily. The nurse would also evaluate the client's and family's ability to use this device accurately and instruct the client to keep a record of blood pressure readings and report very low or high readings to the primary health care provider.

14. D
Hypertensive crisis (or malignant hypertension) is a severe type of elevated BP that rapidly progresses and is considered a medical emergency. A person with this health problem usually has symptoms such as morning headaches, blurred vision, and dyspnea and/or symptoms of uremia (accumulation in the blood of substances ordinarily eliminated in the urine). Clients are often in their 30s, 40s, or 50s with their systolic BP greater than 200 mm Hg.

15. A
Thiazide (low-ceiling) diuretics, such as hydrochlorothiazide, inhibit sodium, chloride, and water reabsorption in the distal tubules while promoting potassium, bicarbonate, and magnesium excretion. Because of the low cost and high effectiveness of thiazide-type diuretics, they are usually the drugs of choice for clients with uncomplicated hypertension.

16. D
Research shows that clients, especially older adults, are more compliant with and able to manage self-care when drug dosages are prescribed once a day. The more frequently doses are scheduled, the more likely a client will be unable to follow the treatment regimen and miss doses of the prescribed drugs.

17. B
Hydrochlorothiazide (HCTZ) is a thiazide diuretic. The most frequent side effect associated with thiazide and loop diuretics is hypokalemia (low potassium level). Monitor serum potassium levels and assess for irregular pulse, dysrhythmias, and muscle weakness, which may indicate hypokalemia.

18. C
Captopril is an angiotensin-converting enzyme inhibitor (ACEI). Antihypertensive drugs all have the potential to cause hypotension. However, the most common side effect of this group of drugs is a nagging, dry cough. The nurse should immediately notify the primary health care provider of this finding. Clients must also be taught to report this problem as soon as possible. If a cough develops, the drug is discontinued and the client is started on another drug therapy to control hypertension.

19. A
ACEIs and ARBs are not as effective in African Americans unless they are taken with diuretics or another drug category such as a beta blocker or calcium channel blocker.

20. A, C, D, F
Health teaching is essential to help clients become successful in managing their BP. Provide oral and written information about the indications, dosage, times of administration, side effects, and drug interactions for antihypertensives. Stress that medication must be taken as prescribed. Teach that suddenly stopping drugs such as beta blockers can result in angina (chest pain), myocardial infarction (MI), or rebound hypertension. Teach clients to obtain an ambulatory BP monitoring (ABPM) device and suggest having a scale in the home for weight monitoring. Remember

316 CHAPTER 33 Concepts of Care for Patients with Vascular Problems

that clients are more compliant with the plan of care when drugs are given once a day. Instruct clients to report unpleasant side effects of antihypertensive drugs so that another drug may be prescribed to minimize those side effects.

21. A, C, E, F

Stage III peripheral arterial pain is also called *rest pain*. Key features include: pain while resting which commonly awakens the client at night; the pain is described as numbness, burning, or toothache-type pain; the pain usually occurs in the distal part of the extremity (toes, arch, forefoot, or heel); and pain is relieved by placing the extremity in a dependent position. Muscle pain, cramping, or burning that occurs with exercise and is relieved with rest is a feature of stage II; and ulcers and blackened tissue occur on the toes, forefoot, and heel, which is characteristic of stage IV.

22. D

Specific findings for PAD depend on the severity of the disease. Assess for loss of hair on the lower calf, ankle, and foot; dry, scaly, dusky, pale, or mottled skin; and thickened toenails. With severe arterial disease, the extremity is cold and gray-blue (cyanotic) or darkened. Pallor may occur when the extremity is elevated.

23. A

The Food and Drug Administration (FDA) approved the drug class, PCSK9 inhibitors, for use in clients with familial hypercholesterolemia or for those who are unable to reduce LDLs with existing therapies. Nicotinic acid (niacin) may lower LDL-C and very-low-density lipoprotein (VLDL) cholesterol levels and increase HDL-C levels but is poorly tolerated due to side effects. Lovaza (omega-3 ethyl esters) is approved by the FDA as an adjunct to diet to reduce TGs that are greater than 500 mg/dL. Caduet is used to decrease blood pressure while decreasing triglycerides (TGs), increasing HDL, and lowering LDL.

24. A, B, C, E, F

Characteristics of venous ulcers include: chronic nonhealing ulcer; no claudication or rest pain; moderate ulcer discomfort; client reports of ankle or leg swelling; location is the ankle area; brown pigmentation; the ulcer bed is pink; the ulcer is usually superficial, with uneven edges; granulation tissue present; ankle discoloration and edema; full veins when leg slightly dependent; no neurologic deficit; pulses present; and may have scarring from previous ulcers.

25. B, C, D, E

Clients at risk for PAD have the same problems or characteristics as those at risk for hypertension. They include people with: low HDL-C, high LDL-C, increased triglycerides, genetic predisposition, diabetes mellitus, obesity, hypertension, sedentary lifestyle, smoking, stress, African American or Hispanic ethnicity, older adult, and diet high in saturated and *trans* fats, cholesterol, sodium, and sugar.

26. D

Most clients initially seek medical attention for a classic leg pain known as **intermittent claudication**. Usually the client can walk only a certain distance before discomfort (e.g., cramping or burning muscular pain) forces them to stop. The pain goes away with rest. When clients resume walking, they walk the same distance and the pain returns. Because of this, the pain is considered reproducible. As the disease progresses, the client can walk only shorter and shorter distances before pain recurs. Ultimately, the pain may occur even while at rest.

27. D

Clients with inflow disease have discomfort in the lower back, buttocks, or thighs. Clients with mild inflow disease have discomfort after walking about two blocks. This discomfort is not severe but causes them to stop walking. The discomfort is relieved with rest.

28. C
Exercise may improve arterial blood flow to the affected leg through buildup of the collateral circulation. Collateral circulation provides blood to the affected area through smaller vessels that develop and compensate for the occluded vessels.

29. C
Instruct all clients with the disease to avoid crossing their legs and avoid wearing restrictive clothing (e.g., garters to hold up nylon stockings commonly used by older women), which interfere with blood flow.

30. A, B, C, E, F
Vasodilation can be achieved by providing warmth to the affected extremity and preventing long periods of exposure to cold (which causes vasoconstriction). Encourage clients to maintain a warm environment at home and to wear socks or insulated shoes at all times. Caution clients to avoid the application of direct heat to the limb with heating pads or extremely hot water because sensitivity in the affected limb is decreased and burns may result. Emotional stress, caffeine, and nicotine also can cause vasoconstriction. Stress that **complete abstinence** from smoking or chewing tobacco is essential to prevent vasoconstriction.

31. A, C, D, E
Clients with chronic peripheral arterial disease are prescribed hemorheologic and antiplatelet agents. Pentoxifylline is a hemorheologic agent that increases the flexibility of red blood cells. It decreases blood viscosity by inhibiting platelet aggregation and decreasing fibrinogen and thus increases blood flow in the extremities. Aspirin and clopidogrel are antiplatelet drugs used to reduce risk for myocardial infarction, stroke, and vascular death. Some clients receive both drugs (dual antiplatelet therapy). Clients who experience disabling intermittent claudication may also benefit from phosphodiesterase inhibitors such as cilostazol because it can help improve symptoms and increasing walking distance. Beta blockers are avoided because they

may have drug-related claudication or a worsening of symptoms. Ezetimibe is a cholesterol-lowering drug.

32. A, B, D, E
A nonsurgical but invasive approach for improving arterial flow is the use of percutaneous vascular intervention (PVI). One or more arteries are dilated with a balloon catheter advanced through a cannula, which is inserted into or above an occluded or stenosed artery. When the procedure is successful, it opens the vessel and improves arterial blood flow. Clients who are candidates for percutaneous procedures must have occlusions or stenoses that are accessible to the catheter. Reocclusion may occur, and the procedure may be repeated. Some clients are occlusion-free for up to 3 to 5 years, whereas others may experience reocclusion within a year. During PVI, intravascular stents (wire meshlike devices) are usually inserted to assure adequate blood flow in a stenosed vessel. Clients often have these procedures in same-day surgery or ambulatory care centers (e.g., very short hospital stays).

33. A, B, D, E, F
All of these actions are appropriate to post procedure care for a client who had a percutaneous transluminal intervention. However, most clients will not need supplemental oxygen, especially at such a high flow rate as 5 L. This flow rate would tend to dry the nasal passages.

34. B
Graft occlusion (blockage) is a postoperative emergency that can occur within the first 24 hours after arterial revascularization. Monitor the client for and report severe, continuous, and aching pain, which may be the first indicator of postoperative graft occlusion and ischemia.

35. D
To assess graft patency after arterial revascularization, monitor the patency of the graft by checking the extremity every 15 minutes for the first hour and then hourly for changes in color, temperature, and pulse intensity. Compare the

operative leg with the unaffected extremity. If the operative leg feels cold; becomes pale, ashen, or cyanotic; or has a decreased or absent pulse, contact the surgeon immediately!

36. B

Acute arterial occlusion is most often caused by an embolus (piece of a clot that travels and lodges in a new area). Emboli originating from the heart are the most common cause of acute arterial occlusions. Most clients with an embolic occlusion have had an acute myocardial infarction (MI) and/or atrial fibrillation within the previous weeks.

37. C

After thrombectomy, monitor for increasing pain, swelling, and tenseness. Report any of these symptoms to the health care provider immediately. These symptoms signal compartment syndrome which occurs when tissue pressure within a confined body space becomes elevated and restricts blood flow. The resulting ischemia can lead to tissue damage and eventually tissue death.

38. A, C, E, F

An aneurysm is a permanent localized dilation of an artery, which enlarges the artery to at least two times its normal diameter. It may be described as fusiform (a diffuse dilation affecting the entire circumference of the artery) or saccular (an outpouching affecting only a distinct portion of the artery). Aneurysms may also be described as true or false. In true aneurysms, the arterial wall is weakened by congenital or acquired problems. False aneurysms occur as a result of vessel injury or trauma to all three layers of the arterial wall. Dissecting aneurysms differ from true aneurysms in that they are formed when blood accumulates within the wall of an artery.

39. B

A saccular aneurysm is an outpouching affecting only a distinct portion of the artery. A fusiform aneurysm is a diffuse dilation affecting the entire circumference of the artery (often appears egg shaped on scans). A dissecting aneurysm is a false aneurysm which occurs when blood accumulates in the wall of an artery.

40. D

Aneurysms tend to occur at specific anatomic sites, most commonly in the abdominal aorta. They often occur at a point where the artery is not supported by skeletal muscles or on the lines of curves or flexion in the arterial tree. Abdominal aortic aneurysms (AAAs) account for most true aneurysms. They are commonly asymptomatic, and frequently rupture. Most of these are located between the renal arteries and the aortic bifurcation (dividing area).

41. B, C, D, E

Assessment findings for a client's AAA include: abdominal, flank, or back pain; pain that is usually described as steady with a gnawing quality, unaffected by movement, and lasting for hours or days; pulsation in the upper abdomen slightly to the left of the midline between the xiphoid process and the umbilicus (a detectable aneurysm is at least 5 cm in diameter); and auscultation of a bruit over the pulsatile mass. **Avoid** palpating the mass because it may be tender and there is risk for rupture of the aneurysm.

42. B, E

To confirm a diagnosis of AAA, computed tomography (CT) scanning with contrast is the standard tool for assessing the size and location of an abdominal or thoracic aneurysm. Ultrasonography is also used.

43. B

The desired outcome of nonsurgical management is to monitor the growth of the aneurysm and maintain the blood pressure at a normal level to decrease the risk for rupture. Clients with hypertension are treated with antihypertensive drugs to decrease the rate of enlargement and the risk for early rupture. Additionally, the client would receive frequent ultrasound or CT scans to monitor the growth of the aneurysm.

44. A, B, C, D, F

Clients with a rupturing AAA are critically ill and at risk for hypovolemic shock caused by hemorrhage. Signs and symptoms include hypotension, diaphoresis, decreased level of consciousness, oliguria (scant urine output), loss of pulses distal to the rupture, and dysrhythmias. Retroperitoneal hemorrhage is manifested by hematomas in the flanks (lower back). Rupture into the abdominal cavity causes abdominal distention. Tachypnea occurs, rather than bradypnea, as a compensation during hypovolemic shock.

45. A, B, D, E, F

The repair of AAAs with endovascular stent grafts is the procedure of choice for almost all clients on an elective or emergent basis. Complications of this procedure include: conversion to open surgical repair; bleeding; aneurysm rupture; peripheral embolization; misplacement of the stent graft; endoleak (a persistent blood flow outside the lumen of an endoluminal graft but within the aneurysm sac or adjacent vascular segment being treated by the device used for endovascular aneurysm repair); and infection.

46. D

The client must follow instructions regarding activity level. Because stair climbing may be restricted initially, he or she may need a bedside commode if the bathroom is inaccessible. Clients may not perform activities that involve lifting heavy objects (usually more than 15 to 20 lb [6.8 to 9.1 kg]) for 6 to 12 weeks after surgery. Advise them to use caution for activities that involve pulling, pushing, or straining. Most clients are restricted from driving a car for several weeks after discharge. Instruct clients to try to walk each day. They should gradually increase and walk a little more each day.

47. A

These findings indicate a ruptured AAA which means that the client is critically ill and at risk for hypovolemic shock caused by hemorrhage. Signs and symptoms include hypotension, diaphoresis, decreased level of consciousness, oliguria (scant urine output), loss of pulses distal to the rupture, and dysrhythmias. The priority action is to notify the Rapid Response Team to intervene and save the client's life.

48. B, C, E, F

When a thoracic aortic aneurysm (TAA) is suspected, assess for back pain and manifestations of compression of the aneurysm on adjacent structures. Signs include shortness of breath, hoarseness, and difficulty swallowing. TAAs are not often detected by physical assessment, but sometimes a mass may be visible above the suprasternal notch. Assess the client with suspected rupture of a thoracic aneurysm for sudden and excruciating back or chest pain. Hypovolemic shock also occurs with TAA.

49. C

This client's symptoms indicate that the client likely has an aortic dissection. The health care provider would prescribe IV morphine sulfate to relieve pain and an IV beta blocker, such as esmolol, to lower heart rate and blood pressure. If this regimen is not effective, nitroprusside or nicardipine hydrochloride may be used. For long-term medical treatment, the recommended target for blood pressure is less than 120/80 mm Hg. Beta blockers (e.g., propranolol) and calcium channel antagonists (e.g., amlodipine) are prescribed to assist with blood pressure maintenance once the client is stabilized.

50. D

The classic signs and symptoms of DVT are calf or groin tenderness and pain, and sudden onset of unilateral swelling of the leg. Examine the painful area, comparing the site with the other limb. Gently palpate the site, observing for induration (hardening) along the blood vessel and for warmth and edema. Redness may also be present.

51. A, B, C, E

Research shows that ambulation with DVT does not increase the risk for pulmonary embolus. The accepted approach is a gradual increase in ambulation as tolerated by the client. Teach clients to elevate the legs when in the bed and chair. To help prevent chronic venous insufficiency, instruct clients with active and resolving DVT to wear knee- or thigh-high sequential or graduated compression stockings for an extended period. Be sure to select the correct stocking size for each client. To prevent the thrombus from dislodging and becoming an embolus, do **not** massage the affected extremity. Anticoagulants are the drugs of choice for actual DVT and for clients at risk for DVT. Venous stasis associated with complete bedrest increases the risk for development of more DVTs.

52. D

Subcutaneous low–molecular-weight heparins (LMWHs) such as enoxaparin or dalteparin have a consistent action and are preferred for prevention and treatment of DVT. Some clients taking LMWH may be safely managed at home with visits from a home care nurse. Candidates for home therapy must have stable DVT or PE, low risk for bleeding, adequate renal function, and normal vital signs. They must be willing to learn self-injection or have a family member, friend, or home care nurse administer the subcutaneous injections.

53. B

Most clients receiving warfarin should have an INR between 1.5 and 2.0 to prevent future DVT and to minimize the risk for stroke or hemorrhage.

54. A, C, E

Characteristics of Raynaud's disease include: painful vasospasms of arteries and arterioles in extremities, especially digits; causes red-white-blue skin color changes on exposure to cold or stress; cause is unknown, but it occurs more in women, and may be autoimmune because it is associated with many rheumatic diseases such as systemic lupus erythematosus (SLE). Claudication and strong association with smoking (young men) refers to Buerger's disease.

55. C

The priority teaching would be to instruct the client about smoking cessation and avoidance of tobacco. Other teaching would include avoiding cold by wearing gloves and warm clothes, managing stress, avoiding caffeine; tell the client taking nifedipine to avoid grapefruit and grapefruit juice to prevent severe adverse effects, including possible death. These substances reduce the enzymes that metabolize nifedipine, allowing blood levels to increase to dangerous levels. Teach a client on vasodilators about side effects such as facial flushing, hypotension, headaches.

56. D

Thoracic outlet syndrome is caused by compression of the subclavian artery by rib or muscle. It is more common in women and clients who have to keep arms moving or above their heads (e.g., golfers, swimmers). The best treatment is physical therapy for an exercise program, avoiding aggravating positions.

57. B

Nifedipine is a calcium channel blocker which acts as a vasodilator for both Raynaud's and Buerger's disease. It will help reverse the vasoconstriction that occurs with these conditions.

58. A

When a client is prescribed a change from UFH to LMWH, the nurse's priority is to discontinue the UFH at least 30 minutes before the first LMWH injection. While the nurse should be familiar with the client's clotting study results, no laboratory values are necessary when the client is receiving LMWH.

59. B, D, E

The primary health care provider may prescribe topical agents, such as Accuzyme, to chemically débride the ulcer, eliminate necrotic tissue and promote healing. Remind clients that they may temporarily feel a burning sensation when the agent is applied. If an infection or cellulitis develops, systemic antibiotics are necessary.

60. B, C, E, F

An Unna boot is used for venous stasis ulcers if the client is ambulatory. An Unna boot dressing is constructed of gauze that has been moistened with zinc oxide. The boot is applied to the affected limb from the toes to the knee after the ulcer has been cleaned with normal saline solution. It is then covered with an elastic wrap and hardens like a cast. This promotes venous return and prevents stasis. The Unna boot also forms a sterile environment for the ulcer. The health care provider changes the boot about once a week. The client is instructed to report increased pain, which indicates that the boot may be too tight.

61. A, C, E

The conservative treatments of choice for managing varicose veins include the three Es: elastic compression hose, **e**xercise, and **e**levation. Graduated compression stockings (GCSs) rely on graduated external pressure to improve venous return by applying pressure to the muscles. Exercise increases venous return by helping the muscles pump blood back to the heart. Teach clients to **avoid** high-impact exercises such as horseback riding and running. Daily walks and ankle flexion exercises while sitting are common exercises that are helpful in promoting circulation. Elevating the extremities as much as possible allows gravity to work with the valves in promoting venous return and prevent reflux.

62. A, B, D, F

Essential teaching for a client being discharged with chronic venous insufficiency includes: elevate your legs for at least 20 minutes four to five times a day; when in bed, elevate your legs above the level of your heart; avoid prolonged sitting or standing; do not cross your legs (crossing at the ankles is acceptable for short periods); and do not wear tight, restrictive pants. Avoid girdles and garters. Compression stocking should be worn during the day but removed at night.

34 CHAPTER

Critical Care of Patients with Shock

1. Which statements about shock are true? **Select all that apply**.
   A. Affects all body organs
   B. Occurs only in the acute care setting
   C. Is a whole-body response to tissue hypoxia
   D. Results in widespread abnormal cellular metabolism
   E. Is classified as a disease rather than a discreet disorder
   F. May occur in older clients in response to urinary tract infections

2. Why are the clinical signs and symptoms of most types of shock the same regardless of what specific events or conditions caused the shock to occur?
   A. The blood, blood vessels, and heart are directly connected to each other so that when one is affected, all three are affected.
   B. Because blood loss occurs with all types of shock, the most common first manifestation is hypotension.
   C. Every type of shock interferes with oxygenation and metabolism of all cells in the same sequence.
   D. The sympathetic nervous system is triggered by any type of shock and initiates the stress response.

3. Which client does the nurse consider to be at **highest risk** for neural-induced distributive shock?
   A. 25-year-old receiving 500 mg of penicillin IV
   B. 47-year-old with sudden-onset severe chest pain and dyspnea
   C. 21-year-old who has received 4 mg of morphine IV for acute pain
   D. 82-year-old who has had severe vomiting and diarrhea for 2 days

4. Which client will the nurse recognize as having a higher risk for obstructive shock?
   A. 32-year-old with a pulmonary embolus
   B. 42-year-old with stable angina
   C. 52-year-old with chronic atrial fibrillation
   D. 72-year-old with a history of heart failure

5. Which conditions will the nurse consider as increasing any client's risk for hypovolemic shock? **Select all that apply**.
   A. Hypoglycemia
   B. Diuretic therapy
   C. Severe head injury
   D. Prolonged diarrhea
   E. Liver failure with ascites
   F. Continuous nasogastric suction
   G. Large draining abdominal wound

6. Which changes in vital signs of a client in the early postoperative period indicates to the nurse that the client may be in the initial stage of hypovolemic shock? **Select all that apply**?
   A. Increased heart rate
   B. Increased respiratory rate
   C. Decreased systolic blood pressure
   D. Decreased urine output
   E. Increased diastolic blood pressure
   F. Increased pulse pressure

7. Which subjective symptom will the nurse expect to find in a client during the compensatory stage of hypovolemic shock?
   A. Thirst
   B. Hunger
   C. Headache
   D. Numbness of the fingers and toes

8. Which body area on a client with darker skin who is at high risk for shock will the nurse examine for indications of pallor and cyanosis?
   A. Oral mucous membranes
   B. Soles of the hands and feet
   C. Earlobes and bridge of the nose
   D. Sclera closest to the inner corner of the eye

9. Which change in laboratory values or clinical symptoms in a client with hypovolemic shock indicates to the nurse that current therapy may need to be changed?
   A. Urine output increases from 5 mL/hr to 6 mL/hr.
   B. Pulse pressure decreases from 28 mm Hg to 22 mm Hg.
   C. Serum potassium level increases from 3.6 mEq/L to 3.9 mEq/L.
   D. Core body temperature increases from 98.2°F (36.8°C) to 98.8°F (37.1°C).

10. Which laboratory values in a client with hypovolemic shock will the nurse associate with the progressive stage of shock? **Select all that apply**.
    A. Arterial blood pH 7.32
    B. Serum lactate 9 mg/dL (1.03 mmol/L)
    C. Sodium 147 mEq/L (mmol/L)
    D. Blood urea nitrogen 15 mg/dL
    E. Potassium 6.3 mEq/L (mmol/L)
    F. Neutrophil count 5,000/mm³ (5 x 10⁹/L)

11. Which actions are **most appropriate** for the nurse to take **first** when a client with blunt trauma to the abdomen who has been NPO for several hours now reports thirst and anxiety? **Select all that apply**.
    A. Obtain an order for a stat hematocrit and hemoglobin.
    B. Get the client a few ice chips or a moistened swab.
    C. Compare current vital signs to baseline.
    D. Check for obvious blood in the urine.
    E. Measure abdominal girth.
    F. Increase the IV rate.

12. Which assessment has the **highest priority** for the nurse to perform to **prevent harm** when caring for a client in hypovolemic shock who is receiving IV sodium nitroprusside?
    A. Asking about chest pain
    B. Determining mental status
    C. Checking blood pressure every 15 minutes
    D. Checking extremities for color and perfusion

13. Which statement made by a client at high risk for hypovolemic shock is of **greatest** concern to the nurse?
    A. "I live alone in my house and my family lives in a different state."
    B. "Do you have any idea when I might go home? No one is feeding my cat."
    C. "Something feels wrong, but I'm not sure what is causing me to feel this way."
    D. "I would usually go golfing with my friends today. I hope they're not worried about me."

14. Which vital sign change in a client with hypovolemic shock indicates to the nurse that the therapy is effective?
    A. Urine output increases from 5 mL/hr to 25 mL/hr.
    B. Pulse pressure decreases from 35 mm Hg to 28 mm Hg.
    C. Respiratory rate increases from 22 breaths/min to 26 breaths/min.
    D. Core body temperature increases from 98.2°F (36.8°C) to 98.8°F (37.1°C).

15. For which change in condition will the nurse teach a client, who is discharged and at continued risk for fluid loss, to check for daily at home?
    A. Elevated temperature and itchiness
    B. Loss of taste sensation and appetite
    C. Numbness of the fingers and toes
    D. Reduced urine output and light-headedness

16. For which client problems associated with hypovolemic shock will the nurse specifically prepare to administer a blood product rather than an IV crystalloid? **Select all that apply**.
    A. Acidosis
    B. Hypoxemia
    C. Dehydration
    D. Hypotension
    E. Hyponatremia
    F. Low hematocrit and hemoglobin levels

17. Which actions are **priorities** for the nurse to perform to **prevent harm** for a client with hypovolemic shock who is receiving an infusion of dobutamine? **Select all that apply**.
    A. Assessing hourly urine output
    B. Assessing for chest pain throughout the infusion
    C. Covering the infusion bag to protect it from light
    D. Measuring blood pressure at least every 15 minutes
    E. Ensuring the drug is infused only with Ringer's lactate
    F. Checking the infusion site every 30 minutes for extravasation

18. Which newly admitted client does the nurse consider to be at **highest risk** for development of sepsis?
    A. 75-year-old with hypertension and early Alzheimer disease
    B. 68-year-old who is 2 days postoperative from bowel surgery
    C. 54-year-old with moderate asthma and severe degenerative joint disease of the right knee
    D. 80-year-old community dweller with no other health problems undergoing cataract surgery

19. Which client parameters will the nurse report to the health care provider as consistent with the quick Sequential Organ Failure Assessment (qSOFA) indicating the possible presence of sepsis or septic shock? **Select all that apply**.
    A. Core body temperature 100°F (37.8°C)
    B. Eyes are open but does not respond to questions
    C. Respiratory rate of 28 breaths/min
    D. SpO_2 is 94% primary
    E. Systolic blood pressure of 92 mm Hg
    F. Urine output of 18 mL/hr

20. Which specific client symptom indicates to the nurse that septic shock (Sepsis-3) may be present?
    A. Hypotension
    B. Pale, clammy skin
    C. Anxiety and confusion
    D. Oozing of blood at the IV site

21. Which specific drug therapy will the nurse anticipate for management of the client who has septic shock?
    A. Antibiotics
    B. Inotropics
    C. Crystalloids
    D. Antidysrhythmics

22. Which complication will the nurse remain alert for in a client who has septic shock?
    A. Psychosis
    B. Skin necrosis
    C. Febrile seizures
    D. Acute respiratory distress syndrome (ARDS)

23. Which symptom in a client with sepsis does the nurse consider a **late** indication of septic shock?
    A. Warm skin
    B. Bounding pulse
    C. Severe hypotension
    D. Decreased urine output

24. How will the nurse interpret a change in the white blood cell (WBC) count of a client with sepsis in which the band neutrophil count is increasing and the segmented neutrophil count is decreasing?
    A. Antibiotic therapy is successful.
    B. The infection is becoming worse.
    C. The client is allergic to the drug therapy.
    D. Disseminated intravascular coagulation (DIC) is now present.

25. When sepsis is diagnosed in a client, when will the nurse initiate the prescribed antibiotic therapy?
    A. Within the first hour after diagnosis
    B. Within the first 24 hours after diagnosis
    C. After the results of blood cultures are known
    D. When blood lactate levels have increased to 9 mg/dL (1.03 mmol/L)

26. Which blood product type does the nurse anticipate will be ordered to infuse **first** in a client who has septic shock with poor clotting and hemorrhage?
    A. Packed red blood cells (PRBCs)
    B. Fresh frozen plasma (FFP)
    C. Clotting factors
    D. Platelets

27. What is the nurse's **best first** action when a client who has sepsis is found to have a blood glucose level of 310 mg/dL?
    A. Check the electronic health record to determine when the last dose of antidiabetic drug was given.
    B. Ask the family how long the client has had diabetes.
    C. Notify the primary health care provider.
    D. Document the finding as the only action.

28. Which changes in condition will the nurse teach a client who is being discharged after successful management of sepsis to check daily as an indicator of a new or ongoing infection? **Select all that apply**.
    A. Shortness of breath
    B. Temperature elevation
    C. Cloudy, foul-smelling urine
    D. New onset of a productive cough
    E. Paleness or blue tinge to mouth membranes
    F. Redness and tenderness of an open skin lesion

Chapter 34 Answer Key

1. A, C, D, F
   Shock is widespread abnormal cellular metabolism that occurs when gas exchange with oxygenation and tissue perfusion needs are insufficient to maintain cell function. It is a condition rather than a disease and is the "whole-body" response that occurs with tissue hypoxia. All body organs are affected by shock and either work harder to adapt and compensate for reduced gas exchange or perfusion or fail to function because of hypoxia. Urinary tract infections that enter the bloodstream (urosepsis) is a common cause of shock in older clients.
   Shock can occur in any setting.

2. D
   Most clinical signs and symptoms of shock are similar regardless of what starts the process or which tissues are affected first. These common changes result from physiologic adjustments (compensatory mechanisms) in the attempt to ensure continued oxygenation of vital organs. These adjustment actions are performed by the sympathetic nervous system triggering the stress response and activating the endocrine and cardiovascular systems.

3. C

    Both acute pain and morphine can lead to neural-induced distributive shock. At first, acute pain stimulates the sympathetic nervous system. However, the parasympathetic system over-rides the sympathetic division. This interference together with morphine acting within the central nervous system result in decreased sympathetic tone to blood vessel smooth muscles, causing widespread vasodilation and reduced mean arterial pressure.

    Option A is incorrect. The type of shock possibly produced by a reaction to penicillin is anaphylactic shock, a type of chemical-induced distributive shock.

    Option B is incorrect. The type of shock associated with sudden-onset severe chest pain and dyspnea is cardiogenic shock from an acute myocardial infarction.

    Option D is incorrect. The type of shock associated with prolonged vomiting and diarrhea is hypovolemic shock with true volume depletion as a result of dehydration.

4. A

    Obstructive shock is caused by problems that impair the ability of the normal heart to pump effectively. The heart itself remains normal, but conditions outside the heart prevent either adequate filling of the heart or adequate contraction of the healthy heart muscle. Although the most common cause of obstructive shock is cardiac tamponade, other causes include arterial stenosis, pulmonary embolism, pulmonary hypertension, pericarditis, thoracic tumor, and tension pneumothorax. The other health problems listed are causes associated with cardiogenic shock.

5. B, D, F, G

    In addition to loss of blood, hypovolemic shock can be caused by dehydration that decreases circulating blood volume. Conditions increasing the risk for dehydration-induced hypovolemic shock include fluid losses resulting from diuretic therapy, diarrhea, continuous nasogastric suction, and excessive wound drainage.

    Hypoglycemia does not result in fluid loss.

    Severe head injury can lead to neural-induced distributive shock, not hypovolemic shock.

Liver failure with ascites is another cause of distributive shock caused by capillary leak.

6. A, B, E

    The initial stage of shock is characterized by sympathetic nervous system compensation with vasoconstriction. Thus, the indicators of the initial stage of hypovolemic shock are subtle and include only increased heart and respiratory rates or a slight increase in diastolic blood pressure.

7. A

    Hormonal compensation for hypovolemic shock includes secretion of antidiuretic hormone (ADH), renin, and aldosterone as a result of decreased tissue perfusion. Subjective changes of this compensation include thirst and anxiety.

8. A

    In dark-skinned clients, pallor or cyanosis is best assessed in the oral mucous membranes. The hands and feet may indicate a temperature change but are not reliable indicators of pallor or cyanosis. Sclera can only indicate the possible presence of jaundice. Although the earlobes and nose can become cyanotic, this would occur much later than changes observed in the oral mucous membranes.

9. B

    A compensatory response to shock is vasoconstriction. Initially, the diastolic pressure increases but systolic pressure remains the same. As a result, the difference between the systolic and diastolic pressures *(pulse pressure)*, is smaller or "narrower." When interventions are inadequate and shock worsens, systolic pressure decreases as cardiac output decreases. This causes the pulse pressure to narrow even further, indicating that shock is progressing. Although an increase in urine output usually signals improvement, a change of 1 1 mL/hr is within the margin of measurement error and is meaningless in this situation.

10. A, B, E

    Laboratory indicators of the progressive stage of hypovolemic shock are a low blood pH, along with rising lactic acid and potassium levels.

The sodium level rises during the compensatory stage. The level listed is only slightly higher than normal.

The BUN is within the normal range.

The neutrophil count is within the normal range.

11. C, E

A client with blunt trauma to the abdomen may have internal bleeding and is at risk for shock. Thirst and anxiety are subjective symptoms of shock. The nurse would assess for other indications of shock or internal bleeding by first assessing vital signs and comparing them to the client's baseline and measure abdominal girth. If the vital signs or abdominal assessment are consistent with shock, the nurse will notify the Rapid Response Team who would order a stat hematocrit and hemoglobin.

Although keeping an IV open and available is important, until the source of bleeding is found and corrected, the IV rate may not be increased in order to slow any hemorrhage.

The kidneys are located on the back wall and not usually directly involved in abdominal trauma.

Until assessment is complete, the client is kept NPO.

12. C

Sodium nitroprusside improves myocardial perfusion by dilating coronary arteries rapidly for a short time. This action also occurs in systemic blood vessels and can result in dangerously low blood pressure. Thus, the nurse assesses blood pressure every 15 minutes while a client is receiving this drug. The drug does not cause chest pain and does not cause peripheral vasoconstriction that could interfere with perfusion of extremities. The drug's effect on mental status is related to blood pressure decreases.

13. C

Anxiety and a sense of impending doom are common changes in mental status that occur with the hypoxemia and sympathetic nervous system associated with shock.

14. A

During shock, the kidneys and baroreceptors sense an ongoing decrease in MAP and trigger the release of renin, antidiuretic hormone (ADH), aldosterone, epinephrine, and norepinephrine to start kidney compensation, which is very sensitive to changes in fluid volume from normal. Renin, secreted by the kidney, causes decreased urine output. ADH increases water reabsorption in the kidney, further reducing urine output. These actions compensate for shock by attempting to prevent further fluid loss. This response is so sensitive that urine output is a very good indicator of fluid resuscitation adequacy. If the therapy was not effective, urine output would not increase.

15. D

Reduced urine output and light-headedness are early indicators of hypovolemia related to fluid loss. The other options are not associated with any problem related to hypovolemia resulting from fluid loss.

16. B, F

Blood products, such as packed red blood cells (PRBCs), are used when shock is caused by blood loss resulting in hypoxemia. PRBCs increase hematocrit and hemoglobin levels along with some fluid volume.

Crystalloid fluids contain only minerals, salts, sugars, and nonprotein substances. They can help restore volume, electrolyte balance, and may buffer lactic acid. However, these fluids neither correct low hematocrit or hemoglobin levels nor correct hypoxemia.

17. B, D, F

Dobutamine is a beta-adrenergic agonist and a positive inotropic agent that can improve cardiac contractility. The increased contractility increases cardiac muscle oxygen consumption, which may not be met during shock, and can lead to angina or myocardial infarction. Although the main action is in the heart muscle, it also acts on blood vessels and can cause a transient hypotension from vascular dilation. When doses are too high, vasoconstriction can occur and is an indication of overdose. In addition, if extravasation occurs local vasoconstriction can cause tissue damage.

The drug is not light sensitive and can be run with other crystalloids, not just Ringer's lactate. Assessing urine output is not the priority when administering dobutamine.

18. B

This client has several risk factors. First, he or she is an older adult. Immune function decreases with age. The greatest risk factor is the recent bowel surgery. Not only does major surgery further reduce the immune response but also the bowel cannot be "sterilized" for surgery. Thus, bacteria in the bowel have the chance to escape the site and enter the bloodstream when the bowel is disrupted.

19. B, C, E

The quick Sequential Organ Failure Assessment (qSOFA) can quickly alert clinicians to the need for further assessment for organ dysfunction. This assessment has three parameters and clients are assigned one point for each abnormal parameter. Abnormal parameters include:
Systolic blood pressure ≤ 100 mm Hg
Respiratory rate ≥ 22 breaths/min
Any change in mental status

20. D

With septic shock, compared to other types of shock, inappropriate clotting occurs with the formation of microthrombi that use available clotting factors and platelets. When these substances are depleted by excessive microclotting, bleeding can occur from any orifice or site of tissue injury. The other symptoms, although present in septic shock, are also present in every other type of shock and are not specific for septic shock.

21. A

Septic shock starts with a localized infection that becomes systemic. Specific therapy for sepsis and septic shock (Sepsis-3) is the use of antibiotics. Inotropics and crystalloids are used for many types of shock, including septic shock. Antidysrhythmics are used whenever life-threatening dysrhythmias are present.

22. D

The lungs are susceptible to damage during septic shock, and the complication of ARDS may occur. ARDS in septic shock is caused by the continued systemic inflammatory response syndrome (SIRS) increasing the formation of oxygen free radicals, which damage lung cells.

23. C

Late in septic shock, the client has hypovolemia and greatly decreased cardiac output with severe hypotension. Decreased urine output is an earlier indicator of shock. Although earlier in sepsis the skin is warm from vasodilation, in late septic shock the skin is cool, clammy, and cyanotic. The pulse is weak and thready.

24. B

When the band neutrophil count is increasing and the segmented neutrophil count is decreasing, a *left shift* is occurring, in which the bone marrow is becoming depleted of mature neutrophils that can fight the infection. The infection is getting worse, indicating that antibiotic therapy is not effective and the client's ability to fight infection is greatly decreased. Changes in these specific WBCs are not associated with an allergic reaction or DIC.

25. A

Antibiotic therapy is initiated as soon as possible, preferably within the first hour after diagnosis, even if blood cultures have not been obtained. It is not delayed until after blood culture results are known. Lactate levels are used to diagnose the condition, not guide the timing of antibiotic therapy.

26. D

In a client with septic shock who has poor clotting and bleeding, it is most likely that disseminated intravascular coagulation (DIC) has occurred and consumed all of the client's available platelets, which are an absolute necessity for appropriate clotting to occur. These are given first.

27. C

Sepsis alone can elevate blood glucose levels in any client. Levels above 180 mg/dL are associated with poor outcomes and management must be started immediately. The nurse's best first action is to notify the primary health care provider immediately.

28. A, B, C, D, E, F

All conditions listed above can be indicators of a new or ongoing infection.

35 CHAPTER

Critical Care of Patients with Acute Coronary Syndromes

1. Which findings would the nurse expect when assessing a client with chronic stable angina? **Select all that apply.**
   A. Chest discomfort that occurs in a pattern that is familiar to the client
   B. Chest discomfort that occurs with moderate to prolonged exertion
   C. Frequency, duration, and intensity of symptoms remain the same over several months
   D. Results in moderate limitation of activity
   E. Usually treated with rest and nitroglycerin (NTG)
   F. Pain lasts less than 15 minutes

2. Which **essential** points would the nurse include when teaching a client with angina about nitroglycerin tablets? **Select all that apply.**
   A. If one tablet does not relieve the chest pain after 5 minutes, put two pills under your tongue.
   B. Keep your nitroglycerin pills with you at all times.
   C. The prescription should last about 7 to 8 months before a refill is needed.
   D. You can tell the tablets are active when you feel a tingling after placing one under your tongue.
   E. Keep the tablets in a glass, light-resistant container.
   F. If no immediate pain relief occurs, just wait because the drug will eventually take effect.

3. A client with chronic stable angina now has chest pressure, cool and clammy skin, blood pressure 150/90 mm Hg, heart rate 100 beats/min, and respiratory rate 32 breaths/min. What are the **priorities** of collaborative care for this client? **Select all that apply.**
   A. Maintain NPO status.
   B. Relieve chest pain.
   C. Improve coronary artery perfusion.
   D. Draw troponin blood samples.
   E. Improve myocardial oxygenation.
   F. Relieve nausea.

4. Which statement by a client indicates to the nurse correct understanding of resuming sexual activity in the presence of angina?
   A. "When I can climb two flights of stairs, it is safe to resume sexual activity."
   B. "It is best to resume sexual activity in the evening before I go to sleep."
   C. "If I am unable to walk at least a mile, it is unsafe for me to resume sexual activity."
   D. "I will discuss alternative methods with my partner as I will no longer be able to resume my previous level of sexual activity."

5. What is the nurse's **next** action 5 minutes after administering a sublingual (SL) nitroglycerin tablet to a client with chest pain?
   A. Apply oxygen at 2 to 4 L by nasal cannula.
   B. Administer morphine sulfate IV push.
   C. Recheck pain intensity and vital signs.
   D. Notify the health care provider and give a chewable aspirin.

6. After administering SL nitroglycerin to a client whose baseline blood pressure is 130/80 mm Hg, for which finding would the nurse **immediately** notify the health care provider?
   A. Client reports a headache.
   B. Systolic pressure is 90 mm Hg.
   C. Anginal pain is somewhat relieved.
   D. Heart rate is 92 beats/min.

7. Which are characteristics the nurse would expect to find in a client with unstable angina (USA)? **Select all that apply.**
   A. Chest pain occurs at rest or with exertion
   B. Pain causes severe limitation of activities
   C. Includes chronic stable angina, vasospastic angina, and new-onset angina
   D. Presents with ECG changes and elevation of troponin levels
   E. Ischemia does not cause myocardial damage or cell death
   F. The pain or pressure is poorly relieved by nitroglycerin

8. Which statements about coronary artery disease and women are accurate? **Select all that apply.**
   A. Postmenopausal women in their 70s have the same incidence of myocardial infarction (MI) as men.
   B. Women have smaller coronary arteries and frequently have plaque that breaks off and travels into the small vessels to form an embolus.
   C. The older a woman is the more likely she is to have coronary artery disease.
   D. More men than women die within a year after a MI.
   E. Women whose parents had CAD are more susceptible to the disease.
   F. Many women experience atypical angina as indigestion, pain between shoulders, aching jaw, and a choking sensation.

9. When would the nurse be sure to hold a beta blocker drug and notify the health care provider?
   A. When a client states he or she woke up with a headache
   B. When a client's respiratory rate is 26 breaths/min on room air
   C. When a client is scheduled for a chest x-ray
   D. When a client's heart rate is less than 50 beats/min and SBP is less than 100 mm Hg

10. Which finding would the nurse expect when a client experiences a non–ST-segment elevation MI (NSTEMI)?
    A. ST depression and T-wave inversion on a 12-lead ECG
    B. Cardiac dysrhythmias
    C. Immediate elevation of troponin levels
    D. ST elevation in two contiguous leads on a 12-lead ECG

11. The nurse would teach a client to seek treatment for symptoms of myocardial infarction (MI) immediately rather than delay, because physical changes occur in how many hours after an MI?
    A. 3 hours
    B. 6 hours
    C. 12 hours
    D. 24 hours

12. Which finding **most** strongly indicates left heart failure in a client when the nurse auscultates heart sounds?
    A. Murmur
    B. Split S_1 and S_2
    C. S_3 gallop
    D. Pericardial friction rub

13. How soon does the nurse expect anginal pain to begin subsiding after administering sublingual nitroglycerin to a client with chronic stable angina?
    A. 1-2 minutes
    B. 5-6 minutes
    C. 10-12 minutes
    D. 15-20 minutes

14. Which indicators of metabolic syndrome would the nurse expect in a client with heart failure? **Select all that apply.**
    A. Blood pressure of 130/86 mm Hg while taking a beta blocker
    B. Large waist of 35 inches (88 cm) or greater for men
    C. HDL-C greater than 40 mg/dL for men
    D. Increased fasting glucose of 100 mg/dL or higher
    E. Increased level of triglycerides of 150 mg/dL or higher
    F. Decreased LDL-C of less than 50 mg/dL for women

15. Which early reaction is **most** common in clients with chest discomfort associated with unstable angina or myocardial infarction (MI)?
    A. Depression
    B. Anger
    C. Fear
    D. Denial

16. Which client does the nurse expect to have the **highest** risk for death related to damage to the left ventricle?
    A. Client with an inferior wall MI (IWMI)
    B. Client with a lateral wall MI (LWMI)
    C. Client with a posterior wall MI (PWMI)
    D. Client with an anterior wall MI (AWMI)

17. Which type of dysrhythmia would the nurse expect to monitor for when a client experiences an inferior wall myocardial infarction (IWMI)?
    A. Premature ventricular complexes (PVCs)
    B. Bradycardia with second-degree heart block
    C. Supraventricular tachycardia
    D. Atrial fibrillation

18. Because many sudden cardiac arrest victims die before reaching the hospital, which **priority** teaching point would the nurse be sure to include in a community presentation about heart disease?
    A. The importance of controlling alcohol consumption and smoking cessation
    B. Modifying risk factors and blood pressure medication compliance
    C. How to operate an automatic external defibrillator (AED) in the workplace
    D. Recognizing unstable angina and when to call for help

19. An alert and oriented client comes to the walk-in clinic with left-sided chest pain, mild shortness of breath, and diaphoresis. What is the nurse's first **priority** action?
    A. Obtain a complete cardiac history for the client.
    B. Place the client in semi-Fowler position with supplemental oxygen.
    C. Instruct the client to go immediately to the nearest full-service hospital.
    D. Immediately alert the health care provider and establish IV access.

20. About which associated symptoms would the nurse ask a client with a history of intermittent episodes of chest pain? **Select all that apply.**
    A. Diarrhea
    B. Nausea
    C. Shortness of breath
    D. Joint pain
    E. Dizziness
    F. Diaphoresis

21. What diagnostic tests would the nurse obtain to determine whether a client admitted with acute-onset chest pain and dyspnea had experienced a myocardial infarction (MI)? **Select all that apply.**
    A. C-reactive protein
    B. 12-lead ECG
    C. Chest x-ray
    D. Serial troponins T and I
    E. Lipid profile
    F. Exercise stress test

22. What **priority** question would the nurse ask before administering SL nitroglycerin to a middle-aged male client with chest pain?
    A. "Have you taken a medication for erectile dysfunction within the past 24 to 48 hours?"
    B. "Do you have a family history of heart disease, especially parents and grandparents?"
    C. "Have you experienced any other symptoms with your chest pain?"
    D. "What were you doing when the chest pain started?"

23. What **priority** action will the nurse take when providing care for a client with chest pain being treated with IV nitroglycerin?
    A. Restrict the client to bedrest with use of a bedpan.
    B. Elevate the head of the bed to 90 degrees.
    C. Monitor blood pressure continuously.
    D. Increase the dose rapidly to achieve pain relief.

24. What is the **best** action for the home health nurse to take when visiting a new client with CAD who is experiencing new-onset chest pain and shortness of breath?
    A. Instruct the client to rest quietly and take slow, deep breaths.
    B. Have the client chew a 325-mg aspirin tablet and call 911.
    C. Apply supplemental home oxygen until the symptoms subside.
    D. Administer a sublingual nitroglycerin tablet and have the family take the client to the emergency room.

25. Which statements about the use of thrombolytic agents for a client with an acute myocardial infarction are accurate? **Select all that apply.**
    A. Clients who cannot receive timely percutaneous coronary intervention (PCI) with indications of ST elevation myocardial infarction (STEMI) should be considered for fibrinolytic therapy.
    B. A client who has received a thrombolytic agent must be carefully monitored before, during, and after the drug is given.
    C. Thrombolytic therapy is indicated for chest pain of less than 15 minutes duration that is relieved by nitroglycerin.
    D. The client must be assessed for absolute and relative contraindications before a thrombolytic agent is administered.
    E. Monitor for bleeding which is a major risk when a client receives thrombolytic therapy.
    F. Indications that the clot has been dissolved and the artery reperfused include sudden onset of ventricular dysrhythmias.

26. Which **absolute** contraindications would the nurse assess for when a client is being considered for thrombolytic therapy? **Select all that apply.**
    A. Any prior intracranial hemorrhage
    B. History of chronic, severe, poorly controlled hypertension
    C. Suspected aortic dissection
    D. Known malignant intracranial neoplasm (primary or metastatic)
    E. Severe uncontrolled hypertension on presentation (SBP >180 mm Hg)
    F. Active bleeding or bleeding diathesis (excluding menses)

27. Which are post-administration nursing responsibilities when caring for a client who received thrombolytic therapy? **Select all that apply.**
    A. Observe all IV sites for bleeding and patency.
    B. Document the client's emotional reaction to the thrombolytic therapy.
    C. Monitor white blood cell (WBC) count and differential.
    D. Test stool, urine, and emesis for occult blood.
    E. Monitor clotting study values.
    F. Observe for signs of internal bleeding (e.g., blood pressure).

28. For which complication does the nurse monitor when a client with chronic stable angina (CSA) is prescribed a calcium channel blocker?
    A. Tachycardia
    B. Wheezes and crackles
    C. Hypotension
    D. Forgetfulness

29. For which manifestations would the nurse monitor when providing care for a client prescribed beta-blocker therapy? **Select all that apply.**
    A. Depression
    B. Bradycardia
    C. Decreased level of consciousness
    D. Increased urine output
    E. Crackles or wheezes in the lungs
    F. Chest discomfort

30. Which diagnostic test is performed after a client's acute stage of an unstable angina episode to determine if there are cardiac changes that are consistent with ischemia?
    A. Electrocardiogram
    B. Echocardiography
    C. Exercise tolerance test
    D. Chest CT scan

31. Which drug therapy would the nurse expect to be prescribed for a client with acute coronary syndrome (ACS) to decrease the risk of recurrent myocardial infarction, stroke, and mortality?
    A. Anti-inflammatory drug
    B. Central vasodilator
    C. High-intensity statin therapy
    D. Anticoagulant therapy

32. Which **essential** points would the nurse include when teaching a client with coronary artery disease how to manage activity at home? **Select all that apply.**
    A. Begin by walking the same distance at home as in the hospital (usually 400 feet) three times each day.
    B. Check your pulse before and after you exercise.
    C. Always carry a bottle of nitroglycerin with you.
    D. Stop your activity if your pulse increases by 10 beats/min.
    E. Exercise outdoors when the weather is pleasant.
    F. Avoid straining (lifting, push-ups, pull-ups, and straining at bowel movements).

33. Which task would the nurse delegate to the assistive personnel (AP) when caring for a client in phase 1 of cardiac rehabilitation?
    A. Assist the client to ambulate 400 feet four times a day.
    B. Assist the client with ambulation to the bathroom.
    C. Assess the client's vital signs and fatigue level with each increase in activity.
    D. Teach the client to notify the health care provider for episodes of chest pain.

34. Which signs and symptoms indicate to the nurse that a client with a myocardial infarction and heart failure is going into cardiogenic shock? **Select all that apply.**
    A. Cold, clammy skin with poor peripheral pulses
    B. Pulmonary congestion and tachypnea
    C. Bradycardia and hypertension
    D. Urine output less than 0.5 to 1 mL/kg/hr
    E. Agitation, restlessness, or confusion
    F. Systolic BP less than 100 mm Hg

35. Which manifestation would the nurse expect with a client labeled class I on the Killip scale for heart failure?
    A. Clear lung sounds and absence of S_3
    B. Crackles in the lower half of the lung fields and possible S_3
    C. Crackles more than halfway up the lung fields and frothy sputum
    D. Systolic blood pressure less than 90 mm Hg and oliguria

36. Which procedure has shown promise for managing clients with cardiogenic shock?
    A. Percutaneous ventricular assistive device
    B. Immediate reperfusion
    C. Intra-aortic balloon pump
    D. Minimally invasive bypass surgery

37. Which clients are potential candidates for coronary artery bypass graft (CABG) surgery? **Select all that apply.**
    A. Client with angina and greater than 50% occlusion of the left main coronary artery that cannot be stented
    B. Client with unstable angina with moderate one-vessel disease appropriate for stenting
    C. Client with valvular disease
    D. Client with coronary vessels unsuitable for percutaneous coronary intervention (PCI)
    E. Client with acute myocardial infarction (MI) that is responding to medical therapy
    F. Client with ischemia or impending MI after angiography or PCI

38. Which interventions would the nurse perform to protect a client from a sternal wound infection after CABG surgery? **Select all that apply.**
    A. Shave the client's body from neck to knees.
    B. Instruct the client to shower with 4% chlorhexidine gluconate.
    C. Prepare the surgical site by clipping hair then applying chlorhexidine with isopropyl alcohol (0.5% or 2 %).
    D. Collect and send urine and sputum samples to the laboratory for culture and sensitivity.
    E. Administer IV antibiotics 1 hour prior to the surgical procedure.
    F. Wear gloves, a gown, and a mask while preparing the client for surgery.

39. Which essential preoperative teaching would the nurse provide to a client scheduled for CABG surgery using the traditional procedure? **Select all that apply.**
    A. There will be a sternal incision.
    B. Coughing will be avoided to keep stress off of the sternal incision.
    C. There will as many as three chest tubes in place after the surgery.
    D. An indwelling urinary catheter will be in place to drain urine.
    E. You will be on bedrest for up to 48 hours after the surgery.
    F. An endotracheal tube will prevent talking immediately after surgery.

40. Following CABG surgery, a client's body temperature is below 96.8°F (36°C). What measures would the nurse take to rewarm the client?
    A. Infuse warm IV fluids.
    B. Do not rewarm because cold cardioplegia is protective.
    C. Place the client in a warm fluid bath.
    D. Use lights and thermal blankets to slowly warm the client.

41. How would the critical care nurse assess for postoperative bleeding in a client who just had CABG surgery?
    A. Measure mediastinal and pleural chest tube drainage at least once an hour and report drainage amount over 150 mL/hr to the surgeon.
    B. Measure mediastinal and pleural chest tube drainage at least once a shift and report drainage amount over 50 mL/hr to the surgeon.
    C. Assess the sternal dressing for bleeding every 4 hours, then reinforce with sterile gauze as needed and report the approximate amount of bleeding to the surgeon.
    D. Assess the vein donor site every 4 hours and report the amount of serous drainage as well as pain to the surgeon.

42. Which statement by the client who had CABG surgery indicates to the nurse that his or her pain is related to the sternotomy and is **not** anginal in origin?
    A. "The pain goes down my arm and sometimes into my jaw."
    B. "My pain increases when I cough or take a deep breath."
    C. "The nitroglycerin helped to relieve my pain."
    D. "I feel nausea and shortness of breath with the pain."

43. Which nursing assessment is **specific** to a client who had CABG surgery with the radial artery used as the graft?
    A. Check the fingertips, hand, and arm for sensation and mobility once a shift.
    B. Take blood pressure every hour on the unaffected arm or use a leg cuff on the legs.
    C. Assess hand color, temperature, ulnar pulse, and capillary refill every hour initially.
    D. Assess for and document expected edema, bleeding, and swelling at the donor site.

44. Which observations would the nurse expect when a client develops mediastinitis after CABG surgery? **Select all that apply.**
    A. Anginal-type chest pain
    B. Fever continuing beyond the first 4 days after surgery
    C. Bogginess of the sternum
    D. Redness and drainage from the suture site
    E. Induration or swelling at the suture site
    F. Decreased white blood cell count

45. Which assessment would the nurse perform to help **prevent harm** from graft collapse after CABG surgery?
    A. Assess for motion and sensation in the donor extremity.
    B. Observe for generalized hypothermia.
    C. Auscultate lungs for crackles or wheezes.
    D. Monitor blood pressure for hypotension.

46. Which finding prompts the nurse to **immediately** contact the surgeon for a client who had a minimally invasive direct coronary artery bypass (MIDCAB)?
    A. Client has difficulty with coughing and deep breathing.
    B. Client has acute incisional pain.
    C. Client has ECG changes including Q waves and ST-segment and T-wave changes in leads V_2 to V_6.
    D. Client has chest tube drainage of 80 mL/hr.

47. Which procedure would the nurse expect to be recommended for a client with discrete, proximal, noncalcified blockage in one coronary artery?
    A. Minimally invasive direct coronary artery bypass (MIDCAB)
    B. Percutaneous coronary intervention (PCI)
    C. Immediate thrombolytic reperfusion therapy
    D. Exercise tolerance test (stress test) on a treadmill

48. Which postprocedure medications would the nurse teach about, before discharge, to a client who had a percutaneous coronary intervention (PCI)? **Select all that apply.**
    A. Furosemide
    B. Clopidogrel
    C. Metoprolol
    D. Isosorbide dinitrate
    E. Docusate
    F. Aspirin

49. Which advantages would the nurse teach a client about with regard to robotic heart surgery? **Select all that apply.**
    A. Shorter surgical time than traditional CABG surgery
    B. Shorter hospital stay of just 2 to 3 days
    C. Decreased pain due to smaller incisions
    D. Shorter time on the heart-lung bypass machine
    E. Chest tubes are never needed
    F. Ability to reach otherwise inaccessible blockage sites

50. Which alternative therapies may be helpful in reducing a client's anxiety about progressive activity postoperatively and during rehabilitation? **Select all that apply.**
    A. Guided imagery
    B. Progressive muscle relaxation
    C. Acupuncture
    D. Music therapy
    E. Pet therapy
    F. Herbal remedies

Chapter 35 Answer Key

1. A, B, C, E, F
   All of these characteristics describe chronic stable angina, except that this condition results in only slight limitation of activity (**not** moderate).

2. B, D, E
   Teach the client to carry NTG at all times. Keep the tablets in a glass, light-resistant container because the drug degrades quickly in light, moisture, and in plastic. The drug should be replaced every 3 to 5 months before it loses its potency or stops producing a tingling sensation when placed under the tongue. Management of chest pain at home includes: keep fresh nitroglycerin available for immediate use; at the first indication of chest discomfort, cease activity and sit or lie down; place one nitroglycerin tablet under your tongue, allowing the tablet to dissolve; wait 5 minutes for relief; if no relief results, call 911 for transportation to a health care facility; while waiting for emergency medical services (EMS), repeat the nitroglycerin and wait 5 more minutes; if there is no relief, repeat and wait 5 more minutes. Be sure to carry a medical identification card or wear a bracelet or necklace that identifies a history of heart problems.

3. B, C, D, E
   This client has experienced a change from chronic stable angina to symptoms that may indicate acute coronary syndrome. The purpose of collaborative care is to decrease pain, decrease myocardial oxygen demand, and increase perfusion (myocardial oxygen supply). Emergency care of the client with chest discomfort includes: assess airway, breathing, and circulation (ABCs); defibrillate as needed; provide continuous ECG monitoring; obtain the client's description of pain or discomfort; obtain the client's vital signs (blood pressure, pulse, respiration); assess/provide vascular access; consult chest pain protocol or notify the cardiac health care provider or Rapid Response Team for specific intervention; obtain a 12-lead

ECG within 10 minutes of report of chest pain; provide pain relief medication and aspirin (non–enteric coated) as prescribed; administer supplemental oxygen therapy to maintain an oxygen saturation > 90%; remain calm and stay with the client if possible; assess the client's vital signs and intensity of pain 5 minutes after administration of medication; remedicate with prescribed drugs (if vital signs remain stable) and check the client every 5 minutes; and notify the cardiac health care provider if vital signs deteriorate. Troponin levels would be sent to the laboratory to check for possible MI.

4. A

In general, a client who can walk one block or climb two flights of stairs without symptoms can usually safely resume sexual activity. Clients can resume sexual intercourse on the advice of the cardiac health care provider, usually after an exercise-tolerance assessment. Suggest that initially clients have intercourse after a period of rest.

5. C

Five minutes after administering a sublingual nitroglycerin tablet, the nurse would check the client's pain level and check his or her blood pressure.

6. B

After administering SL NTG to a client, if the blood pressure (BP) is less than 100 mm Hg systolic or 25 mm Hg lower than the previous reading, lower the head of the bed and notify the cardiac health care provider. If the client is experiencing some, but not complete, relief and vital signs remain stable, another NTG tablet or spray may be used. In 5-minute increments, a total of three doses may be administered in an attempt to relieve anginal pain.

7. A, B, E, F

Unstable angina may last longer than 15 minutes or may be poorly relieved by rest or nitroglycerin. Unstable angina includes new-onset angina, vasospastic angina, and pre-infarction angina. Clients with unstable angina may present with ST segment changes on a 12-lead ECG but do **not** have changes in troponin levels.

Ischemia is present but is not severe enough to cause detectable myocardial damage or cell death.

8. A, B, C, E, F

All of these statements are accurate except that more women than men die within a year after a myocardial infarction.

9. D

The nurse would **not** give beta blockers if the pulse rate was below 50 beats/min or the systolic BP was below 100 mm Hg. He or she would first check with the health care provider. The beta-blocking agent could lead to persistent bradycardia or further reduction of systolic BP, leading to poor peripheral and coronary perfusion.

10. A

Clients with NSTEMI present with ST segment and T-wave changes on a 12-lead ECG. These changes include ST depression and T-wave inversion, which indicate myocardial ischemia. Initially troponin level may be normal, but it elevates over the next 3 to 12 hours (not immediately). ST elevation in two contiguous leads on a 12-lead ECG is characteristic of STEMI. Dysrhythmias may occur with any MI and are not specific to NSTEMI.

11. B

Obvious physical changes do not occur in the heart until 6 hours after the infarction, when the infarcted region appears blue and swollen. These changes explain the need for intervention within the first 4 to 6 hours of symptom onset!

12. C

A client who develops left heart failure would have the presence of an S_3 heart sound as well as crackles. Wheezing, tachypnea, and frothy sputum are noted when a client develops pulmonary edema.

13. A

After administering SL NTG, the nurse expects the client's anginal pain to begin subsiding within 1 to 2 minutes and pain relief should be clearly evident in 3 to 5 minutes. If the client is experiencing some but not complete relief and vital signs remain stable, another NTG tablet or spray may be used. In 5-minute increments, a total of three doses may be administered in an attempt to relieve anginal pain. Angina usually responds to NTG. The client typically states that the pain is relieved or markedly diminished. When simple measures such as taking three sublingual nitroglycerin tablets, in timed increments, one after the other do not relieve chest discomfort, the client may be experiencing an MI.

14. A, D, E, F

Indicators of metabolic syndrome include: blood pressure of 130/85 mm Hg or higher or taking antihypertensive drug(s); HDL-C <40 mg/dL for men or <50 mg/dL for women or taking a cholesterol lowering drug; triglycerides of 150 mg/dL or higher or taking a cholesterol lowering drug; fasting glucose of 100 mg/dL or higher or taking antidiabetic drug(s); and large waist size (excessive abdominal fat causing central obesity) of 40 inches (102 cm) or greater for men or 35 inches (88 cm) or greater for women.

15. D

Denial is a common early reaction to chest pain associated with angina or MI. On average, the client with an acute MI waits more than 2 hours before seeking medical attention. Often, he or she rationalizes that symptoms are caused by indigestion or overexertion. In some situations, denial is a normal part of adapting to a stressful event. However, in this case, denial interferes with identifying a symptom such as chest pain and can be harmful.

16. D

Clients with anterior wall MIs (AWMIs) have the highest mortality rate because they are most likely to have left ventricular failure and dysrhythmias from damage to the left ventricle.

17. B

Typical dysrhythmias for the client with an inferior ACS (includes IWMI) are bradycardias and second-degree atrioventricular (AV) blocks resulting from ischemia of the AV node. These rhythms tend to be intermittent. Monitor the cardiac rhythm and rate and the hemodynamic status. If the client becomes hemodynamically unstable, a temporary pacemaker may be necessary.

18. C

Ninety percent of sudden cardiac arrest victims die before reaching the hospital and many of these deaths are attributed to ventricular fibrillation (v fib). To help combat this problem, automatic external defibrillators (AEDs) are found in many public places, such as workplaces, shopping centers, and on airplanes. Employees are taught how to use these devices if a sudden cardiac arrest occurs.

19. B

The client is likely experiencing an imbalance between oxygen supply and myocardial oxygen demand. Administering supplemental oxygen will help to correct this imbalance and relieve the chest pain symptoms. The nurse would also notify the health care provider, establish IV access, and get a cardiac history, but the **first priority** would be to supply oxygen to the myocardium.

The nurse would not instruct the client to go elsewhere, but with input from the health care provider might call EMS to transport the client to an emergency department if he or she were stable.

20. B, C, E, F

Signs and symptoms associated with anginal chest pain include: nausea, vomiting, diaphoresis, dizziness, weakness, palpitations, and shortness of breath. Diarrhea and joint pain are not associated with anginal pain.

21. B, D

Troponin is specific for MI and cardiac necrosis. Twelve-lead ECGs allow the health care provider to examine the heart from varying perspectives. By identifying the lead(s) in which ECG changes are occurring, the health care provider can identify both the occurrence and the location of ischemia (angina) or necrosis (infarction). Chest x-ray would be useful to rule out aortic dissection, but not diagnose MI. C-reactive protein increases with inflammation or infection. It may rise after MI but is not diagnostic. Elevated lipids are a risk factor but do not diagnose MI. An exercise tolerance test (stress test) on a treadmill is used to assess for ECG changes consistent with ischemia, evaluate medical therapy, and identify those who might benefit from invasive therapy.

22. A

Before administering NTG, ensure that the male client has not taken any phosphodiesterase inhibitors for erectile dysfunction such as sildenafil, tadalafil, avanafil, or vardenafil within the past 24 to 48 hours. Use of NTG at the same time as these inhibitors can cause profound hypotension. Remind clients **not** to take these medications within 24 to 48 hours of one another.

23. C

A serious side effect of nitroglycerin is hypotension, so it is essential that any client receiving this drug by the IV route be continuously monitored for blood pressure. Research has shown that use of bedpans is more stressful to the heart than use of a bedside commode. Elevating the head of the bed at 90 degrees may not be a comfortable position for the client. Increasing the dose too rapidly could rapidly lead to hypotension.

24. B

New-onset angina is a form of unstable angina. Clients with unstable angina may present with ST segment changes on a 12-lead ECG but do **not** have changes in troponin levels. Ischemia is present but is not severe enough to cause detectable myocardial damage or cell death. If the client has new-onset angina at home, he or she should chew aspirin 325 mg (four "baby aspirins" that are 81 mg each) immediately and call 911!

25. A, B, D, E, F

All of the statements about thrombolytic therapy are accurate except option C. A client with chest pain lasting less than 15 minutes that is relieved by nitroglycerin is most likely experiencing chronic stable angina which is not treated with thrombolytics.

26. A, C, D, F

Absolute contraindications to thrombolytic therapy include: any prior intracranial hemorrhage; known structural cerebral vascular lesion (e.g., arteriovenous malformations); known malignant intracranial neoplasm (primary or metastatic); ischemic stroke within 3 months except acute ischemic stroke within 3 hours; suspected aortic dissection; active bleeding or bleeding diathesis (excluding menses); and significant closed-head or facial trauma within 3 months. Relative contraindications include: history of chronic, severe, poorly controlled hypertension and severe uncontrolled hypertension on presentation (SBP >180 mm Hg). See Table 35.4 in the text for additional relative contraindications.

27. A, D, E, F

During and after thrombolytic administration, immediately report any indications of bleeding to the cardiac health care provider or Rapid Response Team. Observe for signs of bleeding by: documenting the client's neurologic status (in case of intracranial bleeding); observing all IV sites for bleeding and patency; monitoring clotting studies; observing for signs of internal bleeding (monitor hemoglobin, hematocrit, and blood pressure.); and testing stools, urine, and emesis for occult blood.

28. C

Calcium channel blockers are prescribed for clients with chronic stable angina to promote vasodilation and myocardial perfusion. The client would be monitored for hypotension because of the vasodilation effect.

29. A, B, C, E, F

During beta-blocker therapy, monitor for: bradycardia; hypotension; decreased level of consciousness (LOC); and chest discomfort. Assess the lungs for crackles (indicative of heart failure) and wheezes (indicative of bronchospasm). Hypoglycemia, depression, nightmares, and forgetfulness are also problems with beta blockade, especially in older clients.

30. C

After the acute stages of an unstable angina episode, the cardiac health care provider often requests an exercise tolerance test (stress test) on a treadmill to assess for ECG changes consistent with ischemia, evaluate medical therapy, and identify those who might benefit from invasive therapy.

31. C

Statin therapy reduces the risk of developing recurrent MI, mortality, and stroke. Before discharge, all clients diagnosed with ACS should be started on high-intensity statin therapy despite results of lipid panel testing. High-intensity statins include atorvastatin 80 mg and rosuvastatin 20 mg to 40 mg daily.

32. A, C, E, F

Teaching about activities at home for clients with CAD would include: begin by walking the same distance at home as in the hospital (usually 400 feet) three times each day; carry nitroglycerin with you; check your pulse before, **during**, and after the exercise; stop the activity for a pulse increase of **more than 20 beats/min**, shortness of breath, angina, or dizziness; make gradual increases in walking distance; exercise outdoors when the weather is good; after an exercise tolerance test and with your health care provider's approval, walk at least three times each week, increasing the distance every other week, until the total distance is 1 mile; and avoid straining (lifting, push-ups, pull-ups, and straining at bowel movements).

33. B

Cardiac rehabilitation is the process of actively assisting the client with cardiac disease to achieve and maintain a vital and productive life while remaining within the limits of the heart's ability to respond to increases in activity and stress. Phase 1 begins with the acute illness and ends with discharge from the hospital. Assisting clients with activities of daily living is within the scope of practice for an AP. Assisting with ambulation is also acceptable, but distractor A suggests the client walk farther and more often than is appropriate for phase 1 of cardiac rehabilitation. Assessing and teaching require additional training and are within the scope of the professional RN.

34. A, B, D, E

Manifestations of cardiogenic shock include: tachycardia; hypotension; systolic BP less than 90 mm Hg or 30 mm Hg less than the client's baseline; urine output less than 0.5-1 mL/kg/hr; cold, clammy skin with poor peripheral pulses; agitation, restlessness, or confusion; pulmonary congestion; tachypnea; and continuing chest discomfort. The nurse would document and report these immediately because undiagnosed cardiogenic shock has a very high mortality.

35. A

The classic Killip system identifies four classes of heart failure based on prognosis. The class I description includes absence of crackles and S_3. See Table 35.5 for descriptions of classes II, III, and IV.

36. B

Immediate reperfusion is an invasive intervention that shows some promise for managing cardiogenic shock. The client is taken to the cardiac catheterization laboratory, and an emergency left-sided heart catheterization is performed. If the client has a treatable occlusion or occlusions, the interventional cardiologist performs a PCI in the catheterization laboratory, **or** the client is transferred to the operating suite for a coronary artery bypass graft (CABG).

37. A, C, D, F

Candidates for CABG surgery are clients who have: angina with greater than 50% occlusion of the left main coronary artery that cannot be stented; unstable angina with severe two-vessel disease, moderate three-vessel disease, or small-vessel disease in which stents could not be introduced; ischemia with heart failure; acute MI with cardiogenic shock; signs of ischemia or impending MI after angiography or percutaneous coronary intervention; valvular disease; and coronary vessels unsuitable for percutaneous coronary intervention (PCI).

38. B, C, E

To decrease risk of a sternal wound infection, the nurse would have the client shower with 4% chlorhexidine gluconate (CHG). This decreases the number of microorganisms on the skin. Surgical sites are prepared by clipping hair and applying CHG with isopropyl alcohol (either 0.5% or 2%). In addition, IV antibiotics are administered 1 hour before the surgical procedure. Research suggests that shaving a client's skin before surgery may raise the risk of an infection; thus, shaving a client's body may not protect against infection nor would sending lab specimens or wearing protective equipment.

39. A, C, D, F

For the traditional surgical procedure, explain that the client will have a sternal incision and possibly a large leg incision also; one, two, or three chest tubes; an indwelling urinary catheter; pacemaker wires; and invasive hemodynamic monitoring. An endotracheal tube will be connected to a ventilator during surgery. The endotracheal tube is removed as soon as the client is awake and stable. Tell the client and family that the client will not be able to talk while the endotracheal tube is in place. Two hours after extubation (removal of the endotracheal tube), clients should be dangled at the bedside as tolerated and turned side to side. Within 4 to 8 hours after extubation, help clients out of bed into a chair. By the first day after surgery, they should be out of bed in a chair and ambulating 25 to 100 feet three times a day as tolerated. Encourage the client to splint, cough, turn, and deep breathe to expectorate secretions.

40. D

Hypothermia is a common problem after CABG surgery. Although warm cardioplegia is now the usual operative procedure used, it is not uncommon for the body temperature to drift downward after the client leaves the surgical suite. Monitor the body temperature and institute rewarming procedures if the temperature drops below 96.8°F (36°C). Rewarming may be accomplished with warm blankets, lights, or thermal blankets. The danger of rewarming clients too quickly is that they may begin shivering, resulting in metabolic acidosis, increased myocardial oxygen consumption, and hypoxia.

41. A

Bleeding after CABG surgery occurs to a limited extent in all clients. Measure mediastinal and pleural chest tube drainage at least hourly. Report drainage amounts **over 150 mL/hr** to the surgeon.

42. B

After CABG, the nurse must distinguish between sternal and anginal pain. Typical sternotomy pain is localized, does not radiate, and often becomes worse when the client coughs or breathes deeply. He or she may describe the pain as sharp, aching, or burning. Pain may stimulate the sympathetic nervous system, which increases the heart rate and vascular resistance while decreasing cardiac output. Administer enough of the prescribed analgesic in adequate doses to control pain. Options A, C, and D are descriptors for anginal pain.

43. C

Monitor the neurovascular status of the donor arm of clients whose radial artery was used as a graft in CABG (usually the nondominant arm is used). Assess the hand color, temperature, pulse (both ulnar and radial), and capillary refill every hour initially. In addition, check the fingertips, hand, and arm for sensation and mobility at least every 4 hours (**not** once a shift).

44. B, C, D, E
After CABG surgery, the nurse would be alert for mediastinitis (infection of the mediastinum) by observing for: fever continuing beyond the first 4 days after CABG; instability (bogginess) of the sternum; redness, induration, swelling, or drainage from suture sites; and an increased white blood cell count (**not** decreased).

45. D
The nurse would monitor for hypotension (systolic BP <90 mm Hg) which is a major problem because it may result in the collapse of the coronary graft. Decreased preload can result from hypovolemia or vasodilation. If the client is hypovolemic, it might be appropriate to increase fluid administration or administer blood. The cardiac health care provider may manage the client with volume replacement followed by vasopressor therapy to increase the BP. However, if hypotension is the result of left ventricular failure, IV inotropes (e.g., dopamine, dobutamine) might be needed.

46. C
After MIDCAB surgery, the nurse assesses for chest pain and ECG changes (Q waves and ST-segment and T-wave changes in leads V_2 to V_6) because occlusion of the internal mammary artery (IMA) graft occurs acutely in only a small percentage of clients. If there is any question of acute graft closure, immediately notify the surgeon.

47. B
Clients who are most likely to benefit from PCI have single- or double-vessel disease with discrete, proximal, noncalcified lesions or clots.

48. B, C, D, F
Clients who undergo PCI are required to take dual antiplatelet therapy (DAPT) consisting of aspirin and a platelet inhibitor (see Table 35.3 in your text). The health care provider also prescribes a long-term nitrate and beta blocker. An angiotensin-converting enzyme (ACE) inhibitor or angiotensin receptor blocker (ARB) is added for clients who have had primary angioplasty after an MI.

49. B, C, F
Robotic heart surgery is a step toward less invasive open-heart surgery. Surgeons operate endoscopically through very small incisions in the chest wall. Other advantages of robotic procedures include shorter hospital stays (average stay is 2 to 3 days), less pain because of smaller incisions, **no need for** heart-lung bypass machine, less anxiety for the client, and greater client acceptance, as well as increased ability to reach otherwise inaccessible blockage sites.

50. A, B, D, E
Additional therapies can aid in reducing the client's anxiety about progressive activity both in the immediate postoperative period and during the rehabilitation phase. Techniques such as progressive muscle relaxation, guided imagery, music therapy, pet therapy, and therapeutic touch may decrease anxiety, reduce depression, and increase adherence with activity and exercise regimens after heart surgery.

36 CHAPTER

Assessment of the Hematologic System

1. Reduced function of which organs will the nurse recognize as possible causes of hematologic problems? **Select all that apply**.
   A. Bone marrow
   B. Brain
   C. Heart
   D. Kidney
   E. Liver
   F. Pancreas
   G. Spleen

2. Which assessment findings on an older adult client will the nurse associate with age-related changes rather than a specific hematologic problem? **Select all that apply**.
   A. Bleeding gums
   B. Dry skin on distal extremities
   C. Pale lips
   D. Smooth tongue
   E. Sparse facial hair
   F. Bright yellow-tinged sclera
   G. Pallor around the mouth
   H. Petechiae on the skin of the abdomen

3. Which substances are essential for proper erythrocyte production? **Select all that apply**.
   A. Cobalt
   B. Copper
   C. Folic acid
   D. Iron
   E. Nickel
   F. Pyridoxine
   G. Vitamin B_{12}

4. Which assessment is **most relevant** for the nurse to perform with a client who reports having undergone a splenectomy several years ago?
   A. Indications of bleeding
   B. Signs of infection
   C. Digestive problems
   D. Jaundice of the skin

5. Which body area on a client with darker skin will the nurse examine for indications of pallor and cyanosis?
   A. Sclera closest to the iris
   B. Oral mucous membranes
   C. General appearance of face
   D. Earlobes and bridge of the nose

6. Which assessment finding will the nurse expect to see in a client who has low serum albumin levels?
   A. Pain
   B. Fever
   C. Edema
   D. Bruising

7. Which subjective symptoms will the nurse expect to be reported by a client with very low hematocrit and hemoglobin levels? **Select all that apply**.
   A. Fatigue
   B. Night sweats
   C. Calf pain
   D. Blood in urine
   E. Shortness of breath
   F. Loss of taste discrimination

8. Which questions are **most relevant** for the nurse to ask a client who has a decrease in hematologic function? **Select all that apply**.
   A. "Do you travel a lot for work or pleasure?"
   B. "Have you ever had any radiation therapy for cancer?"
   C. "Have you ever donated blood or plasma?"
   D. "Does anyone in your family have a blood disorder?"
   E. "What drugs have you used in the past 3 days?"
   F. "Have you ever had a job that exposed you to chemicals?"

9. Which assessment action will the nurse **avoid** to **prevent harm** in a client who is suspected of having a hematologic problem?
   A. Palpating the edge of the liver in the right upper quadrant
   B. Auscultating the heart for abnormal heart sounds or irregular rhythms
   C. Using the fingertips to firmly press over the ribs or sternum
   D. Palpating the left upper quadrant to locate an enlarged spleen

10. With which client will the nurse use the action of applying pressure for 10 minutes at the site of an IV removal to **prevent harm** by reducing the risk for excessive bleeding?
    A. 28-year-old who has a deficiency of protein C
    B. 42-year-old who received a blood transfusion earlier today
    C. 58-year-old with chronic alcoholism and a protein-deficient diet
    D. 62-year-old who is 50 lb overweight and has chronic heart failure

11. For which health problems will the nurse recognize that a client with an antithrombin III deficiency has an increased risk? **Select all that apply**.
    A. Pulmonary embolism
    B. Myocardial infarction
    C. Iron deficiency anemia
    D. Pernicious anemia
    E. Hemolytic anemia
    F. Stroke

12. What action will the nurse take when a client's laboratory results indicate the platelet count is 400,000/mm^3 (400 $\times$ 10^9/L)?
    A. Immediately inform the primary health care provider because of possible spontaneous bleeding.
    B. Instruct assistive personnel (AP) to handle the client gently.
    C. Apply oxygen to improve gas exchange.
    D. Document the result as the only action.

13. Which laboratory value in a client receiving an erythrocyte-stimulating agent (ESA) best indicates to the nurse that the drug is effective?
    A. International normalized ratio of 2.0
    B. Platelet count of 150,000/mm^3 (150 $\times$ 10^9/L)
    C. White blood cell (WBC) count of 9000/mm^3 (9 $\times$ 10^9/L)
    D. Red blood cell (RBC) count of 4.4 $\times$ 10^6/μL (4.4 $\times$ 10^{12}/L)

14. Which increased dietary intake will a nurse suggest to a 35-year-old female client who has heavy menstrual periods?
    A. Red meat and protein sources high in iron
    B. Leafy green vegetables high in vitamin K
    C. Citrus fruit and other food high in vitamin C
    D. Milk and dairy products high in calcium

15. Which instruction is **most important** for the nurse to give to an assistive personnel (AP) to **prevent harm** when providing care to a client who has a low platelet count?
    A. Allow the client to rest between care activities to prevent fatigue.
    B. Report a temperature elevation immediately to identify infection.
    C. Record the client's liquid intake accurately to ensure hydration.
    D. Handle the client gently to avoid bruising.

16. Which assessment finding does the nurse expect to observe in a client who has greatly decreased hematocrit and hemoglobin levels?
    A. Hypotension
    B. Increased bowel sounds
    C. Unilateral swelling of a lower leg
    D. Neck vein distension in the upright position

17. What is the **best** explanation for the nurse to provide to a client with a possible hematologic problem for why a bone marrow aspiration has been ordered?
    A. Establishes whether you are a carrier for sickle cell anemia
    B. Distinguishes between chronic and acute blood loss
    C. Identifies any problems in blood cell production
    D. Determines the source of chronic infection

18. Which of the client's usual activities does the nurse instruct a 50-year-old to **avoid** for about 48 hours to **prevent harm** after a bone marrow biopsy? **Select all that apply**.
    A. Attending a religious service with his family
    B. Playing basketball with his son at the gym
    C. Hanging outdoor Christmas lights
    D. Repairing a neighbor's computer
    E. Taking a low-dose aspirin
    F. Hosting a poker party

Chapter 36 Answer Key

1. A, D, E, G
   The bone marrow is responsible for the production of all blood cells. Decreased functional bone marrow always causes hematologic problems. The kidney secretes erythropoietin, which triggers the bone marrow to produce red blood cells. Anemia is a problem when kidney function is chronically decreased. The liver is responsible for producing the clotting factors and albumin. With decreased liver function, blood clotting problems occur as does a loss of blood viscosity and volume. The spleen stores platelets and degrades old red blood cells. Many spleen problems reduce the number of platelets, which causes bleeding problems. The brain, heart, and pancreas have no direct role in maintaining hematologic function.

2. B, E, G
   Skin on older adults dries with aging and loses color. Color loss makes skin appear pale or slightly yellow-tinged, which is not jaundice; however, bright or dark yellow sclera usually indicate jaundice and should be investigated further. Hair everywhere decreases in thickness and turns gray. Facial hair thinning and pubic hair loss is common. Bleeding gums are never considered normal and can indicate a periodontal or hematologic problem. Although skin becomes more pale, lips should retain a deep red color. The normal tongue has bumps and shallow creases, even in older adults. A smooth tongue is an indicator of some types of anemia. Petechiae, especially if not occurring in response to trauma, is an indicator of a possible hematologic problem and needs to be explored further.

3. A, B, C, D, E, F, G
   Although some substances are only required in trace amounts for adequate erythrocyte production, all are essential for ensuring that sufficient and well-functioning erythrocytes are produced to maintain normal tissue perfusion and gas exchange.

4. **B**

   In addition to having several functions involved in maintaining hematologic function, the spleen also filters antigens and is the site of antibody production. Anyone who has had a splenectomy has reduced immune functions and an increased risk for infection and sepsis.

5. **B**

   Pallor and cyanosis are more easily detected in adults with darker skin by examining the oral mucous membranes and the conjunctiva of the eye, not the sclera closest to the iris. Jaundice can be seen more easily on the roof of the mouth.

6. **C**

   Serum albumin and proteins maintain the osmotic pressure of the blood, preventing the plasma from leaking into the tissues. When clients have low albumin levels, peripheral edema occurs. Low albumin levels alone do not increase the risk for bleeding or fever. Pain is not associated with low albumin levels.

7. **A, E**

   The most common symptom of anemia with low hematocrit and hemoglobin levels is fatigue as a result of decreased oxygen delivery to cells. When blood problems reduce oxygen delivery, the lungs work harder to maintain tissue perfusion, which is manifested as shortness of breath at rest or on exertion. None of the other symptoms are associated with low hematocrit and hemoglobin levels.

8. **B, D, F**

   Radiation for cancer therapy can decrease bone marrow production of blood cells or increase the risk of hematologic malignancies depending on which body area is in the radiation path. Many hematologic disorders have a genetic basis or a familial predisposition. Exposures to a variety of chemical agents can damage the bone marrow and result in many hematologic problems.

   Travel is not known to induce decreases in hematologic function and neither does blood or plasma donation when proper spacing of donations is observed. Although some drugs can reduce hematologic function, longer than a 3-day use is needed for this to occur.

9. **D**

   The normal adult spleen is usually *not* palpable, but an enlarged spleen occurs with many hematologic problems. An enlarged spleen may be detected by palpation, but this is usually performed by the primary health care provider because an enlarged spleen is tender and ruptures easily, which can lead to hemorrhage and death.

10. **C**

    All liver functions are profoundly reduced by chronic alcoholism. Whenever liver function is reduced, such as with liver damage from alcoholism coupled with a low protein diet, the production of clotting factors is below normal and the risk for bleeding greatly increases, even after minor trauma. Receiving a blood transfusion does not increase bleeding risk, neither do obesity and heart failure. Insufficient levels of protein C increases clot formation and does not increase the risk for bleeding.

11. **A, B, F**

    Antithrombin III is a naturally occurring substance that inactivates thrombin and clotting factors IX and X. These actions prevent clots from becoming too large or forming in an area where clotting is not needed. Deficiency of antithrombin III increases clotting and the risk for any problem associated with a venous thromboembolism such as pulmonary embolism, myocardial infarction, and stroke. Anemia of any type is not associated with an antithrombin III deficiency.

12. **D**

    The client's platelet count is within the normal limits and requires no action beyond ensuring documentation.

13. **D**

    ESAs are a synthetic form of erythropoietin, which is a growth factor for specific red blood cells (RBCs, erythrocytes). Its purpose is to raise a client's RBC count to normal or near normal levels ($4.2\text{-}6.1 \times 10^6/\mu L$ ($4.2\text{-}6.1 \times 10^{12}/L$). Although ESAs can increase other cell production somewhat, because its purpose is to increase RBC production, the nurse will assess this laboratory test to evaluate the effectiveness.

14. A

Women have lower red blood cell (RBC) counts than do men. This difference is greater during menstrual years because menstrual blood loss may occur faster than blood cell production. These clients can prevent iron deficiency anemia by increasing their intake of iron-containing foods, such as red meat and proteins. Dairy productions are very low in iron content. Vitamin K does not increase RBCs and hemoglobin levels. Although vitamin C has many roles in good health, it is not the main nutrient needed for RBC and hemoglobin production.

15. D

Clients with low platelet counts are at high risk for bleeding and bruising. These clients must be handled carefully to prevent harm. They are not at particular risk for fatigue, infection, or dehydration.

16. A

Low hematocrit and hemoglobin levels result in blood with a decreased osmotic pressure and low blood pressure. Neck vein distension is more common with hypertension or with right-sided heart failure, not anemia. Unilateral swelling of a lower leg occurs with a venous thromboembolism. Bowel sounds are not directly affected by changes in hematocrit or hemoglobin.

17. C

Bone marrow aspiration and biopsy help evaluate a client's hematologic status when other tests show abnormal findings that indicate a possible problem in blood cell production or maturation. These tests are not used to assess chronicity of blood loss, carrier status for sickle cell disease, or a possible source of chronic infection.

18. B, C, E

After either a bone marrow aspiration or biopsy procedure, the client is advised to avoid any activity that might result in trauma to the site for 48 hours. In addition, aspirin or other drugs that increase the risk for bleeding are avoided. The client is not at risk for contagious infectious diseases as a result of the procedure alone. Thus, instructions for care after the procedure do not include avoiding contact with crowds.

37 CHAPTER

Concepts of Care for Patients with Hematologic Problems

1. Which client does the nurse recognize as most likely to have sickle cell trait?
   A. Parents both have sickle cell disease.
   B. Parents both have two hemoglobin A gene alleles.
   C. Mother has sickle cell disease and father has hemoglobin A gene alleles.
   D. Father has sickle cell trait and mother has hemoglobin A gene alleles.

2. Which questions about the past 48 hours will the nurse ask a client admitted in sickle cell crisis to obtain **relevant** information about the cause of the current crisis? **Select all that apply**.
   A. "Do you have a cough or fever?"
   B. "Have you traveled by airplane?"
   C. "What activities make you short of breath?"
   D. "What physical activity have you performed?"
   E. "Have you consumed alcohol or smoked cigarettes?"
   F. "Do you have any pain or burning when you urinate?"

3. Which fluid will the nurse expect to infuse for a client admitted in sickle cell crisis who is prescribed intravenous hydration therapy?
   A. Half-normal saline (0.45% NaCl)
   B. Lactated Ringer's solution
   C. Normal saline (0.9% NaCl)
   D. Fresh frozen plasma

4. What are the **priority actions** for the nurse to perform when caring for a client in sickle cell crisis? **Select all that apply**.
   A. Managing pain
   B. Ensuring hydration
   C. Preventing malnutrition
   D. Administering platelets
   E. Assessing oxygen saturation
   F. Monitoring for indications of infection

5. Which laboratory value in a client with sickle cell disease (SCD) does the nurse report immediately to the health care provider?
   A. Hematocrit 24%
   B. Hemoglobin S (HbS) 78%
   C. Platelet count 260,000/mm^3
   D. White blood cell (WBC) count 20,000/mm^3

6. Which new assessment finding in a client with sickle cell disease who currently is in crises does the nurse report immediately to the primary health care provider to **prevent harm**?
   A. Facial drooping on the right side
   B. Slow capillary refill in the toes of the right foot
   C. Yellow appearance of the roof of the mouth
   D. Pain in the right hip with limited range of motion

7. Which action will the nurse take to prevent vascular occlusion in the client with sickle cell disease?
   A. Assessing pulse oximetry every 2 hours.
   B. Administering morphine sulfate every 6 hours.
   C. Keeping the room temperature at or below 68°F.
   D. Maintaining an oral fluid intake of at least 4500 mL/day.

8. Which action does the nurse instruct assistive personnel (AP) to **avoid** to **prevent harm** when caring for a client in sickle cell crisis?
   A. Elevating the head of the bed to 25 degrees
   B. Helping to remove any restrictive clothing
   C. Taking blood pressure with an external cuff
   D. Encouraging the client to drink more water

9. Which assessment finding alerts the home care nurse to the possibility of infection in the client with sickle cell disease (SCD) who is recovering from a crisis episode?
   A. Oral temperature of 37.8°C (100°F)
   B. Diminished breath sounds unilaterally
   C. Firm nodular texture to the liver on palpation
   D. Darkened areas of skin on the lower extremities

10. Which signs and symptoms does the nurse expect to find in clients with any type of anemia? **Select all that apply**.
    A. Exercise intolerance
    B. Fatigue
    C. Glossitis
    D. Jaundice
    E. Leukopenia
    F. Microcytic red blood cells
    G. Paresthesias of the hands and feet
    H. Tachycardia
    I. Tachypnea

11. With which member of the interprofessional team will the nurse collaborate when providing instructions for a client who has anemia caused by folic acid deficiency?
    A. Physical therapist
    B. Mental health professional
    C. Registered dietitian nutritionist
    D. Wound care specialty nurse

12. Which common agent(s) will the nurse teach the client newly diagnosed with glucose-6-phosphate dehydrogenase deficiency anemia to **avoid** to **prevent harm**?
    A. Laxatives
    B. Aspirin
    C. Caffeine
    D. Alcohol

13. Which menu selection made by the client with B_{12} deficiency anemia demonstrates to the nurse an adequate understanding of dietary management for this problem?
    A. Fried liver and onions, orange juice, spinach salad
    B. Baked chicken breast, boiled carrots, glass of white wine
    C. Eggplant Parmesan, cream-style cottage cheese, iced tea.
    D. Whole grain pasta with cheese, apple sauce, glass of red wine.

14. Which assessment finding does the nurse expect in a client who has polycythemia vera (PV)?
    A. Elevated temperature
    B. Decreased respiratory rate
    C. Increased blood pressure
    D. Rapid thready pulse

15. Which precautions are **most important** for the nurse to teach the client with polycythemia vera (PV) to **prevent harm**?
    A. Shower or bathe daily.
    B. Use a soft-bristled toothbrush.
    C. Restrict fluids to 2 L/day.
    D. Elevate your feet whenever you are seated.
    E. Wear gloves and socks outdoors in cool weather.
    F. Exercise slowly and only on the advice of your primary health care provider.

16. Which questions are **most relevant** for the nurse to ask when exploring the risk factors for the client newly diagnosed with acute leukemia? **Select all that apply**.
    A. "How many packs of cigarettes per day do you smoke and for how many years have you smoked?"
    B. "Have you ever been treated for a sexually transmitted infection?"
    C. "Have you ever been exposed to radioactive materials?"
    D. "How old was your mother when you were born?"
    E. "Has anyone in your family ever had leukemia?"
    F. "What type of work do your do for a living?"

17. What is the nurse's **best response** when a client newly diagnosed with leukemia asks why infection precautions are needed even though his white blood cell (WBC) count is so high?
    A. "We are preparing you for the decrease in white blood cell when you start chemotherapy."
    B. "The white blood cells you are producing now are too immature to prevent or fight infection."
    C. "Your white blood cell count is falsely high because of the severe dehydration that occurs with leukemia."
    D. "It is the platelets, not your white blood cells, that protect you from infection and your platelet count is low."

18. Which signs and symptoms will the nurse expect on assessment of a client newly diagnosed with acute leukemia before initiation of treatment? **Select all that apply**.
    A. Finger clubbing
    B. Excessive bruising
    C. Bone pain
    D. Dyspnea on exertion
    E. Fatigue
    F. Facial flushing

19. Which collaborative problem will the nurse consider to have the highest **priority** when caring for a client with acute leukemia?
    A. Providing pain control
    B. Helping the client conserve energy
    C. Protecting the client from infection
    D. Minimizing the side effects of chemotherapy

20. Which precautions are **most important** for the nurse to teach a client with leukemia to prevent an infection by autocontamination? **Select all that apply**.
    A. Avoid crowds and people who are ill.
    B. Take antibiotics exactly as prescribed.
    C. Perform mouth care three times daily.
    D. Avoid eating undercooked meat and eggs.
    E. Report any burning on urination immediately.
    F. Shower or wash your armpits and genital area daily.

21. What is the nurse's **best action** when a client being treated for leukemia develops a temperature that is 1°F (0.5°C) above his or her baseline?
    A. Recheck the temperature in 2 hours.
    D. Administer two 325 mg tablets of acetaminophen.
    C. Initiate the unit's standard neutropenic infection protocol.
    D. Document the temperature and other vital signs as the only action.

22. Which laboratory value indicates to the nurse that a client's conditioning regimen before hematopoietic stem cell transplantation (HSCT) for acute leukemia is successful?
    A. Total white blood cell count of 8,000/mm³ (8×10^9/L)
    B. Total white blood cell count of 0/mm³ (0×10^9/L)
    C. Reticulocyte count of 0.5%-2.0% of erythrocytes
    D. Hematocrit of 25% (0.25 volume fraction)

23. For which type of leukemia will the nurse expect to administer imatinib mesylate to the client?
    A. Acute lymphocytic leukemia that has normal chromosomes
    B. Acute myelogenous leukemia that has abnormal chromosomes
    C. Chronic myelogenous leukemia that is Philadelphia chromosome positive
    D. Chronic lymphocytic leukemia that is Philadelphia chromosome negative

24. How will the nurse interpret the laboratory findings of rising white blood cell, erythrocyte, and platelet counts for a client who had a hematopoietic stem cell transplant (HSCT) 4 weeks ago?
    A. Transplant has engrafted.
    B. Client has a systemic infection.
    C. Leukemia is no longer in remission.
    D. Client has graft-versus-host disease.

25. Which care action will the nurse **avoid** to **prevent harm** when caring for a client with leukemia whose platelet count is 50,000/mm^3 (50 × 10^9/L)?
    A. Bathing the client
    B. Administering an enema
    C. Applying pressure to an injection site
    D. Encouraging the use of incentive spirometry

26. Which assessments are a **priority** for the nurse to perform daily to identify the possible presence of sinusoidal obstructive syndrome (SOS) in a client who has had a hematopoietic stem cell transplant (HSCT)? **Select all that apply**.
    A. Weight
    B. Liver size
    C. Joint pain
    D. Abdominal girth
    E. Peripheral vein texture
    F. Color of skin and sclera

27. Which new-onset client health problem will the nurse consider a possible side effect of erythropoiesis-stimulating agent (ESA) therapy?
    A. Loss of taste sensation
    B. Pain on urination
    C. Intense diarrhea
    D. Hypertension

28. Which possible risk factors will the nurse assess for in a client who is newly diagnosed with non-Hodgkin lymphoma (NHL)? **Select all that apply**.
    A. History of an immunosuppressive disorder
    B. Chronic infection with *Helicobacter pylori*
    C. Previous infection with Epstein-Barr virus
    D. Exposure to pesticides and insecticides
    E. Smoking cigars or cigarettes
    F. Chronic alcoholism

29. Which questions are **most relevant** for the nurse to ask a client who has several very enlarged lymph nodes to assess whether any constitutional symptoms of lymphoma are present? **Select all that apply**.
    A. Has your weight changed in the past month?
    B. Do you have any problems with balance?
    C. Is there any blood in your urine or stool?
    D. How often do you have headaches?
    E. Do you sweat heavily at night?
    F. Have you noticed any fever?

30. Which action is **most important** for the nurse to instruct assistive personnel when caring for a client who has thrombotic thrombocytopenic purpura (TTP)?
    A. Handling the client very gently to minimize bruising
    B. Wearing a mask when caring for the client to prevent infection
    C. Encouraging the client to drink fluids to prevent dehydration
    D. Assisting the client to stand to prevent falls related to weakness

31. Which collaborative problem will the nurse consider to have the highest **priority** when caring for a client with multiple myeloma?
    A. Providing pain control
    B. Helping the client conserve energy
    C. Protecting the client from infection
    D. Minimizing the side effects of chemotherapy

32. Which assessment is **most important** for the nurse to perform for the client receiving 1 unit of packed red blood cells from an autologous donation?
    A. Temperature
    B. Blood pressure
    C. Oxygen saturation
    D. IV site assessment for hives

33. What is the nurse's **best first action** to **prevent harm** when an older client, receiving the third unit of packed red blood cells in the past 8 hours, has distended neck veins in the sitting position?
    A. Slow the infusion rate.
    B. Discontinue the transfusion.
    C. Document the observation as the only action.
    D. Check the type of infusing blood with the client's blood type.

34. Which change in a client's laboratory values will the nurse attribute to a blood transfusion?
    A. Blood glucose decrease
    B. Serum sodium 133 mEq/L (mmol/L)
    C. Serum potassium 5.2 mEq/L (mmol/L)
    D. White blood cell count decease to 4,000/mm^3 (4 × 10^9/L)

35. What is the **first priority action** the nurse will take to **prevent harm** when recognizing that a client is having a hemolytic transfusion reaction?
    A. Flushing the blood tubing with normal saline
    B. Initiating the Rapid Response Team
    C. Applying oxygen via face mask
    D. Stopping the transfusion

36. Which type of transfusion reaction does the nurse suspect when a client develops fever, chills, tachycardia, and hypotension during a blood transfusion?
    A. Allergic
    B. Bacterial
    C. Circulatory overload
    D. Graft-versus-host disease

Chapter 37 Answer Key

1. C
   SCD is an autosomal recessive disorder in which clients have two mutated (abnormal) gene alleles for hemoglobin (hemoglobin S) instead of the normal alleles (hemoglobin A). A person who has only one hemoglobin S gene allele and one normal adult hemoglobin A gene allele has sickle cell trait. In option C, the mother can only contribute an S gene allele to her offspring and the father can only contribute a hemoglobin A gene allele. Any offspring of this couple will have sickle cell trait. In option A, any child this couple produces will have two S gene alleles and will have SCD. In option B, any child this couple produces will have two A gene alleles and will have not have either SCD or sickle cell trait. In option D, any offspring this couple produces has a 50% chance of inheriting one gene allele for the trait and no chance for inheriting two alleles for SCD.

2. A, B, C, D, E, F
   All of these questions will obtain relevant information about factors that can reduce gas exchange and oxygenation and increase the risk for a crisis.

3. A
   Usually the client's blood is hypertonic during periods of crisis. To prevent further impeding of blood flow and to correct dehydration, hypotonic fluids are used. Plasma is hypertonic. Normal saline and lactated Ringer's are both isotonic. Half-normal saline (0.45%) is hypotonic.

4. A, B, E, F
Hypoxia is a cause of crises and adequate oxygen therapy is critical. Thus, monitoring oxygen saturation to determine therapy effectiveness is a priority. Pain during crises is severe and usually requires opioid analgesics. Hydration helps reduce the duration of sickling episodes and pain. Clients with SCD are always at risk for infection and the risk is greater during crises. Prevention and early detection monitoring are a priority to protect the patient in sickle cell crisis from infection.

Platelet transfusions are not commonly prescribed.

Ensuring adequate nutrition overall is not a priority during an episode of sickle cell crisis.

5. D
Clients with SCD are usually anemic and the hematocrit level is not critical at this time. The fact that the HbS level is 78% is an expected finding and not one that the health care provider needs to know at this time. The platelet count is lower than normal, but not low enough to lead to uncontrolled bleeding. The WBCs are elevated and indicates the presence of an acute infection. The primary health care provider needs to be notified immediately and the proper interventions instituted.

6. A
All current assessment findings are important. However, the pain in the hip, the slow capillary refill, and the yellow appearance of the roof of the mouth are related to the crises and are expected. The facial drooping as a new finding indicates the possibility of reduced brain perfusion and stroke, which requires immediate attention and intervention.

7. D
Venous stasis causes vascular occlusion. Maintaining hydration prevents venous stasis and vascular occlusion.

8. C
Using an external blood pressure cuff, even for a minute, stops blood flow to the distal arm and causes tissue hypoxia/anoxia in it. The low oxygen tension in that tissue then increases

sickling in that extremity and increases the risk for ischemic injury.

9. B
The client with sickle cell disease (SCD) is more susceptible to infections with encapsulated microorganisms such as *Streptococcus pneumoniae*. Diminished breath sounds, especially if unilateral, indicate possible pneumonia. The other signs and symptoms are expected changes.

10. A, B, H, I
With any type of anemia, the number or quality of red blood cells is low, thus reducing oxygen perfusion to all tissues. This results in fatigue with exercise intolerance. Tachycardia is a compensatory mechanism to help maintain oxygen perfusion, as is the increased respiratory rate of tachypnea. Jaundice is present only when anemia is caused by red blood cell damage and destruction with release of hemoglobin and not by anemia caused by blood loss or deficiencies of iron or B_{12}. Glossitis is associated only with deficiencies of folic acid and B_{12}. Iron deficiency anemia results in microcytic red blood cells, whereas B_{12} deficiency causes macrocytic red blood cells. Red blood cell size is not affected by most other types of anemia. Paresthesias of the hands and feet are associated with B_{12} deficiencies severe enough to alter nerve function.

11. C
Folic acid deficiency anemia is most often caused by poor nutrition, especially a diet lacking green leafy vegetables, liver, yeast, citrus fruits, dried beans, and nuts. This anemia is managed initially with scheduled folic acid replacement therapy and continued nutrition therapy to prevent recurrence.

12. B
Cells with reduced amounts of glucose-6-phosphate dehydrogenase are more susceptible to hemolysis on exposure to aspirin and other drugs.

13. A
Organ meats and leafy green vegetables have the highest content of vitamin B_{12}. Dairy products and most grains are deficient in B_{12}.

14. C

In PV the number of RBCs (and all other blood cells) is greater than normal, making the blood thicker than normal blood. The thick blood moves more slowly and causes hypertension. The pulse is bounding and the respiratory rate is increased because the disorder reduces gas exchange. An elevated temperature is not an expected or common assessment finding in PV unless an infection is present.

15. B, D, E, F

Using a soft-bristled toothbrush minimizes trauma to the gums and prevents bleeding.

Precautions D, E, and F focus on preventing harm from venous stasis, clot formation, and myocardial infarction.

Although showering or bathing daily is a good health plan, clients with PV are not at increased risk for infection from autocontamination.

Fluid intake is recommended to be increased, not decreased to prevent harm.

16. C, E, F

A major risk factor for development of leukemia is exposure to ionizing radiation. Other risk factors include chemical exposures and genetic predisposition.

Cigarette smoking is not a risk factor for leukemia. Neither maternal age nor a history of sexually transmitted infections is associated with leukemia development.

17. B

Leukemia is an overproduction of very immature white blood cells that are nonfunctional. The excessive bone marrow production of these cells limits production of mature leukocytes that are capable of mounting appropriate responses to protect the client from infection. Thus, the risk for infection is greatly increased even before chemotherapy is started. Even if the client is dehydrated, it cannot account for a very high WBC count. Platelets do not protect against infection.

18. B, C, D, E

In acute leukemia, immature white blood cells (WBCs) are overproduced and other blood cell types are low. The rapid production of WBCs in the marrow contributes to bone pain. Low platelet counts cause bleeding and excessive bruising. Low red blood cell counts reduce gas exchange leading to fatigue and dyspnea on exertion.

Finger clubbing is not present because it requires hypoxemia of long duration.

Facial pallor, not flushing, would be present.

19. C

All the listed collaborative problems are important; however, infection prevention has the highest priority because clients are at risk for infection before, during, and for a while after treatment is completed.

20. C, F

Autocontamination is infection through the overgrowth of the client's normal flora (microbiome) that enters his or her internal environment (usually from the mouth or skin). Showering daily helps reduce organisms on the skin. If the client is unable to completely shower, washing the armpits and perineal areas help prevent autocontamination. Meticulous mouth care also prevents autocontamination.

Taking antibiotics does not prevent autocontamination and neither does reporting symptoms of an infection.

Avoiding crowds and people who are will helps prevent cross-contamination (from another person).

21. C

Clients being treated for leukemia are neutropenic and seldom have the typical indications of infection and are at high risk for sepsis and death. This temperature elevation is considered an indication of infection and the standard protocols for obtaining cultures and a chest x-ray, as well as starting antibiotic therapy are performed at once.

22. B

The purpose of pretransplant conditioning is to "wipe out" the client's existing bone marrow cells. A circulating white blood cell count of 0 indicates successful conditioning.

23. C

Imatinib mesylate is targeted therapy for chronic myelogenous leukemia (CML) that is Philadephia chromosome positive. This drug prevents the activation of an enzyme (tyrosine kinase) needed for growth of CML cells that overexpress the *abl* oncogene. This expression is associated with the presence of one or more Philadelphia chromosomes in the leukemia cells. The drug is not effective in leukemia that does not express the Philadelphia chromosome.

24. A

Because the pretransplant conditioning regimen has destroyed the client's own functional bone marrow, rising white blood cell, erythrocyte, and platelet counts indicate that the transplanted marrow has successfully implanted and is reproducing (engraftment).

25. B

The normal range for platelets is 150,000 to 400,000/mm^3 (150 to 400 $\times$ 10^9/L). The client's count is low and bleeding is possible with even slight trauma, such as could occur by administering an enema. The other actions do not increase bleeding risk.

26. A, B, D, F

A complication of HSCT is SOS in which blockage of liver blood vessels by clotting and inflammation (phlebitis) occurs and can be life-threatening. Symptoms include jaundice, pain in the right upper quadrant, ascites, weight gain, and liver enlargement.

Neither the peripheral veins nor the joints are involved in this complication.

27. D

Although ESAs have the intended response of increasing the production of red blood cells, other cell types also have a somewhat increased production. This causes thicker blood that results in hypertension.

28. A, B, C, D

Possible causes of NHL include viral infections (e.g., Epstein-Barr virus [EBV], human T-cell leukemia/lymphoma virus [HTLV], and human immunodeficiency virus [HIV]) and exposure to chemicals, especially pesticides and insecticides. Chronic infection from *Helicobacter pylori* is associated with a type of NHL called mucosa-associated lymphoid tissue (MALT) lymphoma.

Although chronic alcoholism and cigarette smoking are both associated with an increased risk for some types of cancer, this is not true for lymphoma.

29. A, E, F

Some clients with lymphoma have persistent constitutional symptoms that are used to help with diagnosis and prognosis. These include fevers (temperature >101.5°F [>38.6°C]), drenching night sweats, and unplanned weight loss of 10% or more of normal body weight.

Headaches, hematuria, and issues with balance are not part of constitutional symptoms.

30. A

The client with TTP has reduced platelet counts and is at high risk for excessive bleeding with even minor trauma. The client is not at risk for infection, dehydration, or falls related to this health problem.

31. A

All the listed collaborative problems are important; however, pain control has the highest priority for this client. This disorder destroys bone and causes intense pain that interferes with mobility and greatly reduces all aspects of the client's quality of life.

32. A

In an autologous blood transfusion, the client is receiving his or her own blood components. Thus, the chances for an incompatibility reaction do not exist. The main problems that can come from such a transfusion are infection from blood contamination during the collection, storage, or infusion processes and fluid overload. Fluid overload is very unlikely when only 1 unit is being transfused. Contamination and infection are just as likely with an autologous transfusion as they are with a transfusion of donated blood products. Thus, the most important assessment is for signs of infection, including temperature.

33. A

Older clients are at risk for developing fluid overload during transfusion therapy, especially when receiving multiple units of packed red blood cells (which have a high osmotic pressure that draws interstitial fluid into the vascular space). The nurse will slow the infusion rate to as low as possible, even before the client's circulatory status is assessed, to prevent worsening of the problem.

34. C

Red blood cells contain high concentrations of potassium and some cells are broken open during a transfusion. This releases intracellular potassium into the blood, causing hyperkalemia.

35. D

A hemolytic transfusion reaction most often occurs because the client has a different blood type than the blood being transfused. This problem is potentially life threatening and the nurse must prevent more blood from entering the client and increasing the reaction. So, the first priority is to stop the infusion and then apply oxygen while another health care worker notifies the Rapid Response Team. The nurse does not flush the blood tubing with normal saline because this action forces more blood into the client and worsens the reaction.

36. B

Bacterial transfusion reactions occur when the blood product being transfused has been contaminated. Indications include fever, chills, tachycardia, and hypotension.

Assessment of the Nervous System

CHAPTER 38

1. Which are the nurse's **priority** concepts during assessment of a client with a neurologic problem? **Select all that apply.**
   A. Fluid and electrolyte balance
   B. Sensory perception
   C. Perfusion
   D. Cognition
   E. Mobility
   F. Acid-base balance

2. Which type of neuron is the nurse assessing when asking a client to lift one leg and then the other?
   A. Motor
   B. Sensory
   C. Afferent
   D. Synaptic knob

3. Which functions will the nurse assess as cerebellar when checking a client's neurologic status? **Select all that apply.**
   A. Keeping an extremity from overshooting an intended target
   B. Moving from one skilled movement to another in an orderly sequence
   C. Controlling involuntary movement
   D. Maintaining equilibrium
   E. Predicting distance or gauging the speed with which one is approaching an object
   F. Controlling awakeness and awareness

4. Which assessment finding indicates to the nurse that a client's reticular activating system (RAS) is functioning normally?
   A. The client awakens from sleep in response to a loud noise.
   B. The client can move all four extremities.
   C. The client's respirations are within normal range.
   D. The client can sense sharp and dull stimuli.

5. What is the nurse's **priority** concern when a client has an ischemic brainstem stroke with damage to the medulla area of the brain?
   A. Increased intracranial pressure
   B. Seizure activity
   C. Respiratory arrest
   D. Brainstem herniation

6. Which client does the nurse find at the **greatest** disadvantage with regard to the blood-brain barrier (BBB)?
   A. Client with pneumonia who needs supplemental oxygen
   B. Client who is dehydrated and needs IV fluids to correct fluid status
   C. Client in need of major surgery and requires general anesthesia
   D. Client with bacterial meningitis in need of antibiotics

7. Which change will the nurse expect to observe when a client's sympathetic nervous system is stimulated?
   A. Increased salivation
   B. Increased heart rate
   C. Myoclonus in the muscles
   D. Hyperactive deep tendon reflexes

8. Which teaching strategy is best for the nurse to use when instructing an older adult about medications and lifestyle changes?
   A. Relate the information to recent events.
   B. Provide teaching late in the afternoon.
   C. Allow extra time for teaching and questions.
   D. Give limited and simplified information.

9. Which interventions will the nurse employ to **prevent harm** when providing care for an older client who is at risk for falls related to altered balance and decreased coordination? **Select all that apply.**
   A. Instruct the client to move slowly when changing positions.
   B. Encourage the client not to get out of bed unless it is really necessary.
   C. Advise the client to hold on to handrails when ambulating.
   D. Raise all four siderails and place the bed in the lowest position.
   E. Request that a family member or a sitter stay with the client at all times.
   F. Assess the need for an ambulatory aid, such as a cane or walker.

10. What is the **most important** reason that the nurse asks a client whether he or she is right-handed or left-handed during neurologic assessment?
    A. The client may be stronger on the dominant side, which is expected.
    B. The client should be encouraged to strengthen and rely on the dominant side.
    C. Effects of a neurologic event will be worse if the nondominant side is involved.
    D. This information is part of all standard databases for older clients.

11. Which **priority** assessment should be addressed **next** after the emergency department (ED) staff has assessed airway, breathing, and circulation (ABCs) in a client who sustained a head trauma with multiple injuries?
    A. Check for peripheral sensation.
    B. Stabilize long bone fractures.
    C. Rule out cervical spine fracture.
    D. Determine cerebral artery blockage.

12. Which assessment techniques are most relevant for the nurse to use when performing a neurologic examination for cognition on a client? **Select all that apply.**
    A. Give the client a simple command and observe how he or she reacts.
    B. Observe the client walking across the room, turning, and walking back.
    C. Ask the client for his or her name, date of birth, today's date, time, and location.
    D. Observe how well the client follows a topic or attends to an activity.
    E. Show the client a familiar object and ask him or her to state its name and purpose.
    F. Note whether the client responds rapidly and relevantly to questions.

13. Which findings must be reported to the health care provider immediately when the nurse assesses several clients using the Glasgow Coma Scale (GCS)? **Select all that apply.**
    A. A client's GCS decreases by 3 points
    B. A client arouses with supraorbital pressure
    C. A client has fixed nonreactive pupils
    D. A client has extreme flexion of the upper extremities
    E. A client asks for pain medication often before the drug is due
    F. A client is suddenly unable to recall where he or she is now

14. What is the nurse's **first priority** action when assessing a client and finding unilateral loss of motor function and sensation?
    A. Apply oxygen at 2 L per nasal cannula.
    B. Order a stat computed tomography scan.
    C. Place the client in semi-Fowler position.
    D. Immediately notify the health care provider.

15. For which client does the nurse **avoid harm** by **not** performing a sharp and dull sensory for pain assessment?
    A. Client with pulses that are not palpable in the distal extremities
    B. Client who is prescribed anticoagulant therapy and bruises easily
    C. Client who is sensitive to pain and temperature changes
    D. Client who is unable to move the affected or injured side

16. With which interprofessional health care member will the nurse collaborate to assess a client's strength?
    A. Physical therapist
    B. Orthopedic surgeon
    C. Skin care specialist nurse
    D. Neurology technician

17. Which reaction indicates to the nurse that a client has a cerebral or brainstem reason for muscle weakness when asked to close his or her eyes and hold arms perpendicular to the body with palms up for 15 to 30 seconds?
    A. Arms, wrists, and fingers are flexed with internal rotation
    B. Abnormal movement with rigidity and extension of the arms
    C. Arm on client's weak side drifts with the palm turning inward
    D. Dorsiflexion of the thumb and spreading of the other fingers

18. When assessing sensation, why does the nurse make a clinical judgment decision to forgo assessing pain sensation for a client with Guillain-Barré syndrome (GBS)?
    A. The client's temperature sensation is intact.
    B. Sensory function assessment is routinely completed at 4-hour intervals.
    C. Only clients with spinal trauma require completion of this assessment.
    D. Clients with GBS are often too confused to respond appropriately.

19. Which stimuli are recommended for the nurse to apply when a client has not responded to a loud voice or gentle shaking during Glasgow Coma Scale (GSC) assessment? **Select all that apply.**
    A. Supraorbital pressure by placing a thumb under the orbital rim in the middle of the eyebrow and pushing upward
    B. Alternating sharp pin prick with cotton ball on several spots over the hands and feet
    C. Trapezius muscle squeeze by pinching or squeezing the trapezius muscle located at the angle of the shoulder and neck muscle
    D. Mandibular pressure to the jaw by using the index and middle fingers to pinch the lower jaw
    E. Sternal rub by making a fist and rubbing/twisting the knuckles against the sternum
    F. Continuous application of pain for 45 seconds to determine if the client will withdraw from the pain

20. What would be the **priority** concern when the nurse asks a client to stand with arms at the sides, feet and knees close together, and eyes open, then close his or her eyes and maintain position; and the nurse notes client swaying only when the eyes are closed?
    A. Difficulty with performance of activities of daily living
    B. Potential for brainstem injury
    C. Possible falls related to lack of awareness of body position
    D. Functional incontinence due to difficulty with ambulation

21. Which cranial nerve does the nurse suspect is involved when a client reports severe, intermittent facial pain?
    A. Cranial nerve I
    B. Cranial nerve III
    C. Cranial nerve V
    D. Cranial nerve VII

22. Which neurological check finding does the nurse recognize as an **early** indicator of declining neurologic status?
    A. Change in level of consciousness
    B. Nonreactive and dilated pupils
    C. Loss of remote memory
    D. Decorticate posturing

23. Which statement by a client indicates to the nurse **lack** of correct understanding about information provided regarding cerebral angiography?
    A. "I must not have anything to eat or drink for at least 4 to 6 hours before the procedure."
    B. "I will not be able to move my head during the procedure."
    C. "I will feel a warm sensation when the contrast dye is injected into my IV."
    D. "I will not be able to talk to anyone during the procedure."

24. Which actions will the nurse include as follow-up care for a client after cerebral angiography? **Select all that apply.**
    A. Check the dressing for bleeding and swelling around the site.
    B. Apply a heating pad to the site.
    C. Keep the extremity straight and immobilized.
    D. Maintain the pressure dressing for 2 hours.
    E. Check the extremity for adequate circulation.
    F. Monitor for contrast media reactions such as hives or flushing.

25. How will the nurse prepare a client for an electroencephalogram test?
    A. Encourage extra fluids during the evening before the test.
    B. Give the client a sedative before bedtime for sleep.
    C. Give nothing by mouth but ice chips after midnight.
    D. Instruct the assistive personnel to wash the client's hair.

26. Which laboratory result would the nurse notify the radiology department and health care provider about for a client who is scheduled to have a computed tomography (CT) scan with contrast media?
    A. Blood glucose higher than baseline
    B. Decreased white blood cell count
    C. Elevated creatinine level
    D. Abnormal urobilinogen level

27. Which concept is **most directly** related to the nurse's teaching a client about smoking cessation to maintain or improve nervous system health?
    A. Comfort
    B. Perfusion
    C. Mobility
    D. Cognition

28. Which is the **best** interpretation of client neurological assessment documentation that reads PERRLA?
    A. Peripheral nervous system is reactive and responsive when activated.
    B. Parasympathetic nervous system is responsible for reproductive actions.
    C. Pulses are equal in right arm and right leg and client is ambulatory.
    D. Pupils are equal in size, round, regular, and react to light and accommodation.

29. Which are advantages of magnetic resonance imaging (MRI or MR) over computed tomography (CT) in the diagnostic imaging of a client's brain, spinal cord, and nerve roots? **Select all that apply.**
    A. MRI does not use ionizing radiation but instead relies on magnetic fields.
    B. Bony structures are viewed much clearer with MRI.
    C. Multiple sets of images are taken that are used to determine normal and abnormal anatomy.
    D. MRI testing is best for clients who are confused or claustrophobic.
    E. Images may be enhanced with the use of gadolinium, a non–iodine-based contrast medium.
    F. Some facilities have a functional MRI (fMRI) machine that can assess blood flow to the brain.

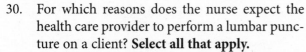

30. For which reasons does the nurse expect the health care provider to perform a lumbar puncture on a client? **Select all that apply.**
    A. To obtain cerebrospinal fluid (CSF) pressure readings with a manometer
    B. To obtain CSF for analysis
    C. To check for spinal blockage caused by a spinal cord lesion
    D. To inject contrast medium or air for diagnostic study
    E. To inject spinal anesthetics
    F. To inject selected drugs

31. For which client would the health care provider **avoid harm** by **not performing** a lumbar puncture?
    A. Client who is unable to ambulate
    B. Client with severe increase in intracranial pressure
    C. Client with hyperactive deep tendon reflexes
    D. Client with muscle weakness in all four extremities

Chapter 38 Answer Key

1. B, D, E
   The priority concepts for neurological assessment are: cognition, mobility, and sensory perception. The interrelated concept for this chapter is perfusion.

2. A
   Some neurons are motor (causing purposeful physical movement or mobility). Sensory neurons result in the ability to perceive stimulation through the sensory organs. Afferent neurons send impulses toward the central nervous system (CNS) and away from the peripheral nervous system (PNS). Synaptic knobs are the enlarged distal ends of each axon.

3. A, B, D, E
   Cerebellar function enables a person to: keep an extremity from overshooting an intended target; move from one skilled movement to another in an orderly sequence; predict distance or gauge the speed with which one is approaching an object; control voluntary (**not** involuntary) movement; and maintain equilibrium. The brainstem (**not** the cerebellum) contains special cells that constitute the reticular activating system (RAS), which controls awareness and alertness.

4. A
   Throughout the brainstem are special cells that constitute the reticular activating system (RAS), which controls awareness and alertness. This tissue awakens a person from sleep when presented with a stimulus such as loud noise or pain or when it is time to awaken.

5. C
   Brainstem functions of the medulla include: respiratory center; cardiac slowing center; and functions of these cranial nerves: cranial nerve nuclei IX (glossopharyngeal), X (vagus), XI (accessory), and XII (hypoglossal) and parts of cranial nerves VII (facial) and VIII (vestibulocochlear). The priority concern for this client is the risk for respiratory arrest which is life threatening.

6. D
   The blood-brain barrier keeps some substances in the bloodstream out of the cerebrospinal circulation and out of brain tissue. Substances that can pass through the BBB include oxygen, glucose, carbon dioxide, alcohol, anesthetics, and water. Large molecules such as albumin, any substance bound to albumin, and many antibiotics are prevented from crossing the barrier.

7. B
   The SNS stimulates the functions of the body needed for "fight or flight" (e.g., increased heart and respiratory rate). It also inhibits certain functions not needed in urgent and stressful situations (e.g., inhibits stomach, pancreas and intestines).

8. C
   Older adults develop slower cognitive time as they age. The nurse provides sufficient time for the affected older adult to respond to questions and/or direction. Allowing adequate time for

processing helps differentiate normal findings from neurologic deterioration. See the box labeled Patient-Centered Care: Older Adult Considerations Changes in the Nervous System Related to Aging in your text.

9. A, C, F

For the older client at risk for falls due to balance alteration and/or decreased coordination, the best care strategies include: instructing the client to move slowly when changing positions; if needed, advising the client to hold on to handrails when ambulating; and assessing the need for an ambulatory aid, such as a cane or walker. The client could be out of bed with assistance from the nursing staff. Most hospitals have policies against having all four siderails in the raised position because clients try to climb over and falls are very much a risk. A sitter or family member could stay with the client, but the client is alert and responsive, so this is not one of the best responses. The client should be instructed to call for assistance whenever he or she needs to get out of bed. See the box labeled Patient-Centered Care: Older Adult Considerations Changes in the Nervous System Related to Aging in your text.

10. A

The nurse asks whether the client is right-handed or left-handed because this information is important for these reasons: the client may be somewhat stronger on the dominant side, which is expected, and the effects of cerebral injury or disease may be more pronounced if the dominant (**not** nondominant) hemisphere is involved.

11. C

When a client has head trauma and multiple injuries, after assessing the ABCs (airway, breathing, and circulation), one of the first priorities is to rule out cervical spine fracture.

12. A, C, D, E, F

Cognition is the complex integration of mental processes and intellectual function for the purposes of reasoning, learning, memory, and personality. All of these responses are appropriate except B. The nurse uses response B to assess

client mobility. See the box labeled Best Practice for Patient Safety and Quality care (QSEN) – Assessment of Cognition in your text for additional methods of assessing cognition.

13. A, C, D, F

The Glasgow Coma Scale (GCS) is a tool used in many acute care settings to establish baseline data for these areas: eye opening, motor response, and verbal response. The client is assigned a numeric score for each of these areas. The lower the score, the lower the client's neurologic function. A decrease of 2 or more points in the Glasgow Coma Scale total is clinically significant and should be communicated to the primary health care provider immediately. Other findings requiring urgent communication with the primary health care provider include a new finding of abnormal flexion or extension, particularly of the upper extremities (decerebrate or decorticate posturing); pinpoint or dilated nonreactive pupils; and sudden or subtle changes in mental status. A change in level of consciousness is the **earliest** sign of neurologic deterioration. Communicate early recognition of neurologic changes to the Rapid Response Team or primary health care provider to prevent complications and preserve CNS function.

14. D

When the nurse discovers a sudden unilateral (one side of the body) loss in motor function and sensation, it is an emergency situation requiring a stroke center and staff with expertise to diagnose and intervene during a stroke or "brain attack." Immediately notifying the health care provider will get the client evaluated by stroke experts and rapid treatment. Oxygen and semi-Fowler position may be of value, but the highest priority is notification of the health care provider and the stroke expert team who will likely order a CT scan and provide rapid treatment.

15. B

Before testing for pain using the dull and sharp method, the nurse must check to determine whether the client is on anticoagulant therapy. If so, the nurse avoids any testing with a sharp object because it can cause bleeding.

16. A

The nurse collaborates with the physical therapist to test the client's strength. When testing strength against resistance, ask the client to resist the examiner's bending or straightening of the arm, hand, leg, or foot being tested. A five-point rating scale is commonly used. Always evaluate and compare strength on each side. Compare previous results with current findings and report all decreases to the primary health care provider. An orthopedic surgeon is not needed to assist in strength testing and nor is a skin care specialist.

17. C

To assess cerebral motor or brainstem integrity, the nurse asks the client to close his or her eyes and hold the arms perpendicular to the body with the palms up for 15 to 30 seconds. If there is a cerebral or brainstem reason for muscle weakness, the arm on the weak side will start to fall, or "drift," with the palm pronating (turning inward). This is called a pronator drift.

18. A

Pain and temperature sensation are transmitted by the same nerve endings. Therefore, if one sensation is tested and found to be intact, it can safely be assumed that the other is intact. Testing temperature sensation can usually be accomplished using a cold reflex hammer and the warm touch of the hand.

19. A, C, D, E

If a client does not respond to a loud voice or shaking during GCS assessment, the nurse could apply one of these methods: supraorbital pressure by placing a thumb under the orbital rim in the middle of the eyebrow and pushing upward; trapezius muscle squeeze by pinching or squeezing the trapezius muscle located at the angle of the shoulder and neck muscle; mandibular pressure to the jaw by using the index and middle fingers to pinch the lower jaw; or sternal (breastbone) rub by making a fist and rubbing/twisting the knuckles against the sternum. If the client does not respond after 20 to 30 seconds, stop applying the painful stimulus.

20. C

The nurse is checking for equilibrium with this assessment. The client is asked to stand with arms at the sides, feet and knees close together, and eyes open. The nurse checks for swaying and then ask the client to close his or her eyes and maintain position. The examiner should be close enough to prevent falling if the client cannot stay erect. If the client sways with the eyes closed but not when the eyes are open (the Romberg sign), the problem is likely related to proprioception (awareness of body position). If the client sways with the eyes both open and closed, the neurologic disturbance is probably cerebellar in origin.

21. C

If the client reports severe, intermittent facial pain, he or she may have trigeminal neuralgia. Trigeminal neuralgia is a persistently painful and debilitating disorder that involves the trigeminal cranial nerve (V). Cranial nerve I is olfactory; cranial nerve III is oculomotor; and cranial nerve VII is facial.

22. A

A change in level of consciousness and orientation is the earliest and most reliable indication that central neurologic function has declined. If a decline occurs, contact the Rapid Response Team or primary health care provider immediately.

23. D

Prior to cerebral angiography, the nurse ensures that the client takes nothing by mouth (NPO) for 4 to 6 hours. Other important points to teach the client include: the head is immobilized during the procedure; the client may not move during the procedure; contrast dye is injected through a catheter placed in the femoral artery and the client will feel a warm or hot sensation when the dye is injected which is normal; and the client will be able to talk to health care professionals during the procedure and should let them know about pain or concerns.

24. A, C, D, E, F

All of these responses are appropriate to post-procedure care for a client with cerebral angiography except response B. Ice should be applied to the site, **not** heat.

25. D

Fasting is avoided before EEG testing because hypoglycemia can alter the test results. Ensure that hair is clean and without conditioners, hair creams, lotions, sprays, or styling gels. Teach the client to avoid the use of sedatives or stimulants in the 12 to 24 hours preceding the EEG.

26. C

Prior to diagnostic test using contrast media, it is essential to evaluate current kidney function. Clients with a serum creatinine greater than or equal to 1.5 mg/dL or a calculated glomerular filtration rate (GFR) of less than 60 mL/min are at **highest risk** for kidney damage from contrast media.

27. B

Practicing a healthy lifestyle can help promote nervous system health. Smoking constricts blood vessels and can lead to decreased perfusion to the brain, resulting in a brain attack or stroke. The nurse teaches clients the importance of smoking cessation.

28. D

Testing pupils is a common cranial nerve test performed by nurses. Pupil constriction is a function of cranial nerve III, the oculomotor nerve. **P**upils should be **e**qual in size, **r**ound, and **r**egular in shape, and react to **l**ight and **a**ccommodation (PERRLA).

29. A, C, E, F

Magnetic resonance imaging (MRI or MR) has advantages over CT in the diagnostic imaging of the brain, spinal cord, and nerve roots. It does not use ionizing radiation but instead relies on magnetic fields. Multiple sets of images are taken that are used to determine normal and abnormal anatomy. Images may be enhanced with the use of gadolinium, a non–iodine-based contrast medium. MRIs of the spine have largely replaced CT scans and myelography for evaluation. Bony structures cannot be viewed with MRI; CT scans are the best way to see bones. Some facilities have a functional MRI (fMRI) machine that can assess blood flow to the brain rather than merely show its anatomic structure. MRI may be contraindicated for clients who are confused, claustrophobic, or unstable.

30. A, B, C, D, E, F

Lumbar puncture (spinal tap) is the insertion of a spinal needle into the subarachnoid space between the third and fourth (sometimes the fourth and fifth) lumbar vertebrae. A lumbar puncture (LP) is used to: obtain cerebrospinal fluid (CSF) pressure readings with a manometer; obtain CSF for analysis; check for spinal blockage caused by a spinal cord lesion; inject contrast medium or air for diagnostic study; inject spinal anesthetics; and inject selected drugs.

31. B

Because of the danger of sudden release of CSF pressure, a lumbar puncture is **not** done for clients with symptoms indicating severely increased intracranial pressure (ICP).

39

CHAPTER

Concepts of Care for Patients with Problems of the Central Nervous System: The Brain

1. Which are microscopic changes that occur in the brain of a client with Alzheimer disease (AD)? **Select all that apply.**
   A. Widening of the cerebral sulci
   B. Neurofibrillary tangles
   C. Decreasing size of the brain
   D. Neuritic plaques
   E. Narrowing of the gyri
   F. Vascular degeneration

2. Which action by a client with Alzheimer disease and documented by the nurse demonstrates the finding of apraxia?
   A. Client is unable to understand or follow a simple command.
   B. Client sustains a burn from a heating pad without realizing it.
   C. Client pushes food on his or her plate with eye glasses.
   D. Client is unable to find words when asked the name of his or her pet dog.

3. For which deficits in cognition does the nurse assess in a client with Alzheimer disease? **Select all that apply.**
   A. Attention and concentration
   B. Judgment and perception
   C. Learning and memory
   D. Aggressiveness and rapid mood swings
   E. Communication and language
   F. Speed of information processing

4. What does the Mini-Mental State Examination (MMSE) measure when the nurse assesses an older adult client with Alzheimer disease?
   A. Level of intelligence
   B. Severity of cognitive impairment
   C. Alterations in communication
   D. Functional ability

5. Which action is **best** for the nurse to take while caring for a client with late-stage advanced Alzheimer disease in a long-term care setting?
   A. Repeating the date, time, and place frequently
   B. Using memory aids such as pill reminders
   C. Reflecting a client's feelings and concerns
   D. Providing puzzles, games, and hands-on activities

6. What is the **priority** for interprofessional care of clients with Alzheimer disease (AD)?
   A. Preserving memory
   B. Promoting functional abilities
   C. Teaching clients and families
   D. Keeping clients safe

7. Which task does the nurse delegate to the assistive personnel (AP) for clients with Alzheimer disease in a long-term care setting?
   A. Assist the client who has incontinence with toileting every 2 hours.
   B. Provide hygienic care for a client who is currently exhibiting agitation.
   C. Encourage the client to consume small amounts of fluid to avoid incontinence.
   D. Give the client a complete bed bath to conserve his or her energy.

8. The nurse will collaborate with which members of the interprofessional team to determine the needs of a client with Alzheimer disease for adaptive devices? **Select all that apply.**
   A. Social services
   B. Occupational therapist
   C. Surgeon
   D. Physical therapist
   E. Registered dietitian nutritionist
   F. Speech language therapist

9. Which statement does the nurse recognize as accurate with regard to drugs used to treat a client with Alzheimer disease?
   A. If started early enough, cholinesterase inhibitors may cure AD.
   B. All clients with AD are treated with antidepressants.
   C. No drugs can cure AD but some may improve symptoms.
   D. A family member should know how to check pulse because of tachycardia.

10. Which actions will the nurse **avoid** when a client with Alzheimer disease is agitated? **Select all that apply.**
    A. Talking softly and calmly to the client
    B. Confronting the client
    C. Attempting to redirect the client
    D. Reasoning with the client
    E. Taking offense at what the client says
    F. Explaining the situation to the client

11. Which does the nurse recognize as cardinal symptoms for a client with Parkinson disease (PD)? **Select all that apply.**
    A. Tremors
    B. Muscle rigidity
    C. Postural instability
    D. Bradykinesia or akinesia
    E. Choreiform movements
    F. Seizure activity

12. What **priority** information does the nurse include when teaching a client with Parkinson disease (PD) about the prescribed drug selegiline, a selective monoamine oxidase type B (MAO-B) inhibitor?
    A. Take the drug with meals.
    B. Avoid driving or operating heavy machinery.
    C. Take the medication daily at bedtime.
    D. Avoid eating aged cheese or cured meats.

13. Which functional assessment is a **priority** when the nurse assesses a client with Parkinson disease and notes masklike face?
    A. Ability to sense pain in the facial area
    B. Ability to hear normal voice tones
    C. Ability to chew and swallow
    D. Ability to see in a dim lighted environment

14. What is the **priority** nursing concern for a client with Parkinson disease (PD) with right-sided trembling and weakness, as well as dizziness when moving from sitting to standing?
    A. Decreased ability to perform activities of daily living
    B. Feelings of isolation and loneliness
    C. Safety related to possible injury due to falls
    D. Poor nutritional and fluid intake

15. To **prevent harm**, which prescribed drug would the nurse question for an older client with Parkinson disease (PD)?
    A. Bromocriptine mesylate
    B. Benztropine
    C. Amantadine
    D. Levodopa-carbidopa

16. Which actions will the nurse expect when a client with Parkinson disease (PD) develops drug toxicity or tolerance? **Select all that apply.**
    A. A reduction in drug dosage
    B. Complete cessation of all drugs used to treat PD symptoms
    C. A change of drug or in the frequency of administration
    D. A drug holiday (particularly with levodopa therapy)
    E. Prescription of additional drugs to help relieve symptoms associated with the disease
    F. Implementation of exercise therapy to maintain functional abilities

17. Which tasks will the nurse delegate to the assistive personnel (AP) when caring for a client with stage 3 moderate Parkinson disease? **Select all that apply.**
    A. Assist client to the bathroom.
    B. Record accurate intake and output.
    C. Teach the client about safety precautions.
    D. Assist client with activities of daily living as needed.
    E. Assess client's gait and posture.
    F. Check and record client's vital signs every 4 hours.

18. Which are signs and symptoms that the nurse will assess in a client with migraine headaches? **Select all that apply.**
    A. Nausea
    B. Throbbing unilateral pain
    C. Transient loss of consciousness
    D. Sensitivity to light
    E. Recurrent episodic headaches
    F. Sensitivity to sound

19. Which action will the nurse consider the highest **priority** when caring for a client who is currently experiencing a migraine headache?
    A. Avoiding environmental triggers of migraine headaches
    B. Providing pain management for client
    C. Assessing the client for visual symptoms
    D. Detecting a pre-migraine aura

20. Which drugs will the nurse expect the health care provider to prescribe for a client with **mild** migraine headaches? **Select all that apply.**
    A. Acetaminophen
    B. Eletriptan
    C. Naproxen
    D. Cafergot
    E. Metoclopramide
    F. Isometheptene combination

21. Which intervention will the nurse implement for a client who has a migraine headache with phonophobia?.
    A. Ensure that the staff knows that the client will need help with ambulation.
    B. Dim the lights in the client's room and close the curtains.
    C. Place the client in a quiet room and instruct the staff to minimize noise.
    D. Increase the amount of ambient light to make it easier for the client to see.

22. What **priority** teaching will the nurse provide for a client on migraine preventive therapy who is taking a beta blocker and a calcium channel blocker drug?
    A. Move slowly when getting out of bed.
    B. Use handrails whenever possible.
    C. Avoid calcium-based foods.
    D. Learn to check your pulse.

23. What is the nurse's **best** action when a client is having a generalized tonic-clonic seizure and becomes cyanotic?
    A. Raise the head of the bed and apply oxygen by nasal cannula.
    B. Suction the client and alert the Rapid Response Team.
    C. Call the health care provider and obtain intubation equipment.
    D. Stay with the client because the cyanosis is usually self-limiting.

24. Which issue does the nurse consider a **priority** when caring for a client diagnosed with atonic (akinetic) seizures?
    A. Possibility of injury related to falls
    B. Limited mobility related to lack of tonicity of muscles
    C. Confusion related to postictal period
    D. Organ ischemia related to decreased perfusion

25. Which medication prescription will the nurse **clarify** before administering it to a client?
    A. Gabapentin for a client who has partial seizures
    B. Diazepam rectal gel for a client with status epilepticus
    C. Carbamazepine for a client with tonic-clonic seizures
    D. Warfarin for a client who takes phenytoin for seizures

26. What equipment will the nurse ensure is in the room of a client being admitted on seizure precautions to **prevent harm**? **Select all that apply.**
    A. Oxygen equipment
    B. Padding for siderails
    C. Suctioning equipment
    D. Saline lock insertion equipment
    E. Padded tongue blade
    F. Neurological assessment flow sheet

27. Which clients will the nurse advise to receive the meningococcal vaccine? **Select all that apply.**
    A. Healthy 18-year-old who has enlisted in the military
    B. 25-year-old who had a splenectomy after an auto accident
    C. Healthy 24-year-old who is interning with a lawyer for the summer
    D. Healthy 20-year-old who plans to live in a university dormitory
    E. Healthy 22-year-old who is unsure about vaccination and plans to visit Asia
    F. 21-year-old who has a summer job with a moving company

28. Which signs and symptoms are commonly assessed by the nurse when a client is diagnosed with meningitis? **Select all that apply.**
    A. Disorientation to person, place, and time
    B. Nuchal rigidity (stiff neck)
    C. Severe, unrelenting headaches
    D. Positive Kernig's sign
    E. Decreased level of consciousness
    F. Generalized muscle aches and pain (myalgia)

29. How does the nurse interpret a serum sodium finding of 126 mEq/L (126 mmol/L) for a client with bacterial meningitis?
    A. An early warning sign that the electrolyte imbalance will potentiate an acute myocardial infarction
    B. Evidence of syndrome of inappropriate antidiuretic hormone which is a complication of bacterial meningitis
    C. Within normal limits considering the diagnosis of bacterial meningitis but test should be repeated looking for downward trend
    D. A protective measure that causes increased urination and therefore reduces the risk of increased intracranial pressure

30. Which diagnostic test does the emergency department nurse anticipate for a client admitted with headache, fever, nausea, and light sensitivity, and who has been living with two people recently diagnosed with meningitis?
    A. Skull x-rays
    B. Myelography
    C. Cerebral angiogram
    D. Lumbar puncture

Chapter 39 Answer Key

1. B, D, F
   While all of these options are changes that occur in the brain with AD, only neurofibrillary tangles, amyloid-rich senile or neuritic plaques, and vascular degeneration are microscopic changes.

2. C
   Apraxia is the inability to use words or objects correctly. In this case the client is attempting to use eye glasses for eating food. Inability to understand or follow simple commands is aphasia. Agnosia is the loss of sensory comprehension so a client may be burned without realizing that it occurs. Anomia is the inability to find words, as when the client is unable to find the word to name his or her pet.

3. A, B, C, E, F
   Deficits in all of these areas of cognition should be assessed. Option D does not assess changes in cognition, but assesses changes in behavior and personality.

4. B
   The Mini-Mental State Examination (MMSE) is an example of a tool used to determine the onset and severity of cognitive impairment. The MMSE, also known as the "mini-mental exam", assesses five major areas—orientation, registration, attention and calculation, recall, and speech-language (including reading).

5. C

For the client in the later stages of AD or another form of dementia, reality orientation does not work and often increases agitation. The interprofessional health care team uses validation therapy for the client with moderate or severe AD. In **validation therapy**, the staff member recognizes and acknowledges the client's feelings and concerns.

6. D

For clients with AD, the priority for interprofessional care is **safety**. Chronic confusion and physical deficits place the client with AD at a high risk for injury, accidents, and elder abuse.

7. A

A client with AD may remain continent of bowel and bladder for a long period of time if taken to the bathroom or given a bedpan or urinal every 2 hours. Toileting may be needed more often during the day and less frequently at night. Assistive personnel (AP) or home caregivers are taught to encourage the client to drink adequate fluids to promote optimal voiding. A client may refuse to drink enough fluids because of a fear of incontinence. The care providers would assure the client that he or she will be toileted on a regular schedule to prevent incontinent episodes.

8. B, D

The nurse would collaborate with the occupational and physical therapists to provide a complete evaluation and assistance in helping the client remain as independent as possible. Adaptive devices, such as grab bars in the bathtub or shower area, an elevated commode, and adaptive eating utensils, may enable him or her to maintain independence in grooming, toileting, and feeding. The physical therapist prescribes an exercise program to improve physical health and functionality.

9. C

There are no drugs that can cure or slow the progression of Alzheimer disease, but a few drugs may improve symptoms associated with the disease for some clients. Cholinesterase inhibitors work to improve cholinergic neurotransmission in the brain by delaying the destruction of acetylcholine (ACh) by the enzyme cholinesterase. This action may slow the onset of cognitive decline in some clients, but none of these drugs alters the course of the disease. Memantine blocks excess amounts of glutamate that can damage in some clients.

10. B, D, E, F

When a client with AD is agitated, actions to **avoid** include raising the voice, confronting, arguing, reasoning, taking offense, or explaining. Talking calmly and softly and attempting to redirect the client to a more positive behavior or activity are **effective** strategies when he or she is agitated.

11. A, B, C, D

Parkinson disease (PD) is a progressive neurodegenerative disease that is one of the most common neurologic disorders of older adults. It is a debilitating disease affecting mobility and is characterized by **four cardinal symptoms**: tremor, muscle rigidity, bradykinesia or akinesia (slow movement/no movement), and postural instability. Huntington disease, a rare hereditary disorder that is characterized by progressive dementia and choreiform movements (uncontrollable rapid, jerky movements) in the limbs, trunk, and facial muscles.

12. D

The nurse would teach clients taking MAOIs about the need to avoid foods, beverages, and drugs that contain **tyramine**, such as cheese and aged, smoked, or cured foods and sausage. Remind them to also avoid red wine and beer to prevent severe headache and life-threatening hypertension. Clients are taught to continue these restrictions for 14 days after the drug is discontinued.

13. C

Changes in facial expression or a masklike face with wide-open, fixed, staring eyes is caused by rigidity of the facial muscles. In late-stage PD, this rigidity can lead to difficulties in chewing and swallowing, particularly if the pharyngeal muscles are involved. As a result, the client may have inadequate nutrition and uncontrolled drooling may occur.

14. C

The nurse's priority concern for this client with PD is related to **safety**. The client has right-sided trembling and weakness, as well as experiencing dizziness when first moving from a sitting to a standing position, all of which increases the risk for injuries due to falls.

15. B

For severe motor symptoms such as tremors and rigidity, one of the older anticholinergic drugs may be prescribed, but they are rarely used as primary drugs of choice for PD. Examples are benztropine, trihexyphenidyl HCl, and procyclidine. These drugs should be **avoided** in older adults because they can cause acute confusion, urinary retention, constipation, dry mouth, and blurred vision. The nurse would be sure to clarify a prescription for this drug written for an older adult with PD.

16. A, C, D, E

When drug tolerance is reached, the drug's effects do not last as long. The treatment of PD drug toxicity or tolerance includes: a reduction in drug dosage; a change of drug or in the frequency of administration; and a drug holiday (particularly with levodopa therapy). During a **drug holiday**, which can last up to 10 days, the client receives no drug therapy for PD and the nurse would carefully monitor the client for symptoms of PD and document assessment findings. Many clients are on additional drugs to help relieve symptoms associated with the disease (e.g., muscle spasms may be relieved by baclofen, drooling can be minimized by sublingual atropine sulfate, and insomnia may require a sleeping aid such as zolpidem tartrate).

17. A, B, D, F

To correctly respond to this question, the nurse must be familiar with the AP's scope of practice which includes assisting clients with ambulation, activities of daily living, recording intake and output, and checking as well as recording vital signs. Assessment and teaching for clients requires the additional training and skills of a professional RN.

18. A, B, D, E, F

All of these signs and symptoms occur with migraine headaches except option C, transient loss of consciousness. Photophobia is sensitivity to light and phonophobia is sensitivity to sound. See the box in your text labeled Key Features of Migraine Headaches for additional manifestations of migraines.

19. B

The priority for care of the client having migraines is **pain** management. This outcome may be achieved by abortive and preventive therapy. Drug therapy, trigger management, and complementary and integrative therapies are the major approaches to managing pain.

20. A, C, E

Drugs commonly prescribed for **mild** migraines include acetaminophen, NSAIDs (e.g., naproxen, ibuprofen), NSAIDs combined with caffeine (e.g., OTC acetaminophen with aspirin and caffeine), and antiemetics for nausea. Metoclopramide may be administered with NSAIDs to promote gastric emptying and decrease vomiting. For more severe migraines, drugs such as triptan preparations, ergotamine derivatives, and isometheptene combinations are needed.

21. C

Phonophobia is sensitivity to sound. The nurse would intervene by placing the client in a quiet room and keeping the noise level to a minimum.

22. D

The nurse will teach clients who take beta-adrenergic blockers or calcium channel blockers how to take their pulse because both drugs lower blood pressure and heart rate. Clients are taught to report bradycardia or adverse reactions such as fatigue and shortness of breath to their primary health care provider as soon as possible. Rising slowly from bed and using handrails are also useful but not the highest priority. The client would not be advised to avoid foods with calcium.

23. D
It is not unusual for a client to become cyanotic during a generalized tonic-clonic seizure. The cyanosis is generally self-limiting, and no treatment is needed so the nurse would remain with the client. Some primary health care providers prefer to give a high-risk client (e.g., older adult, critically ill, or debilitated client) oxygen by nasal cannula or facemask during the postictal (after seizure) phase.

24. A
With an atonic (akinetic) seizure, the client has a sudden loss of muscle tone, lasting for seconds, followed by postictal (after the seizure) confusion. In most cases, these seizures cause the client to fall, which may result in injury.

25. D
Using warfarin together with phenytoin may cause a client to bleed more easily. It may also increase phenytoin levels. Phenytoin levels and prothrombin time or international normalized ratio (INR) should be monitored whenever the dosage is changed or discontinued.

26. A, C, D
Seizure precautions include ensuring that oxygen and suctioning equipment with an airway are readily available. If the client does not have an IV access, a saline lock should be inserted, especially if the client is at significant risk for generalized tonic-clonic seizures. The saline lock provides ready access if IV drug therapy must be given to stop the seizure. Padded siderails may be embarrassing to the client and family. Padded tongue blades do **not** belong at the bedside and should **never** be inserted into the client's mouth because the jaw may clench

down as soon as the seizure begins. Forcing a tongue blade or airway into the mouth is more likely to chip the teeth and increase the risk for aspirating tooth fragments than prevent the client from biting the tongue. Improper placement of a padded tongue blade can also obstruct the airway. The seizure must be documented but a neurological assessment flow sheet is not necessary.

27. A, B, D, E
People aged 16 through 21 years have the highest rates of infection from life-threatening *N. meningitidis* meningococcal infection. The Centers for Disease Control and Prevention (CDC) recommends an initial meningococcal vaccine between ages 11 and 12 years with a booster at age 16 years. Adults are advised to get an initial or a booster vaccine if living in a shared residence (e.g., residence hall, military barracks, group home), or traveling or residing in countries in which the disease is common, or if they are immunocompromised as a result of a damaged or surgically removed spleen or a serum complement deficiency. If the client's baseline vaccination status is unclear and the immediate risk for exposure to *N. meningitidis* infection is high, the CDC recommends vaccination. It is safe to receive a booster as early as 8 weeks after the initial vaccine.

28. A, C, E, F
See the box labeled Key Features of Meningitis in your text for additional common signs and symptoms. The classic nuchal rigidity (stiff neck) and positive Kernig's and Brudzinski's signs have been traditionally used to diagnose meningitis, however, these findings **occur in only a small percentage** of clients with a definitive diagnosis.

29. B
Seizure activity may occur when meningeal inflammation and infection spreads to the cerebral cortex. Inflammation can also result in abnormal stimulation of the hypothalamic area where excessive amounts of antidiuretic hormone (ADH) (vasopressin) are produced. Excess vasopressin results in water retention and

dilution of serum sodium caused by increased sodium loss by the kidneys. This syndrome of inappropriate antidiuretic hormone (SIADH) may lead to further increases in ICP.

30. D

The nurse would anticipate assisting the health care provider with a lumbar puncture. The most significant laboratory test used in the diagnosis of meningitis is the analysis of the cerebrospinal fluid (CSF). Clients older than 60 years, those who are immunocompromised, or those who have signs of increased ICP usually have a CT scan before the lumbar puncture. If there will be a delay in obtaining the CSF, blood is drawn for culture and sensitivity. A broad-spectrum antibiotic should be given before the lumbar puncture. The CSF is analyzed for cell count, differential count, and protein. Glucose concentrations are determined, and culture, sensitivity, and Gram stain studies are performed.

40 CHAPTER

Care of Patients with Problems of the Central Nervous System: The Spinal Cord

1. Which statement about the relapsing-remitting type of multiple sclerosis (RRMS) is accurate?
   A. It involves a steady and gradual neurologic deterioration without remission of symptoms.
   B. It begins with a relapsing-remitting course and later the symptoms becomes steadily and progressively worse.
   C. It is characterized by frequent relapses with partial recovery but not a return to baseline.
   D. It is characterized by symptoms developing and resolving in a few weeks to months, and the client returns to baseline.

2. Which questions will the nurse ask a client, with increased fatigue and stiffness in the extremities, that will assess whether the symptoms may be associated with multiple sclerosis (MS)? **Select all that apply.**
   A. "Has anyone in your family been diagnosed with multiple sclerosis?
   B. "Have your symptoms gotten worse over time?"
   C. "Are you having trouble breathing with slight exertion?"
   D. "Which factors seem to make your symptoms worse?"
   E. "Have your symptoms come and gone over time?"
   F. "Are you having headaches that occur with stress?"

3. What will be the nurse's first intervention when a client states, "I've been dealing with the symptoms of MS for so long. Why won't anyone help me?"
   A. Encourage the client to verbalize his or her feelings and frustrations.
   B. Help the client locate and make an appointment with a specialist.
   C. Ask the client to describe in detail the symptoms and past treatments.
   D. Give the client a brochure about the diagnosis and treatment of MS.

4. Which **priority** teaching point will the nurse be sure to include when instructing a client with MS about the prescribed drug fingolimod?
   A. "You must be carefully monitored for allergic reactions because the level of fingolimod tends to build up in the body."
   B. "We will need to teach you how to check your pulse because fingolimod can cause slowing of your heart rate."
   C. "Fingolimod will improve your ability to walk, but will also increase the risk for seizure activity."
   D. "Fingolimod will decrease the frequency of clinical relapses, but there is an increased risk for stroke."

5. Which nursing assessment findings support a client's diagnosis of multiple sclerosis (MS)? **Select all that apply.**
   A. Intention tremors
   B. Dysmetria
   C. Dysarthria
   D. Nystagmus
   E. Respiratory distress
   F. Tinnitus

6. Which are purposes of the interprofessional team with regard to management of clients with multiple sclerosis (MS)? **Select all that apply.**
   A. To modify the disease's effects on the immune system
   B. To cure the client's illness
   C. To prevent exacerbations
   D. To manage symptoms
   E. To improve function
   F. To maintain quality of life

7. With which member of the interprofessional team will the nurse **collaborate** to improve the symptoms of MS that affect mobility?
   A. Registered dietician nutritionist
   B. Orthopedic surgeon
   C. Physical therapist
   D. Speech-language therapist

8. Which measure will the nurse recommend to **prevent harm** when a client with MS is discharged home?
   A. Avoid exercising outside.
   B. Immediately adapt the home for wheelchair access.
   C. Keep the home free of clutter.
   D. Install a ramp to the door of the home.

9. Which assessment will the nurse perform to monitor a likely **coexisting** complication in a client with MS who has dysarthria?
   A. Check the client's gag reflex and ability to swallow.
   B. Watch the client walk and note smoothness of gait.
   C. Ask the client to use a pencil to write out a sentence.
   D. Have the client stand with eyes closed and observe for swaying.

10. Which is the **best** action for the nurse to take when a client with MS develops diplopia?
    A. Obtain a prescription for referral for corrective lenses.
    B. Teach the client scanning techniques, turning the head from side to side.
    C. Apply an eye patch alternating it from eye to eye every few hours.
    D. Use prophylactic bilateral patches to both eyes during the night hours.

11. Which integrative/complimentary therapies will the nurse recommend to a client with multiple sclerosis? **Select all that apply.**
    A. Reflexology
    B. Herbal therapy
    C. Massage
    D. Conservation therapy
    E. Yoga
    F. Relaxation and meditation

12. Which statement best describes hyperflexion as a cause of a client's spinal cord injury?
    A. Hyperflexion occurs most often in vehicle collisions in which the vehicle is struck from behind or during falls when the client's chin is struck.
    B. Hyperflexion is a sudden and forceful acceleration (movement) of the head forward, causing extreme flexion of the neck.
    C. Hyperflexion results from diving accidents, falls on the buttocks, or a jump in which a person lands on the feet.
    D. Hyperflexion results from injuries that are caused by turning the head beyond the normal range.

13. Which questions will the nurse be sure to ask EMS when an unconscious client with a cervical spinal cord injury (SCI) is brought into the emergency department? **Select all that apply.**
    A. What was the location and position of the client immediately after the injury?
    B. Has the family been notified for permission to begin treatment?
    C. What symptoms occurred immediately after the injury and what changes have occurred since then?
    D. What type of immobilization equipment was used at the site and were there problems with transport?
    E. What treatments were given at the site of injury and during transport?
    F. Does the client have a history of any respiratory problems or difficulties?

14. At what rate does the nurse set the infusion pump for a client with a spinal cord injury (SCI) to receive the prescribed 500 mL of dextran over 4 hours?
    A. 75 mL/hr
    B. 100 mL/hr
    C. 125 mL/hr
    D. 150 mL/hr

15. Which is the initial **priority** action for the nurse when admitting a client with a cervical spinal cord injury?
    A. Spinal cord immobilization
    B. Assessment of client's airway, breathing, and circulation
    C. Evaluation of pulse, blood pressure, and peripheral perfusion
    D. Checking bodily sites for hemorrhage

16. What findings would the nurse expect when caring for a client who is experiencing spinal shock?
    A. Stridor, garbled speech, or inability to clear airway
    B. Bradycardia and decreased urinary output
    C. Hypotension and a decreased level of consciousness
    D. Temporary loss of motor, sensory, reflex and autonomic function

17. What is the **best** term for the nurse to use when documenting a client's paralysis of both lower extremities?
    A. Paraparesis
    B. Paraplegia
    C. Quadriparesis
    D. Quadriplegia

18. Which new-onset symptoms indicate to the nurse that a client with spinal cord injury (SCI) is experiencing autonomic dysreflexia (AD)? **Select all that apply.**
    A. Sudden hypertension with bradycardia
    B. Flaccid paralysis
    C. Blurred vision
    D. Tachypnea
    E. Profuse sweating of face, neck, and shoulders
    F. Severe throbbing headache

19. Which actions will the nurse take when caring for a client with a spinal cord injury who is experiencing autonomic dysreflexia? **Select all that apply.**
    A. Raise the head of the bed.
    B. Check the client's bladder for distention.
    C. Place a condom catheter on male clients as necessary.
    D. Give nifedipine or nitrate as prescribed.
    E. Monitor blood pressure every 10 to 15 minutes.
    F. Check the client for fecal impaction.

20. Which observation indicates to the nurse that a quadriplegic client's spouse understands teaching about performance of assistive coughing (quad cough)?
    A. The spouse assists the client into a wheelchair and coaches deep coughing.
    B. The spouse places hands on the client's lateral chest and pushes inward on exhalation.
    C. The spouse places hands below the client's diaphragm and pushes upward with exhalation.
    D. The spouse assists the client into high-Fowler position and encourage taking a number of deep breaths.

21. What is the nurse's **best first** action when a client with a spinal cord injury suddenly develops an SpO_2 of 92% with stridor, bradycardia with decreased urine output, and a systolic blood pressure of 84 mm Hg?
    A. Apply oxygen at 2 L per nasal cannula.
    B. Place a large-bore IV access.
    C. Insert a urinary catheter.
    D. Notify the Rapid Response Team.

22. Which **priority** teaching points will the nurse provide for a client with a spinal cord injury who is treated with a halo fixator with vest? **Select all that apply.**
    A. Be careful when leaning forward or backward because the weight of the halo device alters balance.
    B. Wear loose clothing, preferably with large openings for head and arms.
    C. Wash under the liner of the vest to prevent rashes or sores.
    D. Support your head with a small pillow when sleeping to prevent unnecessary pressure and discomfort.
    E. Do not drive because you can't turn your head from side to side so peripheral vision is impaired.
    F. Increase fluids and fiber in the diet to prevent constipation.

23. Which **priority** teaching points will the nurse include when teaching a client how to prevent low back pain and injury? **Select all that apply.**
    A. Use good posture when sitting, standing, and walking.
    B. Participate in a regular exercise program that includes daily aerobic workouts
    C. Do not wear high-heeled shoes.
    D. Avoid prolonged sitting or standing.
    E. Ensure adequate calcium and vitamin D intake.
    F. Keep weight within 30% of ideal body weight.

24. When the nurse is taking a history of an adult client who reports acute low back pain (LBP), which question is **most likely** to identify a causative factor?
    A. "Have you recently fallen or been lifting heavy objects?"
    B. "Are you having pain that radiates down your arm?"
    C. "Do you have a family history of neurologic disorders?"
    D. "Are you having trouble with walking or maintaining your balance?"

25. Which technique does the nurse use to assess a client's report of paresthesia in the lower extremities?
    A. Use a Doppler to locate the pedal pulse, the dorsalis pedis pulse, and the popliteal pulse.
    B. Ask the client to identify sharp and dull sensations using a paper clip and a cotton ball.
    C. Use a reflex hammer to test for deep tendon reflexes.
    D. Ask the client to walk across the room and observe for gait and equilibrium.

26. For which client will the nurse question the prescription of ziconotide for severe persistent back pain?
    A. Client with sciatic nerve pain
    B. Client using massage and heat for pain relief
    C. Client with severe mental health problems
    D. Client using NSAIDs and acupuncture for pain relief

27. Which **priority** preoperative teaching about postoperative concerns does the nurse provide for a client scheduled for lumbar surgery? **Select all that apply.**
    A. Bedrest restriction for at least 48 hours
    B. Techniques for getting into and out of bed
    C. Limitations and restrictions for home activities
    D. Expectations for turning and moving in bed
    E. Immediate reporting of any numbness or tingling
    F. Dietary restrictions for sodium and fats

28. Which postoperative assessment finding, for a client who underwent a laminectomy, does the nurse report **immediately** to the surgeon?
    A. Refusal of the client to cough and deep breathe
    B. Swelling or bulging at the operative site
    C. Pain along the operative incision site
    D. Serosanguineous drainage on the dressing

29. What is the **priority** nursing assessment after a client returns from surgery for an anterior cervical discectomy with fusion (ACDF)?
    A. Assess for gag reflex and swallowing ability.
    B. Monitor vital signs and check neurological status.
    C. Check for bleeding and drainage at the incision site.
    D. Assess for airway patency and respiratory effort.

30. Which important points does the nurse teach a client after an anterior cervical discectomy with fusion (ACDF) and prior to discharge? **Select all that apply.**
    A. Information about all prescribed medications
    B. How to care for the surgical incision
    C. A care provider must be with the client for a few days after surgery
    D. Home restriction for lifting and activity
    E. Wear brace or collar as prescribed
    F. Driving is permitted after 3 days

Chapter 40 Answer Key

1. D
   Relapsing-remitting type of multiple sclerosis (RRMS) occurs in most cases of MS. The course of the disease may be mild or moderate, depending on the degree of disability. Symptoms develop and resolve in a few weeks to months, and the client returns to baseline. During the relapsing phase, the client reports loss of function and the continuing development of new symptoms. Option A describes primary progressive MS (PPMS); option B describes secondary progressive MS (SPMS); and option C describes progressive-relapsing MS (PRMS).

2. A, B, D, E
   A complete history is essential for the diagnosis of MS. The nurse asks the client about a history of vision, mobility, and sensory perception changes, all of which are early indicators of MS. Symptoms are often vague and nonspecific in the early stages of the disease and may disappear for months or years before returning. Ask about the progression of symptoms. Pay particular attention to whether they are intermittent or are becoming progressively worse. Document the date (month and year) when the client first noticed these changes. Ask about factors that aggravate the symptoms, such as fatigue, stress, overexertion, temperature extremes, or a hot shower or bath. Ask the client and the family about any personality or behavioral changes that have occurred (e.g., euphoria [very elated mood], poor judgment, attention

loss). Also, ask whether there is a family history of MS or autoimmune disease.

3. A
   The client and family may be relieved to have a definite diagnosis but may also express anger and frustration that it took a long time to start appropriate treatment. The priority at this time is to establish open and honest communication with the client and allow him or her to share frustrations, anger, and anxiety.

4. B
   Fingolimod was the first oral immunomodulator approved for the management of MS. The capsules may be taken with or without food. Teach clients to monitor their pulse every day because the drug can cause bradycardia, especially within the first 6 hours after taking it.

5. A, B, C, D, F
   All options except E are findings that support a diagnosis of MS. Respiratory distress is generally not a symptom of MS. See the Box labeled Key Features Multiple Sclerosis in your text for additional signs and symptoms of MS.

6. A, C, D, E, F
   The purposes of interprofessional management for MS are to modify the disease's effects on the immune system, prevent exacerbations, manage symptoms, improve function, and maintain quality of life. There is no cure for MS.

7. C

The nurse works in collaboration with physical and occupational therapists to plan an exercise program that includes range-of-motion (ROM) exercises and stretching and strengthening exercises to manage spasticity and tremor.

8. C

Before the client is discharged, it is important to assess the client's home for hazards. Any items that might interfere with mobility (e.g., scatter rugs, stacks of magazines) are removed. In addition, care must be taken to prevent injury resulting from vision problems. Teach the client and family to keep the home environment as structured and **free from clutter** as possible.

9. A

If the client experiences dysarthria as a result of muscle weakness, he or she should be evaluated by a speech-language pathologist (SLP). It is **not** unusual for the client with dysarthria to also have dysphagia. The SLP will perform a swallowing evaluation and further diagnostic testing as needed. Monitor the client to determine if there are problems swallowing at meal time that increase the risk of aspiration.

10. C

An eye patch that is alternated from eye to eye every few hours usually relieves **diplopia**.

11. A, C, E, F

Clients with MS report that some complementary therapies are successful in decreasing their symptoms. Integrative therapies used by clients with MS include: reflexology; massage; yoga; relaxation and meditation; acupuncture; and aromatherapy. Conservation strategies (balancing periods of rest and activity) are useful for these clients but this is **not** an integrative therapy.

12. B.

Hyperflexion is a sudden and forceful acceleration (movement) of the head forward, causing extreme flexion of the neck. Option A describes hyperextension; option C describes axial loading or vertical compression; and option D describes excessive rotation.

13. A, C, D, E, F

All of these questions are pertinent to the immediate treatment of the client except option B. While the family must be notified as soon as possible, this is an emergency situation and life-preserving treatment must not be delayed.

14. C

500 mL/4 hr = 125 mL/hr

15. B

For a client with an SCI, the initial and priority assessment focuses on the client's ABCs (airway, breathing, and circulation). After an airway is established, assess the client's breathing pattern. The client with a cervical SCI is at high risk for respiratory compromise because the cervical spinal nerves (C3-5) innervate the phrenic nerve controlling the diaphragm.

16. D

Spinal shock occurs immediately as the cord's response to the injury. The client has complete, but temporary loss of motor, sensory, reflex, and autonomic function that often lasts less than 48 hours but may continue for several weeks.

17. B

The term for bilateral lower extremity paralysis is paraplegia. Paraparesis is weakness of the lower extremities. Paraplegia and paraparesis are seen in lower thoracic and lumbosacral injuries or lesions. Tetraplegia (also called quadriplegia) is paralysis of all four extremities. Quadriparesis refers to weakness involving all four extremities. Quadriplegia and quadriparesis are seen with cervical cord and upper thoracic injury.

18. A, C, E, F

Signs and symptoms of autonomic dysreflexia include: sudden, significant rise in systolic and diastolic blood pressure, accompanied by bradycardia; profuse sweating above the level of lesion, especially in the face, neck, and shoulders; goose bumps above or possibly below the level of the lesion; flushing of the skin above the level of the lesion, especially in the face, neck, and shoulders; blurred vision; spots in the client's visual field; nasal congestion; onset of severe, throbbing headache; flushing about the level of the lesion with pale skin below the level of the lesion; and a feeling of apprehension. See the box labeled Key Features Autonomic Dysreflexia in your text.

19. A, B, D, E, F
All of these actions are appropriate to the care of a client with SCI who has autonomic dysreflexia except option C. If the client requires a catheter, a urinary catheter would be placed, not a condom catheter. See the box labeled Best Practice for Patient Safety & Quality Care Emergency Care of the Patient Experiencing Autonomic Dysreflexia: Immediate Interventions in your text for additional appropriate actions.

20. C
The client is taught by the nurse to coordinate his or her cough effort with an assistant. The spouse, or other assistant, places his or her hands on the upper abdomen over the diaphragm and below the ribs. The client takes a breath and coughs during expiration (exhalation). The assistant locks his or her elbows and pushes inward and upward as the client coughs. This technique is called assisted coughing, quad cough, or **cough assist**. Repeating the coordinated effort, with rest periods as needed, until the airway is clear is important.

21. D
The client with acute spinal cord injury would be monitored at least hourly for indications of neurogenic shock including: pulse oximetry (SpO_2) <95% or symptoms of aspiration (e.g., stridor, garbled speech, or inability to clear airway); symptomatic bradycardia, including reduced level of consciousness and deceased urine output; and hypotension with systolic blood pressure (SBP) <90 mm Hg or mean arterial pressure (MAP) <65 mm Hg. When symptoms of neurogenic shock occur, the **priority** action is to notify the Rapid Response Team or primary health care provider immediately because this problem is an emergency. The other three actions may be applicable, but the priority is to notify the Rapid Response Team of primary health care provider.

22. A, B, C, D, E, F
All of these are important teaching points for a client with a spinal cord injury who is being treated with a halo fixator with vest. The client cannot turn his or her head to check for blind spots, so peripheral vision is limited and it is not safe to drive. See the box labeled Patient and Family Education: Preparing for Self-Management Use of a Halo Fixator with Vest in your text for additional suggested teaching points for this client.

23. A, C, D, E
Important teaching points by the nurse for a client to prevent low back pain (LBP) and injury include: use safe manual handling practices, with specific attention to bending, lifting, and sitting; assess the need for assistance with household chores or other activities; participate in a regular exercise program that promotes back strengthening, such as swimming and walking; do **not** wear high-heeled shoes; use good posture when sitting, standing, and walking; avoid prolonged sitting or standing; use a footstool and ergonomic chairs and tables to lessen back strain; be sure that equipment in the workplace is ergonomically designed to prevent injury; keep weight within 10% of ideal body weight; ensure adequate calcium intake and consider vitamin D supplementation if serum levels are low; and stop smoking (if not able to stop, cut down on the number of cigarettes or decrease the use of other forms of tobacco). Aerobic exercise is not a recommendation for prevention of LBP.

24. A
LBP is most prevalent during the third to sixth decades of life but can occur at any time. Acute and subacute back pain usually result from injury or trauma such as during a fall, vehicular crash, or lifting a heavy object. Options B, C, and D are important questions but do not provide information that helps to identify the cause of the low back pain.

25. B

The nurse asks whether paresthesia (tingling sensation) or numbness is present in the involved leg. Both extremities are checked for sensory perception by using a cotton ball and a paper clip for comparison of light or dull and sharp touch. The client may feel sensation in both legs but may experience a stronger sensation on the unaffected side.

26. C

Ziconotide can be taken with opioid analgesics but should **not** be administered to clients with severe mental health or behavioral health problems because it can cause psychosis. If symptoms such as hallucinations and delusions occur, teach clients and families to stop the drug immediately and notify their primary health care provider.

27. B, C, D, E

The nurse teaches clients preoperatively about postoperative expectations because many clients are discharged to home within 23 to 48 hours after surgery. Priority teaching includes: techniques to get into and out of bed; expectations for turning and moving in bed; reporting immediately any new sensory perceptions, such as numbness and tingling, or new motor impairment that may occur in the affected leg or in both legs; and home care activities or restrictions. Because of the short hospital stay, the nurse teaches family members or other caregivers how to assist the client and

what restrictions the client must follow at home before the surgery occurs.

28. B

The nurse will immediately report bulging at the incision site. This may be due to a cerebrospinal fluid (CSF) leak or a hematoma, both of which should be reported to the surgeon immediately. CSF may be visible as a "halo" around the outer edges of the dressing. The loss of a large amount of CSF may cause the client to report having a sudden headache.

29. D

The priority for care in the immediate postoperative period after an ACDF is maintaining an airway and ensuring that the client has no problems with breathing. Swelling from the surgery can narrow the trachea, causing a partial obstruction.

30. A, B, C, D, E

Important points the nurse will include with discharge teaching include: be sure that someone stays with the client for the first few days after surgery; review drug therapy; teach care of the incision; review activity restrictions including no heavy lifting; no driving until surgeon gives permission and no strenuous activities; walk every day; call the primary health care provider if symptoms of pain, numbness, and tingling worsen or if swallowing becomes difficult; and wear a brace or collar per the primary health care provider's prescription.

41 CHAPTER

Critical Care of Patients with Neurologic Emergencies

1. Which motor symptoms of a transient ischemic attack (TIA) will the nurse recognize when a client experiences this neurologic dysfunction? **Select all that apply.**
   A. Blurred vision
   B. Facial droop
   C. Weakness in hand grasp
   D. Aphasia
   E. Difficulty walking
   F. Lack of balance

2. Which client assessment finding will help the nurse to differentiate a transient ischemic attach (TIA) from a brain attack (stroke)?
   A. Unilateral weakened hand grasp
   B. Slurred speech
   C. Symptoms resolve within 30 to 60 minutes
   D. One-sided numbness of face and arm

3. Which collaborative actions will the nurse expect when a client with TIA is admitted to the hospital? **Select all that apply.**
   A. Performing a carotid angioplasty with stenting to increase perfusion to the brain
   B. Prescribing and teaching about antiplatelet drugs such as aspirin or clopidogrel
   C. Teaching the client about the benefits of taking vitamin supplements
   D. Prescribing and teaching about antihypertensive drugs to lower blood pressure
   E. Promoting lifestyle changes such as smoking cessation, healthy eating, and exercise
   F. Teaching the client to use a cane or walker for stability and balance

4. What actions will the nurse take to determine if an altered level of consciousness (LOC) in a client is a neurologic emergency, or if it represents one of two other conditions that may also lead to altered LOC?
   A. Observe for jaundice and abdominal distention.
   B. Check blood glucose and oxygen saturation.
   C. Observe for jugular vein distention and pitting edema.
   D. Check skin turgor and perform a bladder scan.

5. Which medication will the nurse administer to a client to **prevent harm** from recurrence of a stroke?
   A. Gabapentin
   B. Acetaminophen
   C. Alteplase
   D. Enteric-coated aspirin

6. Which symptoms will the nurse teach the client and family to report to the health care provider immediately after a carotid stent placement procedure, but before discharge? **Select all that apply.**
   A. Severe headache
   B. Muscle weakness
   C. Shortness of breath
   D. Severe neck pain
   E. Difficulty swallowing
   F. Blurred vision

7. What is the nurse's **best first** action when a client with an ischemic stroke now has a systolic blood pressure of 192 mm Hg?
   A. Notify the Rapid Response Team or primary health care provider immediately.
   B. Raise the head of the bed to a position of comfort for the client.
   C. Instruct the client to relax and take several deep breaths.
   D. Position the client supine and recheck the blood pressure every 5 to 10 minutes.

8. Which instruction would the nurse give an assistive personnel (AP) providing morning care for a client with increased intracranial pressure (ICP)?
   A. Give the bath, change the linens, do passive range of motion and then allow the client to rest.
   B. Give the bath, allow rest, change the linen, allow rest, perform passive range of motion, allow rest.
   C. Give the bath, then defer the linen change and range of motion exercises until the client is out of danger.
   D. Look at the client's orders for specifics about activities related to increased ICP that might cause an additional rise in ICP.

9. Which clients will the nurse monitor for increased risk of stroke? **Select all that apply.**
   A. 43-year-old healthy woman who used oral contraceptives
   B. 66-year-old man with type 2 diabetes mellitus
   C. 47-year-old woman who exercises 5 to 6 days a week
   D. 35-year-old man with a history of several transient ischemic attacks
   E. 55-year-old woman with facial muscle weakness due to Bell's palsy
   F. 73-year-old man with chronic alcoholism

10. Within which time frame does the nurse expect administration of intravenous fibrinolytic therapy with alteplase to occur related to a client's stroke symptoms onset?
    A. 24 to 30 hours
    B. 6 to 8 hours
    C. 3 to 4.5 hours
    D. 30 to 60 minutes

11. What is the nurse's **best** action when a client seems to have difficulty with swallowing?
    A. Limit the diet to clear liquids given only through a straw.
    B. Withhold food and fluids until swallowing is assessed and tested.
    C. Observe the client while eating and note which foods are problematic.
    D. Monitor the client's weight and food intake, then compare current trends to baseline.

12. Which guiding principles will the nurse use to **best** determine actions that will help with communications for a stroke client with aphasia? **Select all that apply.**
    A. Present just one idea or thought in a sentence.
    B. Use simple one-step commands.
    C. Speak slowly and loudly avoiding the use of cues.
    D. Avoid yes and no questions for a client with sensory aphasia.
    E. Use alternative forms of communication such as a communication board.
    F. Do not rush the client when speaking.

13. Which actions will the nurse delegate to the assistive personnel (AP) providing care for a client with right cerebral hemisphere damage? **Select all that apply.**
    A. Suggest that the family bring in familiar family photos.
    B. Move the client's bed so that his or her unaffected side faces the door.
    C. Place a patch over the client's affected eye and remove it every 2 hours.
    D. Remind the client to wash both sides of his or her face.
    E. Remove clutter to ensure a safe environment.
    F. Assess the client for memory deficits.

14. Which cardiac dysrhythmia does the nurse expect to see when a client with an embolic stroke is placed on a cardiac monitor?
    A. Sinus bradycardia
    B. Atrial fibrillation
    C. Sinus tachycardia
    D. Ventricular fibrillation

15. What condition does the nurse suspect when a client reports **sudden** onset of a severe headache associated with nausea and vomiting, and photophobia?
    A. Brain tumor
    B. Ischemic stroke
    C. Migraine headache
    D. Cerebral aneurysm

16. What is the nurse's **best first** action when the assistive personnel (AP) reports that a client scheduled for discharge has suddenly developed slurred speech and left-sided weakness?
    A. Assess the client within 10 minutes for signs and symptoms of brain attack.
    B. Instruct the client to follow-up with his or her primary care provider tomorrow.
    C. Call the health care provider to obtain a delay for the discharge.
    D. Instruct the client to stay in bed and initiate neurologic checks every 2 hours.

17. Which are the **best** actions for the nurse to take when caring for a client with a stroke who develops increased intracranial pressure (ICP)? **Select all that apply.**
    A. Provide oxygen therapy to prevent hypoxia for clients with oxygen saturation less than 94%.
    B. Maintain the head in a midline, neutral position to promote venous drainage from the brain.
    C. Elevate the head of the bed to improve perfusion pressure.
    D. Cluster nursing care together and then allow the client to rest.
    E. Avoid sudden and acute hip or neck flexion during positioning.
    F. Maintain a quiet environment for the client experiencing a headache.

18. Which is the **first** sign of increased intracranial pressure (ICP) that the nurse will notice in a client at risk for this condition?
    A. Decrease in level of consciousness
    B. Increase in systolic blood pressure
    C. Changes in pupil size and response
    D. Abnormal posturing of extremities

19. What is the nurse's **next best** action when caring for a client with an epidural hematoma who had decreased level of consciousness, then experienced a period of alert lucidity and was able to talk with the family?
    A. Document the client's exact behaviors, comparing them to previous assessments and continue with neurologic assessments every 2 hours.
    B. Stay with the client and have the charge nurse alert the health care provider because this is an ominous sign for the client.
    C. Monitor the client for the next 48 hours to 2 weeks because a subacute condition may be slowly developing.
    D. Instruct the family that the dangerous period has passed but encourage them to leave to avoid tiring the client excessively.

20. Which drug does the nurse expect will be prescribed to control cerebral vasospasm when a client is diagnosed with subarachnoid hemorrhage (SAH)?
    A. Phenytoin
    B. Clopidogrel
    C. Nimodipine
    D. Dexamethasone

21. Which questions are essential for the nurse to ask when getting an accurate history of a client's traumatic brain injury (TBI)? **Select all that apply.**
    A. When, where, and how did the injury occur?
    B. Did the client lose consciousness? If so, for how long?
    C. Was drug or alcohol consumption related to the TBI?
    D. Does the client have a history of seizure disorders?
    E. Precisely how did the older client fall to cause the TBI?
    F. Has there been a change in the client's level of consciousness?

22. Which signs and symptoms indicate to the nurse that a client's traumatic brain injury (TBI) will be diagnosed as **mild? Select all that apply.**
    A. Client appears dazed or stunned
    B. Loss of consciousness (if any occurred) was between 30 to 60 minutes
    C. Nausea and vomiting
    D. Headache
    E. Difficulty with gait or balance
    F. Sensitivity to noise

23. Why does the health care provider prescribe a ventilator setting to maintain partial pressure of arterial carbon dioxide ($Paco_2$) between 35 and 38 mm Hg for a client with a traumatic brain injury (TBI)?
    A. Lower levels of arterial carbon dioxide are essential for gas exchange.
    B. Carbon dioxide is a waste product that must be eliminated from the body.
    C. Lower levels of arterial carbon dioxide facilitate brain oxygenation.
    D. Carbon dioxide is a vasodilator that can cause increased intracranial pressure.

24. What is the nurse's **best** interpretation when a client with traumatic brain injury and increased intracranial pressure (ICP) develops severe hypertension with widened pulse pressure and bradycardia?
    A. The client needs an emergency craniotomy.
    B. Intravenous antihypertensive drugs will be administered.
    C. This is a late sign of increased ICP and death is imminent.
    D. A cardiac monitor should be placed followed by IV atropine.

25. What is the nurse's **best** action when providing care for a client with a traumatic closed head injury, with no history of respiratory problems, when the health care provider has prescribed oxygen at 2 L by nasal cannula?
    A. Apply pulse oximetry and administer oxygen to the client if the saturation drops below 90%.
    B. Clarify the prescription because oxygen therapy is unnecessary for this client.
    C. Place the client on oxygen as prescribed because hypoxemia may increase intracranial pressure.
    D. Apply the nasal cannula oxygen and wean the client off it over 12 to 24 hours.

26. What is the nurse's **best** interpretation when assessing a client with a traumatic brain injury and finding that the right pupil appears more ovoid in shape than the left?
    A. An ovoid pupil is not significant unless the client has severe hypertension, changes in level of consciousness, and respiratory distress.
    B. An ovoid pupil is assumed to signal brain herniation in progress with a poor prognosis.
    C. An ovoid pupil is considered a normal variation for a small percentage of clients who sustain minor head injuries.
    D. An ovoid pupil is regarded as the mid-stage between a normal pupil and a dilated pupil and must be reported immediately.

27. Which action does the nurse use **to prevent harm** by further increasing ICP when an intubated client with a traumatic head injury needs to be suctioned?
    A. Providing 100% oxygen before and after each pass of the endotracheal suction catheter
    B. Aggressively hyperventilating with 100% oxygen before endotracheal suctioning
    C. Performing oral suctioning often but avoiding endotracheal suctioning
    D. Obtaining an arterial blood gas sample before suctioning the client

28. Which actions will the nurse include when caring for a trauma client in the emergency department (ED) for whom the health care provider prescribes spinal precautions? **Select all that apply.**
    A. Avoiding neck flexion with a pillow or a roll
    B. Placing client on bedrest with bathroom privileges
    C. Using log roll procedure when repositioning the client
    D. Avoiding reverse Trendelenburg positioning
    E. Using a hard, rigid cervical collar to maintain cervical spine precautions
    F. Avoiding thoracic or lumbar flexion

29. Which position does the nurse use for a client who had an infratentorial craniotomy?
    A. High-Fowler position and turned toward the operative side
    B. Head of bed raised to 30 degrees and turned toward nonoperative side
    C. Flat in bed except elevation of head 30 degrees for meals
    D. Flat in bed and positioned side-lying, alternating sides every 2 hours

30. Which are common signs and symptoms of brain tumors a nurse will assess in a client? **Select all that apply.**
    A. Headaches that are more severe in the mornings on waking
    B. Loss of balance and dizziness
    C. Difficulty thinking and speaking
    D. Apraxia and alexia
    E. Nausea and vomiting
    F. Hearing loss

31. Which actions will the nurse delegate to the assistive personnel (AP) when caring for a client after craniotomy to remove a tumor? **Select all that apply.**
    A. Assess the head dressing for signs of drainage.
    B. Remind the client to take deep breaths every 2 hours.
    C. Reposition the client every 2 hours avoiding pressure on the operative site.
    D. Teach the client to report headaches.
    E. Apply intermittent sequential pneumatic devices.
    F. Record accurate intake and output.

32. What is the nurse's **best first** action when a client who had a craniotomy develops periorbital edema and ecchymosis?
    A. Immediately notify the surgeon.
    B. Apply cold compresses.
    C. Check pupillary response.
    D. Perform a focused neurologic assessment.

33. Which statement by a client indicates understanding of the use of a disc-shaped wafer (carmustine) as part of treatment for a brain tumor?
    A. "I'll place the wafer under my tongue and allow it to completely dissolve."
    B. "The wafer must be dissolved in water and taken with my morning meals."
    C. "The wafer will be placed directly into the cavity created during removal of my tumor."
    D. "The wafer will be taped to my chest and the drug absorbed through my skin."

34. What is the nurse's **best** action when caring for a client after craniotomy and finding the dressing is saturated and the Hemovac drainage is 100 mL over 8 hours?
    A. Notify the surgeon immediately.
    B. Reinforce the dressing with sterile gauze.
    C. Record the Hemovac drainage on the intake and output sheet.
    D. Check the drainage on the dressing for a halo effect.

Chapter 41 Answer Key

1. B, C, E, F

   Mobility (motor) symptoms of TIA include weakness (facial droop, arm or leg drift, hand grasp), and ataxia (lack of muscle control and coordination that affects gait, balance, and the ability to walk). Blurred vision is a visual sensory symptom of TIA and aphasia is a speech symptom, **not** a motor symptom of TIA.

2. C

   A TIA is a temporary neurologic dysfunction resulting from a **brief** interruption in cerebral blood flow. Typically, symptoms of a TIA resolve within 30 to 60 minutes, but may last as long as 24 hours.

3. A, B, D, E

   Depending on the client, collaborative interventions may include: performing traditional or minimally invasive surgery to remove atherosclerotic plaque buildup within the carotid artery and increase perfusion to the brain; performing a carotid angioplasty with stenting to increase perfusion to the brain; prescribing antiplatelet drugs, typically aspirin or clopidogrel, to prevent thrombotic or embolic strokes (may be placed on a combination of both drugs); reducing high blood pressure (the most common risk factor for stroke) by adding or adjusting drugs to lower blood pressure; controlling diabetes (if present) and keeping glucose levels in a target range, typically 100 to 180 mg/dL; and promoting lifestyle changes, such as smoking cessation, eating more heart-healthy foods, and increasing mobility and physical activity.

4. B

   When LOC is suddenly decreased or altered, the nurse will immediately determine if the client has hypoglycemia or hypoxia because these conditions may mimic emergent neurologic disorders. Hypoglycemia and hypoxia are easily treated and reversed, unlike brain injury from inadequate perfusion or trauma.

5. D

   Antiplatelet drugs include the use of aspirin and/or clopidogrel and are the standard of care for treatment following acute ischemic strokes and for preventing future strokes. Aspirin is an antiplatelet drug that prevents further clot formation by reducing platelet adhesiveness (clumping or "stickiness").

6. A, B, D, E

   Before discharge after carotid stent placement, the nurse teaches the client and family to report these symptoms to the primary health care provider immediately: severe headache; change in LOC or cognition (e.g., drowsiness, new-onset confusion); muscle weakness or motor dysfunction; severe neck pain; swelling at neck incisional site; and hoarseness or dysphagia (difficulty swallowing) due to nerve damage.

7. A

   For ischemic strokes, if the client's SBP is more than 185 mm Hg, the nurse notifies the Rapid Response Team or primary health care provider immediately and expects possible prescription of an IV antihypertensive medication. Monitoring the client's BP and mean arterial pressure (MAP) (normal MAP is 70-100 mm Hg; need at least 60 mm Hg to perfuse major organs) should be done every 5 minutes until the SBP is adequate to maintain brain perfusion.

8. B

   The nurse would instruct the AP to **avoid** the clustering of nursing procedures (e.g., giving a bath followed immediately by changing the bed linen). When multiple activities are clustered in a narrow time period, the effect on ICP can be a dramatic elevation.

9. A, B, D, F

   The leading causes of stroke include smoking, obesity, hypertension, diabetes mellitus, and elevated cholesterol. Other risk factors for stroke include substance use disorder (especially cocaine and heavy alcohol consumption) and use of oral contraceptives for women who are at risk for cardiovascular adverse effects.

10. C

    The most important factor in determining whether or not to give alteplase is the time between symptom onset and time seen in the stroke center. The U.S. Food and Drug Administration (FDA) approves administration of alteplase within 3 hours of stroke onset. The American Stroke Association endorses extension of that time frame to 4.5 hours to administer this intravenous fibrinolytic drug.

11. B
Clients who have stroke symptoms are at risk for aspiration due to impaired swallowing as a result of muscle weakness. The best practice for all suspected and diagnosed stroke clients is to maintain NPO status until swallowing ability is assessed and tested. Follow agency guidelines for screening or use an evidence-based bedside swallowing screening tool to determine if dysphagia is present. Refer the client to the speech-language pathologist (SLP) for a swallowing evaluation per stroke protocol as needed.

12. A, B, E, F
To help communication for the client with aphasia, the nurse uses these guiding principles: present one idea or thought in a sentence; use simple one-step commands rather than ask clients to do multiple tasks; speak slowly but **not** loudly; use cues or gestures as needed; avoid "yes" and "no" questions for clients with **expressive** aphasia; use alternative forms of communication if needed, such as a computer, handheld mobile device, communication board, or flash cards (often with pictures); and do not rush the client when speaking.

13. B, D, E
Clients with right hemisphere brain damage typically have difficulty with visual-perceptual or spatial-perceptual tasks. They often have problems with depth and distance perception and with discrimination of right from left or up from down. Because of these problems, clients can have difficulty performing routine ADLs. Caregivers can help the client adapt to these disabilities by using frequent verbal and tactile cues and by breaking down tasks into discrete steps. The AP's scope of practice includes activities of daily living, and reminding clients what has already been taught. The nurse instructs the AP about positioning the client with

the unaffected side toward the room door and the AP follows through. Removal of clutter makes the client's environment safer by decreasing the risk of falls. Options A, C, and F are appropriate to the care of a client with left hemisphere brain damage.

14. B
An embolic stroke is caused by a thrombus or a group of thrombi that break off from one area of the body and travel to the cerebral arteries via the carotid artery or vertebrobasilar system. The usual source of emboli is the heart. Emboli can occur in clients with **atrial fibrillation**, heart valve disease, mural thrombi after a myocardial infarction (MI), a prosthetic heart valve, or endocarditis (infection within the wall of the heart).

15. D
The client with a subarachnoid hemorrhage (SAH), particularly when the hemorrhage is from a ruptured (leaking) cerebral **aneurysm**, often reports the onset of a sudden, severe headache described as "the worst headache of my life." Additional symptoms of SAH or cerebral aneurysmal and arterial-venous malformation (AVM) bleeding are nausea and vomiting, photophobia (sensitivity to light), cranial nerve deficits, stiff neck, and change in mental status.

16. A
Before calling the health care provider (HCP) or Rapid Response Team (RRT), the nurse gathers information. The priority action is to assess this client as soon as possible, preferably within 10 minutes. With this assessment, the next action will be to notify the HCP or RRT. The five most common symptoms are: sudden confusion or trouble speaking or understanding others; sudden numbness or weakness of the face, arm, or leg; sudden trouble seeing in one or both eyes; sudden dizziness, trouble walking, or loss of balance or coordination; and sudden severe headache with no known cause.

17. A, B, C, E, F
All responses are correct except D. Nursing activities should **not** be clustered because this

practice tires the client and can cause increased ICP. Best practices for managing increased ICP for clients experiencing a stroke include: elevate the head of the bed per agency or primary health care provider protocol to improve perfusion pressure; provide oxygen therapy to prevent hypoxia for clients with oxygen saturation less than 94% or per agency or primary health care provider protocol or prescription; maintain the head in a midline, neutral position to promote venous drainage from the brain; **avoid** sudden and acute hip or neck flexion during positioning because extreme hip flexion may increase intrathoracic pressure, leading to decreased cerebral venous outflow and elevated ICP, extreme neck flexion also interferes with venous drainage from the brain and intracranial dynamics; **avoid** the clustering of nursing procedures because when multiple activities are clustered in a narrow time period, the effect on ICP can be dramatic elevation; hyperoxygenate the client before and after suctioning to avoid transient hypoxemia and resultant ICP elevation from dilation of cerebral arteries; provide airway management to prevent unnecessary suctioning and coughing that can increase ICP; maintain a quiet environment for the client experiencing a headache, which is common with a cerebral hemorrhage or increased ICP; keep the room lights low to accommodate any photophobia the client may have; and closely monitor blood pressure, heart rhythm, oxygen saturation, blood glucose, and body temperature to prevent secondary brain injury and promote positive outcomes after stroke.

18. A

The nurse must be alert for symptoms of increased ICP. The first sign of increased ICP is a declining level of consciousness (LOC). Any deterioration in a client's neurological status must be reported immediately to the health care provider or Rapid Response Team immediately.

19. B

Clients with epidural hematomas have "lucid intervals" that last for minutes, during which time the client is awake and talking. This follows a momentary unconsciousness that can occur within minutes of the injury. After the initial interval, symptoms of neurologic impairment from hemorrhage can progress very quickly, with potentially life-threatening ICP elevation and irreversible structural damage to brain tissue. Monitor the client suspected of epidural bleeding frequently (every 5 to 10 minutes) for changes in neurologic status. The client can become rapidly and increasingly symptomatic. A loss of consciousness from an epidural hematoma is a neurosurgical emergency. Notify the primary health care provider or Rapid Response Team immediately.

20. C

The nurse will expect a calcium channel blocking drug that crosses the blood-brain barrier, such as nimodipine, may be given to treat or prevent cerebral vasospasm after a subarachnoid hemorrhage. Vasospasm, which usually occurs between 4 and 14 days after the stroke, slows blood flow to the area and causes ischemia. Nimodipine works by relaxing the smooth muscles of the vessel wall and reducing the incidence and severity of the spasm. In addition, this drug dilates collateral vessels to ischemic areas of the brain. Phenytoin is an antiseizure drug; clopidogrel is an antiplatelet drug, and dexamethasone is a corticosteroid hormone with anti-inflammatory and anti-inflammatory properties.

21. A, B, C, D, E, F

All of these questions are important when getting an accurate history of a TBI. In addition, other concerns would include hand dominance, any diseases of or injuries to the eyes, and any allergies to drugs or food. The nurse asks about a history of alcohol or drug use because these substances may interfere with the neurologic baseline assessment. The nurse would also gather information about whether the client is a victim of violence, if he or she lives in residential care or has a caregiver.

22. A, C, D, E, F

All of these signs and symptoms indicate **mild** TBI except option B. If a client had loss of consciousness, with mild TBI it would be less than 30 minutes. See the box labeled Key Features Mild Traumatic Brain Injury in your text for additional signs and symptoms of a mild TBI.

23. D
Hypercarbia ($Paco_2$ greater than 40 to 45 mm Hg or increased partial pressure of carbon dioxide in arterial blood) can cause cerebral vasodilation and contribute to elevated ICP. Keeping the $Paco_2$ low prevents increased ICP.

24. C
The nurse recognizes Cushing's triad, a classic but very late sign of increased ICP. It is manifested by severe hypertension, a widened pulse pressure (increasing difference between systolic and diastolic values), and bradycardia. This triad of cardiovascular changes usually indicates imminent death.

25. C
Hypotension and hypoxemia, defined as a partial pressure of arterial oxygen (Pao_2) less than 80 mm Hg, restrict the flow of blood to vulnerable brain tissue, also contributing to cerebral edema which leads to increased ICP.

26. D
An ovoid pupil is regarded as the mid-stage between a normal-size and a dilated pupil. Asymmetric (uneven) pupils, loss of light reaction, or unilateral or bilateral dilated pupils are treated as herniation of the brain from increased ICP until proven differently and must be reported to the health care provider immediately.

27. B
Avoid overly aggressive hyperventilation with endotracheal suctioning because of the potential for hypocarbia. Cerebral ischemia caused by even transiently decreased oxygen and either high or low carbon dioxide levels contributes to secondary brain injury.

28. A, C, E, F
Spinal precautions are maintained until the primary health care provider indicates that it is safe to bend or rotate the cervical, thoracic, and lumbar spine. Spinal precautions include: (1) complete bedrest; (2) no neck flexion with a pillow or roll; (3) no thoracic or lumbar flexion; (4) manual control of the cervical spine anytime the rigid collar is removed; and (5) using a "log roll" procedure to reposition the client. A hard, rigid cervical collar is used to maintain cervical spine precautions and immobilization with a confirmed cervical injury.

29. D
Keep the client with an *infratentorial* (brainstem) craniotomy flat or at 10 degrees, depending on the primary health care provider's prescription. Position the client side-lying, alternating sides every 2 hours, for 24 to 48 hours or until ambulatory. This position prevents pressure on the neck-area incision site. It also prevents pressure on the internal tumor excision site from higher cerebral structures. Make sure that the client remains on NPO status until awake and alert because edema around the medulla and lower cranial nerves may also cause vomiting and aspiration.

30. A, B, C, E
Common symptoms of a brain tumor include: headaches that are usually more severe on awakening in the morning; nausea and vomiting; seizures (also called convulsions); impaired sensory perception, such as facial numbness or tingling and visual changes; loss of balance or dizziness; weakness or paralysis in one part or one side of the body (hemiparesis or hemiplegia); difficulty thinking, speaking, or articulating words; and changes in cognition, mentation, or personality. Apraxia and alexia are signs of stroke.

31. B, C, E, F
The AP's scope of practice includes recording intake and output, repositioning clients, and reminding clients what has already been taught. The AP will be familiar with application of sequential pneumatic devices and this could also be delegated. Assessing and teaching clients requires the additional skills and education of a professional RN.

32. B

For periorbital edema and ecchymosis (bruising) around one or both eyes, the nurse will manage this condition with cold compresses to decrease swelling.

33. C

Disc-shaped drug wafers, such as carmustine, may be placed directly into the cavity created during surgical tumor removal (interstitial chemotherapy). This therapy is usually given for newly diagnosed high-grade malignant tumors, but recurrent tumors may also be treated with this method.

34. A

After craniotomy, monitor the client's dressing for excessive amounts of drainage. Report a saturated head dressing or drainage greater than 50 mL over 8 hours **immediately** to the surgeon. Monitor frequently for signs of increasing ICP.

42

CHAPTER

Assessment and Concepts of Care for Patients with Eye and Vision Problems

1. When the medial rectus muscle is not functioning correctly, which eye movement will the nurse note the client has difficulty with?
   A. Looking upward
   B. Looking downward
   C. Gazing in toward the nose
   D. Gazing out toward the ear

2. Which cranial nerve is the nurse assessing when asking a client to open and close the eyelids?
   A. Cranial nerve II (optic)
   B. Cranial nerve III (oculomotor)
   C. Cranial nerve V (trigeminal)
   D. Cranial nerve VII (facial)

3. Which error in refraction does the nurse recognize when a client reports difficulty seeing objects at a distance?
   A. Myopia
   B. Hyperopia
   C. Emmetropia
   D. Astigmatism

4. Which age-related changes in eyes and vision will the nurse expect for an older adult client? **Select all that apply.**
   A. Cornea flattens which blurs vision
   B. Ocular muscle strength is decreased
   C. Decreased discrimination among colors green, blue, and violet
   D. Tear production is decreased resulting in dry eyes
   E. Lens elasticity increases
   F. Eyes appear sunken

5. How does the nurse expect a decreased ability of the iris and pupil to dilate to affect an older client's vision?
   A. Difficulty with tear production resulting in dry eyes
   B. Increased difficulty with vision in dark environments
   C. Difficulty seeing objects that are close
   D. Difficulty with vision because of cataract formation

6. Which specific **priority** teaching for eye protection will the nurse provide for a client who spends a great deal of time in the sun?
   A. Use sunscreen whenever you are in the sun for longer than 30 minutes.
   B. Wear a large hat when you are working in your yard.
   C. Sit in the shade whenever you can.
   D. Use sunglasses that filter UV light when outdoors.

7. When the nurse is instilling ophthalmic drops in a client's eyes, which steps are included in the correct procedure? **Select all that apply.**
   A. Check the eyedrop name, strength, expiration date, color, and clarity.
   B. Wash hands and remove the cap from the bottle.
   C. Instruct the client to tilt the head backward, open eyes, and look down at the floor.
   D. Gently pull the lower lid down against the client's cheek, forming a small pocket.
   E. Hold the eyedrop bottle (with the cap off) like a pencil, with the tip pointing down.
   F. Without touching any part of the eye or lid with the tip of the bottle, gently squeeze and release the prescribed number of drops into the pocket.
   G. Gently release the lower lid and tell the client to close the eye gently.
   H. Gently blot away any excess drug or tears with a tissue.
   I. Ask the client to keep eyes closed for about 1 minute.

8. For which client situation will the nurse contact the eye health care provider **immediately**?
   A. Client whose intraocular pressure by tonometry is 14 mm Hg
   B. Client scheduled for CT scan to assess the eyes and the bony structures around the eyes
   C. Client scheduled for MRI whose eye was injured by a piece of metal
   D. Client scheduled for ultrasonography to assess the orbit and eye

9. Which statements about vision testing of a client by the nurse are accurate? **Select all that apply.**
   A. The Snellen eye chart measures distance vision.
   B. The light perception test determines if a client is unable to identify the presence or absence of light.
   C. A Rosenbaum Pocket Vision Screener or a Jaeger card tests far vision.
   D. Visual field testing determines the degree of a client's peripheral vision.
   E. Color vision is usually tested using Ishihara color plates.
   F. The six cardinal positions of gaze are used to assess muscle function.

10. Which assessment findings will the nurse consider normal when assessing a client's eyes? **Select all that apply.**
    A. Nystagmus in the lateral gaze
    B. Presbyopia in a 35-year-old client
    C. Yellow sclera with small pigmented dots in a dark-skinned person
    D. Ptosis of the eyelids
    E. Pupil constriction within 1 minute in response to light
    F. Head tilting or squinting

11. Which assessment does the nurse use to determine if a client documentation will include PERRLA?
    A. Assess for presence, relief, or decrease in pain.
    B. Assess size, shape, and reactivity of pupils.
    C. Assess pupils, retina, and light refraction.
    D. Assess for signs of presbyopia or retinal detachment.

12. For which diseases or conditions will the nurse monitor clients carefully because they can adversely affect eyes and vision? **Select all that apply.**
    A. Inflammatory bowel disease
    B. Pregnancy
    C. Diabetes
    D. Hypertension
    E. Osteoarthritis
    F. Thyroid problems

13. How frequently will the nurse recommend a basic eye examination for a 50-year-old African-American client?
    A. Every 2 to 4 years
    B. Every 3 to 5 years
    C. Every 1 to 3 years
    D. Every 1 to 2 years

14. What **priority** information would the nurse include when documenting a client's intraocular pressure (IOP)?
    A. Client's body position during IOP measurement
    B. IOP measurement completed in a dark room
    C. Time of mydriatic drops and response to IOP measurement
    D. Type and time of IOP measurement

15. Which predisposing factors will the nurse ask about when taking a history of a client at risk for cataracts? **Select all that apply.**
    A. Recent or past trauma to the eyes
    B. Presence of diabetes or hypertension
    C. History of excessive alcohol intake
    D. Family history of cataracts
    E. Prolonged use of corticosteroids or beta blockers
    F. Recent or past history of cancer

16. Which signs and symptoms will the nurse expect when a client is in the **early** stage of cataract development? **Select all that apply.**
    A. Photophobia
    B. Decreased color perception
    C. Double vision
    D. Blurred vision
    E. Decreased depth perception
    F. Pain and eye redness

17. Which finding does the nurse expect to see when examining a client with a mature cataract using an ophthalmoscope?
    A. Dilated pupil
    B. Bluish-white pupil
    C. Yellow tinge to sclera
    D. Enlarged retina

18. Which priority topics would the nurse teach the client and family for postoperative care after cataract surgery? **Select all that apply.**
    A. Proper instillation of antibiotic and steroid ointments
    B. Remind the client that mild eye itching and "bloodshot appearance" is normal
    C. Apply cool compresses for mild eyelid swelling
    D. Use acetaminophen or aspirin for mild discomfort
    E. Report yellow or green drainage to the eye health care provider immediately
    F. Final best vision will not occur until 4 to 6 weeks after surgery

19. Which activities will the nurse instruct a client receiving discharge teaching after cataract surgery are acceptable?
    A. Vacuuming or mopping are OK, but do not bend over to scrub.
    B. Driving during the day is acceptable, but do not drive at night.
    C. Having sexual intercourse with a familiar partner is acceptable.
    D. Meal preparation and washing dishes are acceptable activities.

20. Which signs and symptoms will the nurse instruct the client and family to **immediately** report to the eye health care provider after cataract surgery? **Select all that apply.**
    A. Mild eye itching
    B. Sharp sudden pain in the eye
    C. Bleeding or increased discharge from the eye
    D. Flashes of light or floating shapes seen in the eye
    E. Decreased vision in the eye that had surgery
    F. Green or yellow, thick drainage from the eye

21. Which **first** sign will the nurse expect when evaluating a client for primary open-angle glaucoma (POAG)?
    A. Brow pain with nausea and vomiting
    B. Gradual loss of visual fields
    C. Seeing halos and floaters
    D. Sudden severe pain around the eyes

22. Which interprofessional collaboration will the nurse seek to assist a client diagnosed with glaucoma to cope who expresses anxiety over the possibility of sight loss?
    A. Mental health professional
    B. Eye health care provider
    C. Home health nurse
    D. Occupational therapist

23. Which statements about drugs administered by the nurse for treatment of increased intraocular pressure (IOP) in a client with glaucoma are accurate? **Select all that apply.**
    A. The prostaglandin agonist drugs reduce IOP by dilating blood vessels in the trabecular mesh, which then collects and drains aqueous humor at a faster rate.
    B. Teach clients prescribed cholinergic agonists that eye color darkens, and eyelashes elongate, over time in the eye receiving the drug.
    C. Cholinergic agonists reduce IOP by limiting the production of aqueous humor and making more room between the iris and the lens, which improves fluid outflow.
    D. Carbonic anhydrase inhibitors directly and strongly inhibit production of aqueous humor.
    E. Teach clients prescribed adrenergic agonists to wear dark glasses outdoors and also indoors when lighting is bright.
    F. Teach clients prescribed beta blockers to check their pulse at least twice per day and to notify the eye health care provider if the pulse is consistently below 60 beats/min.

24. Which **priority** instruction does the nurse teach a client with glaucoma who is prescribed eyedrops to decrease intraocular pressure (IOP)?
    A. Wait 15 minutes between eyedrop drug instillations.
    B. Perform punctal occlusion after using eyedrops for glaucoma therapy.
    C. If a dose is missed, skip it and administer the next dose when it is due.
    D. Blink several times after each eyedrop installation.

25. What is the **next** management action the nurse expects when a client with glaucoma does not respond to prescribed eyedrops with a decrease in intraocular pressure (IOP)?
    A. Insertion of an implanted shunt
    B. A scleral buckling procedure
    C. A laser trabeculoplasty
    D. Visual field testing

26. Which instruction will the nurse teach a client with bilateral eye infections and two bottles of the same antibiotic solution are prescribed?
    A. Obtain one bottle from the pharmacy and return for the second bottle if the infection does not clear.
    B. Obtain one bottle for both eyes because a second bottle is not necessary.
    C. Obtain both bottles and label one for the right eye and the other for the left eye.
    D. Obtain both bottles but save the second because the infection will likely recur.

27. What will the nurse teach the client to **prevent harm** postoperatively after keratoplasty (corneal transplant)? **Select all that apply.**
    A. Do not use an ice pack on the eye.
    B. Wear an eye shield at night for the first week after surgery.
    C. Avoid jogging and any other activity that promotes rapid or jerky head motions for several weeks after surgery.
    D. Lie on the operative side to reduce intraocular pressure (IOP).
    E. Report the presence of purulent discharge immediately to the surgeon.
    F. Examine the eye daily for the presence of infection or graft rejection.

28. With which **specific** interprofessional team member, would the nurse collaborate to **manage** a client's dry, age-related macular degeneration for which there is no cure?
    A. Registered dietitian nutritionist
    B. Eye health care provider
    C. Mental health professional
    D. Speech-language pathologist

29. To **avoid harm** after a scleral buckling procedure for retinal detachment, which instruction does the nurse provide the client?
    A. Turn your head from side to side once an hour to ensure the effects of gravity are distributed equally.
    B. Avoid reading, writing, and work that requires close vision in the first week after surgery.
    C. Keep your head in the horizontal position for at least 12 hours daily.
    D. Place a patch over your eye at night only and apply ice beneath the patch.

30. Which sign or symptom does the nurse expect when a client has **early** retinitis pigmentosa (RP)?
    A. Cataracts
    B. Headache
    C. Night blindness
    D. Poor distance vision

31. Which activity will the nurse expect a client with myopia to have difficulty with when he or she has forgotten to bring glasses to the hospital?
    A. Eating lunch
    B. Looking at an informational brochure
    C. Using a cell phone
    D. Watching the television

32. What is the nurse's **best** response when a young athletic client who suffered a traumatic eye injury with enucleation states, "What's the point of learning about how to take care of this empty hole in my face?"
    A. "Would you like information about joining a support group?"
    B. "Let's take things one step at a time. I'll come back later."
    C. "You seem frustrated. Tell me about how this accident will affect your life."
    D. "Preventing infection will prevent further disfigurement and problems."

33. Which issue will the nurse consider a **priority** when caring for a client with cataracts and impaired vision?
    A. Self-care needs
    B. Safety
    C. Mobility
    D. Communication

Chapter 42 Answer Key

1. C
   When the medial rectus muscle is working correctly and contracts alone, it turns the eye toward the nose. Thus, when it is not functioning, the client would have difficulty gazing toward the nose.

2. D
   The nurse is assessing the facial nerve (CN VII), which innervates the lacrimal glands and muscles for eyelid closure, when asking a client to open and close the eyelids.

3. A
   Myopia (nearsightedness) occurs when the eye overbends the light and images converge in front of the retina. Near vision is normal, but distance vision is poor. Myopia is corrected with a concave lens in eyeglasses or contact lenses. With hyperopia (farsightedness), the client has poor near vision; emmetropia is the perfect refraction of the eye in which light rays from a distant source are focused into a sharp image on the retina; and astigmatism is caused by unevenly curved surfaces on or in the eye, especially the cornea. These uneven surfaces distort vision.

4. A, B, C, D, F
   Options A, B, C, D, and F are correct. Option E is incorrect because there is decreased elasticity in the lens which requires corrective lenses to read.

5. B

Decrease in ability to dilate results in small pupil size and poor adaptation to darkness. The nurse teaches the client that good lighting is needed to avoid bumping into objects, tripping, and falling.

6. D

The risks for cataract formation and for cancer of the eye (ocular melanoma) increase with exposure to ultraviolet (UV) light. The nurse teaches adults to protect the eyes by using sunglasses that filter UV light whenever they are outdoors, at tanning salons, and when work involves UV exposure.

7. A, B, D, E, F, G, H, I

All of these steps for instilling eyedrops into the eyes of a client are correct except option C. The client is instructed to tilt the head backward, open the eyes, and look up at the ceiling.

8. C

MRI is often used to examine the orbits and the optic nerves and to evaluate ocular tumors. It cannot be used to evaluate injuries involving metal in the eyes. Metal in the eye is an absolute contraindication for MRI because the metal could move during the procedure and cause more damage. The nurse must contact the eye health care provider immediately.

9. A, B, D, E, F

All statements about vision testing are accurate except option C. A Rosenbaum Pocket Vision Screener or a Jaeger card tests near (not far) vision.

10. A, B, C,

Nystagmus, an involuntary and rapid twitching of the eyeball, is a normal finding for the far lateral gaze. Presbyopia is an age-related problem in which the lens loses its elasticity and is less able to change shape to focus the eye for close work. As a result, images fall behind the retina. This problem usually begins in adults in their 40s. In dark-skinned adults, the normal sclera may appear yellow, and small, pigmented dots may be visible. The pupil should immediately constrict when a light is directed at it (e.g., a brisk response). If the pupil takes more than 1 *second* to constrict, the response is sluggish. Ptosis, head tilting, and squinting are not normal. Head tilting or squinting often indicate that the client is trying to attain clear vision.

11. B

The abbreviation "PERRLA" stands for **p**upils **e**qual, **r**ound, **r**eactive to **l**ight, and **a**ccommodation.

12. B, C, D, F

Diseases and conditions that commonly affect the eyes and vision include: diabetes mellitus; hypertension; lupus erythematosus; sarcoidosis; thyroid problems; acquired immune deficiency syndrome; cardiac disease; multiple sclerosis; and pregnancy.

13. A

The nurse recommends that a client of any race between the ages of 40 and 64 years have a basic eye examination every 2 to 4 years. African-American clients are recommended to have a basic eye examination every 2 to 4 years from the age of 20 to 64 years. Adults over the age of 65 (any race) are recommended to have this examination every 1 to 2 years.

14. D

IOP varies throughout the day and typically peaks at certain times of the day. Therefore, the nurse will be sure to document the type and time of IOP measurement.

15. A, B, D, E

While age is important because cataracts are most prevalent in the older adult, the nurse asks about other predisposing factors including: recent or past trauma to the eye; exposure to radioactive materials, x-rays, or UV light; prolonged use of corticosteroids, chlorpromazine, or beta blockers; presence of intraocular disease (e.g., recurrent uveitis); presence of systemic disease (e.g., diabetes mellitus, hypoparathyroidism, hypertension); previous cataract, or family history of cataracts; and history of smoking.

16. B, D

Early signs and symptoms of cataracts are slightly blurred vision and decreased color perception. As lens cloudiness continues, blurred vision worsens and double vision occurs. The client may have difficulty with ADLs. Clients commonly report increasing difficulty seeing at night, especially while driving. **No** pain or eye redness is associated with age-related cataract formation.

17. B

As a cataract matures, the opacity makes it difficult to see the retina, and the red reflex may be absent. When this occurs, and the nurse examines the client with an ophthalmoscope, the pupil is bluish white.

18. A, B, C, E, F

All of these teaching points are taught by the nurse to the client and family except option D. Aspirin is avoided because it affects bleeding. If the client's pain is more severe, then acetaminophen with oxycodone may be prescribed.

19. D

The nurse teaches the client about activity restrictions after cataract surgery. Cooking and light housekeeping are permitted, but vacuuming is avoided for several weeks because of the forward flexion involved and the rapid, jerky movements required. Advise the client to refrain from driving until vision is clear. The client is taught to avoid activities that increase IOP such as having sexual intercourse. For additional activities to avoid, see Table 42.5 in your text.

20. B, C, D, E, F

All of these signs and symptoms must be reported to the eye health care provider except option A. Mild eye itching is a normal and expected finding after a client's cataract surgery.

21. B

Primary open-angle glaucoma (POAG), the most common form of primary glaucoma, usually affects both eyes and has no signs or symptoms in the early stages. It develops slowly, with gradual loss of visual fields that may go unnoticed because central vision at first is unaffected.

22. A

The possibility or reality of the loss of vision can be distressing for clients. For clients who experience anxiety or depression related to changes in their sight, the nurse collaborates with a mental health professional. The nurse supports the client at regular visits, and the mental health professional can provide ongoing counseling and support to the client during this time of transition.

23. A, C, D, E, F

All statements about drugs used to treat IOP in glaucoma are correct except option B.

Prostaglandin agonists are the only drugs for glaucoma that cause eye color to darken and eyelashes to elongate over time in the eye or eyes receiving the drug.

24. B

The nurse teaches the client the technique of punctal occlusion (placing pressure on the corner of the eye near the nose) immediately after eyedrop instillation to prevent systemic absorption of the drug. The time between drugs should be 5 to 10 minutes. To decrease IOP, it is essential that the client does not miss doses. After each dose, the client is instructed to close the eyes but not blink them several times.

25. C

Surgery can be performed when drugs for open-angle glaucoma are not effective at controlling IOP. Two common procedures are laser trabeculoplasty and trabeculectomy. A laser trabeculoplasty burns the trabecular meshwork, scarring it and causing the meshwork fibers to tighten. Tight fibers increase the size of the spaces between the fibers, improving outflow of aqueous humor and reducing IOP. Trabeculectomy is a surgical procedure that creates a new channel for fluid outflow. Both are ambulatory surgery procedures.

26. C

   If both eyes are infected, separate bottles of drugs are needed for each eye. The nurse teaches the client to clearly label the bottles "right eye" and "left eye" and not to switch the drugs from eye to eye.

27. A, C, E, F

   All options are correct except B and D. The client is taught to wear a protective shield over the eye at night for a month (not a week) after surgery. The nurse teaches the client to lie on the **non**operative side to decrease IOP.

28. A

   Dry AMD has no cure. Management in the community setting is focused on slowing the progression of the vision loss and helping the client maximize remaining vision and quality of life. The risk for dry AMD can be reduced by increasing long-term dietary intake of vitamins C and E, zinc oxide, copper, and the carotenoids lutein and zeaxanthin. The registered dietitian nutritionist is best equipped to collaborate with the nurse to increase dietary intake of the crucial elements.

29. B

   The nurse instructs the client to avoid reading, writing, and work that requires close vision in the first week after surgery because these activities cause rapid eye movements and detachment. The client is taught about restricted activity and head movement before surgery to prevent further tearing or detachment. An eye patch is placed over the affected eye to reduce eye movement. The client's head does not need to be flat or horizontal for 12 hours daily and ice packs are avoided.

30. C

   The earliest symptoms of RP are usually noticed in childhood. The client may report night blindness and loss of peripheral vision. Over time, decreased acuity progresses to total blindness.

31. D

   Myopia is nearsightedness, in which the eye over-refracts the light and the bent images fall in front of, not on, the retina. Distance vision is poor, so watching television from a distance will be difficult.

32. C

   In option C, the nurse indicates to the client willingness to be attentive and listen to his or her concerns. The other options are not focused on the client's concerns at this time.

33. B

   The priority problem for the client with cataracts is impaired visual *sensory perception*, which is a safety risk. Clients often live with reduced vision for years before the cataract is removed.

43

CHAPTER

Assessment and Concepts of Care for Patients with Ear and Hearing Problems

1. Which questions will the nurse ask to assess a client's auditory sensory perception? **Select all that apply.**
   A. "Are you having any pain or itching in your ears?"
   B. "What kind of music do you prefer to listen to?"
   C. "Do you have a hearing problem now?"
   D. "Have you had any ear trauma or surgery?"
   E. "Have you been exposed to loud noises in your work?"
   F. "Have you had problems with excessive ear wax?"

2. What actions will the nurse take to enhance communication with a hearing-impaired client? **Select all that apply.**
   A. Talk with the client in a quiet room with minimal distractions.
   B. Sit side by side to access the client's better ear.
   C. Sit in adequate light.
   D. Face the client while speaking.
   E. Use short, simple language.
   F. Stand in front of a bright light or a window.

3. Which action by a client indicates to the nurse the **highest** likelihood of hearing impairment?
   A. Client sits and stares out the window at the sky.
   B. Client tilts the head to one side and leans forward.
   C. Client uses an over-the-ear headset to better listen to music.
   D. Client responds to a whispered question.

4. Which **priority** teaching points will the nurse be sure to include when instructing a client about how to irrigate his or her ears for cerumen removal? **Select all that apply.**
   A. Use tap water that feels just barely warm to you.
   B. If the earwax is thick and sticky, place drops of mineral oil into the ear an hour or so before irrigating the ear.
   C. The safest type of ear syringe to use is one that has a right angle or "elbow" in the tip.
   D. Insert the syringe tip only about an inch into your ear canal.
   E. Apply gentle but firm continuous pressure, allowing the water to flow against the top of the canal.
   F. Use blasts or bursts of sudden pressure to irrigate the cerumen out of the ear.

5. For which client does the nurse forgo using an otoscope to examine the ears?
   A. Client with pain during an otoscopic examination
   B. Client who has excess cerumen in the ear canals
   C. Client who is confused and unable to sit still
   D. Client with grey, flaky cerumen in the ear canals

6. Which structure does the nurse expect to be impaired in a client who has a sensorineural hearing loss?
   A. Mobility of the bony ossicles
   B. First cranial nerve
   C. Patency of external ear canal
   D. Eighth cranial nerve

7. When administering which drug to a client will the nurse be sure to monitor carefully for ototoxicity?
   A. Furosemide
   B. Digoxin
   C. Levothyroxine
   D. Vitamin B$_{12}$

8. Which are age-related changes in the ears and hearing that the nurse would expect in an older adult client? **Select all that apply.**
   A. Tympanic membrane loses elasticity and may appear dull and retracted
   B. Cerumen is drier and impacts more easily, reducing hearing function
   C. Pinna becomes shortened and thickened due to increased elasticity
   D. Hair in the ear canal becomes very sparse or may be absent
   E. All older adults experience some hearing loss
   F. The ability to hear high-frequency sounds is lost first

9. Which techniques will the nurse use to perform an otoscopic assessment on a client?
   A. The client's head is tilted slightly toward the nurse.
   B. The nurse holds the otoscope upside down like a large pen.
   C. The pinna is pulled downward and backward.
   D. The internal ear is visualized while the speculum is slowly inserted.

10. Which hearing test will the nurse use to compare a client's hearing by air conduction with hearing by bone conduction?
    A. Audioscopy
    B. Weber test
    C. Rinne test
    D. Voice test

11. Which signs and symptoms will the nurse recognize as indicators that a client has otitis media? **Select all that apply.**
    A. Intense ear pain
    B. Nausea and vomiting
    C. Headache
    D. Blurred vision
    E. Tinnitus
    F. Dizziness

12. What is the nurse's **best** interpretation when a client with otitis media states that the affected ear feels better, but on assessment pus and blood are found?
    A. The infection is worsening.
    B. The ear is permanently damaged.
    C. The eardrum has perforated.
    D. Antibiotics are resolving the infection.

13. Which nonsurgical actions does the nurse expect to perform when caring for a client with otitis media? **Select all that apply.**
    A. Administering oral opioid drugs for mild to moderate pain
    B. Allowing the client to rest
    C. Applying low heat to help relieve pain
    D. Providing a quiet environment
    E. Administering antihistamines to decrease fluid in the middle ear
    F. Giving systemic antibiotic therapy

14. Which priority teaching points will the nurse include for a client after myringotomy surgery? **Select all that apply.**
    A. Avoid straining when having a bowel movement.
    B. Use a straw for consumption of any liquids.
    C. Avoid excessive coughing for 2 to 3 weeks.
    D. Leave the ear dressing in place until the office visit with your health care provider.
    E. Avoid people with respiratory illnesses or infections.
    F. Report excessive drainage immediately to your health care provider.

15. Which action must the nurse teach a client to **avoid to prevent harm** after recovering from the inflammation of external otitis?
    A. Using earplugs during swimming or other water sports
    B. Inserting cotton-tipped applicators into the ears after bathing
    C. Dropping diluted alcohol into the ear to prevent recurrence
    D. Using analgesics and warm compresses for pain relief

16. What is the nurse's **best** rationale for irrigating an older adult's cerumen impaction with fluid that is at body temperature?
    A. It reduces the chance of stimulating the vestibular sense.
    B. Evidence-based practice guides the selection of the temperature.
    C. It is much less painful than irrigation with hotter or colder temperatures.
    D. It potentiates the melting and mobilization of the client's cerumen.

17. Which action does the nurse expect **next** when a client with mastoiditis does not respond to IV antibiotics?
    A. Cultures of the ear drainage
    B. Surgical removal of the infected tissue
    C. Prescription for pain relief drugs
    D. Application of heat to decrease pain

18. Which condition does the nurse suspect when assessment of a client reveals lymph node tenderness behind the ears?
    A. Cerumen impaction
    B. Otosclerosis
    C. Mastoiditis
    D. Ménière disease

19. When the nurse is completing a client's history, which associated factors may contribute to the development of tinnitus? **Select all that apply.**
    A. Otosclerosis
    B. Irrigating the ears too often
    C. Drugs such as aspirin and NSAIDs
    D. Ménière disease
    E. Tophi of the pinna
    F. Continuous exposure to loud noise

20. For which client will the nurse recommend playing soft music during sleeping hours?
    A. Client who reports an odd sensation of "whirling in space"
    B. Client with a hearing aid who reports excessive loud background noise
    C. Client with frequent episodes of acute otitis media
    D. Client with continuous tinnitus

21. Which are the **classic** symptoms of Ménière disease that the nurse recognizes in a client?
    A. Excessive drainage from the affected ear
    B. Hearing loss
    C. Unpredictable episodes of vertigo
    D. Painful uric acid crystal deposits in the pinna
    E. Tinnitus
    F. Buildup of dry, grey cerumen in the affected ear

22. What **priority** teaching will the nurse provide to an assistive personnel (AP) who will help with morning care for a client with vertigo episodes?
    A. "Noise from the television and hallway should be minimized."
    B. "The client's condition may escalate, so report any discomfort."
    C. "Face the client with good light whenever you speak with him or her."
    D. "There is a high risk of falls, so follow fall precautions with this client."

23. Which question will the nurse ask a client with Ménière disease who is prescribed meclizine to determine if the drug is providing the desired **therapeutic** effect?
    A. "On a scale of 1 to 10, which number represents your current level of pain?"
    B. "Has the medication helped to relieve your dizziness and nausea?"
    C. "Do you think the medication has decreased the buzzing in your ears?"
    D. "Has the medication improved your hearing since you started taking it?"

24. Which **priority** teaching points will the nurse include when instructing a client about home management of Ménière disease? **Select all that apply.**
    A. Teach the client to move or turn the head slowly.
    B. Remind the client to take daily vitamin supplements.
    C. Tell the client about the importance of reducing intake of dietary salt.
    D. Instruct the client to avoid caffeinated beverages.
    E. Discuss smoking cessation programs with the client.
    F. Teach the client to avoid standing on ladders or chairs.

25. Which response indicates to the nurse that a client understands information provided about the diagnosis of acoustic neuroma?
    A. "The tumor is benign so I do not need to worry about it."
    B. "I'm not sure if I want to have chemotherapy and radiation."
    C. "The tumor is benign but possible neurological damage sounds scary."
    D. "Hearing loss in one ear is not too bad if that's the worst complication."

26. With which condition must the nurse be **extra** vigilant and cautious if a client is prescribed an ototoxic drug?
    A. Chronic heart failure
    B. Chronic pancreatitis
    C. Chronic obstructive pulmonary disease
    D. Chronic glomerulonephritis

27. Which information will the nurse include when teaching a client how to use a hearing aid? **Select all that apply.**
    A. Avoid exposing the hearing aid to extreme temperatures.
    B. Turn the hearing aid off when not in use.
    C. Avoid using hair spray and cosmetics that might come into contact with the receiver.
    D. Keep extra batteries on hand and change the battery as needed.
    E. Avoid using soap and water when cleaning the hearing aid.
    F. Adjust the volume to the lowest setting that allows you to hear.

28. Which precaution will the nurse remind the client about after stapedectomy surgery?
    A. You will be on bedrest for 2 to 3 days after the surgery.
    B. Improvement in hearing may not occur until 6 weeks after surgery.
    C. You may have difficulty with swallowing for a while.
    D. Getting up to the bathroom will require a bedside commode.

29. Which step is a correct part of the procedure the nurse uses to instill eardrops into a client's ears?
    A. Perform hand hygiene and wear sterile gloves during the procedure.
    B. Place the eardrops bottle in a bowl of hot water for 5 minutes.
    C. Gently irrigate the ear canal if the membrane is not intact.
    D. Tilt the client's head in the opposite direction of the affected ear.

30. Which **specific** assessment will the health care provider look for in a client, after asking the nurse to obtain a pneumatic otoscope?
    A. Mobility of the eardrum
    B. Patency of the eardrum
    C. Gently elicit pain or discomfort
    D. Infection or inflammation

31. Which sounds would the client report to the nurse as **most** difficult to hear when just beginning to notice some hearing loss?
    A. Toddler angry and screaming
    B. Cell phone ringing with low-frequency tones
    C. Woman singing in a soprano range
    D. Gunfire shots on a television show

32. Which client will the nurse expect has the **highest** risk for developing hearing loss related to occupation?
    A. Nurse who works night shift in a Level I trauma center
    B. Bus driver who picks up and drops off elementary school children
    C. Coach who works with a high school swim team
    D. Bartender who works in a night club with live music

Chapter 43 Answer Key

1. A, C, D, E, F
   The nurse would begin by asking if a client has a hearing problem now. Personal history includes past or current signs and symptoms of ear pain, ear discharge, **vertigo** (spinning sensation), **tinnitus** (ringing), decreased hearing, and difficulty understanding people when they talk. Clients would be asked about: ear trauma or surgery; past ear infections; excessive cerumen; ear itch; any invasive instruments routinely used to clean the ear (e.g., Q-tip, match, bobby pin, key); type and pattern of ear hygiene; exposure to loud noise or music during work or leisure activities; air travel (especially in unpressurized aircraft); swimming habits and the use of ear protection when swimming; history of health problems that can decrease the blood supply to the ear, such as heart disease, hypertension, or diabetes; history of vitiligo (a pigment disorder that may include a loss of melanin-containing cells in the inner ear, resulting in hearing loss); history of smoking; and history of vitamin B_{12} and folate deficiency. Option B is incorrect because the important issue is the loudness of the music, not its specific type.

2. A, C, D, E
   During the interview, the nurse sits in adequate light and faces the client to allow him or her to see the nurse speak. Use short, simple language with which the client is comfortable rather than long medical terms. A quiet room with minimal distraction is the best setting to enhance communication with a hearing-impaired client.

3. B
   A client's posture and response provide information about hearing acuity. For example, actions such as tilting the head to one side or leaning forward when listening to another person speak may indicate the presence of a hearing problem. Staring out the window does not indicate hearing impairment, nor does using an over-the-ear headset to listen to music. Correctly responding to a whispered comment indicates normal hearing acuity.

4. A, B, C, D, E
   All responses are correct and appropriate for teaching a client to irrigate his or her ears to remove cerumen except response F. The client and family are taught **not** use blasts or bursts of sudden pressure, but to apply gentle, firm, continuous pressure.

5. C
   The purpose of a brief otoscopic examination is to assess the patency of the external canal, identify lesions or excessive cerumen in the canal, and assess whether the tympanic membrane (eardrum) is intact or inflamed. The nurse avoids using an otoscope to examine the ears of any client who is unable to hold his or her head still during the examination or who is confused, because of the risk for trauma to the ear structures especially the eardrum.

6. D
   Sensorineural hearing loss results from a defect in the cochlea, the **eighth cranial nerve**, or

the brain. (Exposure to loud noise or music causes this type of hearing loss by damaging the cochlear hair.)

7. A

Many drugs are **ototoxic** (having a toxic effect on the inner ear structures), especially many antibiotics, some diuretics (e.g., furosemide), NSAIDs, and many chemotherapy agents.

8. A, B, F

Options A, B, and F are expected age-related changes in older adults. Option C is incorrect. The pinna becomes elongated because of loss of subcutaneous tissues and decreased elasticity. Option D is incorrect. Hair in the canal becomes coarser and longer, especially in men. Option E is incorrect. While many older adults experience hearing loss, not all do. The nurse must **not** assume that all older adults have a hearing loss.

9. B

The nurse tilts the client's head slightly away and holds the otoscope upside down, like a large pen. This position permits the nurse's hand to lie against the client's head for support. If the client moves, both nurse's hand and the otoscope also move, preventing damage to the canal or eardrum. The nurse holds the otoscope in his or her dominant hand and gently pulls the pinna up and back with the other hand to straighten the canal, then views the external ear canal while slowly inserting the speculum.

10. C

The Rinne tuning fork test compares hearing by air conduction with hearing by bone conduction. Sound is normally heard twice as long by air conduction than by bone conduction. The nurse performs this test by placing the vibrating tuning fork stem on the mastoid process (bone conduction) and asking the client to indicate when the sound is no longer heard. When the client no longer hears the sound, the fork is quickly brought in front of the pinna (air conduction) without touching the client. The client is instructed to indicate when this sound is no longer heard. The client normally continues to hear the sound twice as long in front of

the pinna after not hearing it with the tuning fork touching the mastoid process.

11. A, B, C, E, F

A client with acute or chronic otitis media will present with ear pain. Other signs and symptoms can include tinnitus, headaches, malaise, fever, nausea, vomiting, and dizziness. Blurred vision is not a sign of otitis media.

12. C

When otitis media worsens and progresses, the eardrum spontaneously perforates, and pus or blood drains from the ear. The client usually has a marked decrease in pain as the pressure on middle ear structures is relieved.

13. B, C, D, E, F

All of these actions are appropriate for nonsurgical management of otitis media except option A. Opioid drugs would only be prescribed for severe pain.

14. A, C, E, F

Instructions the nurse provides for the client and family after myringotomy include: avoid straining with a bowel movement; avoid drinking through a straw for 2 to 3 weeks; avoid air travel for 2 to 3 weeks; avoid excessive coughing for 2 to 3 weeks; avoid people with respiratory infections; when blowing your nose, blow gently, without blocking either nostril and with your mouth open; avoid getting your head wet or washing your hair for several days; you may shower but before doing so, place a ball of cotton coated with petroleum jelly (e.g., Vaseline) in the ear or use a waterproof earplug; avoid rapidly moving the head, bouncing, and bending over for 3 weeks; if you have a dressing, change it every 24 hours or as directed; and report excessive drainage immediately to your health care provider.

15. B

The nurse teaches the client to avoid the use of cotton swabs inserted into the ear to clean the ears or remove cerumen. Use of these swabs can push the wax deeper into the ear canal and might also seriously damage sensitive ear canal skin or the eardrum.

16. A

When irrigating an older adult's cerumen impaction, the nurse must ensure that the fluid is at body temperature (about 98.6°F or 37°C) to reduce the chance for stimulating the vestibular sense which can lead to dizziness and lack of balance.

17. B

When a client has mastoiditis, interventions focus on halting the infection before it spreads to other structures. IV antibiotics are used but do not easily penetrate the infected bony structure of the mastoid. Cultures of the ear drainage are taken to determine which antibiotics should be most effective. Surgical removal of the infected tissue is needed if the infection does not respond to antibiotic therapy within a few days. A simple or modified radical mastoidectomy with tympanoplasty is the most common treatment. All infected tissue must be removed so the infection does not spread to other structures.

18. C

The signs and symptoms of mastoiditis include swelling behind the ear and pain when moving the ear or the head. Cellulitis develops on the skin or external scalp over the mastoid process, pushing the ear sideways and down. The eardrum is red, dull, thick, and immobile. Lymph nodes behind the ear are tender and enlarged. Clients may have low-grade fever, malaise, and ear drainage.

19. A, C, D, F

Factors that contribute to tinnitus include age, sclerosis of the ossicles, Ménière disease, certain drugs (aspirin, NSAIDs, high-ceiling diuretics, quinine, aminoglycoside antibiotics), exposure to loud noise, and other inner ear problems.

20. D

When no cause can be found or the disorder is untreatable, therapy focuses on ways to mask the tinnitus with background sound, noise-makers, and music during sleeping hours.

21. B, C, E

Ménière disease is a condition that includes a **classic trio** of symptoms – episodic **vertigo** (the sensation of whirling or turning in space), tinnitus, and hearing loss.

22. D

Institute and teach fall precautions to all clients with Ménière disease, as vertigo may result in falls. The nurse teaches the AP to follow fall precautions to prevent falls due to vertigo.

23. B

Meclizine is an antivertiginous drug used to treat vertigo and nausea. The therapeutic effect of the drug is improvement or relief of vertigo and nausea. It does not relieve pain or tinnitus nor does it improve hearing.

24. A, C, D, E, F

Teach clients to move the head slowly to prevent worsening of the vertigo. Tell clients about nonpharmacologic treatment for Ménière disease which includes diet and lifestyle adjustments because clients with this condition are often sensitive to triggers such as high salt intake, caffeine, monosodium glutamate (MSG), alcohol, nicotine, stress, and allergens. Instruct clients to avoid activities that place them at risk of experiencing vertigo and falls, such as standing on chairs or ladders. While taking a vitamin supplement is a good idea, it is not specific to Ménière disease.

25. C

An acoustic neuroma is a benign tumor of the vestibulocochlear nerve (cranial nerve VIII) that often damages other structures as it grows. Depending on the size and exact location of the tumor, damage to hearing, facial movements, and sensation can occur. An acoustic neuroma can cause many neurologic signs and symptoms as the tumor enlarges in the brain. Radiation may be part of the treatment, but chemotherapy is not.

26. D

The nurse must be extra cautious when ototoxic drugs are prescribed for clients with reduced kidney function (e.g., glomerulonephritis). Increased ototoxicity can occur because drug elimination is slower, especially among older patients.

27. A, B, C, D, F
Important points the nurse will teach when instructing a client about use of a hearing aid include: keep the hearing aid dry; clean the ear mold with mild soap and water while avoiding excessive wetting; use a toothpick to clean debris from the hole in the middle of the part that goes into the ear; turn off the hearing aid when not in use; check and replace the battery frequently; keep extra batteries on hand; keep the hearing aid in a safe place; avoid dropping the hearing aid or exposing it to temperature extremes; adjust the volume to the lowest setting that allows you to hear to prevent feedback squeaking; avoid using hair spray, cosmetics, oils, or other hair and face products that might come into contact with the receiver; if the hearing aid does not work: change the battery, check the connection between the ear mold and the receiver, check the on/off switch; clean the sound hole; adjust the volume; and take the hearing aid to an authorized service center for repair.

28. B
After this surgery, the nurse reminds the client that improvement in hearing may not occur until 6 weeks after surgery. The client will need assistance with getting out of bed slowly, using the bathroom, and activities of daily living. A bedside commode is not necessary. Vertigo, nausea, and vomiting usually occur after surgery because of the nearness to inner ear structures. The surgical procedure is performed in an area where cranial nerves VII, VIII, and X

can be damaged by trauma or by swelling after surgery. The nurse assesses for facial nerve damage or muscle weakness. Indications include an asymmetric appearance or drooping of features on the affected side of the face. Ask the patient about changes in facial perception of touch and in taste.

29. D
The steps the nurse uses to instill eardrops into a client's ear include: gather the solutions to be administered; check the labels to ensure correct dosage, time, and expiration date; wear clean gloves to remove and discard any ear packing; wash hands; perform a gentle otoscopic examination to determine whether the eardrum is intact; irrigate the ear if the eardrum **is** intact; place the bottle of eardrops (with the top on tightly) in a bowl of **warm** water for 5 minutes; tilt the patient's head in the opposite direction of the affected ear and place the drops in the ear; with his or her head tilted, ask the patient to gently move the head back and forth five times; insert a cotton ball into the opening of the ear canal to act as packing; and wash your hands again.

30. A
The purpose of a pneumatic otoscope is to detect decreased eardrum mobility.

31. B
Hearing loss occurs first with the low-frequency tones; in some patients, it progresses to include all levels and eventually becomes permanent.

32. D
Clients whose occupations involve chronic exposure to loud noise or music are at **high** risk to develop hearing loss related to occupation.

44 CHAPTER

Assessment of the Musculoskeletal System

1. Which body minerals are stored almost exclusively in bones and contribute to bone density? **Select all that apply.**
   A. Calcium
   B. Chloride
   C. Magnesium
   D. Phosphorus
   E. Potassium
   F. Sodium

2. Which client will the nurse assess **most closely** for indications of osteoporosis based on race or ethnicity?
   A. 40-year-old Chinese-American female
   B. 50-year-old Irish-American female
   C. 60-year-old African-American female
   D. 66-year-old African-American male

3. Which bone problem will the nurse expect in a client who has a tumor that secretes excessive amounts of parathyroid hormone (PTH)?
   A. Increased osteoclastic activity with osteoporosis
   B. Increased osteoblastic activity and foot enlargement
   C. Decreased growth hormone levels and thinning of facial bones
   D. Decreased bone phosphorus levels resulting in bone spur formation

4. Which nutrient will the nurse suspect is deficient in a client who has bowing of the bones in both lower limbs?
   A. Iron
   B. Protein
   C. Vitamin C
   D. Vitamin D

5. Which hormones are important in promoting bone mass and density in an adult client? **Select all that apply.**
   A. Calcitonin
   B. Estrogen
   C. Glucocorticoids
   D. Growth hormone
   E. Insulin
   F. Parathyroid hormone
   G. Testosterone
   H. Thyroxine

6. Which assessment findings will the nurse expect in an older female client who has osteoporosis? **Select all that apply.**
   A. Gait changes
   B. Inability to bear weight
   C. Muscle atrophy
   D. History of fractures
   E. Swelling in the finger joints
   F. Spinal curvature with postural changes

7. How will the nurse document the assessment observation in which the client's spinal thoracic vertebrae curve sideways to the right and then return to midline?
   A. Dextrosis
   B. Lordosis
   C. Kyphosis
   D. Scoliosis

8. Which client will the nurse recognize as having the greatest risk for developing chronic osteomyelitis?
   A. 25-year-old who performs heavy manual labor
   B. 35-year-old who stepped on a rusty nail 10 years ago
   C. 45-year-old with diabetes who has a recurrent foot ulcer
   D. 55-year-old with osteoporosis who has sprained the same wrist twice

9. Which actions will the nurse suggest to a 72-year-old female client to **prevent harm** by reducing the rate of osteoporosis? **Select all that apply.**
   A. Walking one mile 5 to 7 days per week
   B. Eating a diet high in fruits and vegetables
   C. Swimming for 30 minutes three times weekly
   D. Performing isometric and isotonic exercises daily
   E. Taking a calcium supplement that contains vitamin D
   F. Performing range-of-motion exercises for the arm while sitting

10. Which assessment information obtained from a 60-year-old male client with severe osteoarthritis of the right knee will the nurse consider the greatest contributing factor?
    A. Is 10 lb (4.5 kg) overweight
    B. Has ridden a motorcycle for 35 years
    C. Has worked laying carpet for the past 20 years
    D. Has a 25 pack-year history of cigarette smoking

11. Which additional electrolyte change will the nurse expect to find in a client who has hypercalcemia?
    A. Hyponatremia
    B. Hyperkalemia
    C. Hypochloremia
    D. Hypophosphatemia

12. Which laboratory changes will the nurse expect to find with a client who suffered extensive soft-tissue damage from a crush injury of the thighs? **Select all that apply.**
    A. Serum potassium 5.2 mEq/L (mmol/L)
    B. Creatine kinase 280 units/L (345 IU/L)
    C. Serum calcium 11.5 mg/dL (2.68 mmol/L)
    D. Alkaline phosphatase 90 units/L (120 IU/L)
    E. Aspartate aminotransferase 50 units/L (57 IU/L)
    F. White blood cell (WBC) count 11,000/mm^3 (11 × 10^9/L)

13. How will the nurse interpret the physical therapist's report that a client has 70 degrees of flexion based on goniometry measurement on the left knee?
    A. Flexion is reduced
    B. Flexion is increased
    C. Extension is unaffected
    D. Range of motion is normal

14. Which action will the nurse perform **next** when an obese client's popliteal pulse on one side cannot be palpated?
    A. Palpating the popliteal pulse on the opposite side
    B. Attempting to assess the pedal pulse on the same side
    C. Notifying the primary health care provider immediately
    D. Using a Doppler to assess blood flow in that popliteal space

15. Which activity does the nurse ask a client to perform when assessing range of motion (ROM) in the hand?
    A. Gripping the nurse's hand as hard as possible
    B. Rapidly rotating the hand from palm up to palm down
    C. Apposing each finger to thumb and then making a fist
    D. Waving the hand from side to side as though waving goodbye

16. Which aspects will the nurse include when assessing the neurovascular status of a client's right limb after diagnostic arthroscopy 1 hour ago? **Select all that apply.**
    A. Presence of pain
    B. Gait and balance
    C. Distal pulses
    D. Capillary refill
    E. Sensation
    F. Skin temperature

17. What is the nurse's **best** response when a client who is scheduled for an ultrasound to identify whether osteomyelitis is present states that she is afraid of the pain the procedure will cause?
    A. "This procedure does not involve needles or incisions and is usually painless."
    B. "There would only be pain with this procedure if you don't remain perfectly still."
    C. "A small amount of numbing medicine will be applied to the skin before the procedure."
    D. "The same medication your dentist uses will be injected 10 minutes before the needle is inserted."

18. Which is the **priority** action for the nurse to perform when caring for a patient who just had a needle bone biopsy under local anesthesia?
    A. Administering pain medication
    B. Assessing for bleeding
    C. Checking the gag reflex
    D. Assessing the distal pulse

Chapter 44 Answer Key

1. **A, D**
   Bone is the only significant storage site for calcium and phosphorus, although there is some phosphorus in some other body cells for metabolism and energy production. These two minerals are responsible for maintenance of bone density. All other cells store potassium. The major storage site of sodium and chloride is the kidney. Magnesium is present in higher concentrations in muscle cells.

2. **A**
   Chinese Americans of either gender are most at risk for osteoporosis because of racial differences in bone size and density. Bones are smaller and less dense. The density difference increases the risk for osteoporosis. African Americans have greater bone density than most other races. Although Irish Americans have less bone density than do African Americans, they are taller than and have greater bone density than Chinese Americans.

3. **A**
   PTH is a hormone normally secreted by the parathyroid glands to prevent serum calcium levels from becoming too low. One of its action is moving calcium out of the bones (calcium resorption) and into the blood by increasing osteoclastic activity. When osteoclastic activity is prolonged and not balanced by osteoblastic activity, bone density is lost and osteoporosis occurs.

4. **D**
   A deficiency of vitamin D can result in osteomalacia, which is softening of the bones. When osteomalacia occurs in weight-bearing bones, such as those in the lower legs, the bones can bend or bow.

5. A, B, D, E, G, H
Except for glucocorticoids and parathyroid hormone, all of the listed hormones play important roles in maintaining bone density and balancing osteoblastic activity with osteoclastic activity for bone health. Glucocorticoids and parathyroid hormone promote bone density loss and do not help maintain healthy bone matrix.

6. A, D, F
Osteoporosis occurs with severe osteopenia in which there is great loss of bone density. Less dense bones, especially in the spine, result in kyphosis with postural changes, and gait changes. The loss of bone density increases the risk for fragile factures even with minimal trauma. Clients usually can still weight bear. Osteoporosis is not directly responsible for muscle atrophy and does not cause joint swelling.

7. D
Scoliosis is an abnormal lateral curvature of the spine. In lordosis, the abnormal spinal curvature is inward and occurs in the lumbar spinal area. Kyphosis is an outward curvature of the thoracic spine causing a "humped back" appearance. Dextrosis is not a spinal curvature.

8. C
Clients who have diabetes have poor wound healing and a high risk for infection in any open wound. An injury to the foot is difficult to heal and can progress inward through the soft tissue to the bone. Infection can spread to the bone this way, resulting in chronic osteomyelitis.

9. A, D, E
Performing weight-bearing exercises, such as walking, and muscle-strengthening exercises can reduce bone density loss and slow osteoporosis. Ensuring adequate intake of calcium and vitamin D is critical to bone density maintenance. Swimming, although an aerobic activity, is not a weight-bearing exercise. Fruits and vegetables are not major sources of either calcium or vitamin D. Arm range-of-motion exercises can maintain arm muscle function and shoulder joint flexibility, but do not prevent bone density loss.

10. C
Laying carpet requires extensive time in the kneeling position and carpet layers also use their dominant knee to push a device that stretches the carpet and places it under the baseboard. Both actions are repetitive and cause force injuries to the involved joints that can reduce articulating cartilage. Being 10 lb (5 kg) overweight is not usually sufficient in a male to cause osteoarthritis of the knee. A smoking history increases the risk for osteopenia but not arthritis. Riding a motorcycle may cause some musculoskeletal problems, but not osteoarthritis of the knees.

11. D
Blood calcium and phosphorus levels exist in a balanced reciprocal relationship that causes one level to rise as the other one decreases. Elevations of serum calcium levels above normal cause a corresponding decrease in serum phosphorus levels. High levels of serum calcium do not change the serum levels of sodium, potassium, or chloride.

12. A, B, D, E
All the laboratory values are elevated. The only ones that are associated with probable skeletal muscle trauma are an elevated serum potassium level (because cells have high levels of potassium, which is released when cells are damaged or destroyed), and the other substances that are present in higher concentrations in skeletal muscle than in the blood, creatine kinase, alkaline phosphatase, and aspartate aminotransferase. Skeletal muscle damage does not directly increase the serum calcium concentration or the white blood cell count.

13. A
The minimum normal knee joint flexion is 90 degrees. Therefore, this client's range of motion in the left knee is reduced. There is not enough information in the question to draw a conclusion about the extension of the left knee.

14. D
The popliteal pulse may be difficult to palpate in an obese client. The next best action is to assess this pulse using a Doppler device.

Although other assessment findings on that limb, such as checking for a pedal pulse, can help determine whether general blood flow is adequate, it does not establish whether or not there is a problem in that specific artery.

15. C
A quick way to assess range of motion in the hand is by asking the client to perform two separate maneuvers. One is making a fist. The other is bringing each fingertip separately to appose the thumb. Gripping is a way to assess strength but not ROM. Waving and rotating the hand palm up and palm down assesses some ROM of the wrist but not of the fingers.

16. A, C, D, E, F
After arthroscopy for either diagnostic or surgical intervention purposes, the nurse assesses the neurovascular status on a regular basis to prevent harm from poor circulation in the extremity or any possible nerve damage. Assessment includes monitoring distal pulses, warmth, color, capillary refill, pain, movement, and sensation of the affected extremity. Neurovascular assessment does not include gait and balance.

17. A
Ultrasonography is noninvasive and involves rolling a probe on the skin over the area to be imaged. Ultrasound jelly is applied to the skin over the site to be examined to reduce the friction of the probe and make movement smoother. Although clients report a cold sensation, pain is not expected, and no special preparation necessary.

18. B
Bone is very vascular and can bleed excessively after a biopsy. Although pain management is also important, the medication can be administered after first assessing whether excessive bleeding is present. The gag reflex is not affected by local anesthesia. Pulses distal to the biopsy area are not likely to be affected by the procedure. They should be assessed but not as the first or priority action.

45 CHAPTER

Concepts of Care for Patients with Musculoskeletal Problems

1. Which assessment findings will the nurse recognize as modifiable risk factors when planning strategies to **prevent harm** from progression of a client's osteopenia? **Select all that apply.**
   A. Has rheumatoid arthritis
   B. Mother has osteoporosis
   C. Is 11 lb (5 kg) underweight for height
   D. Smokes one pack of cigarettes per day
   E. Drinks one glass of red wine with dinner nightly
   F. Takes a calcium supplement containing vitamin D daily

2. How will the nurse interpret the risk for osteoporosis in a client whose T-score is -3?
   A. Osteopenia is present.
   B. Osteoporosis is present.
   C. Risk for osteopenia is increased.
   D. Score is normal and does not indicate a risk for osteoporosis.

3. Which client will the nurse determine has the **highest** risk for osteoporosis?
   A. 30-year-old female who drinks 48 oz (~1250 mL) of diet cola daily and uses high-protection sunscreen
   B. 40-year-old male who is 72 inches (1.8 m) tall, eats a vegan diet, and participates in competitive martial arts
   C. 50-year-old male with type 1 diabetes mellitus who lifts weights for exercise
   D. 60-year-old female who is 15 lb (6.8 kg) overweight and walks 2 miles daily

4. Which client risk factors or health problems will the nurse associate with osteoporosis? **Select all that apply.**
   A. Muscle cramps
   B. Sedentary lifestyle
   C. Back pain relieved by rest
   D. Fracture
   E. Urinary or renal stones
   F. High-cholesterol diet

5. Which activity will the nurse recommend that a client with regional osteoporosis of the vertebrae **avoid** to **prevent harm**? **Select all that apply.**
   A. Jogging
   B. Jumping rope
   C. Riding horses
   D. Participating in yoga
   E. Riding a stationary bicycle
   F. Performing water aerobics

6. Which client will the nurse assess for the possibility of regional osteoporosis?
   A. 40-year-old who has been in a long leg cast for 10 weeks
   B. 45-year-old on long-term corticosteroid therapy for a chronic inflammation
   C. 55-year-old who is being managed for hyperparathyroidism
   D. 60-year-old who is postmenopausal with a history of falls

7. Which condition or factor will the nurse consider as the most likely cause of a client's loss of bone density in the L-1 to L-5 vertebrae?
   A. Swims an hour every day at an indoor pool
   B. Has worked as a data entry technician 40 hours weekly for the past 25 years
   C. Takes 1300 mg of acetaminophen daily for pain relief from osteoarthritis of the left knee
   D. Has had five epidural injections of cortisol into the lower back during the past year for severe pain

8. Which clients will the nurse collaborate with a registered dietitian nutritionist to assist in modifying their nutritional risk for osteoporosis? **Select all that apply.**
   A. 25-year-old female who drinks six cups of coffee daily
   B. 30-year-old female who is overweight for height
   C. 35-year-old male who is on the high-protein Atkins diet
   D. 45-year-old female who drinks unfortified almond milk
   E. 55-year-old male who drinks one carbonated beverage every day
   F. 65-year-old male with chronic alcoholism

9. How will the nurse instruct a client to prepare for a dual x-ray absorptiometry (DXA) scan?
   A. "Blood and urine specimens will be taken immediately before the test."
   B. "Leave metallic objects such as jewelry, coins, and belt buckles at home."
   C. "Be sure to have someone come with you to drive you home after the test."
   D. "Bring a comfortable loose nightgown without buttons or snaps, and a pair of slippers."

10. Which foods will the nurse suggest to increase calcium and vitamin D intake for a client who is lactose intolerant?
    A. Fresh apples and pears
    B. Whole-grain bread and pasta
    C. Fortified soy or rice products
    D. Skim milk and fat-free yogurt

11. Which MRI report/finding indicates to the nurse that the client has significant generalized bone density loss?
    A. Red blood cell production is increased above normal.
    B. Perfusion of the wrist and elbow joints is greater than expected.
    C. Percentage of bone marrow adipose tissue is higher than expected.
    D. Osteoblastic activity appears equal to or greater than osteoclastic activity.

12. Which exercise will the nurse suggest for the client with kyphosis to improve lung capacity?
    A. Swimming and yoga
    B. Deep breathing and pectoral stretching
    C. Range of shoulder and hip movements
    D. Walking or jogging 30 minutes three times weekly

13. Which dietary changes will the nurse in collaboration with the registered dietitian nutritionist reinforce to the client who has osteoporosis to treat the disorder. **Select all that apply.**
    A. Increasing fiber
    B. Limiting caffeinated beverages
    C. Increasing leafy green vegetables
    D. Increasing low-fat dairy products
    E. Reducing high carbohydrate-containing fruit
    F. Eliminating eggs and other animal-sourced proteins

14. Which drugs belong to the estrogen agonist/antagonist class? **Select all that apply.**
    A. Alendronate
    B. denosumab
    C. estrogen/bazedoxifene
    D. ibandronate
    E. raloxifene
    F. risedronate
    G. zoledronic acid

15. Which instruction is **most** appropriate for the nurse to teach a client prescribed to take alendronate 10 mg daily?
    A. "Be sure to rotate injection sites every week."
    B. "Be sure to take the drug 1 hour before or at least 2 hours after a meal."
    C. "Remain in the upright position for at least 30 minutes after taking the drug."
    D. "Report any headaches you experience to your primary health care provider immediately."

16. For which client with osteoporosis will the nurse question the primary health care provider's prescription for calcium and vitamin D supplementation?
    A. 40-year-old with diabetes mellitus
    B. 50-year-old with urinary stones
    C. 55-year-old with esophageal ulcers
    D. 65-year-old with venous thromboembolism

17. What is the nurse's **best** response when a client who has been treated for 4 weeks for osteomyelitis asks why the disease is so difficult to cure?
    A. "Bones have a poor blood supply and are located so deep in the body that it is hard for antibiotics to reach them."
    B. "There are no early symptoms of osteomyelitis, so by the time it is detected the infection is widespread."
    C. "After a bone abscess forms, it gets covered with a new layer of bone that is difficult for drugs to penetrate."
    D. "The most common organisms that cause osteomyelitis are usually drug-resistant."

18. Which client condition will the nurse recognize as increasing the risk for osteomyelitis of facial bones?
    A. Chronic sinusitis as a result of persistent allergies
    B. Poor dental hygiene and periodontal infection
    C. Untreated pharyngeal streptococcal infection
    D. Presence of chronic diabetic foot ulcers

19. Which assessment findings will the nurse expect in a client who is admitted with acute osteomyelitis of the left lower leg?
    A. Temperature greater than 101°F, swelling, tenderness, erythema, and warmth in the area
    B. Ulceration resulting with sinus tract formation, localized pain, and drainage
    C. Aching pain, poorly described, deep, and worsened by pressure and weight bearing
    D. Shortening of the extremity with pain during weight bearing or palpation

20. With which client will the nurse remain **most alert** for indications of acute hematogenous osteomyelitis?
    A. 30-year-old male with a leg fracture and external skeletal pins
    B. 50-year-old female in an ICU with pneumonia
    C. 65-year-old female with MRSA infection
    D. 72-year-old male with a catheter-related urinary tract infection

21. A client is being evaluated for bone pain in the lower extremity. Which laboratory result indicates to the nurse a possible malignant bone tumor?
    A. Low vitamin D level
    B. Decreased serum calcium level
    C. Elevated serum alkaline phosphatase
    D. Decreased erythrocyte sedimentation rate

22. Which assessment findings will the nurse caring for a client who had an allograft for a large bone defect that resulted from tumor removal **report immediately** to the surgeon to **prevent harm**? **Select all that apply.**
    A. Pain at the surgical site
    B. Signs of infection
    C. Hemorrhage
    D. Fracture
    E. Difficulty ambulating
    F. Loss of muscle tone

23. What is the nurse's best response to a 50-year-old male client scheduled for a bunionectomy with wire placement who states "Since this is ambulatory surgery and I won't have to spend the night, I can plan on participating in a 10 K race next month."?
    A. "You may have to change your plans and only run a 5 K next month."
    B. "This is ambulatory surgery but the healing time is usually at least 6 to 12 weeks."
    C. "After this surgery, it is unlikely you will ever be able to run more than a mile again."
    D. "If you wear the orthopedic boot, you can run again as soon as you can tolerate the pain."

24. Which instruction will the nurse give to the client with plantar fasciitis about self-management to reduce pain?
    A. Use rest, elevation, and warm packs.
    B. Perform gentle jogging exercises.
    C. Strap the foot to maintain the arch.
    D. Wear loose or open shoes, such as sandals.

Chapter 45 Answer Key

1. C, D
    Two common modifiable risk factors for osteopenia progressing to osteoporosis are being underweight and cigarette smoking. Although having rheumatoid arthritis and having a parent with osteoporosis are also risk factors, they are not modifiable. Taking a calcium supplement containing vitamin D is a prevention strategy. Excessive alcohol consumption is a risk factor and one glass of wine nightly is not excessive.

2. B
    The T-score represents the standard deviations above or below the average bone marrow density (BDM) for young healthy adults. A T-score of -1 to -2.5 indicates osteopenia. A T-score lower than -2.5 (-3) indicates osteoporosis.

3. A
    Risk factors for osteoporosis include being female, consuming excessive amounts of phosphorus (which is a major component of carbonated soft drinks), and being deficient in vitamin D. Not only does the amount of soft drinks consumed daily increase the blood levels of phosphorus, it may well be consumed in place of calcium and vitamin D containing dairy products. The use of high-protection sunscreen limits the amount of vitamin D activated in the skin by exposure to sunlight.

4. B, C, D
    A sedentary lifestyle with little weight-bearing activity contributes to the development of osteoporosis. Health problems that can result from osteoporosis include back pain relieved by rest and fragile fractures. Muscle cramps and urinary stones do not result in or from osteoporosis. Although poor nutrition is associated with osteoporosis, no evidence suggests that a high-cholesterol diet increases the risk for osteoporosis.

5. A, B, C
    Clients with regional osteoporosis of the spine (vertebrae) are at risk for harm from vertebral compression fractures. To reduce this risk, clients are advised to avoid activities that jar the spine. Riding a stationary bicycle, performing water aerobics, and participating in yoga are not "jarring" activities.

6. A
    Regional osteoporosis results from conditions that affect only one body region or area. Having a leg in a long leg cast for 10 weeks can result in bone density loss from reduced mobility and disuse. The other conditions can cause generalized osteoporosis rather than regional problems.

7. D
Cortisol, a corticosteroid, causes bone density loss generally when taken orally or given parenterally. When it is administered in an epidural, it is present in a high concentration surrounding the vertebrae in the area for weeks with each administration. This high local concentration causes local bone density loss without inducing loss anywhere else.

8. A, C, D, F
High caffeine intake increases calcium loss and increases the risk for osteoporosis. High-protein diets reduce the levels of free calcium in the blood by keeping it bound to plasma proteins. Almond milk may contain calcium but if it is unfortified, it does not also contain vitamin D, which is needed to absorb calcium in the GI tract. Chronic alcoholism often results in a variety of nutritional deficits that increase the risk for osteoporosis. Drinking one carbonated beverage daily or being overweight does not increase osteoporosis risk.

9. B
DXA scans are painless and do not require medications or blood and urine specimens. The client remains dressed, but is required to have no metallic objects on them. Metal can interfere with the test.

10. C
Fortified soy and rice products are good sources of calcium and vitamin D. A client who is lactose intolerant would not be able to use dairy products as a calcium source. The other items listed do not contain significant amounts of calcium and vitamin D.

11. C
Bone marrow adipose tissue (BMAT) or fat is present in higher than expected levels in clients who have bone marrow loss. The other findings listed are not associated with bone marrow loss or osteoporosis.

12. B
Kyphosis reduces chest expansion and lung capacity. Exercises that can specifically improve lung capacity include abdominal tightening, deep breathing, and pectoral stretching.

13. B, D
The specific dietary treatment for osteoporosis is the same as prevention. This focuses on increasing intake of calcium and vitamin D (dairy products) and reducing dietary intake of substances that can reduce blood levels of the mineral and vitamin (i.e., caffeine). Eggs and other proteins are needed to maintain good bone health, as are fruits and vegetables.

14. C, E
Alendronate, ibandronate, risedronate, and zoledronic acid all belong to the bisphosphonate class of drugs. Denosumab is a monoclonal antibody. Estrogen/bazedoxifene and raloxifene are from the estrogen agonist/antagonist class of drugs.

15. C
This drug, along with all others in the bisphosphonate class, greatly increases the risk for esophagitis, esophageal ulcers, and gastric ulcers. The drug must be taken with food and not on an empty stomach. Having the client remain in the upright position after taking the drug helps prevent stomach contents from refluxing back into the esophagus and irritating it.

16. B
Increasing serum calcium levels can exacerbate the development of urinary stones in a client who has a history of stone formation.

17. C
Bone infections can easily damage bone tissue leading to tissue necrosis and abscess formation. Because bone is a dynamic tissue and attempts to heal itself, osteoblasts often lay new bone tissue over the infected tissue making it difficult for drug therapy to penetrate into the infected bone. Although some organisms may be drug-resistant, even when the organism is sensitive to the antibiotic, the real problem is drug penetration. Higher doses and longer duration of drug therapy are needed to eradicate the infection and prevent complications such as chronic osteomyelitis and sepsis.

18. B

    Often, osteomyelitis develops as a result of infection in adjacent tissues that spreads directly to nearby bone. These are known as contiguous osteomyelitis infections. Poor dental hygiene and periodontal (gum) infection can be causative factors in contiguous osteomyelitis in facial bones.

19. A

    The most common symptom of acute osteomyelitis is pain. Fever, usually with temperature greater than 101° F (38.3° C) also is present. As the area around the infected bone swells, tenderness on palpation occurs. Erythema (redness) and heat may also be present.

20. D

    Acute hematogenous infection results from bacteremia, underlying disease, or nonpenetrating trauma. Urinary tract infections, particularly in older men, tend to spread to the lower vertebrae.

21. C

    Most often, the presence of a malignant bone tumor causes an elevated serum alkaline phosphatase (ALP) levels, regardless of specific tumor type. Elevation of this enzyme results from the body's attempt to form new bone by increasing osteoblastic activity.

22. B, C, D

    Hemorrhage, infection, and fracture represent serious complications of the allograft surgery and can result in graft loss, as well as an increased risk for sepsis. To prevent harm and possible limb loss, indications of these problems need to be reported to the surgeon or Rapid Response Team immediately.

23. B

    Recovery from any surgery on the foot is quite slow compared with that in any other body region because it is so far away from the heart. Complete healing may take longer than 6 to 12 weeks. Only partial weight-bearing is permitted. Walking is difficult with an orthopedic boot and running is very unlikely. This client needs to have an in-depth discussion with his surgeon for exactly what the surgery entails and what is expected after surgery. The length of time for the surgery and the fact that it usually does not require an overnight stay have no bearing on the length of healing time required.

24. C

    Plantar fasciitis is an inflammation of the fascia that holds foot bones in place to form the foot's arch. Supporting the arch by wearing shoes with a good arch support or an orthotic insert can help prevent the fascia from pulling and irritation. Strapping the center of the sole of the foot, which can be performed by the client, also helps maintain the arch and reduce the pain.

46
CHAPTER

Concepts of Care for Patients with Arthritis and Total Joint Arthroplasty

1. Which clients will the nurse be sure to assess as having an increased risk for developing osteoarthritis (OA)? **Select all that apply.**
   A. 30-year-old woman with a family history of rheumatoid arthritis
   B. 35-year-old man who is 10 lb (4.5) underweight and has never smoked
   C. 40-year-old woman with multiple knee injuries from playing soccer in high school
   D. 45-year-old man who worked construction for 25 years
   E. 50-year-old man who is 10 lb (4.5 kg) overweight and plays golf twice weekly
   F. 65-year-old obese woman who lives alone after working as a hairdresser for 40 years

2. Which client statement indicates to the nurse the possibility of osteoarthritis (OA)?
   A. "When I stand too long in one place, my back hurts although walking doesn't bother it."
   B. "I noticed that my third finger joint seems to be tilting inward toward my other fingers."
   C. "My knees hurt so much that I end up taking a lot of acetaminophen or aspirin."
   D. "There is a lot of osteoarthritis in my family. What can I do to prevent it?"

3. How will the nurse document the assessment finding of a grating sound and grating feeling when moving the knee joint through range of motion on a client who reports pain in that knee?
   A. Crepitus
   B. Osteophytosis
   C. Secondary synovitis
   D. Subcutaneous emphysema

4. When interviewing a client who is suspected to have osteoarthritis (OA), which question is **most important** for the nurse to ask?
   A. "Can you tell if your pain and mobility are worse after eating certain foods?"
   B. "In looking at your family, who has more arthritis, the men or the women?"
   C. "What activities would you like to do but don't because of your joint pain?"
   D. "When pain is present, is it usually accompanied by a headache?"

5. What lifestyle changes does the nurse suggest to help slow joint degeneration for a client who has been newly diagnosed with osteoarthritis (OA)? **Select all that apply.**
   A. Avoiding direct sunlight and other sources of ultraviolet light
   B. Keeping body weight appropriate for height and body type
   C. Quitting smoking, vaping, or using nicotine in any form
   D. Avoiding any participation in outdoor activities
   E. Avoiding activities that may result in trauma
   F. Engaging in low-impact exercises daily

6. Which associated problem will the nurse assess for in a client with osteoarthritis who has a large effusion of the left knee?
   A. Corresponding symptoms in the right knee
   B. Atrophy of the muscles above the left knee
   C. Presence of Heberden nodules on the right knee
   D. Joint hardness on palpation of the left knee

7. Which responses, from a client with advanced osteoarthritis, alert the nurse that the client may be having a problem coping with the image and role changes related to disease progression? **Select all that apply**.
   A. "It seems that I am getting younger. I used to tie my shoes; now I am using Velcro closures just like my grandkids."
   B. "Washing dishes in very warm water makes my hands feel so good that I don't use the dishwasher much."
   C. "I used to be a playground assistant; now I contribute by working with children who need help with reading."
   D. "Because my joints hurt so much, I just look out the window instead of working in my garden."
   E. "I no longer wear my rings so I don't draw attention to how awful my hands look."
   F. "Although I can no longer play the piano, I really enjoy going to concerts."

8. What health problem does the nurse suspect when the laboratory results of the fluid around a client's painful, swollen joint show urate crystals?
   A. Gout
   B. Osteoarthritis
   C. Psoriatic arthritis
   D. Rheumatoid arthritis

9. Which assessment findings will the nurse expect in a client who has osteoarthritis that affects the spine?
   A. Localized pain at T6-12, inflexibility, and muscle asymmetry
   B. Localized pain at L3-4, bone spurs, stiffness, and muscle atrophy
   C. Radiating pain throughout the spine, stiffness, and muscle weakness
   D. Radiating pain at L3-4 and C4-6, stiffness, muscle spasms, and bone spurs

10. Which precaution is **most appropriate** for the nurse to teach a client with osteoarthritis (OA) who is prescribed to take acetaminophen for mild to moderate pain?
    A. "Avoid alcoholic beverages while taking this drug."
    B. "Avoid coffee and other caffeinated drinks while taking this drug."
    C. "Do not drive or operate dangerous machinery until you know how this drug affects you."
    D. "If any decrease in vision occurs, stop the drug and notify your primary health care provider immediately."

11. Which statement by a client with osteoarthritis (OA) indicates to the nurse the need for more education about health promotion to **prevent harm**?
    A. "My children gave me a gift certificate for paraffin dips for my feet."
    B. "When my joints are really stiff, I try to stay in bed most of the day."
    C. "I find that my knees hurt less when I wear shoes with firm soles rather than slippers."
    D. "Keeping my knees bent on a large pillow while sleeping at night helps reduce my pain."
    E. "Even on days when I have more severe symptoms, I try to walk short distances outside."
    F. "I read that avoiding eating tomatoes, potatoes, and eggplant can help reduce arthritis pain."

12. For which client with osteoarthritis (OA) will the nurse question a prescription for celecoxib?
    A. 40-year-old with asthma
    B. 45-year-old with type 2 diabetes
    C. 50-year-old with cardiovascular disease
    D. 55-year-old with irritable bowel syndrome

13. Which health problems or assessment findings in a client with osteoarthritis who reports that he has been taking glucosamine for joint pain causes the nurse to have concern about this complementary therapy?
    A. Client is 20 lb (9.9 kg) overweight
    B. Blood pressure is 150/90
    C. Resting pulse is 90 beats/min
    D. A light red rash is present
    E. Client has type 2 diabetes
    F. Morning stiffness lasts 2 hours

14. Which assessment findings in a client with osteoarthritis scheduled to have a total joint replacement (TJR) will the nurse report to the surgeon immediately? **Select all that apply.**
    A. Reports having an abscessed tooth
    B. Has asthma symptoms with seasonal allergies
    C. Had a dental implant placed about 3 years ago
    D. Repeat blood pressure readings are consistently higher than 160/90
    E. Pain rating in affected joint is 9 on a 0 to 10 pain rating scale
    F. Has type 2 diabetes and today's fasting blood glucose level is 102 mg/dL (5.7 mmol/L)

15. With which surgical approach for total hip replacement does the nurse expect that clients will have fewer problems with pain or postoperative joint displacement?
    A. Anterior approach
    B. Direct lateral approach
    C. Posterolateral approach
    D. Indirect lateral approach

16. For which side effect will the nurse **most closely** monitor an older client receiving an opioid drug for pain control after total hip replacement surgery?
    A. Sudden-onset hypertension
    B. Urinary retention
    C. Acute confusion
    D. Dark, tarry stools

17. Which question is **most important** for the nurse to ask a client who is about to receive a prescribed preoperative dose of IV cefazolin before total joint replacement surgery to **prevent harm**?
    A. "Did you shower with chlorhexidine gluconate this morning?"
    B. "When did you last take aspirin or any other NSAID?"
    C. "Do you have a sulfa drug allergy?"
    D. "Do you have a penicillin allergy?"

18. Which new-onset symptoms in a client who is 2 days postoperative after total hip arthroplasty (THA) suggests to the nurse that hip dislocation may have occurred? **Select all that apply.**
    A. Agitation
    B. Loss of appetite
    C. Increased pain intensity
    D. Clear drainage on dressing
    E. Inability to dorsiflex the foot
    F. Leg shortening on the operative side

19. Which actions will the nurse take to **prevent harm** from surgical site infection (SSI) in clients who have undergone total joint arthroplasty? **Select all that apply.**
    A. Culturing drainage when a change is observed
    B. Washing hands thoroughly when caring for clients
    C. Encouraging early ambulation along with leg exercises
    D. Using aseptic technique for wound care and emptying of drains
    E. Administering low–molecular-weight heparin every 12 hours as prescribed
    F. Assessing the incision every 4 to 8 hours for increasing redness or purulent drainage

20. Which actions will the nurse take for a client after a left total knee arthroplasty (TKA) to **prevent harm** from venous thromboembolism (VTE)? **Select all that apply.**
    A. Encouraging early ambulation
    B. Instructing the client to keep the legs straight
    C. Administering the prescribed anticoagulant therapy
    D. Removing antiembolic stockings for 1 hour every 4 hours
    E. Ensuring the sequential compression device is in place and functional
    F. Helping the client to perform dorsiflexion and plantar flexion exercises hourly

21. Which action will the nurse take to prevent subluxation after surgery in a client who had total shoulder arthroplasty?
    A. Maintaining the wrist and fingers in a slightly flexed position
    B. Maintaining the wrist and fingers in a slightly extended position
    C. Placing the arm on the surgical side in an abduction immobilizer
    D. Wrapping the arm on the surgical side in elastic roller bandages in a figure-eight pattern from the fingers to the shoulder

22. Which client with persistent joint pain and stiffness will the nurse suspect has rheumatoid arthritis rather than any other type of arthritis?
    A. 36-year-old white woman with bilateral wrist swelling
    B. 40-year-old black woman whose mother has osteoarthritis
    C. 45-year-old white man with a history of kidney stones
    D. 50-year-old black man who played professional football

23. Which statement made by the client taking hydroxychloroquine for rheumatoid arthritis (RA) does the nurse report immediately to the rheumatologist to **prevent harm**?
    A. "If I take the medication with food, my stomach bothers me less."
    B. "My vision is getting blurry. I think I must need new glasses."
    C. "Could you give me another pain pill just for muscle pain?"
    D. "I get kind of light-headed when I stand up too quickly."

24. Which statements by a client who has arthritis indicates to the nurse the possibility of Sjögren syndrome? **Select all that apply**.
    A. "Lately, my eyes have felt gritty by the end of the day."
    B. "Ice sometimes helps my joint pain better than heat does."
    C. "If I don't use a vaginal lubricant, intercourse is painful."
    D. "Some little bumps have appeared on my arm, but they don't hurt."
    E. "When my arthritis gets worse in one joint, the pain seems worse in all my joints."
    F. "It's kind of crazy but I have had more cavities in the past 2 years than in all the rest of my life."

25. An elevation in which laboratory value **most specifically** indicates to the nurse that a client has rheumatoid arthritis (RA)?
    A. Antinuclear antibodies
    B. Total leukocyte count
    C. Erythrocyte sedimentation rate
    D. Anti-cyclic citrullinated peptide

26. Which laboratory test result is **most important** for the nurse to know before administering the first dose of a biological response modifier (BRM) to a client with rheumatoid arthritis?
    A. Complete blood count
    B. Tuberculosis skin test
    C. Immunoglobulin E level
    D. Hepatitis B and C antibody levels

27. Which precautions are **most important** for the nurse to stress to **prevent harm** when teaching about drug therapy to a 32-year-old female client who is prescribed to take oral methotrexate? **Select all that apply**.
    A. Do not drink alcohol while taking this medication.
    B. Be sure to use a reliable form of contraception.
    C. If the drug causes you nausea, take it at bedtime.
    D. Avoid crowds of people and those who are ill.
    E. If you miss a dose, call your rheumatology health care provider immediately.
    F. This drug may require weeks to months before a full effect is seen.

28. What is the nurse's **best first** action when the client with rheumatoid arthritis has one knee that is much more swollen than any other joint, and is both reddened and hot to the touch?
    A. Comparing the range of motion for this joint with that of the opposite knee
    B. Asking the client whether any recent injury has occurred to this joint
    C. Notifying the rheumatology health care provider immediately
    D. Elevating the affected knee and applying ice

29. Which is the **priority** action for the nurse to take when caring for a client with rheumatoid arthritis who just had an arthrocentesis?
    A. Assessing for return of the client's gag reflex
    B. Assessing for postprocedural pain to ensure optimal pain relief
    C. Placing the client in a prone position and elevating the extremity
    D. Monitoring the insertion site for bleeding or leakage of synovial fluid

30. What is the nurse's **best first** action when a client with rheumatoid arthritis appears to have experienced a subluxation of the first and second vertebrae?
    A. Assessing respiratory status, and applying oxygen as needed
    B. Notifying the rheumatology health care provider or Rapid Response Team
    C. Performing neurovascular checks in all extremities
    D. Assessing for pain that radiates down the arm and changes in mental status

Chapter 46 Answer Key

1. C, D, F
   Obesity is an independent risk factor for OA in men and women. Although more men than women usually have OA as a result of sports injuries, women who sustained significant joint injuries when younger also have an increased risk for OA in those previously injured joints. Working at jobs that require heavy manual labor or remaining in one position for long periods of time increase the risk. A family history of rheumatoid arthritis does not increase the risk for OA and neither does participating in lower impact activities such as golf.

2. C
   Persistent and specific joint pain is the most common reason that clients with OA seek health care.

3. A
   Crepitus is a grating sensation heard or felt on palpation when moving a joint through range of motion. It is caused by loosened bone and cartilage present in a synovial joint.

4. C
   Assessing how much the pain affects the client's quality of life and ability to participate in ADLs, as well as home care, work, and pleasurable activities, is important in planning interventions and client education materials for management of the disorder.

5. B, C, E, F
   Increased weight both causes OA and worsens damage to existing OA. Nicotine causes vasoconstriction and reduces blood flow to joints,

which may result in ischemia and necrosis of already damaged joints. Activities that may result in trauma put stress on uninjured joints and intensify the damage to joints already affected by OA. Engaging in daily, low-impact exercises helps prevent muscle atrophy around affected joints, taking some stress off those joints.

Avoiding sunlight or any ultraviolet light does not prevent problems with OA and, because exposure to sunlight activates vitamin D in the skin and contributes to bone density maintenance, limited sun exposure may increase the risk for osteopenia. There is no orthopedic benefit to avoiding the outdoors.

6. B
Decreased mobility is common when clients have pain from joint effusions, which results in muscle atrophy above the affected joint. With OA, the disorder is usually unilateral. Heberden nodules appear on the fingers (distal joints), not on the knees. Joint effusions fill the joint with fluid, making them soft on palpation.

7. D, E
The responses about missing an activity without replacing it and the one about how awful the hands look shows a negative body image. All of the other responses demonstrate positive changes or adaptations that the client uses in adapting to disease progression.

8. A
Gout, or gouty arthritis, is a systemic metabolic disorder in which an error in protein metabolism causes excessive urate crystals to form. These crystals deposit in joints causing severe joint inflammation. Although some other forms of arthritis may result in effusions, the fluid does not contain urate crystals.

9. D
OA of the spine tends to most often occur in the lumbar region at the L3-4 level or the cervical region at C4-6. In the neck, compression of spinal nerve roots may occur as a result of vertebral facet bone spurs. Common symptoms include radiating pain, stiffness, and muscle spasms in one or both extremities.

10. A
Acetaminophen can cause severe liver damage and even liver failure when taken at high doses or too often. This adverse reaction is much more likely to occur in clients who drink alcoholic beverages while on acetaminophen therapy.

11. B, D
Staying in bed can lead to muscle atrophy and other problems that worsen mobility. Keeping the knees bent on a large pillow while sleeping can lead to flexion contractures that reduce mobility.
Options A, C, and E are good health promotion actions for clients with OA. Although there is no evidence that avoiding certain foods can help reduce pain and other problems from OA, the avoidance of the listed foods does not cause harm to the client.

12. C
All COX-2 NSAIDs, including celecoxib, increase the risk for cardiovascular events, especially myocardial infarctions. These drugs are either not recommended or are used with extreme caution in clients with cardiovascular disease.

13. B, E
Glucosamine can increase blood glucose levels and raise blood pressure. It is contraindicated for clients who are hypertensive or have diabetes mellitus. The other problems or findings have no significance with glucosamine therapy.

14. A, D
Before TJR can proceed, the client needs to be infection free and have other chronic health problems well controlled. The client has a current infection and hypertension is not controlled. The diabetes is controlled. None of the other client issues are contraindications for TJR surgery.

15. A
The anterior approach does not cut through muscle and tendons, as the posterolateral and direct lateral approaches do. This approach not only results in less pain, but it also holds the prosthesis more tightly in place, reducing the

risk for displacement postoperatively. The indirect lateral approach is not a common or valid surgical technique for total hip replacement.

16. C

Although any client can become confused as a result of opioid drugs, older clients are much more likely to have this side effect.

17. D

The most commonly used antibiotic prescribed to be administered within an hour of initiation of surgery is cefazolin. This drug is structurally similar to penicillin and if the client is allergic to penicillin, he or she will also be allergic to cefazolin.

18. A, C, F

Signs and symptoms specific to hip dislocation include report of sudden intense pain, sudden agitation for the patient who is unable to communicate, and affected leg rotation, and/or leg shortening.

19. A, B, D, F

Encouraging ambulation and administering heparin help prevent venous thromboembolism but do not prevent SSI. All other actions listed help prevent SSI or identify it early so management can prevent failure to heal or sepsis.

20. A, B, C, E, F

With the exception of option D, all actions help prevent VTE. Antiembolic stockings remain in place throughout the 24-hour day except for a short period during which the stockings are removed to allow inspection of the limb and application of fresh stockings.

21. C

Excessive movement of the shoulder joint can cause subluxation of the head of the humerus from the glenoid cavity after shoulder replacement surgery. Placing the arm on the surgical side in an abduction immobilizer can help prevent shoulder movement that promotes subluxation. The position of the wrists and fingers does not contribute to shoulder subluxation.

22. A

Rheumatoid arthritis is an autoimmune disease with the highest incidence in young- to middle-age women. Unlike osteoarthritis, it is usually bilateral and often includes non–weight-bearing joints.

23. B

A dangerous side effect of hydroxychloroquine is central retinitis that can lead to total blindness. Any change in vision requires immediate follow-up. If the change is related to hydroxychloroquine, the drug must be discontinued immediately.

24. A, C, F

The three hallmarks of Sjögren syndrome are dry eyes, dry mouth, and (in women) vaginal dryness. Dry mouth greatly increases the risk for and incidence of dental cavities.

25. D

Elevations in all of these tests are associated with RA. However, most are also elevated with other inflammatory disorders. Only the anti-cyclic citrullinated peptide (anti-CCP) is very specific and sensitive in detecting early RA. Its presence is also a marker for aggressive and erosive late-stage disease.

26. B

BRMs lower overall immunity and increase the risk for infection and are not given if an active infection is present. If the client has ever had tuberculosis (TB), the microorganism remains in her or his body and is dormant. The use of BRMs can reactivate the dormant organism and cause active TB. Therefore, a positive TB test is a contraindication to BRM therapy.

27. A, B, D

This drug induces liver toxicity and clients are taught not to drink alcohol while on this drug. The drug is known to increase the risk for birth defects and is contraindicated during pregnancy. Methotrexate lowers immunity and increases the risk for infection. The client is taught to avoid crowds and people who are ill. Although the drug may require an extensive period of time before symptoms are reduced, this information does not prevent harm and neither does the suggestion to take it at bedtime. The drug is only taken once per week. If the client misses a dose on the regularly scheduled day, he or she is taught to take it as soon as it is remembered. The health care provider does not need to be notified.

28. C
The presence of only one hot, swollen, painful joint (out of proportion to the other joints) is considered infected until proven otherwise. The condition requires immediate assessment and treatment by the rheumatology health care provider to prevent harm from more serious infection and sepsis.

29. D
The first priority is assessing the insertion site for bleeding or leakage. The procedure is performed under local anesthesia and the client's gag reflex is not affected. Often the client's pain after the procedure is reduced as the pressure of the effusion is decreased when fluid is removed.

30. A
Subluxation of the first and second cervical vertebrae may be life threatening because branches of the phrenic nerve that supply the diaphragm are compressed and respiratory function may be compromised. The nurse assesses the client's respiratory status first and applies oxygen if there is any indication of respiratory impairment. Then the rheumatology health care provider or the Rapid Response Team is notified. The nurse also keeps the client's neck straight in a neutral position to prevent permanent damage to the spinal cord or spinal nerves.

47
CHAPTER

Concepts of Care for Patients with Musculoskeletal Trauma

1. Which clients with fractures will the nurse recognize as being at **increased risk** for delayed or slow bone healing? **Select all that apply.**
   A. 28-year-old male with multiple long-bone fractures
   B. 35-year-old female with diet-induced osteopenia
   C. 45-year-old female semiprofessional tennis player
   D. 58-year-old female taking corticosteroids daily for an autoimmune disorder
   E. 65-year-old male with arteriosclerosis
   F. 75-year-old male chronic obstructive pulmonary disease

2. Clients with which problems or factors will the nurse assess **most frequently** for development of acute compartment syndrome? **Select all that apply.**
   A. Lower legs caught between the bumpers of two cars
   B. Massive infiltration of IV fluid into the forearm
   C. Bivalve cast on the lower leg
   D. Multiple insect bites to lower legs
   E. Daily use of oral corticosteroids
   F. Severe burns to the upper extremities

3. Which assessment finding in a client who has a fracture of the right wrist alerts the nurse to a possible *early* indication of a complication?
   A. Wiggling fingers causes pain.
   B. Client reports numbness and tingling.
   C. Fingers are cold and pale; pulses are impalpable.
   D. Pain is severe and seems out of proportion to injury.

4. Which client will the nurse assess **most frequently** for indications of venous thromboembolism (VTE)?
   A. 25-year-old weightlifter with a fracture of the right femur
   B. 45-year-old with metastatic cancer and a spinal compression fracture
   C. 55-year-old car crash victim with multiple facial fractures
   D. 65-year-old with a broken elbow and hypertension

5. Which assessment findings in a client with a complete and displaced fracture of the femur indicates to the nurse possible fat embolism syndrome (FES)? **Select all that apply.**
   A. Increased swelling over the fracture site
   B. Petechiae on the neck and chest
   C. Decreased platelet count
   D. Dry mucous membranes
   E. Sudden-onset confusion
   F. $PaO_2 = 72$ mm Hg

6. Which suggestion will the nurse make to help a client who has complex regional pain syndrome (CRPS) in the right arm weeks after an open reduction was required to repair a broken elbow and fractured radius to reduce the discomfort?
   A. Take pain medications around the clock even when the pain is not present.
   B. When the sensations occur, immobilize and ice the limb until they pass.
   C. Use a dry wash cloth and rub the skin on the arm several times daily.
   D. Wrap the arm in warm, wet compresses as soon as the pain starts.

7. Which assessments are a **priority** for the nurse to perform to **prevent harm** on a client who was hit by a motorcycle and has a suspected pelvic fracture? **Select all that apply.**
   A. Checking vital signs
   B. Asking about opioid use
   C. Examining urine for presence of blood
   D. Asking the client to rate his or her pain
   E. Determining the level of consciousness
   F. Performing neurovascular checks of the lower limbs

8. Which assessment is the **priority** for the nurse to perform on a client admitted to the emergency department with multiple rib fractures?
   A. Pulses in all four extremities
   B. Pulse rate and rhythm
   C. Oxygen saturation
   D. Pain intensity

9. Which assessment finding on a client who has a closed fracture of the lower femur with extensive swelling and bruising **best** indicates to the nurse that perfusion in the affected limb is adequate?
   A. Pulse oximetry on the right forefinger is 98%.
   B. Pedal pulse of the affected limb is easily palpated and strong.
   C. Femoral pulse of the affected limb is easily palpated and strong.
   D. Capillary refill on great toe of the affected limb is about 4 seconds.

10. After ensuring airway, breathing, and circulation along with a head-to-toe assessment, which action will the nurse take **next** in the emergency care of a client with an extremity fracture?
   A. Checking the neurovascular status of the area distal to the injury: temperature, color, sensation, movement, and distal pulses by comparing the affected and unaffected limbs
   B. Elevating the affected area on pillows, applying an ice pack that is wrapped to protect the skin, and obtaining a prescription for pain medication
   C. Immobilizing the extremity by splinting; include joints above and below the fracture site, followed by rechecking the circulation

   D. Removing or cutting the client's clothing to inspect the affected area while supporting the injured area above and below the injury

11. Which assessment finding on an older client who fell while getting out of bed indicates to the nurse a possible fracture?
   A. The client is extremely confused and trying to get up.
   B. The client cries out when the nurse attempts to examine him.
   C. One leg is shorter than the other and has a protruding bump on the side.
   D. The skin of both legs is cooler and darker than that of the upper extremities.

12. What is the nurse's **best** response when a client who had a long-leg plaster cast applied an hour ago reports that the cast feels "hot?"
   A. "Plaster gives off heat as it dries, and the heat does not mean anything is wrong."
   B. "It is likely that you have an infection and will need to be started on antibiotics immediately."
   C. "This means you are having an allergic reaction and this cast will have to be removed immediately."
   D. "Don't worry. This heat is normal and I will apply a cooling blanket over it for your comfort."

13. A client who had a plaster splint applied to the ankle at 7 a.m. and received pain medication at 9 a.m. now at 11 a.m. reports that the pain is getting worse, not better. What is the nurse's **best first** action to **prevent harm**?
   A. Assessing the pulses and skin temperature distal to the splint
   B. Loosening the splint and reassessing the client's pain in 15 minutes
   C. Requesting a prescription to administer the pain medication IV
   D. Repositioning the extremity on a pillow and placing an ice pack

14. Which action will the nurse perform **first** when a client in a body cast reports a painful "hot spot" underneath the cast and an unpleasant odor?
    A. Requesting a cast change
    B. Offering the client a PRN pain medication
    C. Assessing the client's temperature and other vital signs
    D. Elevating the extremity and applying an ice pack over the spot

15. Which precautions or care information are appropriate for the nurse to include when teaching a client going home with a synthetic forearm cast?
    A. "Be sure to change the stockinette at least once a week."
    B. "Limit movement of the fingers and wrist joints to prevent pain."
    C. "Keep your hand and arm elevated above the level of your heart to reduce swelling."
    D. "Use an ice pack on the cast for the first 6-8 hours, and cover the pack with a towel."
    E. "When upright, wear the sling so that it distributes over your shoulders and not just your neck."
    F. "Call your primary health care provider immediately if numbness and tingling occur in your hand or fingers."

16. What is the nurse's **best** response to a young adult client who says "How will I ever walk on that?" on seeing his pale and thin leg after removal of a long-leg cast that has been in place for 7 weeks?
    A. "Fractures can heal but the bones are never as strong as they were before the break."
    B. "The leg will be weak at first, but will regain muscle strength and size as you exercise."
    C. "The bone will thicken as healing continues and make this leg as large as your other one."
    D. "The color changed because the plaster in the cast rubbed off on it and will improve when you are able to shower."

17. Which actions are appropriate for the nurse to perform when caring for a client who is placed in Buck's traction after a hip fracture? **Select all that apply.**
    A. Ensuring that the weights never rest on the floor
    B. Removing the boot or belt every 8 hours to assess skin integrity
    C. Comparing the amount of weights applied with the amount prescribed
    D. Removing the weights every 8 hours for 30 minutes to prevent muscle spasms
    E. Assessing circulation distal to the traction device every hour for the first 24 hours
    F. Instructing all personnel and visitors to not touch or change the position of the weights

18. Which question is **most appropriate** for the nurse to ask a client who has been receiving scheduled and PRN opioids for severe pain with multiple fractures who now has a distended abdomen and hypoactive bowel sounds?
    A. "Did you use opioids or other recreational drugs before your injury?"
    B. "What specific foods have you eaten in the past 2 days?"
    C. "How would you rate your pain on a 0 to 10 scale?"
    D. "When was your last bowel movement?"

19. A client expresses concern over the presence of external pins and external devices used to manage her fracture and says she wishes it all could have been placed internally so it wouldn't be visible. What advantages will the nurse tell the client that external fixation has over internal fixation of fractures? **Select all that apply.**
    A. The risk for infection is reduced.
    B. You lost less blood than you would have with an internal fixation.
    C. This device allows you to move and walk earlier than an internal device.
    D. You will not need surgery to remove these devices after healing is complete.
    E. Most people have less pain with the external devices than with internal devices.
    F. This device replaces the need for the use of any other device, such as a cast or a boot, later.

20. What is the **most appropriate** action for the nurse to take when assessment on a client with external fixation reveals crusts have formed around the pin sites?
    A. Assessing the client's temperature
    B. Notifying the surgeon immediately
    C. Documenting the finding as the only action
    D. Removing the crusts and culturing the drainage

21. Which client with a nonhealing fracture of the humerus will the nurse recognize as having a contraindication for use of electrical bone stimulation?
    A. 30-year-old with a seizure disorder
    B. 40-year-old smoker with hypertension
    C. 50-year-old with an implanted cardiac pacemaker
    D. 60-year-old with reduced immunity from corticosteroid use

22. Which precaution or care information will the nurse teach a client prescribed low-intensity pulsed ultrasound treatments for a very slow-healing fracture of the lower leg specific for this treatment?
    A. Use a reliable form of birth control until treatment is complete.
    B. The treatment cannot be used if you have any type of diabetes mellitus.
    C. The device should not be used in the same room with a microwave oven.
    D. Expect to dedicate approximately 20 minutes each day for the treatment.

23. Which client will the nurse consider to be at **highest risk** for nonunion after a fracture?
    A. 40-year-old who is 20 lb overweight and has a Colles fracture of the wrist
    B. 50-year-old female with comminuted fracture of the humerus
    C. 60-year-old male with multiple fractured ribs
    D. 70-year-old female with a "tib-fib" fracture

24. Which assessment findings on a client being prepared for a vertebroplasty for a compression fracture of the lumbar vertebrae will the nurse report immediately to the orthopedic surgeon? **Select all that apply.**
    A. Platelet count is 40,000/mm³ (40 × 10⁹/L)
    B. White blood cell count is 9000/mm³ (9 × 10⁹/L)
    C. Client reports taking the prescribed dose of an antihypertensive this morning
    D. Client reports taking the prescribed dose of rivaroxaban this morning
    E. Pain rating is an 8 on a 0 to 10 scale
    F. Sensation to pinprick stimulation is reduced on the right leg

25. Which client will the nurse determine requires the **most** assistance with performance of ADLs?
    A. 28-year-old with bilateral below-the-knee amputations
    B. 40-year-old with amputation of the dominant hand
    C. 50-year-old with an above-the-knee amputation of the dominant leg
    D. 70-year-old with amputations of all the toes on the left foot

26. Which actions will the nurse take to prevent a flexion contracture in a client who is postoperative from an above-the-knee amputation low on the femur? **Select all that apply.**
    A. Applying the elastic wraps on the stump distal to proximal in a figure-eight pattern
    B. Using aseptic technique when irrigating the wound or changing the dressing
    C. Instructing the client to perform gluteal muscle contraction exercises hourly while awake
    D. Assisting the client to a prone position for 20 to 30 minutes every 3 to 4 hours
    E. Keeping the remaining part of the extremity positioned above the level of the heart
    F. Encouraging the client to spend as much time as possible in a chair while awake

27. Which instructions for handling the amputated digit will the nurse provide to a caller to the emergency department who reports that a friend just sustained an amputation of a finger while cleaning his lawn mower?
    A. "Place the finger in a glass of milk and keep it cold while transporting it."
    B. "Seal the finger in a plastic bag and pack with the cut side up in a cup of ice."
    C. "Wrap the finger in a clean cloth, seal it in a plastic bag, and place the bag in ice water."
    D. "Place the finger back on your friend's hand and wrap it tightly with an elastic bandage."

28. What is the nurse's **best** response to a client with a lower limb amputation who says "I think I am going crazy. I know my foot is gone but I still feel my big toe burning and itching."?
    A. "Are you sure you were awake? Sometimes people dream this pain as part of hoping that the missing body part will grow back."
    B. "You are not crazy; many people continue to feel pain and other sensations in a limb that was amputated. How severe is this pain?"
    C. "This complication is usually seen in a person who has not accepted the fact that the limb is gone. A psychologist can help you cope with this."
    D. "This problem is very common and although nothing can be done about it, we can give you pain medication for the pain you feel at the surgical site."

29. Which points and actions will the nurse include when teaching a client and family after a below-the-knee amputation about care of the residual limb? **Select all that apply.**
    A. Demonstrating how to apply a figure-eight elastic wrap
    B. Reviewing the signs and symptoms of wound infection
    C. Reminding the client and family to rewrap the limb several times each day
    D. Obtaining a return demonstration of the elastic wrap application
    E. Reviewing positioning and exercises for prevention of flexion contractures
    F. Informing the client that after the incision is healed, it can be cleaned during bathing or showering with soap and water

30. Which client assessment findings or factors indicate to the nurse the possible presence of carpal tunnel syndrome (CTS)? **Select all that apply.**
    A. Client has been taking calcium and vitamin D supplements for osteopenia.
    B. Numbness and pain are reported on performance of the Phalen maneuver.
    C. Muscle pad below the thumb is flat and atrophied.
    D. Client's favorite hobby is knitting and crocheting.
    E. Wrist and hand pain awaken the client at night.
    F. Lifestyle is very sedentary.

Chapter 47 Answer Key

1. B, D, E, F
   Risk factors for delayed or slow bone healing after a fracture include age older than 70 years, presence of bone density loss, such as with osteopenia or chronic use of corticosteroids, and poor circulation, such as would be present with arteriosclerosis. Unless there are complications, multiple fractures do not increase delayed healing risk.

2. A, B, D, F
   Acute compartment syndrome is a serious limb-threatening condition in which increased pressure within one or more compartments (that contain muscle, blood vessels, and nerves) reduces circulation to a lower leg or forearm. Common health problems leading to this condition include crush injuries to the extremities, extravasation and infiltration of IV fluids, and

severe inflammatory responses with excessive swelling in an extremity, such as with burn injuries or release of toxins from multiple insect stings or bites.

3. B
Numbness and tingling are *early* indications of nerve entrapment or impingement. Moving the fingers below a wrist injury is expected to cause some pain. Cold, pale fingers in which pulses cannot be palpated is a late indication of a complication, as is pain that grows worse out of proportion to the injury.

4. A
VTE is the most common complication of lower extremity fracture resulting from trauma. Immobilization of the limb also contributes to the risk.

5. B, C, E, F
Decreased arterial oxygen level, acute confusion, and a decreased platelet count are common indicators of FES. Although the presence of a petechial rash is a late manifestation, it is a classic finding of FES. Swelling over the fracture site and dry mucous membranes are not symptoms associated with FES.

6. C
CRPS is a dysfunction of the central and peripheral nervous systems in areas of bone fractures with soft-tissue damage that leads to severe, persistent burning pain, muscle spasms, and changes in skin color, temperature, and sensitivity among other symptoms. To facilitate soft-tissue healing and prevent CRPS, clients are told to frequently apply a variety of objects with varying surface types directly to the skin to desensitize it. These objects can be rough, smooth, hard, soft, sharp (but not enough to damage the skin), or dull.

7. A, C, E
Injuries that cause pelvic fractures often also cause significant damage to the abdomen and can cause internal hemorrhage, as well as damage to the bladder. Assessing vital signs and

level of consciousness have the highest priority to rule out whether hemorrhage and shock are present. Assessing for bladder injury is also a priority. Although the other assessments are important, they are not the immediate priority.

8. C
Rib fractures are painful and the client may be breathing too shallowly to maintain gas exchange. In addition, if there are sharp edges on the ribs, the lungs can be punctured. After respiratory assessment, cardiac assessment would be the next priority.

9. B
Measures of perfusion adequacy in the affected limb must be made on the affected limb, distal to the injury. Although capillary refill can provide an indication of perfusion adequacy, it is not as reliable as a pedal pulse.

10. D
Before any appropriate intervention action can be taken, the nurse must first visually inspect the area to adequately assess the trauma. This entails removing or cutting away clothing in the affected area without causing more harm.

11. C
Strong indicators of lower limb fracture or joint dislocation is a change in the length (usually shorter) of the affected limb and abnormal protrusions or obvious deformities. In an older client, the skin of the legs is cooler and darker than that of the arms. Confusion may be a cause or a consequence of the fall but does not indicate a fracture or bone injury. Pain is nonspecific.

12. A
Plaster is applied as a wet and easily deformed substance. As plaster dries, it gives off heat as part of this normal chemical reaction. The client is reassured that the heat is normal. Because plaster is easily deformed until it dries completely, it cannot be covered with a cooling blanket.

13. A
The ankle could be swelling under the cast and impinging on circulation, leading to increased pain from tissue hypoxia or anoxia. The nurse's best first action is performing neurovascular assessments to determine if a circulatory problem is present. If circulation is compromised, the nurse would then loosen the splint and notify the primary health care provider.

14. C
A hot spot coupled with an unpleasant odor are indications of a possible infection under the cast. Before notifying the primary health care provider or taking any other action, the nurse will assess the client's temperature and other vital signs for other indications of infection.

15. C, D, E, F
A synthetic cast dries quickly and is not deformed by handling it. A fresh fracture is likely to swell and applying ice to the cast, as well as keeping the hands and arms elevated above the level of the heart can help limit the swelling. The swelling can still cause impingement of a nerve, and the client is instructed to report numbness and tingling as soon as possible to prevent harm. Slings, although partially supported by the neck, should have the greater support resting on the shoulders and trunk to prevent damage to the neck. The stockinette is not changed separately from the cast. The client is instructed to move the wrist and fingers to maintain range of motion and prevent muscle atrophy or contractures.

16. B
With immobilization in a cast, leg muscles atrophy and become thin. Skin becomes pale, dry, and flaky from lack of exposure to air and water. Both of these conditions improve when the cast is off. How much strength returns to the leg depends on the degree of exercise and use it gets, not on the thickness of the bone.

17. A, B, C, E, F
Traction weights are prescribed at a specific weight and are not removed without an order. They are not to be lifted manually, allowed to rest on the floor, and must hang freely at all times. The belt or boot used for skin traction is removed every 8 hours to inspect the skin under the device. The client's circulation is monitored every hour for the first 24 hours after traction is applied and at least every 4 hours thereafter.

18. D
Severe fractures are very painful and usually require opioid pain medications for some time regardless of whether the client has ever used opioids in the past. A major side effect of opioids is decreased peristalsis and constipation (opioid-induced constipation [OIC]). The first question to ask is when did the client last have a bowel movement. The client usually requires a bowel regimen to relieve constipation and prevent a possible paralytic ileus.

19. B, C, D, E
The use of external fixation devices results in less blood loss and less pain than internal fixation devices. Moving, walking, and exercising can occur much earlier. The infection risk with external fixation devices is greater than with internal devices because there is a continuing disruption of skin integrity with the presence of pins. Other devices may still be needed after fractures are stabilized with external fixation devices.

20. C
Drainage of clear fluid (weeping) is expected in the first 72 hours around pin sites. The drainage forms crusts that are believed to protect the site from infection and are not removed.

21. C
Any type of electrical bone stimulation on an arm is contraindicated for clients who have implanted pacemakers.

22. D
There are no specific adverse effects or contraindications for the use of this therapy.

23. D
This client has three major risk factors for nonunion: older age, female, and lower limb fracture.

24. A, D

Although a vertebroplasty is considered a type of minimally invasive surgery, there is a danger of bleeding into the spinal area. Contraindications to the procedure are a platelet count lower than $100,000/mm^3$ ($100 \times 10^9/L$) and/or having taken an anticoagulant drug, such as rivaroxaban, within 48 hours. The other assessment findings are either normal or expected as a response to spinal compression fractures.

25. B

Clients who have any part of an upper extremity amputated, especially of the dominant hand are much more likely to become less independent in ADLs. A 70-year-old client who has been independent in ADLs is likely to remain independent after amputation of all toes on the left foot although balance and mobility may be changed.

26. C, D

Gluteal muscles are extensors of the hip joint. Contraction exercises of these buttocks muscles straighten the leg and make the extensor muscles stronger to help prevent flexion contractures. Having the client assume a prone position for 20 to 30 minutes every 3 to 4 hours also helps keep the upper leg in an extended position and prevents flexion contractures. Sitting in a chair requires flexion and promotes flexion contractures.

27. C

Current recommended guidelines for maintaining viability of an amputated finger (or other digit) are to wrap the completely severed finger in a dry clean cloth, place the finger in a watertight, sealed plastic bag, and then put the bag in ice water, never directly on ice.

28. B

Phantom limb pain (PLP) is a real physiologic problem for many people after amputation. The pain is real and requires appropriate management. Telling the client that the limb cannot be hurting because it is missing is not therapeutic and will not reduce this client's expressed concern that he may be "crazy." Drug therapy for PLP varies with the type of sensation felt as well as the intensity. Although some clients may need a mental health care professional to assist with coping, immediate pain management is the priority for this client, along with allaying his anxiety.

29. A, B, C, D, E, F

All of the listed points and actions are appropriate for the nurse to include when teaching a client and family about care of the residual limb at home.

30. B, C, D, E

CTS is most commonly caused by repetitive motions of the hand and wrist, such as would occur with knitting and crocheting. Muscle atrophy of hand muscles often results from CTS. Pain and numbness with the Phalen maneuver are strong indicators of CTS as is the increased presence of these symptoms at night. Neither osteopenia nor a sedentary lifestyle predispose a person to CTS.

48 CHAPTER

Assessment of the Gastrointestinal System

1. About which pancreatic functions will the nurse teach a client with a gastrointestinal (GI) disorder? **Select all that apply.**
   A. Breaking down amino acids
   B. Producing glucagon from the endocrine part of the organ
   C. Detoxifying potentially harmful compounds
   D. Secreting enzymes for digestion from the exocrine part of the organ
   E. Producing enzymes that digest carbohydrates, fats, and proteins
   F. Beta cells producing insulin

2. What does the nurse expect when a client's parietal cells do not produce enough intrinsic factor?
   A. Reflux of GI contents
   B. Poor regulation of metabolism
   C. Buildup of harmful substances
   D. Development of pernicious anemia

3. When the nurse collects a client's gastrointestinal (GI) history, which substances are **most likely** to be risk factors for peptic ulcer disease or GI bleeding? **Select all that apply.**
   A. Caffeine
   B. Furosemide
   C. Aspirin
   D. Desmopressin
   E. Alcohol
   F. Ibuprofen

4. Based on the nurse's knowledge of gastrointestinal (GI) changes that occur with age, for which disorder in an older client will the nurse vigilantly monitor related to decreased peristalsis?
   A. Loss of appetite for favorite foods
   B. Constipation with possible impaction
   C. Vomiting that occurs after eating
   D. Indigestion related to consuming spicy foods

5. For which finding does the nurse alert the health care provider **immediately** after assessing a client's abdomen?
   A. Bulging, pulsating mass
   B. Borborygmus
   C. Unintentional weight loss
   D. Reflux with dyspepsia

6. Which findings will the nurse be sure to document after inspecting a client's abdomen during assessment? **Select all that apply.**
   A. Overall asymmetry of the abdomen
   B. Size of percussed abdominal organs
   C. Discoloration or scarring
   D. Abdominal distention and skin folds
   E. High-pitched musical sounds
   F. Location and size of pressure injuries

7. For what **priority** information will the nurse ask **next** after a client reports decreased appetite, decreased nutritional intake, and episodes of nausea over the past 2 months?
   A. Usual bowel pattern
   B. Baseline blood pressure
   C. Preferred favorite foods
   D. Usual weight and weight loss

8. Which important information will the nurse gather when a client reports a change in bowel habits? **Select all that apply.**
   A. Presence of abdominal distention or gas
   B. Intentional weight gain
   C. Occurrence of diarrhea or constipation
   D. Color and consistency of feces
   E. Occurrence of heartburn or reflux
   F. Presence of bloody or tarry stools

9. What is the nurse's **best** action when assessment of a client 2 hours after abdominal surgery reveals hypoactive bowel sounds?
   A. Documenting the finding and continue to monitor
   B. Notifying the surgeon immediately
   C. Putting a nasogastric (NG) tube in place
   D. Obtaining an immediate abdominal x-ray

10. What type of bowel sounds will the nurse expect to auscultate when a client reports having diarrhea for the past 2 days?
    A. Decreased or diminished sounds
    B. Increased sounds in the left lower quadrant only
    C. Increased loud and gurgling sounds
    D. Decreased sounds in the right upper quadrant only

11. For which abnormal laboratory findings will the nurse monitor when providing care for a client with acute pancreatitis? **Select all that apply.**
    A. Increased prothrombin time
    B. Increased serum lipase
    C. Increased unconjugated bilirubin
    D. Increased aspartate transaminase
    E. Increased serum amylase
    F. Increased serum ammonia

12. What instructions will the nurse provide to a client with a gastrointestinal problem who is scheduled for an abdominal x-ray?
    A. "Wear a hospital gown and remove any jewelry or belts."
    B. "You will have nothing to eat or drink until after the procedure."
    C. "A nasogastric tube will be placed to decompress your stomach."
    D. "You will receive a laxative to clear stool out of your bowel."

13. What is the nurse's **first priority** when providing care for a client after an esophagogastroduodenoscopy (EGD)?
    A. Monitoring the client's vital signs every 15 minutes
    B. Auscultating the client's breath sounds for crackles
    C. Keeping the client NPO until the gag reflex returns
    D. Recording accurate intake and output

14. Which diagnostic procedure does the nurse expect will be ordered by the health care provider to view a client's liver, gallbladder, bile ducts, and pancreas for identification of the location of an obstruction?
    A. Upper gastrointestinal radiographic series
    B. Percutaneous transhepatic cholangiography
    C. Endoscopic retrograde cholangiopancreatography
    D. Esophagogastroduodenoscopy

15. Which teaching points will the nurse include when instructing a client about preparation for a colonoscopy? **Select all that apply.**
    A. "Avoid taking aspirin, NSAIDs, or anticoagulants for several days before the test."
    B. "Drink lots of red, orange, or purple beverages the day before the test."
    C. "Do not eat or drink for 4 to 5 hours before the test."
    D. "After the bowel-cleansing solutions, you may develop constipation for 1 to 2 days."
    E. "Drink only clear liquids the day before the colonoscopy."
    F. "An IV will be placed to give medication to help you relax during the procedure."

16. Which actions will the nurse include when providing care for a client after a colonoscopy procedure? **Select all that apply.**
    A. Checking vital signs every 15 to 30 minutes until the client is alert
    B. Keeping client in left lateral position to promote passing of flatus
    C. Assessing for signs and symptoms of bowel perforation, including severe abdominal pain and guarding
    D. Preventing the client from taking anything by mouth until sedation wears off
    E. Keeping the top side rails up until the client is alert
    F. Holding the client 6 to 8 hours before allowing him or her to drive home

17. For which gastrointestinal diagnostic test does the nurse teach a client to expect mild gas pain, flatulence, and a small amount of bleeding after the procedure if a biopsy was obtained?
    A. Endoscopic retrograde cholangiopancreatography
    B. Esophagogastroduodenoscopy
    C. Barium swallow
    D. Proctosigmoidoscopy

18. What is the nurse's **priority** assessment when a client is given IV midazolam hydrochloride before a colonoscopy?
    A. Monitoring the rate and depth of respirations
    B. Auscultating for bowel sounds in all four quadrants
    C. Monitoring the client for cardiac dysrhythmias
    D. Suctioning secretions as needed to prevent aspiration

19. The nurse reviews a client's laboratory values and discovers a serum potassium level of 3.1 mEq/L. Which gastrointestinal condition could cause this value?
    A. Malabsorption
    B. Gastric suctioning
    C. Acute pancreatitis
    D. Liver disease

20. Which gastrointestinal condition does the nurse suspect a client is at increased risk for, when she reports emotional distress about her family situation and whether she will be able to return to work?
    A. Hiatal hernia
    B. Exacerbation of irritable bowel syndrome
    C. Nausea accompanied by vomiting and diarrhea
    D. Esophageal ulcers

21. What procedural teaching will the nurse provide for a client scheduled for an abdominal CT scan with contrast? **Select all that apply.**
    A. The test will take about 30 to 45 minutes.
    B. An IV line will be placed for injection of the contrast.
    C. You may experience loud and gurgling sounds from your belly.
    D. The CT technician may ask you to hold your breath while images are taken.
    E. You may feel warm and flushed, and may experience a metallic taste with the injection.
    F. If you are claustrophobic, you can be given a mild sedative before the procedure.

22. Which gastrointestinal (GI) changes will the nurse expect in an older client with a GI problem? **Select all that apply.**
    A. Increased hydrochloric acid secretion
    B. Decreased absorption of iron and vitamin B_{12}
    C. Decreased peristalsis with constipation
    D. Increased cholesterol synthesis
    E. Decreased lipase with decreased fat digestion
    F. Decreased drug metabolism with risk of toxicities

Chapter 48 Answer Key

1. B, D, E, F
The nurse teaches the client about two major cellular bodies (exocrine and endocrine) within the pancreas that have separate functions. The exocrine part consists of cells that secrete enzymes needed for digestion of carbohydrates, fats, and proteins (proteases, amylase, and lipase). The endocrine part of the pancreas is made up of the *islets of Langerhans*, with alpha cells producing glucagon and beta cells producing insulin.

2. D
Parietal cells produce intrinsic factor, a substance that aids in the absorption of vitamin B_{12}. Absence of the intrinsic factor leads to decreased absorption of vitamin B_{12} and causes pernicious anemia.

3. A, C, E, F
Large amounts of aspirin or NSAIDs (e.g., ibuprofen) can predispose a client to peptic ulcer disease (PUD) and GI bleeding. Alcohol and caffeine consumption are of concern because both substances are associated with many GI disorders, such as gastritis and peptic ulcer disease.

4. B
As clients age, peristalsis decreases and GI nerve impulses are dulled. This leads to decreased sensation for defecation and can result in postponement of bowel movements, which can lead to constipation and impaction.

5. A
If a bulging, pulsating mass is present during assessment of the abdomen, the nurse does not touch the area because the client may have an abdominal aortic aneurysm which is a life-threatening problem. The nurse notifies the health care provider of this finding **immediately**!

6. A, C, D, F
After inspecting a client's abdomen, the nurse documents these findings: overall asymmetry of the abdomen; discoloration or scarring; abdominal distention; bulging flanks; taut, glistening skin; skin folds; subcutaneous fat; and location, size, and description of any pressure injuries. Percussion and auscultation are not parts of abdominal inspection.

7. D
The next important information the nurse asks about is the client's usual weight and whether he or she has experienced a weight loss (especially unintentional). It is important to inquire about unintentional weight loss because some GI cancers may present in this manner.

8. A, C, D, F
Changes in bowel habits are commonly reported by clients. Important information for the nurse to gather from the client includes: pattern of bowel movements, color and consistency of the feces, occurrence of diarrhea or constipation, effective action(s) taken to relieve diarrhea or constipation, presence of frank blood or tarry stools, and presence of abdominal distention or gas.

9. A
Bowel sounds are characterized as normal, hypoactive, or hyperactive. They are diminished (hypoactive) or absent after abdominal surgery. The most reliable way of knowing that peristalsis has returned is when the client passes flatus or stool. After surgery this may take a few hours. The nurse's best action is to document the finding and continue to monitor for flatus or stool.

10. C
Increased bowel sounds, especially loud, gurgling sounds (borborygmus), result from increased motility of the bowel. These sounds are usually heard when a client has diarrhea, gastroenteritis, or a complete intestinal obstruction (sounds will be heard above the obstruction).

11. B, E
Elevations in serum amylase and lipase may indicate acute pancreatitis, a serious inflammation of the pancreas characterized by a sudden onset of abdominal pain, nausea, and vomiting.

Serum amylase levels begin to elevate within 24 hours of onset and remain elevated for up to 5 days. The values listed in options A, C, D, and F are more commonly seen with liver disease.

12. A

The nurse teaches the client that no preparation is required except to wear a hospital gown and remove any jewelry or belts, which may interfere with the film.

13. C

After an EGD, the nurse's priority of care is to prevent aspiration. The client is kept NPO until the gag reflex returns (usually in 30 to 60 minutes) because an absent gag reflex increases the risk for aspiration. Clients must not be offered fluids or food by mouth until the gag reflex is intact!

14. C

Endoscopic retrograde cholangiopancreatography (ERCP) includes visual and radiographic examination of the liver, gallbladder, bile ducts, and pancreas to identify the cause and location of obstruction. After a cannula is inserted into the common bile duct, a radiopaque dye is instilled, and several x-ray images are obtained. The health care provider may perform a papillotomy (a small incision in the sphincter around the ampulla of Vater) to remove gallstones. If a biliary duct stricture is found, plastic or metal stents may be inserted to keep the ducts open. Biopsies of tissue are also frequently taken during this test.

15. A, C, E, F

Clients are instructed to avoid aspirin, anticoagulants, and antiplatelet drugs for several days before the procedure. The health care provider will prescribe the specific method of preparation of the bowel which begins the night before the procedure. Drinkable solutions can be chilled to improve taste. Teach the client to have a clear liquid diet the day before the scheduled colonoscopy. The nurse instructs him or her to avoid red, orange, or purple (grape) beverages or gelatin. The client should be NPO for several hours before the procedure, based on the health care provider's

instructions. Watery diarrhea usually begins about an hour after starting the bowel preparation process. In some cases, the client may also require laxatives, suppositories (e.g., bisacodyl), or one or more small-volume cleansing enemas. Intravenous access is necessary for the administration of moderate sedation. The health care provider prescribes drugs to aid in relaxation during the procedure.

16. A, B, C, D, E

All of these options must be included in the care provided to the client after colonoscopy except option F. If the procedure is performed in an ambulatory care setting, another person must drive the client home because of the action of IV drugs given to help with relaxation during the procedure.

17. D

The nurse informs the client that after proctosigmoidoscopy, mild gas pain and flatulence may be experienced from air instilled into the rectum during the examination. If a biopsy was obtained, a small amount of bleeding may be observed. The client is instructed to report excessive bleeding to the health care provider immediately.

18. A

Midazolam is commonly used for sedation with procedures such as colonoscopy. These drugs can depress the rate and depth of respirations. Thus, the nurse's priority assessment is checking the client's rate and depth of respirations. If the client's respiratory rate is below 10 breaths/min or the exhaled carbon dioxide level falls below 20%, the nurse uses a stimulus such as a sternal rub to encourage deeper and faster respirations.

19. B

Gastrointestinal causes of decreased potassium include vomiting, gastric suctioning, diarrhea, and drainage from intestinal fistulas.

20. B

The nurse must ask a client about experiencing stressful events because stress has been associated with the development or exacerbation (flare-up) of irritable bowel syndrome (IBS).

21. B, D, E, F

    The nurse instructs the client that an IV access is required for injection of the contrast medium. Advise the client that he or she may feel warm and flushed, or experience a metallic taste, on or after the injection. A client who has claustrophobia may require a mild sedative to tolerate the study. The CT technician will instruct the client to lie still and to hold his or her breath when asked, as a series of images are taken. The test takes about 10 minutes and the client is not likely to experience gurgling bowel sounds.

22. B, C, E, F

    The nurse understands that as people age, and after 65 years of age, physiologic changes occur in the GI system. Options B, C, E, and F are expected changes that occur with aging. For additional changes, see the box titled Patient-Centered Care: Older Adult Considerations: Changes in the Gastrointestinal System Associated With Aging in your text.

49 CHAPTER

Concepts of Care for Patients with Oral Cavity and Esophageal Problems

1. Which clients will the nurse carefully assess for high risk of oral cavity disorders? **Select all that apply.**
   A. Clients who are homeless or live in institutions
   B. Clients with sexually transmitted infection
   C. Clients who are developmentally disabled
   D. Clients who consume an unhealthy diet
   E. Clients who work in coal mines
   F. Clients who regularly use tobacco or alcohol

2. Which important information will the nurse include when teaching clients how to maintain healthy oral cavities? **Select all that apply.**
   A. Perform a monthly self-examination of the mouth looking for changes.
   B. Eat a well-balanced diet and stay hydrated by drinking water.
   C. If you wear dentures, make sure that they are in good repair and fit properly.
   D. Thoroughly brush and floss your teeth (or brush dentures) consistently twice daily.
   E. Use mouthwashes that contain alcohol to destroy organisms that live in the mouth.
   F. See the dentist regularly and have dental problems repaired as soon as possible.

3. For which reason will the nurse carefully examine the mouth of an older adult for candidiasis?
   A. Older clients are more likely to wear dentures which increases the risk for candidiasis.
   B. Older adults on fixed incomes consume fewer fresh vegetables and fruits.
   C. Older adults' immune systems decline with aging increasing their risk for candidiasis.
   D. Older clients are less likely to see a dentist and have healthy oral hygiene.

4. Which oral disorder does the nurse suspect when assessment findings reveal white plaquelike lesions that when wiped away show an underlying red and sore surface?
   A Leukoplakia
   B. Candidiasis
   C. Erythroplakia
   D. Kaposi's sarcoma

5. Which actions will the nurse assign to the assistive personnel (AP) who will be helping to care for a client with stomatitis? **Select all that apply.**
   A. Providing oral care every 2 hours or more if stomatitis is not controlled
   B. Teaching the client to use a soft toothbrush or gauze, and to avoid commercial mouthwashes and lemon-glycerin swabs which can irritate mucosa
   C. Encouraging frequent rinsing of the mouth with warm saline, sodium bicarbonate (baking soda) solution, or a combination of these solutions
   D. Applying topical analgesics or anesthetics as prescribed by the primary health care provider and documenting effectiveness
   E. Instructing the client on how to select soft, bland, and nonacidic foods
   F. Removing dentures if the client has severe stomatitis or oral pain

6. Which **priority** teaching will the nurse provide to **prevent harm** when a client with an oral problem is prescribed viscous lidocaine?
   A. "Lidocaine causes an anesthetic effect so you may not feel burns from hot liquids."
   B. "You should avoid drinking either cool or cold liquids which can damage the tongue."
   C. "When you take viscous lidocaine, you should swish it around your mouth then spit it out."
   D. "Viscous lidocaine will decrease the pain in your mouth when you use it regularly."

7. What does the nurse suspect when assessing a client's mouth and finding an oral cavity tumor that appears as a red, velvety lesion on the tongue, palate, floor of the mouth, or mandibular mucosa?
   A. Kaposi's sarcoma
   B. Basal cell carcinoma
   C. Erythroplakia
   D. Leukoplakia

8. Which question will the nurse be sure to ask a client suspected of having leukoplakia?
   A. "Do you smoke, dip, or chew tobacco products?"
   B. "How much alcohol do you drink each day?"
   C. "Do you consume many of fast food meals?"
   D. "How often do you have dental checkups?"

9. Which signs and symptoms will the nurse assess when a client is diagnosed with oral cancer? **Select all that apply.**
   A. Bleeding from the mouth
   B. Painful oral lesions that are red, raised, or eroded
   C. Difficulty chewing or swallowing
   D. Unplanned weight gain
   E. Thick or absent saliva
   F. Thickening or lump in cheek

10. What is the nurse's **best** response when a client asks which diagnostic test will determine if an oral tumor is cancerous?
    A. "MRI is the only test that you will need at this time."
    B. "No single test will make the diagnosis on its own."
    C. "Aqueous toluidine blue will be absorbed by malignancies."
    D. "Biopsy is the definitive method for diagnosing oral cancer."

11. Which action is the **priority** for the nurse to take when caring for clients with oral cancers?
    A. Providing pain control
    B. Maintaining the airway
    C. Promoting tissue integrity
    D. Enhancing nutrition

12. Which are the **most common** symptoms of gastroesophageal reflux disease (GERD) reported to the nurse by a client? **Select all that apply.**
    A. Eructation
    B. Water brash
    C. Dyspepsia
    D. Regurgitation
    E. Odynophagia
    F. Flatulence

13. Which actions will the nurse teach a client with severe GERD that causes pain after each meal, lasts for at least 45 minutes, and worsens when he or she lies down? **Select all that apply.**
    A. "Drink fluids right away."
    B. "When you lie down, try lying on your side."
    C. "Take an antacid as prescribed by the health care provider."
    D. "Eat something bland such as a slice of white bread."
    E. "Maintain an upright position for at least an hour after you eat."
    F. "Try pressing over your abdomen to mobilize the food in your stomach."

14. Which **most** accurate diagnostic test will the nurse expect to be ordered for a client to verify the diagnosis of GERD?
    A. Esophagogastroduodenoscopy (EGD)
    B. Esophageal manometry
    C. Ambulatory esophageal pH monitoring
    D. Motility testing

15. Which drug does the nurse expect to administer to a client in order to decrease hydrochloric acid secretion in the stomach?
    A. Famotidine
    B. Gaviscon
    C. Mylanta
    D. Antibiotic

16. Which **priority** teaching will the nurse provide to an older client with GERD who is prescribed omeprazole for symptom relief?
    A. "Older adults taking this drug may be at increased risk for hip fracture because it interferes with calcium absorption."
    B. "Because of this drug's side effect of decreasing potassium, you may be prescribed a potassium supplement."
    C. "This drug causes sodium retention, so you may be prescribed a dietary sodium restriction."
    D. "A pacemaker may be necessary because this drug changes magnesium levels which can lead to life-threatening dysrhythmias."

17. Which actions will the nurse teach a client with GERD to use to **prevent harm? Select all that apply.**
    A. Do not consume caffeinated or carbonated beverages.
    B. Avoid peppermint, chocolate, and fried foods.
    C. Eat slowly and chew food thoroughly.
    D. Consume four to six small meals each day.
    E. Do not eat for 3 hours before going to bed.
    F. Sleep on your side to prevent regurgitation.

18. Which signs and symptoms will the nurse expect to assess when a client is diagnosed with a paraesophageal hernia? **Select all that apply.**
    A. Regurgitation
    B. Feeling of fullness (after eating)
    C. Dyspepsia
    D. Breathlessness (after eating)
    E. Dysphagia
    F. Chest pain that mimics angina

19. Which diagnostic test will the nurse expect the client to undergo to **best** identify a hiatal hernia?
    A. Esophagogastroduodenoscopy (EGD)
    B. 24-hour ambulatory pH monitoring
    C. Esophageal manometry
    D. Barium swallow with fluoroscopy

20. Which postoperative instructions will the nurse provide for a client after laparoscopic Nissen fundoplication (LNF)? **Select all that apply.**
    A. Consume a soft diet for about a week; avoid carbonated beverages, tough foods, and raw vegetables that are difficult to swallow.
    B. You will no longer need to take antireflux medications after your surgery is over.
    C. You must not drive for a week after surgery; especially do not drive after taking an opioid pain medication.
    D. Walk every day but do not do any heavy lifting.
    E. Remove the small dressings and closure strips 2 days after surgery and then you may shower.
    F. Report fever above 101°F (38.3°C), nausea, vomiting, or uncontrollable bloating or pain.

21. How does the nurse expect a client's nasogastric (NG) tube drainage to appear immediately after Nissen fundoplication surgery?
    A. Bright red mixed with brown
    B. Dark brown
    C. Yellowish to green
    D. Green to clear

22. Which actions will the nurse teach a client to **avoid** to **prevent harm** after Nissen fundoplication surgery when gas bloat syndrome occurs? **Select all that apply.**
    A. Drinking carbonated beverages
    B. Passing flatus or belching
    C. Eating gas-producing foods
    D. Chewing gum
    E. Drinking through a straw
    F. Changing positions frequently

23. Which client does the nurse assess as at **highest** risk for development of esophageal cancer?
    A. 45-year-old on a high-fiber diet
    B. 50-year-old with a sedentary lifestyle
    C. 55-year-old who smokes and is 25 lb overweight
    D. 60-year-old who is prescribed famotidine for reflux

24. What is the **most common** symptom the nurse expects clients with esophageal cancer to report?
    A. Difficulty with swallowing
    B. Shortness of breath
    C. Reflux especially at night
    D. Productive cough

25. What manifestation of esophageal cancer does the nurse recognize when a client describes experiencing a dull and steady substernal pain after drinking cold liquids?
    A. Angina
    B. Aspiration
    C. Dysphagia
    D. Odynophagia

26. Which nonsurgical treatment options for cancer of the esophagus will the nurse discuss with the client? **Select all that apply.**
    A. Swallowing therapy
    B. Smoking cessation programs
    C. Nutritional therapy
    D. Chemoradiation
    E. Photodynamic therapy
    F. Esophageal dilation

27. Which nonsurgical treatment will the nurse expect the client with esophageal cancer to receive for immediate relief of dysphagia?
    A. Photodynamic therapy
    B. Esophageal dilation
    C. Radiation therapy
    D. Swallowing therapy

28. After esophagectomy for esophageal cancer, what is the nurse's **priority** for client care?
    A. Wound care
    B. Nutrition management
    C. Respiratory care
    D. Hydration status

29. Which cause does the nurse recognize as a potential intentional cause for a client's esophageal trauma?
    A. Nasogastric (NG) tube placement
    B. Esophageal ulcers
    C. Struck by a foreign object
    D. Chemical injury

30. Which drugs will the nurse expect the health care provider to prescribe for a client after esophageal trauma? **Select all that apply.**
    A. Broad-spectrum antibiotics
    B. Loop diuretics
    C. Corticosteroids
    D. Antacids
    E. Pain medications
    F. Viscous lidocaine

Chapter 49 Answer Key

1. A, C, D, F
   The nurse would carefully assess clients for increased risk of oral cavity disorders with these conditions: having developmental delays or mental health disorders, having limited access to care due to homelessness or health disparities, residing in institutions, using tobacco and/or alcohol, consuming an unhealthy diet, having a type of oral cancer, and consuming dietary excess.

2. B, C, D, F
   See the box in your text titled Patient and Family Education: Preparing for Self-Management Maintaining of a Healthy Oral Cavity for additional teaching points on how to maintain a healthy oral cavity. Option A is not correct. The nurse teaches the client to examine the mouth weekly and report any changes to the HCP. Option E is not correct. Mouthwashes containing alcohol are avoided because they can cause tissue damage.

3. C
   Older adults are at high risk for candidiasis because the immune system naturally declines as people age.

4. B
   When a client develops oral candidiasis, white plaquelike lesions appear on the tongue, palate, pharynx (throat), and buccal mucosa (inside the cheeks). When these patches are wiped away, the underlying surface is red, sore, and painful, and tissue integrity is compromised.

5. A, C, F
   See the box in your text entitled Best Practice for Patient Safety & Quality Care **QSEN** Care of the Patient With Problems of the Oral Cavity for appropriate client safety and quality care for a client's oral cavity problem. The nurse must also be familiar with the scope of practice for an AP which includes assisting with personal care and oral care. Teaching and instructing clients are within the scope of the professional nurse, but the AP may reinforce what has already been taught to the client. Administering medications is also appropriate to the professional nurse, but application of topical drugs could be assigned to an LPN/LVN. Lemon-glycerin swabs and commercial mouthwashes with alcohol can cause more damage and are avoided.

6. A
   The nurse teaches the client to use viscous lidocaine with extreme caution. Lidocaine causes a topical anesthetic effect so the client may not easily feel burns from hot liquids. As sensation in the mouth and throat decreases, the risk for aspiration increases.

7. C
   Erythroplakia, which is considered precancerous, appear as red, velvety mucosal lesions on the floor of the mouth, tongue, palate, and mandibular mucosa.

8. A
   Tobacco use increases the chance of development of leukoplakia. The nurse asks the client about any current or historical tobacco use.

9. A, C, E, F
   Signs and symptoms that the nurse will monitor for when a client has oral cancer include: bleeding from the mouth; poor appetite, compromised nutrition status; difficulty chewing or swallowing; unplanned weight loss; thick or absent saliva; painless oral lesions that are red, raised, or eroded; and thickening or lump in the cheek.

10. D
    The best diagnostic test for oral cancer is a biopsy. A needle-biopsy specimen, or an incisional biopsy, of the abnormal tissue will be obtained by the health care provider to assess for malignant or premalignant changes. In very small lesions, an excisional biopsy can permit complete tumor removal.

11. B
    While all of these concerns are important, airway maintenance to facilitate gas exchange is the priority of care for clients with oral cancer.

12. C, D
Dyspepsia, also known as indigestion, and re-gurgitation are the main symptoms of GERD, although symptoms may vary in severity. With severe GERD, these sensations generally occur after each meal and last for 20 minutes to 2 hours.

13. A, C, E
When a client experiences GERD, drinking fluids, taking antacids as prescribed, or main-taining an upright posture usually provides prompt relief.

14. C
Ambulatory esophageal pH monitoring is the most accurate method of diagnosing GERD. With this procedure, a transnasally placed catheter or wireless, capsule-like device is affixed to the distal esophageal mucosa. The client is asked to keep a diary of activities and symptoms over 24 to 48 hours (depending on diagnostic method), and the pH is continu-ously monitored and recorded.

15. A
Famotidine is a histamine receptor antagonist (histamine blocker). This drug works by inhib-iting gastric acid (e.g., hydrochloric acid) secre-tion, which relieves the dyspepsia and other symptoms of GERD.

16. A
Omeprazole is a proton pump inhibitor (PPI). These drugs may increase the risk for hip frac-ture, especially in older adults. PPIs can inter-fere with calcium absorption and protein diges-tion and therefore, reduce available calcium to bone tissue. Decreased calcium makes bones more brittle and likely to fracture, especially as adults get older.

17. A, B, C, D, E
All of these recommendations are appropriate for the nurse to teach a client to avoid the harmful effects of GERD, except option F. The client is taught to sleep propped up to promote gas exchange and prevent regurgitation. This can be done by placing blocks under the head of

the bed or by using a large, wedge-style pillow instead of a standard pillow.

18. B, D, F
Signs and symptoms of paraesophageal hernias include: feeling of fullness (after eating), breath-lessness (after eating), feeling of suffocation (after eating), chest pain that mimics angina, and worsening of symptoms in a recumbent position. Regurgitation, dyspepsia, and dys-phagia are symptoms of sliding hiatal hernias.

19. D
The barium swallow study with fluoroscopy is the most specific diagnostic test for identifying a hiatal hernia. Rolling hernias are usually clearly visible, and sliding hernias can often be observed when the client moves through a se-ries of positions that increase intra-abdominal pressure.

20. A, C, D, F
See the box entitled Patient and Family Educa-tion: Preparing for Self-Management Postop-erative Instructions for Patients Having Lapa-roscopic Nissen Fundoplication (LNF) or Paraesophageal Repair via Laparoscope in your text for additional teaching points. Option B is not correct because the client may take anti-reflux medications for a month after surgery. Option E is not correct because the closure strips are kept in place for 10 days after surgery.

21. B
Initially the nurse expects the NG drainage to be dark brown with old blood. The drainage should become normal yellowish green within the first 8 hours after surgery.

22. A, C, D, E
After Nissen fundoplication surgery, some cli-ents develop gas bloat syndrome, in which they cannot voluntarily eructate (belch). Teach the client to avoid drinking carbonated beverages and eating gas-producing foods (especially high-fat foods), chewing gum, and drinking with a straw. Frequent position changes and ambulation are often effective interventions for eliminating air from the GI tract. If gas pain is

still present, clients may be recommended to take simethicone, which relieves gas pressure.

23. C

The client in option C has two major risk factors for esophageal cancer, tobacco use and obesity. Primary risk factors associated with the development of esophageal cancer include: alcohol intake, diets chronically deficient in fresh fruits and vegetables, diets high in nitrates and nitrosamines (found in pickled and fermented foods), malnutrition, obesity (especially with increased abdominal pressure), smoking, and untreated GERD.

24. A

One of the most common symptoms of esophageal cancer that clients report is dysphagia (difficulty with swallowing). This symptom may not be present until the esophageal opening has narrowed significantly.

25. D

Odynophagia is defined as painful swallowing. Odynophagia occurs with the original cancer and may recur because of stricture, reflux, or cancer recurrence. It should be reported to the health care provider promptly.

26. A, C, D, E, F

All of these options are nonsurgical treatments for esophageal cancer except option B, smoking cessation programs. See the list of nonsurgical options in your text for additional suggestions.

27. B

Esophageal dilation may be performed as necessary throughout the course of the disease to achieve temporary but immediate relief of dysphagia. It is usually performed in an ambulatory care setting. Dilators are used to tear soft tissue, thereby widening the esophageal lumen (opening).

28. C

Respiratory care is the highest postoperative priority for clients having an esophagectomy. For those who undergo traditional surgery, intubation with mechanical ventilation is necessary for at least the first 16 to 24 hours. Pulmonary complications include atelectasis and pneumonia. The risk for postoperative pulmonary complications is increased in the client who has received preoperative radiation. Once the client is extubated, the nurse supports deep breathing, turning, and coughing every 1 to 2 hours. The nurse assesses the client for decreased breath sounds and shortness of breath every 1 to 2 hours. Incisional support is provided along with adequate analgesia to enhance effective coughing.

29. D

Chemical injury is usually a result of the accidental or intentional ingestion of caustic substances. The damage to the mouth and esophagus is rapid and severe. Acid burns tend to affect the superficial mucosal lining, whereas alkaline substances cause deeper penetrating injuries. Strong alkalis can cause full perforation of the esophagus within 1 minute. Additional complications may include aspiration pneumonia and hemorrhage. Esophageal strictures may develop as scar tissue forms.

30. A, C, E, F

To prevent sepsis, the health care provider prescribes broad-spectrum antibiotics. High-dose corticosteroids may be administered to suppress inflammation and prevent strictures (esophageal narrowing). Opioid and nonopioid analgesics may be prescribed for pain management. When caustic burns involve the mouth, topical agents such as viscous lidocaine may be used.

50 CHAPTER

Concepts of Care for Patients with Stomach Disorders

1. Which finding does the nurse understand is an early pathologic manifestation when a client is diagnosed with acute gastritis?
   A. Thickened, reddened mucous membrane with prominent rugae
   B. Patchy, diffuse inflammation
   C. *H. pylori* infection
   D. Thin, atrophied wall and lining of the stomach

2. Which risk factors will the nurse assess for when taking a history of a client suspected of having gastritis? **Select all that apply.**
   A. Use of alcohol
   B. Excessive caffeine intake
   C. Smoking cigarettes
   D. Life stressors
   E. Prescribed steroids
   F. Ingestion of corrosive substances

3. Which condition or symptom does the nurse associate with a client who has chronic gastritis?
   A. Hematemesis
   B. Pernicious anemia
   C. Dyspepsia
   D. Epigastric burning

4. What **priority** teaching points will the nurse include when instructing a client and family about how to prevent gastritis? **Select all that apply.**
   A. Eat a well-balanced diet and exercise regularly.
   B. Do not take large doses of aspirin, other NSAIDs (e.g., ibuprofen), and corticosteroids.
   C. Decrease the amount of smoking and/or use of other forms of tobacco.
   D. Manage stress levels using complementary and integrative therapies such as relaxation and meditation techniques.
   E. Use over-the-counter (OTC) proton pump inhibitors if you experience symptoms of esophageal reflux.
   F. Protect yourself against exposure to toxic substances in the workplace such as lead and nickel.

5. Which diagnostic test does the nurse expect will be ordered for a client with suspected gastritis?
   A. Computed tomography (CT) scan
   B. Upper gastrointestinal (GI) series
   C. Esophagogastroduodenoscopy (EGD)
   D. Barium swallow

6. Which drugs will the nurse expect to give a client with acute gastritis that are antisecretory agents? **Select all that apply.**
   A. Famotidine
   B. Omeprazole
   C. Sucralfate
   D. Pantoprazole
   E. Nizatidine
   F. Calcium carbonate

7. What **priority** teaching will the nurse provide to **prevent harm** when a client with gastritis reports taking ibuprofen regularly for discomfort related to arthritis?
   A. "Do not take ibuprofen more than twice a day."
   B. "Ibuprofen can interfere with the action of the drugs you take for gastritis."
   C. "This drug is excellent for pain relief related to arthritis."
   D. "Avoid taking ibuprofen because it can cause gastritis."

8. Which types of ulcers does the nurse teach a client about when discussing peptic ulcer disease (PUD)? **Select all that apply.**
   A. Pressure ulcers
   B. Gastric ulcers
   C. Duodenal ulcers
   D. Stress ulcers
   E. Esophageal ulcers
   F. Colon ulcers

9. Which statement by a client indicates to the nurse that teaching about the action of sucralfate has been successful?
   A. "The main side effect of sucralfate is diarrhea."
   B. "I will take my sucralfate with each meal."
   C. "Sucralfate will work to heal my ulcer."
   D. "I will take my sucralfate with my antacid."

10. From where does the nurse suspect a client with PUD is bleeding when massive coffee-ground emesis occurs?
    A. Colon
    B. Rectum
    C. Small intestine
    D. Upper GI system

11. Which signs and symptoms does the nurse expect to assess when a client experiences an upper GI bleed? **Select all that apply.**
    A. Decreased blood pressure
    B. Decreased heart rate
    C. Dizziness or light-headedness
    D. Melena (tarry or dark sticky) stools
    E. Weak peripheral pulses
    F. Increased hemoglobin and hematocrit levels

12. Which complication does the nurse suspect when a client with PUD suddenly develops sharp epigastric pain that spreads over the entire abdomen?
    A. Gastric erosion
    B. Perforation
    C. Hemorrhage
    D. Gastric cancer

13. What is the nurse's **best first** action when a client with a gastric ulcer is found lying in the knee-chest (fetal) position with a rigid, tender, and painful abdomen?
    A. Notify the primary health care provider.
    B. Administer opioid pain medication.
    C. Reposition the client supine.
    D. Measure the abdominal circumference.

14. Which simple, noninvasive tests will the nurse expect to be ordered to detect *H. pylori* in a client with PUD? **Select all that apply.**
    A. Serologic testing for antibodies
    B. Abdominal ultrasound
    C. Urea breath test
    D. Computerized tomography scan
    E. Stool antigen test
    F. Magnetic resonance imaging

15. Which drugs will the nurse expect to administer to a client with PUD, caused by an *H. pylori* infection, who is prescribed PPI–triple therapy?
    A. A proton pump inhibitor, two antibiotics, and bismuth
    B. A proton pump inhibitor and two antibiotics
    C. An opioid drug, proton pump inhibitor, and an antibiotic
    D. An H_2 histamine blocker, an antibiotic, and a proton pump inhibitor

16. Which priority actions will the nurse take to manage a client's active upper GI bleeding? **Select all that apply.**
    A. Administering oxygen
    B. Starting two large-bore IV lines
    C. Infusing 0.9% normal saline solution as prescribed
    D. Collecting a urine sample for urinalysis
    E. Inserting a nasogastric tube (NGT)
    F. Monitoring serum electrolytes

17. Which **priority** teaching will the nurse provide to a client who is prescribed bismuth for peptic ulcer disease (PUD)?
    A. "Take this drug with an aspirin."
    B. "You may experience dyspepsia between doses."
    C. "Bismuth may cause your tongue and stool to appear black."
    D. "Be sure to take this drug before each meal and snack."

18. For which reasons will the nurse insert a large-bore nasogastric tube (NGT) in a client with active upper GI bleeding or possible obstruction? **Select all that apply.**
    A. To provide nutritional supplements
    B. To determine the presence or absence of blood in the stomach
    C. To assess the rate of bleeding
    D. To administer medications
    E. To prevent gastric dilation
    F. To administer gastric lavage

19. When providing discharge teaching, for which symptoms will the nurse teach a client with peptic ulcer disease (PUD) to seek immediate medical attention? **Select all that apply.**
    A. Bloody or black stools
    B. Dyspepsia or reflux
    C. Bloody vomit or vomit that looks like coffee grounds
    D. Odynophagia with nausea
    E. Sharp, sudden, persistent, and severe epigastric or abdominal pain
    F. Loss of appetite with dysphagia

20. Which food will the nurse recommend a client **avoid** when he or she reports fear of stomach cancer?
    A. Foods that cause reflux
    B. Pickled or processed foods
    C. Large, heavy meals
    D. Spicy foods that cause gas

21. Which signs and symptoms does the nurse expect to assess when a client has early gastric cancer? **Select all that apply.**
    A. Nausea and vomiting
    B. Feeling of fullness
    C. Weakness and fatigue
    D. Epigastric, back, or retrosternal pain
    E. Palpable gastric mass
    F. Abdominal discomfort initially relieved with antacids

22. For which client with gastric cancer does the nurse expect that minimal invasive surgery (MIS) plus radiation therapy or chemotherapy may be curative?
    A. 45-year-old with advanced disease
    B. 50-year-old with early disease
    C. 60-year-old with liver metastases
    D. 65-year-old with invasion of the stomach muscle

23. What complication does the nurse suspect when a client who had a gastrectomy develops tachycardia, syncope, and a desire to lie down 30 minutes after eating?
    A. Fluid overload
    B. Early dumping syndrome
    C. Late dumping syndrome
    D. Vitamin B_{12} deficiency

24. Which actions will the nurse take to manage a client's dumping syndrome? **Select all that apply.**
    A. Providing smaller, more frequent meals
    B. Eliminating ingestion of fluids with meals
    C. Providing a high-carbohydrate diet
    D. Administering acarbose as prescribed
    E. Increasing fat and protein in the diet
    F. Administering subcutaneous octreotide three times a day before meals

25. What does the nurse suspect when assessment of a client after gastric resection reveals a tongue that is smooth, shiny, and appears "beefy"?
    A. Inadequate nutrition
    B. Hypovolemia
    C. Anemia
    D. Atrophic glossitis

Chapter 50 Answer Key

1. A
   The early pathologic manifestation of acute gastritis is a thickened, reddened mucous membrane with prominent rugae, or folds, in the stomach. Options B, C, and D are signs and symptoms of chronic gastritis.

2. A, B, C, D, E, F
   All of these options are potential factors that increase the risk for a client to develop gastritis.

3. B
   With chronic gastritis, progressive gastric atrophy from chronic mucosal injury occurs. The function of the parietal (acid-secreting) cells decreases, and the source of intrinsic factor is lost. Intrinsic factor is critical for absorption of vitamin B_{12}. When body stores of vitamin B_{12} are eventually depleted, pernicious anemia results.

4. A, B, D, F
   See the box entitled Patient and Family Education: Preparing for Self-Management Gastritis Prevention in your text for additional points for preventing gastritis. Option C is not correct because the client should stop smoking and using tobacco products. Option E is not correct because the client should seek medical care for symptoms of reflux and not use OTC drugs.

5. C
   Esophagogastroduodenoscopy (EGD) via an endoscope with biopsy is the gold standard for diagnosing gastritis. The primary health care provider performs a biopsy to establish a definitive diagnosis of the type of gastritis.

6. B, D
   H_2-receptor antagonists, such as famotidine and nizatidine, are typically used to block gastric secretions. Sucralfate, a mucosal barrier fortifier, may also be prescribed. Antisecretory agents (proton pump inhibitors [PPIs]), such as omeprazole or pantoprazole, are prescribed to suppress gastric acid. Calcium carbonate (chewable or liquid) is also a potent antacid.

7. D
   Ibuprofen is a nonsteroidal anti-inflammatory drug (NSAID). The nurse teaches the client that long-term NSAID use creates a high risk for acute gastritis. NSAIDs inhibit prostaglandin production in the mucosal barrier. Use of this drug may have caused the gastritis and continued use will cause it to worsen.

8. B, C, D

Three types of peptic ulcers may occur in PUD: duodenal ulcers, gastric ulcers, and stress ulcers (less common). Duodenal ulcers are most common, gastric ulcers occur in the antrum of the stomach, and stress ulcers are acute gastric mucosal lesions occurring after an acute medical crisis or trauma, such as sepsis or a head injury.

9. C

Sucralfate is a mucosal barrier fortifier. It helps ulcers to heal by coating and protecting the inner lining of the stomach. It should be given 1 hour before and 2 hours after meals and at bedtime because food may interfere with drug's adherence to mucosa. Sucralfate is not given within 30 minutes of giving antacids or other drugs because antacids may interfere with its effects.

10. D

With massive bleeding, the client vomits bright red or coffee-ground blood (hematemesis). Gastric acid digestion of blood typically results in the coffee-ground appearance. Hematemesis usually indicates bleeding at or above the duodenojejunal junction (e.g., upper GI bleeding).

11. A, C, D, E

See the box labeled Key Features Upper GI Bleeding in your text for a list of what signs and symptoms to expect when this occurs. Option B is not correct because heart rate is increased, and option F is not correct because hemoglobin and hematocrit levels are decreased when upper GI bleeding occurs.

12. B

Gastric and duodenal ulcers can perforate and bleed. Perforation occurs when the ulcer becomes so deep that the entire thickness of the stomach or duodenum is worn away. The stomach or duodenal contents can then leak into the peritoneal cavity. Sudden, sharp pain begins in the mid-epigastric region and spreads over the entire abdomen.

13. A

When the client's abdomen is tender, rigid, and board-like, this is likely an infection (peritonitis).

The client often assumes a "fetal" position to decrease the tension on the abdominal muscles. He or she can become severely ill within hours. Bacterial septicemia and hypovolemic shock can follow. Peristalsis diminishes, and paralytic ileus develops. Peptic ulcer perforation is a surgical emergency and can be life threatening. The nurse's best first action is to notify the primary health care provider or the Rapid Response Team (RRT).

14. A, C, E

There are three simple, noninvasive tests to detect *H. pylori* in the client's blood, breath, or stool. Although the breath and stool tests are considered more accurate, serologic testing for *H. pylori* antibodies is the most common method used to confirm *H. pylori* infection.

15. B

A common drug regimen for *H. Pylori* infection is PPI–triple therapy, which includes a proton pump inhibitor (PPI), such as lansoprazole, plus two antibiotics such as metronidazole and tetracycline or clarithromycin and amoxicillin for 10 to 14 days.

16. A, B, C, E

The nurse understands that a client with an active GI bleed has a life-threatening emergency and needs supportive therapy to prevent hypovolemic shock and possible death. The priority for care of this client is to maintain airway, breathing, and circulation (ABCs). Collecting urine for urinalysis is not a priority at this time, nor is monitoring serum electrolytes. Options A, B, C, and E are appropriate actions for this emergency situation. See the section in your text entitled Emergency: Upper GI Bleeding for more information.

17. C

The nurse teaches the client that bismuth may cause the stools and/or tongue to turn black. This discoloration is temporary and harmless.

18. B, C, E, F

Upper GI bleeding or obstruction often requires the primary health care provider or nurse to insert a large-bore NGT in order to:

determine the presence or absence of blood in the stomach, assess the rate of bleeding, prevent gastric dilation, and administer gastric lavage.

19. A, C, E

The nurse teaches a client with PUD to seek immediate medical attention for these symptoms: sharp, sudden, persistent, and severe epigastric or abdominal pain; bloody or black stools; or bloody vomit or vomit that looks like coffee grounds.

20. B

Stomach cancer seems to be positively correlated with eating excessive pickled foods, nitrates from processed foods, and salt added to food. The ingestion of these foods over a long period can lead to atrophic gastritis, which is a precancerous condition.

21. B, D, F

Although clients with early gastric cancer may be asymptomatic, dyspepsia and abdominal discomfort are the most common symptoms. A feeling of fullness and epigastric, back, or retrosternal pain are also early symptoms. Nausea and vomiting, weakness and fatigue, and a palpable gastric mass are late symptoms of gastric cancer.

22. B

In early stages of gastric cancer, laparoscopic surgery (minimally invasive surgery [MIS]) plus adjuvant chemotherapy or radiation may be curative.

23. B

These are early manifestations of dumping syndrome, which typically occur within 30 minutes of eating. Symptoms include vertigo, tachycardia, syncope, sweating, pallor, palpitations, and the desire to lie down. The nurse reports these manifestations to the surgeon and encourages the client to lie down.

24. A, B, D, E, F

All of these actions will help with management of a client's dumping syndrome, except option C. The nurse teaches the client to eat a high-protein, high-fat, low- to moderate-carbohydrate diet.

25. D

After gastrectomy the nurse assesses for the development of atrophic glossitis secondary to vitamin B_{12} deficiency. In atrophic glossitis, the tongue takes on a shiny, smooth, and "beefy" appearance.

51 CHAPTER

Concepts of Care for Patients with Noninflammatory Intestinal Disorders

1. When the nurse is teaching a client about bowel obstructions, which conditions will be described as mechanical bowel obstructions? **Select all that apply.**
   A. Adhesions
   B. Paralytic ileus
   C. Tumors
   D. Functional obstruction
   E. Crohn disease
   F. Absent peristalsis

2. Which acid-base imbalance does the nurse expect when a client experiences a bowel obstruction high in the small intestine?
   A. Respiratory acidosis
   B. Respiratory alkalosis
   C. Metabolic acidosis
   D. Metabolic alkalosis

3. Which potential causes will the nurse be sure to ask about when taking a history from an older client suspected of having a mechanical obstruction? **Select all that apply.**
   A. Fecal impaction
   B. Strictures from previous radiation therapy
   C. Fibrosis related to endometriosis
   D. Recent bowel surgery
   E. Benign tumor
   F. Diverticulitis

4. Which condition will the nurse **most likely** suspect as the cause of a client's symptoms of obstipation and failure to pass flatus?
   A. Complete obstruction
   B. Partial obstruction
   C. Colorectal cancer
   D. Singultus

5. Which assessment findings will the nurse expect to find when a client is experiencing early mechanical small bowel obstruction? **Select all that apply.**
   A. Absence of bowel sounds
   B. Abdominal distention
   C. Visible peristaltic waves
   D. High-pitched bowel sounds
   E. Abdominal rigidity
   F. Cramping

6. What does the nurse suspect has occurred when a client with a bowel obstruction starts passing flatus and has a small bowel movement?
   A. Blockage is complete.
   B. Peritonitis has occurred.
   C. Peristalsis has returned.
   D. Client is rehydrated.

7. Which actions will the nurse include when providing care for a client with a nasogastric tube (NGT) in place? **Select all that apply.**
   A. Assessing for NGT placement every 8 hours
   B. Keeping the client in a semi-Fowler position
   C. If the NGT is repositioned, confirming placement with an x-ray
   D. Instructing the client that feeling nausea is due to the NGT placement
   E. Monitoring the contents and drainage from the NGT
   F. Irrigating the NGT with 30 mL of normal saline as prescribed

8. How will the nurse know that the drug alvimopan, given to a client with postoperative ileus, is working and providing its intended action?
   A. Gastrointestinal (GI) motility is increased.
   B. The client has a large, formed bowel movement.
   C. Indications of infection are gone.
   D. Nausea and vomiting are no longer present.

9. Which nursing care action will the nurse assign to the assistive personnel (AP) when caring for a client with a bowel obstruction?
   A. Discussing surgical procedures with the client
   B. Checking the client's abdomen for distention
   C. Assessing the client's level of discomfort
   D. Providing mouth care every 2 hours as needed

10. What **priority** teaching points will the nurse include when teaching a group of older adults about prevention of fecal impaction? **Select all that apply.**
    A. "Eat high-fiber foods including raw fruits and vegetables."
    B. "Consume adequate fluids, especially water."
    C. "Use a laxative daily as needed to foster bowel regularity."
    D. "Walking every day is an excellent exercise for promoting intestinal motility."
    E. "Use natural foods to stimulate peristalsis, such as warm beverages and prune juice."
    F. "Avoid bulk-forming products to ease bowel elimination."

11. Which are the **major** risk factors for development of colorectal cancer that the nurse will be sure to ask about when taking a client's history? **Select all that apply.**
    A. Age older than 50 years
    B. Personal or family history of cancer
    C. History of intestinal blockage
    D. Crohn disease
    E. Ulcerative colitis
    F. Duodenal ulcers

12. Which are the **most common** symptoms of colorectal cancer that clients are likely to report to nurses?
    A. Constipation and fatigue
    B. Rectal bleeding and change in stool consistency
    C. Weight loss and abdominal fullness
    D. Abdominal pain and diarrhea

13. Which location of a tumor in the colon does the nurse suspect when a client presents with passage of red blood via the rectum?
    A. Transverse colon
    B. Ascending colon
    C. Descending colon
    D. Rectosigmoid colon

14. Which diagnostic test will the nurse prepare a client for to confirm the diagnosis of colorectal cancer (CRC)?
    A. Fecal occult blood test (FOBT)
    B. Carcinoembryonic antigen (CEA)
    C. Colonoscopy with biopsy
    D. CT-guided virtual colonoscopy

15. What is the **next best** action for the nurse to take after assessing a client who returned to the care unit with a colostomy by minimally invasive surgery (MIS) that is covered by a petrolatum gauze dressing under a dry sterile dressing?
    A. Reinforcing the dressing and leave it in place until the surgeon changes it the next morning
    B. Collaborating with the certified wound, ostomy, continence nurse (CWOCN) to place a pouch system as soon as possible
    C. Teaching the client how to use the patient-controlled anesthesia (PCA) machine to control his or her pain
    D. Notifying the surgeon that the colostomy stoma is pink, moist, slightly edematous, and protrudes 2 cm from the abdominal wall

16. Which dietary change suggestions will the nurse make to a client to decrease the risk of colorectal cancer (CRC)? **Select all that apply.**
    A. Decrease fat intake
    B. Increase fiber foods
    C. Decrease proteins
    D. Decrease refined carbohydrates
    E. Increase brassica vegetables
    F. Increase intake of red meat

17. What is the nurse's **best** response when a client asks which kind of stool to expect from a colostomy in the descending colon?
    A. "Your stool will be solid and similar to what you expelled from your rectum."
    B. "It will be very watery and similar to diarrhea stool."
    C. "You should expect your stool to be somewhat thin and gelatin-like."
    D. "Most likely your stool will have the consistency of paste and be thick."

18. What advice will the nurse give when a client expresses concern about gas and odor from a colostomy?
    A. "Place an aspirin in the colostomy bag once a day to help eliminate gas."
    B. "Empty the bag often, especially when it is about half full."
    C. "Adding a breath mint to the pouch can help to eliminate odors."
    D. "Cutting a small hole in the top of the bag will allow for the release of excess gas."

19. Which potential causes will the nurse monitor for when a client is suspected of having irritable bowel syndrome? **Select all that apply.**
    A. Stress
    B. Caffeinated beverages
    C. Sugary deserts
    D. Anxiety
    E. Red meats
    F. Dairy products

20. What action does the nurse expect to occur after administration of the drug linaclotide to a client with irritable bowel syndrome (IBS)?
    A. Control of symptoms of diarrhea
    B. Elimination of pain associated with bowel movement
    C. Reduction of anxiety and stress
    D. Increased fluid in the intestines to promote bowel elimination

21. Which alternative or complimentary therapies will the nurse teach a client may be helpful in managing irritable bowel syndrome (IBS)? **Select all that apply.**
    A. "Probiotics can help decrease bacteria and IBS symptoms."
    B. "Ginkgo can be used for abdominal discomfort and to expel gas."
    C. "Meditation may help decrease stress and help eliminate IBS symptoms."
    D. "Regular exercise will help decrease stress and lead to regular bowel movements."
    E. "Peppermint oil has been used to expel gas and relax spastic intestinal muscles."
    F. "Hydrotherapy may help decrease IBS symptoms."

22. What type of hernia does the nurse suspect when assessing a client and discovering these findings: abdominal pain, nausea, vomiting, pain, heart rate 118 beats/min, and temperature 101°F (38.3°C)?
    A. Incisional
    B. Strangulated
    C. Incarcerated
    D. Umbilical

23. Which **priority** points will the nurse include when providing discharge teaching for a client who had a minimally invasive inguinal hernia repair (MIIHR)?
    A. "Limit your oral fluid intake to between 1000 and 1200 mL per day."
    B. "Avoid strenuous activity for several days before returning to work and normal activities."
    C. "Take your prescribed stool softener regularly to prevent the occurrence of constipation."
    D. "You will need to learn how to insert a straight urinary catheter for the first week after your surgery."
    E. "Observe your incisions and report any signs of infection to your surgeon immediately."
    F. "This procedure is fairly painless so you will not need a prescription for pain medications."

24. Which conditions or actions will the nurse expect to worsen the presence and symptoms of a client's hemorrhoids? **Select all that apply.**
    A. Pregnancy
    B. Straining with constipation
    C. Weight lifting
    D. Prolonged bedrest
    E. Strenuous exercise
    F. Obesity

25. Which statement by a client to the nurse indicates correct understanding of the management of hemorrhoids after surgical removal?
    A. "It will take 10 to 14 days for the rubber band used on the hemorrhoid to fall off."
    B. "After surgery, I will need to consume a low-fiber, low-fluid diet."
    C. "My first bowel movement after the surgery may be very painful."
    D. "Stool softeners and laxatives are avoided after hemorrhoid surgery."

Chapter 51 Answer Key

1. A, C, E
   When the nurse describes mechanical bowel obstructions, they include conditions where the bowel is physically blocked by problems outside the intestine (e.g., adhesions), in the bowel wall (e.g., Crohn disease), or in the intestinal lumen (e.g., tumors).

2. D
   An obstruction high in the small intestine causes a loss of gastric hydrochloric acid, which can lead to metabolic alkalosis.

3. A, B, C, E, F
   In people aged 60 years or older, the nurse asks about diverticulitis, tumors, and fecal impaction, which are the most common causes of obstruction. Causes of mechanical obstruction also include: adhesions (scar tissue from surgeries or pathology); benign or malignant tumors; complications of appendicitis; hernias; fecal impactions (especially in older adults); strictures due to Crohn disease (a chronic inflammatory bowel disease) or previous radiation therapy; intussusception (telescoping of a segment of the intestine within itself); volvulus

(twisting of the intestine); and fibrosis due to disorders such as endometriosis. Option D is incorrect because surgery that involves handling the bowel causes a nonmechanical obstruction.

4. A
   Obstipation (no passage of stool) and failure to pass flatus are associated with complete obstruction. Singultus is hiccups.

5. B, C, D, F
   On examination of the abdomen, the nurse observes for abdominal distention which is common in all forms of intestinal obstruction. Peristaltic waves may also be visible. The nurse auscultates for proximal (above the obstruction) high-pitched bowel sounds (borborygmi), which are associated with cramping early in the obstructive process as the intestine tries to push the mechanical obstruction forward. Absent bowel sounds and abdominal rigidity occur in later stages of the obstruction.

6. C
   When a client with a bowel obstruction has been treated and begins to pass flatus and have

bowel movements, these signs indicate a return of peristalsis and that the bowel is no longer blocked.

7. B, C, E, F
When managing a client who has a nasogastric tube (NGT) in place, these nursing care actions are included: monitoring drainage, ensuring tube patency, checking tube placement every 4 hours; irrigating tube as prescribed (usually 30 mL normal saline), maintaining the client on NPO status, providing frequent mouth and nares care, and maintaining the client in a semi-Fowler position. If the NGT is repositioned or replaced, confirmation of proper placement is obtained by x-ray before using it.

8. A
When administered to a client with a postoperative ileus (POI), alvimopan is given short-term. This drug is an oral, peripherally acting mu opioid receptor antagonist that increases GI motility. The nurse expects to auscultate increased bowel sounds.

9. D
To choose the best response to this question, the nurse must be familiar with the scope of practice for an AP. APs are assigned care tasks that are within their scope of practice such as assisting clients with ADLs and personal care such as mouth care. Discussing surgical procedures, checking for abdominal distention, and assessing a client's level of comfort are skills that require the additional training of the professional RN.

10. A, B, D, E
See the box in your text entitled Nursing Focus on the Older Adult Preventing Fecal Impaction for priority teaching points about preventing fecal impaction, which include: teaching the client to eat high-fiber foods, including plenty of raw fruits and vegetables and whole-grain products; encouraging the client to drink adequate amounts of fluids, especially water; avoiding routinely taking a laxative; teaching the client that laxative abuse decreases abdominal muscle tone and contributes to an atonic colon; encouraging the client to exercise regularly, if

possible; walking every day is an excellent exercise for promoting intestinal motility; using natural foods to stimulate peristalsis, such as warm beverages and prune juice; and taking bulk-forming products to provide fiber and stool softeners to ease bowel elimination.

11. A, B, D, E
The major risk factors for the development of colorectal cancer (CRC) include being older than 50 years, genetic predisposition, personal or family history of cancer, and/or diseases that predispose the client to cancer such as familial adenomatous polyposis (FAP), Crohn disease, and ulcerative colitis.

12. B
The most common signs of CRC are rectal bleeding, anemia, and a change in stool consistency or shape. Stools may contain microscopic amounts of blood that are occult (hidden), or the client may have mahogany-colored (dark), or bright red stools.

13. D
Tumors in the transverse and descending colon result in symptoms of obstruction as growth of the tumor blocks the passage of stool. The client may report "gas pains," cramping, or incomplete evacuation. Tumors in the rectosigmoid colon are associated with hematochezia (the passage of red blood via the rectum), straining to pass stools, and narrowing of stools.

14. C
A colonoscopy provides views of the entire large bowel from the rectum to the ileocecal valve. As with sigmoidoscopy, polyps can be seen and removed, and tissue samples can be taken for biopsy. Colonoscopy with biopsy is the definitive test for the diagnosis of colorectal cancer.

15. B
Option A is not correct because the nurse collaborates with the certified wound, ostomy, continence nurse (CWOCN) to place a pouch system as soon as possible (option B). The colostomy pouch system, also called an appliance, allows more convenient and suitable collection

of stools than a dressing does. Option C is not correct because a client who has an open colon resection may need PCA for 24 to 36 hours postoperative, but a client who undergoes MIS has less pain and usually does **not** require PCA. Option D is not correct because it describes a healthy stoma. This must be documented, but **not** be reported to the surgeon.

16. A, B, D, E

The nurse teaches adults at risk for colorectal cancer to modify their diets as needed to decrease fat, refined carbohydrates, and low-fiber foods. Encourage baked or broiled foods, especially those high in fiber and low in animal fat. Remind adults to eat increased amounts of brassica vegetables, including broccoli, cabbage, cauliflower, and sprouts.

17. A

The colostomy should start functioning in 2 to 3 days after surgery. Stool is liquid immediately after surgery but becomes more solid, depending on where in the colon the stoma was placed. For example, stool from an ascending colon colostomy continues to be liquid, stool from a transverse colon colostomy becomes pasty, and stool from a descending colon colostomy becomes more solid (similar to stool expelled from the rectum).

18. C

Charcoal filters, pouch deodorizers, or placement of a breath mint in the pouch helps eliminate odors. The client should be cautioned to **not** put aspirin tablets in the pouch because they may cause ulceration of the stoma. Pouches with vents that allow release of gas from the ostomy bag through a deodorizing filter are available and may decrease the client's level of self-consciousness about odor.

19. A, B, D, F

The cause of IBS remains unclear. Research suggests that a combination of environmental, immunologic, genetic, hormonal, and stress factors plays a role in the development and course of the disorder. Examples of environmental factors include foods and fluids such as caffeinated or carbonated beverages and dairy products. Considerable evidence relates the role of stress and mental or behavioral illness, especially anxiety and depression, to IBS.

20. D

Linaclotide is a drug for IBS-C (IBS constipation). It works by simulating receptors in the intestines to increase fluid absorption and promote bowel transit time. The drug also helps relieve pain and cramping that are associated with IBS. The nurse teaches the client to take this drug once a day about 30 minutes before breakfast.

21. A, C, D, E

Probiotics have been shown to be effective for reducing bacteria and successfully alleviating GI symptoms of IBS. There is also evidence that peppermint oil capsules may be effective in reducing symptoms for clients with IBS. Relaxation techniques, meditation, and/or yoga may help the client decrease GI symptoms. The nurse teaches the client that regular exercise is important for managing stress and promoting regular bowel elimination.

22. B

A hernia is strangulated when the blood supply to the herniated segment of the bowel is cut off by pressure from the hernial ring (the band of muscle around the hernia). If a hernia is strangulated, there is ischemia and obstruction of the bowel loop. This can lead to necrosis of the bowel, sepsis, and possibly bowel perforation. Signs of strangulation are abdominal distention, nausea, vomiting, pain, fever, and tachycardia.

23. B, C, E

The nurse teaches the client to avoid strenuous activity for several days before returning to work and a normal routine. A stool softener may be needed to prevent constipation. Clients who are taking oral opioids for pain management are cautioned not to drive or operate heavy machinery. Clients are instructed to observe their incisions for redness, swelling, heat, drainage, and increased pain and promptly report these occurrences to the surgeon. The nurse reminds clients that soreness and discomfort (rather than severe, acute pain) are common after MIIHR.

24. A, B, C, E, F
All of these actions or conditions can cause worsening of hemorrhoids except option D. Prolonged sitting or standing may worsen hemorrhoids, but bedrest does **not**.

25. C
The nurse tells the client who has had a surgical intervention for hemorrhoids that the first postoperative bowel movement may be very painful. The client is also instructed to be sure that someone is with or nearby when this happens, because some clients become lightheaded and diaphoretic, and may have syncope (temporary loss of consciousness) related to a vasovagal response.

52

CHAPTER

Concepts of Care for Patients with Inflammatory Intestinal Disorders

1. Which cardinal signs will the nurse expect to assess in a client diagnosed with peritonitis?
   A. Fever with headache and confusion
   B. Dizziness with nausea and vomiting
   C. Loss of appetite with nausea and weight loss
   D. Abdominal pain with distention and tenderness

2. Which important information will the nurse include when teaching a client about peritonitis? **Select all that apply.**
   A. Peritonitis is caused by contamination of the peritoneal cavity by bacteria or chemicals.
   B. Respiratory problems associated with peritonitis are related to increased abdominal pressure against the diaphragm.
   C. White blood cell counts are often decreased when a client is diagnosed with peritonitis.
   D. Chemical peritonitis is caused by leakage of pancreatic enzymes or gastric acids.
   E. Fairly common causes of peritonitis include invasive tumors and continuous ambulatory peritoneal dialysis (CAPD).
   F. When the peritoneal cavity is contaminated by bacteria, the body begins an inflammatory reaction, walling off a localized area to fight the infection.

3. Which surgical client will the nurse recognize as having the highest risk for development of peritonitis?
   A. 35-year-old having a laparoscopic appendectomy
   B. 45-year-old having a vaginal hysterectomy
   C. 60-year-old having a traditional cholecystectomy for cholelithiasis
   D. 72-year-old having a bowel resection for colon cancer

4. Which interventions will the nurse include when care of a client with peritonitis is focused on restoring fluid volume balance? **Select all that apply.**
   A. Administering IV isotonic fluids and broad-spectrum antibiotics
   B. Assigning the assistive personnel (AP) to weigh the client daily and record intake and output
   C. Providing nasogastric tube (NGT) care and keeping the stomach decompressed
   D. Administering opioid pain medications as prescribed by the primary health care provider
   E. Maintaining the client on NPO status while the NGT is in place to low suction
   F. Assessing whether the client retains fluid used for irrigation by comparing and recording the amount of fluid returned with the amount of fluid instilled

5. In which position will the nurse place a client with peritonitis to promote comfort and **prevent harm** from potential complications?
   A. Semi-Fowler
   B. Left side-lying with knees to chest
   C. Right side-lying with knees to chest
   D. Supine flat with hips and knees flexed

6. Which assessment findings on a client with peritonitis indicate to the nurse the probability that the fluid shift into the peritoneal cavity is continuing? **Select all that apply.**
   A. Weight loss
   B. Tachycardia
   C. Hypertension
   D. Decreasing urine output
   E. Hyperactive bowel sounds
   F. Skin tenting over the forehead and sternum

7. Which complication will the nurse suspect when a client with peritonitis reports increased pain in the upper left abdominal quadrant and in the left shoulder, especially during inhalation?
   A. Sepsis
   B. Pneumonia
   C. Localized abscess
   D. Bacterial hepatitis

8. When the nurse is providing discharge instructions for a client recovering from peritonitis, which essential findings will the client and family be instructed to report immediately to the primary health care provider? **Select all that apply.**
   A. Completion of broad-spectrum antibiotics as prescribed
   B. Unusual or foul-smelling drainage
   C. Signs of wound dehiscence or ileus
   D. Swelling, redness, warmth, or bleeding from the incision site
   E. A temperature higher than 101°F (38.3°C)
   F. Abdominal pain or board-like stiffness in the abdomen

9. To **prevent harm** after a surgical procedure for peritonitis, which action will the nurse teach a client to **avoid**?
   A. Taking additional acetaminophen to prevent liver toxicity
   B. Lifting for at least 6 months after an open surgical procedure
   C. Resuming normal activities for at least 3 to 4 days after the procedure
   D. Using stool softeners and laxatives to prevent diarrhea

10. What does the nurse suspect when a client comes into the emergency department (ED) with right lower quadrant cramping pain, nausea, vomiting, and guarding with rigidity of the abdomen?
    A. Gastroenteritis
    B. Ulcerative colitis
    C. Appendicitis
    D. Crohn disease

11. Which laboratory finding will the nurse expect to see in a client who is suspected of having an acute, uncomplicated appendicitis?
    A. Decreased serum potassium level
    B. Increased international normalized ratio (INR)
    C. Increased white blood cell (WBC) count
    D. Decreased erythrocyte sedimentation rate

12. Which actions will the nurse perform when caring for a client with acute appendicitis before surgical management? **Select all that apply.**
    A. Maintaining the client on NPO status
    B. Administering IV fluids as prescribed
    C. Providing laxatives and enemas to clear the bowel
    D. Advising the client to maintain semi-Fowler position
    E. Giving adequate medications to control the client's pain
    F. Applying hot compresses to the right lower quadrant

13. Which care actions does the nurse expect to perform when caring for a client who had an appendectomy with an abscess? **Select all that apply.**
    A. Providing care for wound drains inserted during the surgery
    B. Administering IV antibiotics as prescribed by the surgeon
    C. Providing the client with a clear liquid diet
    D. Assessing the nasogastric tube (NGT) position and drainage
    E. Providing nonsteroidal anti-inflammatory drugs (NSAIDs) for pain control
    F. Helping the patient out of bed on the evening of surgery

14. Which common signs and symptoms will the nurse expect to find on assessment of a 60-year-old client who has had gastroenteritis for the past 2 days? **Select all that apply.**
    A. Weight loss
    B. Elevated temperature
    C. Dry mucous membranes
    D. Hypotension
    E. Oliguria
    F. Poor skin turgor

15. Which statement by a client with gastroenteritis due to infection with the norovirus indicates that the nurse's teaching about this illness has been successful?
    A. "I got this infection from being around my grandchildren when they had respiratory illnesses."
    B. "It is most likely that I got this infectious illness from either contaminated food or water."
    C. "I may have gotten sick when I was travelling last month to Florida."
    D. "It's really important that I don't go to restaurants for at least a month after I am well."

16. Which actions will the nurse teach a client to take to prevent the spread of gastroenteritis? **Select all that apply.**
    A. Washing hands well for at least 30 seconds
    B. Using easily accessible hand sanitizers
    C. Taking broad-spectrum antibiotics prophylactically
    D. Testing all food preparation employees
    E. Sanitizing all surfaces that may be contaminated
    F. Properly preparing food and beverages

17. Which drug will the nurse be sure to question to **prevent harm** when prescribed for an older adult with gastroenteritis?
    A. Azithromycin
    B. Protective skin barrier cream
    C. Ciprofloxacin
    D. Diphenoxylate hydrochloride with atropine sulfate

18. Which serum laboratory value is **most important** for the nurse to monitor when caring for an older client with gastroenteritis who has an irregular heart rate and reports "feeling weak?"
    A. Albumin
    B. Sodium
    C. Potassium
    D. Leukocyte count

19. Which client with symptoms of chronic abdominal pain and frequent bowel movements will the nurse consider at **highest risk** for a diagnosis of ulcerative colitis (UC)?
    A. 26-year-old white woman of Jewish ancestry who has an identical twin sister with the disorder
    B. 40-year-old black man who has just returned home from a business trip to southeast Asia
    C. 50-year-old Latino man with liver cirrhosis whose uncle died of colon cancer
    D. 65-year-old obese Asian woman who has chronic inflammatory cystitis

20. Which laboratory assessment findings will the nurse expect in a client who is diagnosed with ulcerative colitis?
    A. Increased albumin
    B. Decreased hemoglobin
    C. Increased sodium
    D. Decreased potassium
    E. Elevated white blood cell (WBC) count
    F. Elevated erythrocyte sedimentation rate

21. What is the **most important** assessment for the nurse to perform before administering the first dose of sulfasalazine to a client diagnosed with ulcerative colitis?
    A. Obtaining an accurate weight
    B. Asking whether he or she has an allergy to sulfa drugs
    C. Measuring heart and respiratory rate and blood pressure
    D. Determining the number of times the client has had a stool today

22. In collaboration with the registered dietitian nutritionist, which nutrients and substances will the nurse instruct a client with ulcerative colitis (UC) to **avoid** to reduce symptoms? **Select all that apply.**
    A. Eggs
    B. Corn
    C. Caffeine
    D. Vitamin C
    E. Dried fruits
    F. Carbohydrates
    G. Dairy products
    H. Pepper-based spices

23. For which client assessment finding will the nurse withhold the scheduled monthly dose of a prescribed parenteral biologic for management of ulcerative colitis (UC)?
    A. 5 lb (2.3 kg) weight gain
    B. Increased number of diarrhea stools per day
    C. Presence of occult blood in today's stool sample
    D. Cough and fever of 102°F (38.9°C)

24. Which action is appropriate for the nurse to take to **prevent harm** when caring for a client with ulcerative colitis who has undergone a total proctocolectomy with placement of a permanent ileostomy?
    A. Irrigating the ileostomy to maintain patency
    B. Using a skin barrier to prevent excoriation
    C. Monitoring the client for nausea due to decreased intestinal motility
    D. Giving small, frequent feedings to compensate for malnutrition from short-gut syndrome

25. What is the nurse's **best first** action when the stoma of a client who had a permanent ileostomy placed 2 days ago now has a dark bluish-purple appearance?
    A. Notifying the surgeon immediately
    B. Applying oxygen by nasal cannula
    C. Placing the client in a high-Fowler position
    D. Documenting the finding as the only action

26. Which disease features will the nurse commonly associate with a client who has Crohn disease (CD) that are rare or absent in a client with ulcerative colitis (UC)? **Select all that apply.**
    A. The problem first appears in the rectum and proceeds in a continuous manner toward the cecum.
    B. Fistulas commonly develop.
    C. Clients have five to six soft, loose, nonbloody stools per day.
    D. There is a greatly increased risk for colon cancer.
    E. Many clients have one or more extraintestinal problems such as arthritis, ankylosing spondylitis, and erythema nodosum.
    F. The appearance of the affected intestine areas resemble "cobblestone."

27. Which new-onset assessment finding in a client with Crohn disease (CD) indicates to the nurse the possibility of fistula development?
    A. Anorexia
    B. Pyuria with fever
    C. Smooth, beefy red tongue
    D. Decreased serum albumin

28. Which lunch food selection made by a client with diverticulosis indicates to the nurse the correct understanding of the necessary dietary modifications for management of the problem?
    A. A turkey sandwich on whole wheat bread, steamed carrots, and a raw apple
    B. Roasted chicken, potato salad, and a glass of milk
    C. Chicken salad sandwich on white bread, creamed soup, and hot tea
    D. Fried shrimp, lettuce and tomato salad, and a dinner roll

29. Which action will the nurse instruct a client with celiac disease to perform to reduce symptoms?
    A. Limiting caffeine
    B. Drinking more liquids
    C. Reading labels on prepared foods
    D. Avoiding raw fruits and vegetables

Chapter 52 Answer Key

1. D
   The nurse expects to assess these cardinal signs of peritonitis: abdominal pain, tenderness, and distention. In the client with localized peritonitis, the abdomen is tender on palpation in a well-defined area with rebound tenderness in this area. With generalized peritonitis, tenderness is widespread.

2. A, B, D, F
   Options A, B, D, and F are correct statements about peritonitis. Option C is in not correct because white blood cell counts increase (not decrease) with peritonitis. Option E is not correct because tumors and CAPD are not common causes of peritonitis.

3. D
   A client of any age having open bowel surgery is always at greater risk for peritonitis because the bowel is difficult to disinfect. This client is older and likely to have reduced immunity, placing him or her at even higher risk for peritonitis following bowel resection surgery.

4. A, B, C, E, F
   All of these options are important in the care of a client with peritonitis with a focus on restoring fluid volume balance, except option D. Administering opioid pain drugs would be part of the care focused on eliminating pain for this client.

5. A
   The client with peritonitis is placed in a semi-Fowler position to promote drainage to the lower abdominal region. Also, this position prevents abscess formation under the diaphragm and promotes lung expansion. Most clients also find this position comfortable.

6. B, D, F
   When fluid shifts from the vascular space into the peritoneal cavity, the client experiences central dehydration with hypovolemia. Symptoms include tachycardia and hypotension (not hypertension). Weight is not lost because the fluid has changed places in the body but it is not lost from the body. With hypotension, urine output decreases and skin turgor is poor. Bowel motility decreases further.

7. C
   Peritonitis can cause a localized abscess to form. Indications of this problem are more pain in one area of the abdomen than in the rest of the abdomen. An abscess in the upper right

abdomen often causes referred pain to the right shoulder.

8. B, C, D, E, F
Before being discharged home, the nurse assesses the client's ability for self-management and provides the client and family with written and oral instructions to report the following problems to the primary health care provider immediately: unusual or foul-smelling drainage; swelling, redness, warmth, or bleeding from the incision site; a temperature higher than 101°F (38.3°C); abdominal pain; and signs of wound dehiscence or ileus.

9. A
The nurse teaches the client to avoid taking additional acetaminophen to prevent liver toxicity. Clients are instructed to refrain from any lifting for at least 6 weeks (not months) after an open surgical procedure. Other activity limitations are based on individual need and the primary health care provider's recommendation. Patients who have laparoscopic surgery can resume activities within a week or two and may not have any major restrictions. Stool softeners are often prescribed to prevent constipation.

10. C
Cramping abdominal pain followed by nausea and vomiting can indicate appendicitis. When the nurse or emergency health care provider finds muscle rigidity and guarding on palpation of the abdomen, peritonitis is suspected.

11. C
With an acute uncomplicated appendicitis, the white blood cell count is usually elevated above normal but remains below 20,000/mm^3 (20 × 10^9/L). The potassium level and INR are unaffected. The inflammation associated with the infection may or may not cause an elevation of the erythrocyte sedimentation rate, but would not cause it to decrease.

12. A, B, D, E
The client with suspected or known appendicitis is kept NPO to prepare for the probability of surgery. IV fluids are administered to maintain fluid and electrolyte balance and replace fluid

volume. The client is instructed to maintain a semi-Fowler position so abdominal drainage can be contained in the lower abdomen. Once the diagnosis of appendicitis is confirmed and surgery is scheduled, opioid analgesics and antibiotics are administered as prescribed. The client with suspected or confirmed appendicitis must not receive laxatives or enemas, which can cause perforation of the appendix. Heat is not applied to the abdomen because this may increase circulation to the appendix and result in increased inflammation and perforation!

13. A, B, D, F
If complications such as peritonitis or abscesses are found during open traditional surgery, the nursing care is more complex and includes caring for wound drains and a nasogastric tube that may be placed to decompress the stomach and prevent abdominal distention. The nurse administers IV antibiotics and opioid analgesics as prescribed. The client is helped out of bed on the evening of surgery to help prevent respiratory complications, such as atelectasis.

14. A, B, C, D, E, F
After 2 days of vomiting and diarrhea with gastroenteritis, the client would have some degree of dehydration with all of the signs and symptoms listed.

15. B
Norovirus is transmitted (spread) through the fecal-oral route from person to person and from contaminated food and water. Infected individuals can also contaminate surfaces and objects in the environment. Vomiting may cause the virus to become airborne.

16. A, B, E
The nurse teaches clients and families to prevent the spread of gastroenteritis by using these strategies: washing hands well for at least 30 seconds with an antibacterial soap, especially after a bowel movement, and maintaining good personal hygiene; restricting the use of glasses, dishes, eating utensils, and tubes of toothpaste for his or her own use (in severe cases, disposable utensils may be used); maintaining

clean bathroom facilities to avoid exposure to stool; informing the primary health care provider if symptoms persist beyond 3 days; and not preparing or handling food that will be consumed by others.

17. D

Diphenoxylate hydrochloride with atropine sulfate reduces GI motility but is used sparingly because of its habit-forming ability. The drug is not recommended for older adults because it also causes drowsiness and could contribute to falls.

18. C

In clients who are older, the diarrhea of gastroenteritis can cause significant potassium loss along with fluid loss, which can cause cardiac dysrhythmias and skeletal muscle weakness.

19. A

UC is most common among younger white women. The disorder has a higher prevalence in adults with Ashkenazi Jewish heritage and has some degree of genetic predisposition. Thus, presence in an identical twin or other first-degree relative increases the risk.

20. B, D, E, F

Hematocrit and hemoglobin are often low from chronic blood loss. The inflammatory nature of the disease results in an increased WBC count and erythrocyte sedimentation rate. Sodium, potassium, and albumin levels are low from loss of these substances in the frequent diarrheal stools and malabsorption through the diseased bowel.

21. B

Although all assessment information is appropriate and important, the most important data to obtain is determining whether the client has a sulfa allergy. The drug sulfasalazine contains significant amounts of sulfa and if the client has a sulfa allergy, he or she is likely to have an allergic reaction to this drug.

22. B, C, E, G, H

Although each client with UC may have different foods that trigger diarrhea, common nutrients and substances that cause problems in most clients with UC include caffeine, alcohol, raw vegetables, dried fruits, dairy products, pepper, corn, nuts, carbonated beverages, and any high-fiber foods. The client is instructed to reduce or eliminate the intake of these items and any other that are known to increase his or her symptoms. Carbohydrates, protein, and vitamin C are needed in the diet.

23. D

"Biologics" (biological response modifiers) all cause some degree of immunosuppression and are not given when a client has indications of an infection. The weight gain would indicate a positive response to the drug. The presence of diarrhea stools and occult blood in the stool are the reasons why the drug is given.

24. B

Prevention of harm from skin problems (irritation, excoriation) is a nursing priority for these clients. The contents of the small intestine contain proteolytic enzymes and bile salts that are very irritating to the skin. Therefore, the priority action is to use a skin barrier.

25. A

A healthy stoma has a pink to bright red color. A dark bluish-purple appearance indicates inadequate blood flow to the stoma and the intestine behind it. The nurse notifies the surgeon immediately to take action to restore circulation to the area and prevent necrosis.

26. B, C, F

The affected intestinal areas in CD are not continuous and usually have normal tissue in between lesions ("skip lesions") that often have a cobblestone appearance. Fistula development is very common and serious. Although colon cancer can occur in clients with CD, it is much more common in clients with UC. Extraintestinal symptoms, bloody stools, and development from the rectum toward the cecum are characteristics of ulcerative colitis, not CD.

27. B
Pyuria, white blood cells or pus in the urine, is a strong indicator of an enterovesical fistula between the bowel and the bladder. Anorexia is nonspecific and can be a chronic problem because of the discomfort associated with CD. A smooth, beefy red tongue is common with vitamin B_{12} deficiency. Decreased albumin levels can indicate worsening of the disorder but is not specific to fistula development.

28. A
Dietary recommendations to prevent problems in a client with diverticulosis include a high-fiber diet with protein, root vegetables, whole grain breads and cereals, and fruit with the skin on.

29. C
Celiac disease results in inflammatory intestinal responses when gluten, especially wheat, is eaten. Clients are instructed to avoid obvious gluten sources such as breads, cereals, and food made with most types of flour. Many prepared or packaged foods contain some wheat or other gluten as a minor ingredient that can still cause symptoms. Clients are taught to read packaged food labels carefully for possible "hidden" gluten content.

53
CHAPTER

Concepts of Care for Patients with Liver Problems

1. Which client's previous health history will the nurse most associate with a risk for developing postnecrotic cirrhosis of the liver?
   A. 28-year-old woman who had gallstones 1 year ago and has recently lost 20 lb (9 kg) on a low-calorie, low-fat diet
   B. 45-year-old man with hepatitis C infection and chronic use of acetaminophen
   C. 50-year-old man who has many years of excessive alcohol consumption
   D. 55-year-old woman who has chronic biliary obstruction

2. What liver problem does the nurse suspect in a client whose liver is hard with a nodular texture and the hepatic enzymes remain normal?
   A. Prenecrotic inflammation
   B. Postnecrotic inflammation
   C. Compensated cirrhosis
   D. Decompensated cirrhosis

3. What will the nurse recognize as the cause of splenomegaly in a client who has cirrhosis?
   A. Increased pressure in the portal vein causing backflow of blood into the spleen
   B. The loss of cellular regulation in the liver spreading to the spleen and causing extensive scarring
   C. Chronic inflammation and infection increasing the spleen's maturation and release of white blood cells
   D. Direct destruction of spleen cells from alcohol or other toxins causing replacement with scar tissue formation

4. Which activities are **most important** for the nurse to teach a client with esophageal varices to **prevent harm** from bleeding or hemorrhage? **Select all that apply.**
   A. Avoid alcoholic beverages.
   B. Eat soft foods and cool liquids.
   C. Do not engage in strenuous exercise or heavy lifting.
   D. Try to eat six smaller meals daily instead of three larger ones.
   E. Be sure to keep your mouth open when sneezing or coughing.
   F. Cross your legs only at the ankles when sitting, rather than the knees.

5. Which essential nutrient will the nurse expect to be deficient in a client who has liver cirrhosis and ascites?
   A. Sodium
   B. Potassium
   C. Vitamin C
   D. Vitamin K

6. Which signs and symptoms will the nurse expect to find on assessment of a client with chronic liver disease who has an elevated serum bilirubin level? **Select all that apply**.
   A. Pruritus
   B. Icterus
   C. Hypertension
   D. Jaundice
   E. Pale, clay-colored stools
   F. Dark, coffee-colored urine

7. Which common factors will the nurse recognize as contributing to or worsening of hepatic encephalopathy in clients with liver cirrhosis? **Select all that apply**.
   A. Anorexia
   B. Infection
   C. Opioids
   D. Diarrhea
   E. GI bleeding
   F. High-protein diet
   G. Diabetes mellitus
   H. Chronic confusion

8. Which client will the nurse recognize as having the **greatest risk** for nonacoholic fatty liver disease (NAFLD)?
   A. 45-year-old Latino man who is 30 lb (13.9 kg) overweight and has type 2 diabetes
   B. 50-year-old white woman who drinks one glass of wine daily and has breast cancer
   C. 60-year-old black woman who is hypertensive and takes a diuretic daily
   D. 70-year-old Asian man who has gastroesophageal reflux disease (GERD)

9. Which assessment technique will the nurse use to **most** accurately determine increasing ascites in a client with advanced liver cirrhosis and portal hypertension?
   A. Interpreting the serum albumin value
   B. Measuring the client's abdominal girth
   C. Testing stool for the presence of occult blood
   D. Weighing the client daily at the same time of the day

10. Which neuromuscular assessment change indicates to the nurse that a client who has late-stage liver cirrhosis now has encephalopathy?
    A. Asterixis
    B. Positive Chvostek sign
    C. Increased deep tendon reflex responses
    D. Decreased deep tendon reflex responses

11. Which new-onset assessment findings in a client with Laennec cirrhosis indicates to the nurse that the client may be starting to have delirium tremens (DTs) from alcohol withdrawal? **Select all that apply.**
    A. Anxiety
    B. Tachycardia
    C. Hypotension
    D. Hypertension
    E. Cool, clammy skin
    F. Psychotic behavior

12. What is the nurse's **priority** action when a client with ascites reports increased abdominal pain and chills?
    A. Applying oxygen and making the client NPO
    B. Notifying the primary health care provider immediately
    C. Assessing for abdominal rigidity and taking the client's temperature
    D. Applying a heating blanket and raising the head of the bed to a 45-degree angle

13. Which assessment findings will the nurse expect in a client with late-stage liver cirrhosis whose total serum albumin level is low? **Select all that apply**.
    A. Ascites
    B. Hypotension
    C. Hyperkalemia
    D. Hyponatremia
    E. Dependent edema
    F. Decreased serum ammonia levels

14. Which actions are appropriate for the nurse to perform to **prevent harm** in a client with cirrhosis and ascites who has just undergone an esophagogastroduodenoscopy (EGD)? **Select all that apply.**
    A. Measuring oxygen saturation
    B. Checking for leakage from the site
    C. Assessing for return of the gag reflex
    D. Monitoring heart rate and blood pressure
    E. Auscultating bowel sounds in all four quadrants
    F. Comparing weight with that obtained before the procedure

15. Which serum electrolyte value in a client with early-stage ascites from chronic liver disease who is taking spironolactone will the nurse report immediately to the primary health care provider?
A. Sodium 133 mEq/L (mmol/L)
B. Potassium 6.4 mEq/L (mmol/L)
C. Chloride 101 mEq/L (mmol/L)
D. Calcium 8.9 mg/dL (2.2 mmol/L)

16. Which actions will the nurse perform when preparing a client for paracentesis? **Select all that apply.**
A. Obtaining informed consent
B. Maintaining the client on NPO status
C. Asking the client to void before the procedure
D. Placing the client in the flat supine position
E. Weighing the client before the procedure
F. Assessing the respiratory rate and blood pressure

17. Which symptoms in a client with cirrhosis and encephalopathy indicate to the nurse that the prescribed lactulose therapy is effective? **Select all that apply.**
A. Decreased confusion
B. Increased urine output
C. Musty odor to the breath
D. Two to three soft stools daily
E. Lower serum bilirubin levels
F. Lower serum ammonia levels

18. Which precaution is **most important** for the nurse to instruct a client with cirrhosis and his or her family about continuing care in the home?
A. Avoid taking acetaminophen or drinking alcohol.
B. Maintain one-floor living to prevent excessive fatigue.
C. Use cool baths to reduce the sensation of itching.
D. Report any change in cognition to the health care provider.

19. For clients with which types of hepatitis will the nurse teach about prevention of infection spread through the oral-fecal contamination route? **Select all that apply.**
A. Hepatitis A (HAV)
B. Hepatitis B (HBV)
C. Hepatitis C (HCV)
D. Hepatitis D (HDV)
E. Hepatitis E (HEV)
F. Toxic hepatitis

20. What is the nurse's **best** response to a client who fears he may have been exposed to hepatitis A while attending a banquet last week after which three restaurant workers were diagnosed with hepatitis A?
A. "Which types of food did you eat at the banquet?"
B. "If you have no symptoms at this time, you are probably safe."
C. "You can receive an immunoglobulin injection to prevent the infection."
D. "Contact your primary health care provider about receiving the hepatitis A vaccine."

21. Which actions are most effective for nurses and other health care workers to prevent occupational transmission of viral hepatitis? **Select all that apply.**
A. Washing hands before and after contact with all clients
B. Using needleless systems for parenteral therapy
C. Using Standard Precautions with all clients regardless of age or sexual orientation
D. Obtaining an immunoglobulin injection after exposure to hepatitis A
E. Being fully vaccinated with the hepatitis B vaccine
F. Wearing gloves during direct contact with all clients

22. Which clients will the nurse suggest to be immunized against hepatitis B (HBV)? **Select all that apply.**
    A. People who have unprotected sex with more than one partner
    B. Men who have sex with men
    C. Any client scheduled for a surgical procedure
    D. Firefighters
    E. Health care providers
    F. Clients prescribed immunosuppressant drugs

23. How will the nurse interpret a client's laboratory finding of the presence of immunoglobulin G antibodies directed against hepatitis A (HAV)?
    A. Active, infectious HAV is present.
    B. Permanent immunity to HAV is present.
    C. This is the client's first infection to HAV.
    D. The risk for infection if exposed to HAV is high.

24. Which precaution is **most** important for the nurse to instruct clients with hepatitis C (HCV) who are receiving drug therapy with **any** second-generation protease inhibitor?
    A. Avoid crowds and people who are ill.
    B. Do not touch these drugs with your bare hands.
    C. Alternate periods of activity with periods of rest.
    D. Be sure to take vitamin K supplements with this drug.

25. What is the nurse's **best first** action when a client who just had a liver transplant develops oozing around two IV sites as well as has some new bruising?
    A. Applying pressure to the IV sites
    B. Checking the client's platelet levels
    C. Notifying the surgeon immediately
    D. Documenting the findings as the only action

Chapter 53 Answer Key

1. B
   Postnecrotic cirrhosis of the liver is caused by viral hepatitis, especially hepatitis C, and drugs that are liver toxic, such as acetaminophen. Cirrhosis caused by chronic alcoholism is Laennec cirrhosis. Chronic biliary obstruction can result in biliary cirrhosis. Gallstones are not associated with cirrhosis unless chronic biliary obstruction is also present.

2. C
   In compensated cirrhosis, the liver is scarred with physical changes and cellular regulation is impaired, but the organ can still perform essential functions, including maintaining normal liver enzyme levels without causing major symptoms. In decompensated cirrhosis, liver function is impaired with obvious signs and symptoms of liver failure, including elevated liver enzymes.

3. A
   Portal hypertension caused by stiffened liver tissue results from increased resistance to or obstruction (blockage) of the flow of blood through the portal vein and its branches. This increased portal vein pressure causes backflow of blood into the spleen, resulting in splenomegaly.

4. B, C
   Esophageal varices are thin-walled blood vessels that bleed easily with mechanical irritation or any increase in pressure within the portal system. Clients must avoid any activity that increases intra-abdominal pressure such as strenuous exercise and heavy lifting. Hard or rough foods can mechanically open the varices and cause bleeding. Avoiding alcohol may prevent worsening of the liver problems but does not directly prevent bleeding or hemorrhage. None of the other activities alter intra-abdominal pressure or prevent direct injury to the varices.

5. D
   Clients with advanced liver disease, such as cirrhosis with ascites, are unable to metabolize fats and absorb fat-soluble vitamins from the GI tract. As a result, vitamin K is deficient. (Vitamin C is water-soluble.)

6. A, B, D, E, F

Bilirubin is a bile pigment. Elevated serum bilirubin levels stain the skin yellow (jaundice) and the eyes yellow (icterus). Jaundice is accompanied by intense itching. The excess bilirubin is excreted in the urine, turning it dark and coffee-colored. With liver disease and reduced function, the bilirubin does not reach the intestinal system where it is normally broken down to give stool its dark brown color. Because the bilirubin does not reach the GI tract, stools are light with a gray or clay color.

7. B, C, E, F

Factors that may contribute to or worsen hepatic encephalopathy in patients with cirrhosis include high-protein diet, infection, hypovolemia (decreased fluid volume), hypokalemia (decreased serum potassium), constipation, GI bleeding (causes a large protein load in the intestines), and some drugs, especially hypnotics, opioids, sedatives, analgesics, diuretics, illicit drugs.

8. A

Obesity and type 2 diabetes with metabolic syndrome are risk factors for NAFLD. In addition, a genetic variation in the *PNPLA3* gene increases the risk. This variation is much more common among Latinos.

9. D

Although measuring abdominal girth can show increases in girth that can be interpreted as more ascites, weighing the client provides more accurate information of water retention in the abdominal and dependent areas.

10. A

A late finding in clients who have late-stage liver cirrhosis and encephalopathy is asterixis, which is a coarse tremor that is characterized by rapid, nonrhythmic extensions and flexions in the wrists and fingers (hand-flapping).

11. A, B, D, F

Alcohol withdrawal occurs sometimes as soon as 6 to 8 hours after stopping alcohol intake after heavy and prolonged use and can lead to DTs. Cognitive, behavioral, and autonomic changes that occur may include acute confusion, anxiety, and psychotic behaviors, such as delusions and hallucinations, along with autonomic changes of tachycardia, elevated blood pressure, and diaphoresis.

12. C

Increasing abdominal pain and the presence of chills in a client who has ascites indicate possible spontaneous bacterial peritonitis. The nurse would perform a complete abdominal assessment and assess for a temperature elevation before notifying the primary health care provider.

13. A, B, D, E

Serum albumin maintains plasma oncotic pressure and sodium levels in the normal range. When albumin levels are low, plasma volume decreases as fluid leaks into the abdomen and dependent areas, forming ascites and dependent edema. Sodium follows the albumin, making serum sodium levels low. The decreased plasma volume results in hypotension.

14. A, C, D

A client with cirrhosis and ascites is at risk for bleeding and hemorrhage as a result of reduced blood clotting factor synthesis. The endoscope placement for an EGD can irritate or rupture any varices in the esophagus, stomach, or duodenum and lead to hemorrhage. The client must be closely monitored for indications of bleeding and hemorrhage by examining for changes in oxygen saturation, heart rate, and blood pressure. In addition, the procedure is performed under local anesthesia or light sedation and the client's gag reflex is affected.

15. B

Although the sodium and calcium levels are slightly low, they do not pose a significant risk at this time. The serum potassium level is well above normal, which may be related to the spironolactone therapy because it causes sodium excretion and potassium retention, and must be reported to the primary health care provider immediately. The serum chloride level is normal.

16. C, E, F

Vital signs, including weight, are taken before the procedure to use as a baseline for changes after the procedure. Weight is important because it can help determine the volume of fluid removed (clients are expected to weigh less after a paracentesis). Having the client void before procedure helps prevent injury to the bladder. The health care provider performing the paracentesis is responsible for obtaining informed consent, not the nurse. The client does not need to be NPO before the procedure. The client is positioned with the head of the bed elevated.

17. A, D, F

Lactulose helps reduce encephalopathy by increasing stools, which causes the loss of some nitrogen-producing bacteria in the intestinal tract. This loss reduces ammonia levels and helps decrease confusion. Lactulose does not affect serum bilirubin levels or increase urine output. A musty odor of the breath (fetor hepaticus) is an indication of worsening encephalopathy.

18. A

Although all of the listed precautions are important, the most important is the avoidance of acetaminophen and alcohol. These substances are toxic to the liver and will worsen the client's liver disease.

19. A, E

HAV and HEV are spread by the oral-fecal route from contaminated food and water sources. HBV, HCV, and HDV are spread primarily by the parenteral route although sexual contact can also result in infection spread. Toxic hepatitis is not infectious and is caused by exposure to hepatotoxic chemicals.

20. C

Receiving immunoglobulin with a high concentration of antihepatitis A antibodies within 2 weeks of exposure can prevent an exposed person from developing the infection. Receiving the vaccination at this time takes too long to develop sufficient immunity to prevent an infection from this exposure.

21. A, B, C, D, E

With the exception of F, all actions are effective in preventing or reducing transmission of infectious hepatitis among health care workers as a result of occupational exposure (see the Best Practices for Patient Safety and Quality Care: Prevention of Viral Hepatitis in Health Care Workers box). Wearing gloves during direct contact with all clients may give a false sense of security and does not prevent transmission if gloves are contaminated and then come into contact with another person. Gloves are not needed for all client contact.

22. A, B, D, E, F

HBV can be spread by both the parenteral and sexual routes. Exposures are more likely to result in infection in clients who are immunosuppressed for any reason. Individuals who are exposed to blood and other bodily fluids in the workplace are at risk for exposure.

23. B

Immunoglobulin G (IgG) directed against HAV are antibodies that indicate the client was previously exposed to HAV and developed immunity against it.

24. A

All of these drugs cause some degree of immunosuppression and increase the client's risk for infection.

25. C

Bleeding around the IV sites is a strong indicator of clotting problems. Such problems are an indicator of impaired function of the transplanted liver and may be an early sign of transplant rejection. Immediate action is needed to prevent harm in the form of graft loss.

54 CHAPTER

Concepts of Care for Clients with Problems of the Biliary System and Pancreas

1. Which signs and symptoms will the nurse expect to find on assessment of a client who is admitted with obstructive jaundice? **Select all that apply**.
   A. Pruritus
   B. Hypertension
   C. Pale, clay-colored stools
   D. Dark, coffee-colored urine
   E. Pink discoloration of sclera
   F. Bright red bleeding from the gums

2. Which client will the nurse recognize as having the **most** risk factors for cholelithiasis?
   A. 25-year-old white female athlete who is 10 lb (4.5 kg) underweight and had an appendicitis 2 months ago
   B. 35-year-old African-American male who is 10 lb (4.5 kg) overweight and is hypertensive
   C. 50-year-old Mexican-American female who has three children and takes hormone replacement therapy
   D. 60-year-old Asian-American male who had coronary artery bypass graft surgery 4 weeks ago

3. Which statement indicates to the nurse that a client who is experiencing frequent episodes of "indigestion" and flatulence may have cholecystitis?
   A. "My stools are sometimes very dark and tarry looking."
   B. "Sometimes at night I have bad-tasting fluid in my mouth."
   C. "Usually about a half hour after I eat, I become sweaty and nauseated."
   D. "My right arm and shoulder always seem to hurt after I eat fried foods."

4. Which signs or symptoms will the nurse assess for in a client who is suspected of having chole-cystitis? **Select all that apply**.
   A. Anorexia
   B. Jaundice
   C. Ascites
   D. Steatorrhea
   E. Eructation
   F. Rebound tenderness

5. What is the nurse's **priority** action when caring for a client with acute cholecystitis who now has severe abdominal pain, diaphoresis, heart rate of 118 beats/min, BP 95/70, respirations 32 breaths/min, and temperature 101°F (38.3°C)?
   A. Initiating the Rapid Response Team
   B. Assisting the client to a semi-Fowler position
   C. Administering the prescribed opioid analgesic
   D. Auscultating the client's abdomen in all four quadrants

6. What instruction will the nurse provide to a client to prepare him or her to undergo ultrasonography of the right upper abdominal quadrant to diagnose gallstones?
   A. Do not eat or drink for at least 6 hours before the test.
   B. Shower with an antibacterial soap the morning before the test.
   C. Be sure to have someone come with you who can drive you home.
   D. A small instrument will be rolled over your upper abdomen and there will be no pain.

7.   For which client will the nurse expect extracorporeal shock wave lithotripsy (ESWL) as treatment for gallstones to be *contraindicated*?
   A.   30-year-old who is 70 inches (1.75 m) tall and weighs 325 lb (147.2 kg)
   B.   35-year-old who has cholesterol-based stones
   C.   45-year-old who has a shellfish allergy and uses hormone replacement therapy
   D.   55-year-old who has bilateral total knee replacements

8.   Which advantages of minimally invasive surgery (MIS) laparoscopic cholecystectomy will the nurse reinforce to a client after the surgeon has provided information for informed consent? **Select all that apply.**
   A.   Bile duct injuries are rare.
   B.   Complications are uncommon.
   C.   Postoperative pain is less severe.
   D.   Mortality is about equal to that of traditional cholecystectomy.
   E.   IV antibiotics are not needed because infection does not occur.
   F.   Depending on the nature of the job, some clients can return to work within 1 to 2 weeks.

9.   What action will the nurse take when, 12 hours after a traditional cholecystectomy, a client's Jackson-Pratt (JP) drain shows serosanguineous drainage stained with bile?
   A.   Placing the client to the left lateral Sims' position
   B.   Clamping the drain intermittently for 30 minutes every hour
   C.   Measuring the drainage and documenting the findings
   D.   Disconnecting the suction device and gently irrigating the drain with sterile saline

10.   A client has postcholecystectomy syndrome (PCS) with persistent abdominal pain accompanied by vomiting for several weeks after removal of the gallbladder. Which possible causes or complications will the nurse remain alert for in this client? **Select all that apply.**
   A.   Pseudocyst
   B.   Common bile duct leak
   C.   Dumping syndrome
   D.   Diverticular compression
   E.   Ductal stricture or obstruction
   F.   Sphincter of Oddi dysfunction
   G.   Primary sclerosis cholangitis
   H.   Retained or new gallstones

11.   Which nursing assessment has the **highest priority** for the nurse to perform on a client admitted in severe pain with acute pancreatitis?
   A.   Asking the client to rate the level of pain
   B.   Measuring heart rate, blood pressure, and oxygen saturation
   C.   Auscultating bowel sounds in all four abdominal quadrants
   D.   Determining the amount of alcoholic beverages the client consumes daily

12.   Which action will the nurse take **first** when an 80-year-old client with acute pancreatitis has no breath sounds in the left lower lung lobe?
   A.   Apply oxygen.
   B.   Assess the breath sounds on the right.
   C.   Notify the primary health care provider.
   D.   Document the finding as the only action.

13.   Which serum laboratory values will the nurse expect to be elevated in a client who has acute pancreatitis? **Select all that apply.**
   A.   Amylase
   B.   Bilirubin
   C.   Calcium
   D.   Lipase
   E.   Magnesium
   F.   Glucose

14. Which clients will the nurse recognize as having a **higher risk** for development of acute pancreatitis? **Select all that apply.**
    A. 26-year-old woman who is a marathon runner
    B. 34-year-old man with Stage II HIV disease
    C. 40-year-old woman who has had cholelithiasis for 3 years
    D. 56-year-old man who drinks alcohol heavily and is underweight
    E. 62-year-old woman with gastroesophageal reflux disease
    F. 70-year-old man who has type 2 diabetes

15. Which actions will the nurse take to help relieve the severe pain in a client with acute pancreatitis? **Select all that apply.**
    A. Maintaining the client on NPO status
    B. Administering oral NSAIDs around the clock
    C. Inserting a nasogastric (NG) tube to low suction
    D. Providing opioids by patient-controlled analgesia
    E. Administering pancreatic enzyme replacement therapy
    F. Assisting the client to a side-lying position with knees drawn up to the chest

16. Which change in electrolyte values will the nurse expect in a client with acute pancreatitis who reports numbness around the mouth and leg muscle twitching?
    A. Hyponatremia
    B. Hypokalemia
    C. Hypocalcemia
    D. Hypochloremia

17. Which complication in a client with acute necrotizing pancreatitis who develops a temperature spike to 104°F (40°C) will the nurse suspect?
    A. Pancreatic pseudocyst
    B. Pancreatic abscess
    C. Chronic pancreatitis
    D. Pancreatic cancer

18. Which is the **most effective** action for the nurse to take to assess adequate bowel function in a client with acute pancreatitis who is at risk for the development of paralytic (adynamic) ileus?
    A. Observing contents of the nasogastric drainage
    B. Listening for bowel sounds in all four abdominal quadrants
    C. Asking the client if he or she has passed flatus or had a stool
    D. Interpreting the report of a CT scan of the abdomen with contrast medium

19. Which statements about eating habits and diet therapy indicate to the nurse that the client recovering from acute pancreatitis understands the recommendations made in collaboration with the registered dietitian nutritionist? **Select all that apply.**
    A. "Now I can go back to my usual three meals a day."
    B. "Replacing carbohydrates with protein will speed my recovery."
    C. "Although they do not contain fat, I will avoid chocolate and caffeine."
    D. "If vomiting or diarrhea occur, I will call my primary health care provider."
    E. "I can't wait to have some good, spicy Mexican food after all this hospital food."
    F. "I am planning on joining Alcoholics Anonymous and giving up drinking altogether."

20. Which actions and precautions will the nurse educate a client with chronic pancreatitis about when starting pancreatic enzyme replacement therapy (PERT)? **Select all that apply.**
    A. Do not crush or chew the capsules.
    B. Take these drugs with all meals and snacks.
    C. Sit in an upright position for at least 30 minutes after taking the drug.
    D. Wear sunscreen and protective clothing outdoors to prevent severe sunburn.
    E. Check your stools for amount and presence of fat to assess whether the drugs are working.
    F. If you are too nauseated to eat or to take the drug, go to an emergency department for an injectable form of the drug.

21. Which client will the nurse recognize as having the highest risk for pancreatic cancer?
    A. 27-year-old man who is underweight and has opioid use disorder
    B. 35-year-old woman who is overweight and uses oral contraceptives
    C. 50-year-old woman who has ductal breast cancer and receiving radiotherapy
    D. 60-year old man who smokes two packs of cigarettes daily and has liver cirrhosis

22. Which signs and symptoms will the nurse expect to see in a client who is diagnosed with advanced pancreatic cancer? **Select all that apply.**
    A. Light-colored urine and dark-colored stools
    B. Anorexia and weight loss
    C. Splenomegaly
    D. Ascites
    E. Leg or calf pain
    F. Weakness and fatigue

23. In which position will the nurse place a client after an open Whipple procedure for treatment of pancreatic cancer?
    A. Semi-Fowler position to reduce tension on the suture line
    B. Prone position to prevent acute respiratory distress syndrome
    C. Left lateral Sims' position with knees drawn up to the chest to reduce pain
    D. Right lateral Sims' position with knees drawn up to the chest to reduce pain

24. Which fluid and electrolyte balance assessment action will the nurse perform **most often** for a client with pancreatic cancer after surgery with a traditional Whipple procedure?
    A. Using a reflex hammer to check deep tendon reflexes
    B. Pinching up skin over the sternum and checking for tenting
    C. Applying a blood pressure cuff and assessing for a Trousseau sign
    D. Asking the client whether he or she has noticed tingling or numbness around the mouth

Chapter 54 Answer Key

1. A, C, D
   Jaundice is a yellow discoloration of the skin and mucous membranes from excessive bilirubin in these structures and blood. Jaundice is accompanied by intense itching. The excess bilirubin is excreted in the urine, turning it dark and coffee-colored. The obstruction prevents bilirubin from reaching the intestinal system where it is broken down and gives stool its dark brown color. Because the bilirubin does not reach the GI tract, stools are light with a gray or clay color.

2. C
   Cholelithiasis has a higher incidence among Mexican-Americans, especially women who have had multiple pregnancies, and among those who are taking estrogen/progesterone hormone replacement therapy.

3. D
   Cholecystitis and cholelithiasis can cause referred pain to the right shoulder area, including under the right shoulder blade. Dark, tarry stools are associated with GI bleeding. Bad-tasting fluid or vomitus in the mouth at night is related to gastroesophageal reflux disease. Becoming sweaty and nauseated after a meal is associated with dumping syndrome, not gallbladder disease.

4. A, B, D, E, F
   Characteristic signs and symptoms of cholecystitis include episodic or vague upper abdominal pain or discomfort that can radiate to the right shoulder, pain triggered by a high-fat or high-volume meal, anorexia, nausea and/or vomiting, dyspepsia, eructation, flatulence, feeling of abdominal fullness, rebound tenderness (Blumberg's sign), and fever. Additional symptoms include jaundice and fatty stools (streatorrhea).

5. A
   The client is exhibiting the symptoms associated with biliary colic and possible shock. This

is an emergency and, if the client's primary health care provider is not immediately available, initiating the Rapid Response Team is a priority.

6. D

An ultrasound is performed with an electronic probe lubricated and rolled on the skin over the area to be examined. It causes no pain, does not require the client to be NPO or to be sedated, and special cleansing of the area is not needed.

7. A

Some clients who have small, cholesterol-based stones and good gallbladder function may undergo extracorporeal shock wave lithotripsy (ESWL) to break up the stones. This procedure can be used only for patients who have a normal weight.

8. A, B, C, F

Injuries and complications are much lower than with traditional cholecystectomy and the postoperative pain is less severe. Many clients can resume their normal activies within 1 week. The mortality rate is very low, much lower than traditional cholecystectomy. Although the infection rate is low, there is still an infection risk anytime an incision is made.

9. C

Serosanguineous drainage stained with bile is expected and normal during the first 24 hours after traditional cholecystectomy. The drain is not to be clamped or irrigated. Placing the client in left lateral Sims' position can be done but is not related to drainage from the JP.

10. A, B, D, E, F, G, H

PCS most commonly indicates possible problems in the biliary tract, such as pseudocyst, common bile duct leak, diverticular compression, ductal stricture or obstruction, sphincter of Oddi dysfunction, primary sclerosis cholangitis, and retained or new gallstones. Dumping syndrome is not part of the problems associated with PCS. Further testing is needed to identify the cause and provide interventions to prevent even more serious complications.

11. B

The client with acute pancreatitis is at high risk for death from hemorrhage and shock as a result of necrotic blood vessels destroyed by enzymatic digestion. Although all the above assessments are appropriate, the priority is to determine whether any indications of internal hemorrhage and shock are present.

12. A

Left lower lung effusions, atelectasis, and pneumonia often develop in clients with acute pancreatitis, especially in older adults, and can lead to pulmonary failure and death. The nurse would first apply oxygen and then immediately notify the primary health care provider.

13. A, B, D, F

With acute pancreatitis, the pancreatic enzymes amylase and lipase are elevated. Bilirubin also is usually elevated as a result of biliary dysfunction or obstruction. Blood glucose levels are often elevated because pancreatic secretion of insulin is reduced. Most often, magnesium and calcium levels are decreased.

14. B, C, D

Although the cause of acute pancreatitis is often unknown, risk factors include viral infection with HIV, long-term cholelithiasis that can lead to obstruction, and alcoholism. Being thin and active is not directly associated with pancreatitis. Neither gastroesophageal reflux disease nor type 2 diabetes increase the risk for acute pancreatitis.

15. A, D, F

Pain can be reduced by preventing pancreatic stimulation by keeping the client NPO. Opioids are needed for severe pain and are best provided by PCA. Clients may obtain some pain relief from a side-lying position with the knees drawn closely to the chest. NSAIDs are not used and pancreatic enzyme replacement therapy would only make the pancreatitis worse at this time. NG tube placement is reserved for only those clients who have continuous vomiting or biliary obstruction.

16. C
The free or unbound serum calcium level is usually low in clients who have acute pancreatitis as a result of fat necrosis and the inability of the body to use protein-bound calcium.

17. B
A sudden temperature elevation in a client with acute necrotizing pancreatitis is a strong indicator of pancreatic abscess that develops as a secondary bacterial infection with suppuration and pus formation of the necrotic pancreatic tissue. This condition can lead to sepsis and multiple organ dysfunction syndrome (MODS).

18. C
The best indicator of bowel function and adequate motility is the actual passage of flatus or stool. Bowel sounds may still be present in the presence of an adynamic ileus. A CT scan is static and does not indicate motility. Gastric contents cannot indicate bowel motility.

19. C, D, F
Recommendations for diet therapy during recovery from acute pancreatitis includes small, frequent, moderate- to high-carbohydrate, high-protein, low-fat meals with bland, non-spicy food; avoidance of alcohol; and avoidance of GI stimulants such as caffeine-containing food (tea, coffee, cola, and chocolate). If clients start to have nausea, vomiting, or diarrhea after eating, he or she is instructed to notify the primary health care provider.

20. A, B, E
PERT is used to assist in the digestion of foods. Thus, it must be taken orally only whenever the client eats a meal or snack. Capsules are not to be opened, crushed, or chewed for maximum benefit. The amount of fat in the stools, as well as the amount and consistency of stools are used to evaluate PERT effectiveness. It is not necessary to remain upright, and the drug does not cause or increase photosensitivity.

21. D
Although the exact cause of pancreatic cancer is not known, the older man who smokes and has liver cirrhosis has four risk factors.

22. A, B, C, D, E, F
All of the signs and symptoms listed are associated with pancreatic cancer.

23. A
After a radical pancreatectomy, the client is kept in a semi-Fowler position to reduce tension on the suture line and anastamosis site.

24. B
Clients are at extreme risk for dehydration during and after a traditional Whipple surgical procedure for pancreatic cancer because of variety of factors. These factors include exposure of the bowel during surgery, extensive NPO status, the presence of drainage tubes, and protein malnutrition resulting in poor osmotic/oncotic pressure.

55 CHAPTER

Concepts of Care for Patients with Malnutrition: Undernutrition and Obesity

1. Which set of energy balance factors leads to body weight loss?
   A. Energy intake and energy use are balanced.
   B. Energy use and energy intake are both zero.
   C. Energy intake exceeds energy use.
   D. Energy use exceeds energy intake.

2. Which foods will the nurse expect a client who follows a lacto-ovo vegetarian diet to select as menu items for breakfast? **Select all that apply.**
   A. Milk
   B. Toast
   C. Cereal
   D. Sausage
   E. Tuna fish
   F. Scrambled eggs

3. Indications of which vitamin deficiency will the nurse be sure to assess for in a client who follows a strict vegan diet?
   A. Vitamin A
   B. Vitamin B_{12}
   C. Vitamin C
   D. Vitamin D_3

4. Which symptom reported by a client after eating eggs indicates to the nurse a possible allergy to eggs rather than an egg intolerance?
   A. Diarrhea
   B. Excessive flatulence
   C. Throat itching and swelling
   D. Nausea when smelling eggs

5. Which assessment findings in an older client indicate to the nurse that this client is at increased risk for developing undernutrition? **Select all that apply.**
   A. Male
   B. Is of Jewish ethnicity
   C. Reports chronic diarrhea
   D. Receiving oxygen after surgery
   E. Does not consume pork products
   F. Has chronic obstructive pulmonary disease
   G. Presence of chronic draining pressure injury
   H. Presence of swollen gums and many missing teeth

6. With which client will the nurse **avoid** relying on body mass index (BMI) as an indicator of nutrition status?
   A. 25-year-old female with anorexia
   B. 35-year-old male weight-lifter who works out daily
   C. 55-year-old female runner who is post-menopausal
   D. 65-year-old male who plays golf twice a week and walks 5 miles daily

7. Which changes in a 60-year-old client's assessment findings over the past 4 weeks indicate to the nurse the need for a nutrition status evaluation? **Select all that apply.**
   A. Sprained a wrist 2 weeks ago
   B. Initiation of a strict vegan diet
   C. Unintentional weight loss of 6%
   D. Initiation of a regular exercise program
   E. Reports starting counseling for depression
   F. Reduced cigarette smoking from two packs/day to one pack/day

8. Which activity of a nutritional screening will the nurse assign to an assistive personnel (AP)?
   A. Obtaining an accurate height and weight
   B. Asking about the client's usual food intake
   C. Reviewing the client's laboratory results
   D. Performing a psychosocial assessment

9. Which client will the nurse identify as **most at risk** for the marasmic-kwashiorkor form of protein-energy malnutrition (PEM)?
   A. 48-year-old with rheumatoid arthritis who has worn dentures for 6 years
   B. 58-year-old who suffered a traumatic amputation of the left arm 15 years ago
   C. 68-year-old vegan who is 10 lb (4.5 kg) underweight and has bacterial pneumonia with a high fever
   D. 78-year-old who has type 2 diabetes mellitus and lives with his 50-year-old daughter

10. Which signs/symptoms in an older client admitted for a medical problem indicate to the nurse the possibility of "failure to thrive?" **Select all that apply.**
   A. Weakness
   B. Exhaustion
   C. Poor skin turgor
   D. Reduced hearing
   E. Stress incontinence
   F. Slow walking speed
   G. Low physical activity
   H. Unintentional weight loss

11. Which assessment will the nurse use as the **most reliable** indicator of a client's fluid status?
   A. Intake and output
   B. Trends in weight
   C. Changes in skin turgor
   D. Presence of dependent edema

12. Which action will the nurse take **first** to promote adequate intake in a client who is malnourished?
   A. Asking the client about his or her food preferences
   B. Providing the client with high-calorie, high-protein food
   C. Offering frequent snacks or protein shakes between meals
   D. Obtaining serial weights on a weekly basis to monitor progress

13. Which actions will the nurse take to enhance an older client's desire to eat? **Select all that apply.**
   A. Assisting the client to make menu selections and substitutions to match his or her food preferences
   B. Removing any items from sight that reduce appetite such as emesis basins, urinals, and bedpans
   C. Eliminating distractions, such as turning down the volume of the television
   D. Offering the client the opportunity to toilet before the meal arrives
   E. Opening cartons and condiment packages for the client
   F. Bringing the client's medications to take with the meal
   G. Ensuring the food served is at appropriate temperature
   H. Asking all of the client's visitors to leave

14. Which assessment findings will the nurse expect in a client with chronic a vitamin D deficiency?
   A. Swollen, bleeding gums
   B. Reddened and dry conjunctiva
   C. Osteomalacia, bone pain, and rickets
   D. Enlargement of the liver and spleen

15. What nutritional deficiency does the nurse suspect when a client reports recent onset of alopecia?
   A. Zinc
   B. Vitamin A
   C. Riboflavin
   D. Vitamin C

16. Which techniques will the nurse instruct the family who will be caring for an 88-year-old female client who has severe osteoarthritis, muscle weakness, and dementia to use to improve nutrition and prevent harm? **Select all that apply.**
    A. "Be sure to keep her in bed while eating to prevent her from becoming over tired."
    B. "Let her feed herself as much as possible even if she uses her fingers."
    C. "Always include some foods that you know she likes for every meal."
    D. "Withhold her pain medications before meals to prevent nausea."
    E. "If she doesn't finish a meal in 20 minutes, take the food away."
    F. "During meals, be sure she has her glasses and hearing aid on."

17. Which clients will the nurse expect to be prescribed total enteral nutrition (TEN) to help attain or maintain an adequate nutrition status? **Select all that apply.**
    A. 28-year-old who remains comatose 10 days after a head injury
    B. 38-year-old with esophageal strictures and an intestinal blockage
    C. 48-year-old who eats all meals but remains 22 lb (10 kg) underweight
    D. 58-year-old who has lung cancer and cachexia
    E. 68-year-old with no teeth or dentures
    F. 78-year-old who cannot swallow after a stroke

18. What is the nurse's **best action** to **prevent harm** for a client who is receiving enteral feedings by nasogastric (NG) tube when stomach contents cannot be aspirated and the client is coughing continuously?
    A. Notify the primary health care provider to request an order for a chest x-ray.
    B. Use a piston-style syringe and gentle pressure to instill 30 mL of water.
    C. Reposition the client on his or her right side and apply oxygen.
    D. Remove the tube.

19. Which actions will the nurse take to **prevent harm** when caring for a client receiving continuous enteral tube feeding? **Select all that apply.**
    A. Checking the residual volume at least every 6 hours
    B. Changing the feeding bag and tubing every 12 hours
    C. Keeping the head of the bed elevated at least 30 degrees
    D. Using clean technique when changing the feeding system
    E. Discarding unused open enteral products after 24 hours
    F. Warming the enteral products before infusion

20. Which complication does the nurse suspect when a client in a starvation state receiving enteral feedings has shallow respirations, weakness, acute confusion, and oozing from the IV site?
    A. Sepsis
    B. Aspiration
    C. Hypoglycemia
    D. Refeeding syndrome

21. Which electrolyte imbalance will the nurse assess for most frequently in a client who is receiving total parenteral nutrition with a solution that contains both glucose and insulin?
    A. Hypochloremia
    B. Hyperchloremia
    C. Hypokalemia
    D. Hyperkalemia

22. Which action will the nurse take to **prevent harm** when a client's total parenteral nutrition (TPN) bag has only 20 mL left in it and the next bag will not be delivered for at least 1 hour?
    A. Capping the TPN line until the next TPN solution is available
    B. Infusing 10% dextrose/water until the TPN solution is available
    C. Preparing to treat the client for hypoglycemia
    D. Notifying the primary health care provider

23. Which health problem will the nurse assess for in an obese client who has a 40-inch waist circumference and a waist-to-hip ratio of 0.90?
    A. Rheumatoid arthritis
    B. Chronic kidney disease
    C. Cardiovascular disease
    D. Type 1 diabetes mellitus

24. Which precaution to **prevent harm** is most important for the nurse to teach an overweight client who is prescribed to take orlistat?
    A. "Take a multivitamin daily because this drug prevents absorption of some vitamins."
    B. "Notify your primary health care provider if you have any thoughts about hurting yourself."
    C. "Be sure to use a reliable method of contraception because this drug can cause birth defects."
    D. "Watch for feelings of light-headedness and jitteriness because this drug can cause hypoglycemia."

25. Which assessment is the **priority** for the nurse to make in the immediate postoperative period for a client after bariatric surgery?
    A. Asking the client to rate his or her pain
    B. Checking oxygen saturation and respiratory effort
    C. Examining the wound for indications of infection or dehiscence
    D. Monitoring skinfold areas for cleanliness and indications of breakdown

26. What is the nurse's **best first** action when assessment findings on a client after gastric bypass surgery reveal increased back pain, restlessness, heart rate of 126 beats/min, and a urine output of only 15 mL for the past 2 hours?
    A. Increasing the IV infusion rate
    B. Inserting a fresh nasogastric tube
    C. Listening for bowel sounds in all abdominal quadrants
    D. Notifying the surgeon or Rapid Response Team immediately

27. Which actions will the nurse take when caring for a client after bariatric surgery to **prevent harm** from complications? **Select all that apply**.
    A. Monitoring oxygen saturation
    B. Applying an abdominal binder
    C. Placing the client in semi-Fowler position
    D. Applying sequential compression stockings
    E. Assessing skinfolds for redness and excoriation
    F. Maintaining the client on bedrest for 24 to 48 hours

28. Which problem does the nurse suspect in a client who is 4 weeks postoperative from gastric bypass surgery and reports that after a meal her heart races, she is nauseated, and has abdominal cramping with diarrhea?
    A. Hyperglycemia
    B. Intestinal obstruction
    C. Possible peritonitis
    D. Dumping syndrome

Chapter 55 Answer Key

1. D
   Energy balance is the relationship between energy use and energy intake. When energy used is greater than energy taken in or stored, weight loss occurs.

2. A, B, C, F
   An adult who follows a lacto-ovo vegetarian diet eats a primarily plant-based diet that also includes eggs and dairy products. Meat, poultry, and fish are avoided.

3. B
   A strict vegan diet is plant-based only. All animal sources of protein, such as meat, poultry, fish, seafood, eggs, and dairy products are avoided as are any complex foods that contain these products. Vitamin B_{12} is highest in red meats.

4. C
   A true food allergy is an immune and inflammatory response that can occur as a systemic

response, as well as in tissues that came into direct contact with the allergen in the food. A food intolerance is seen as a physiologic change in gastrointestinal responses that indicate a problem with digesting the food item. The nausea after smelling the odor of eggs is a learned behavior that is neither a food allergy nor a physiologic food intolerance.

5. C, F, G, H
The risk for malnutrition is not particularly associated with ethnicity or gender. Conditions that increase nutrient loss, such as chronic wounds and chronic diarrhea contribute to undernutrition risk. Poor dentition interferes with a client's ability to consume adequate nutrients. Health problems that increase energy expenditure, such as COPD, greatly increase caloric need and promote undernutrition. Although pork is an animal protein source, its elimination from the diet does not alone contribute to undernutrition. Receiving oxygen after surgery is common and not an indicator of undernutrition risk.

6. B
BMI is an unreliable indicator of overnutrition or undernutrition in adults who are very athletic and muscular. When muscle mass is significantly greater than average, the client will weigh more even though the percentage of body fat is low.

7. B, C, E
The changes that could alter nutrition status the most for this 60-year-old client are the start of a strict vegan diet, unintentional weight loss greater than 5% in a month, and the presence of depression. Many people who decide to begin a strict vegan diet are unaware of what types of plant-based foods will be needed to maintain an adequate intake of micronutrients and protein. Many, but not all, people with depression often lose interest in maintaining an adequate nutritional intake.

8. A
Accurately measuring height and weight are within the AP's scope of practice. Collecting information about a client's nutrition history,

reviewing laboratory findings, and performing a psychosocial assessment require greater knowledge and skill and are not within an AP's scope of practice.

9. C
Marasmus is an energy (caloric) malnutrition with some degree of starvation in which body fat and muscle proteins are wasted although serum proteins may be normal. The client appears thin. Kwashiorkor malnutrition occurs with a severe protein deficiency although overall caloric intake may be adequate to maintain a normal weight, but serum proteins are low. Marasmic-kwashiorkor is a more severe malnutrition in which both protein and caloric intake are inadequate and the client is seriously underweight. It is most common when a client already is malnourished and develops a health problem that greatly increases the metabolic need for nutrients.

10. A, B, F, G, H
"Failure to thrive" in older clients is a combination of any three of these five symptoms: weakness, slow walking speed, low physical activity, unintentional weight loss, and exhaustion.

11. B
Weight change is the most reliable indicator of fluid status. A liter of water weighs 1 kg (2.2 lb). An actual weight gain or loss can account for a daily change of only about a half lb (~240 g). More than that indicates increased fluid and less than that indicates fluid loss.

12. A
Regardless of a dietary intervention for malnutrition, if the client does not eat the food provided or recommended, malnutrition will continue. Incorporating the client's food preferences into a planned dietary intervention increases the likelihood of the intervention's success.

13. A, B, C, D, E, G
Although it is not possible to increase a client's appetite, actions that make the client more comfortable, reduce unpleasant thoughts, and

make food more appetizing can improve a client's interest or desire to eat. These include toileting before meals, removing objects that evoke unpleasant thoughts, providing food that the client likes at the right temperatures, making it easier for the client to access food items on the tray, and avoiding interruptions with medication administration. Visitors do not have to leave and may, in fact, make the dining experience more pleasant. Visitors are only asked to leave if they hamper a client's desire to eat.

14. C

    Activated vitamin D is needed to absorb and use calcium, an element that contributes to bone density. When a client is chronically deficient in vitamin D, bones become soft (osteomalacia), bend (rickets), and bone pain increases.

15. A

    Hair loss is one of the first indicators of a zinc deficiency.

16. B, C, F

    Clients are more likely to eat when they enjoy the experience and have some control over the process. Clients are encouraged to feed themselves whenever it is possible and to eat food that they like. Wearing prescribed glasses and hearing aids increase sensory perception, which can help hold the client's interest in eating. Having the client up in a chair for meals, rather than in bed, improves movement through the GI tract, reduces the risk for aspiration, and helps keep the client awake. Clients are more likely to eat if they are not in pain. Giving prescribed pain medication an hour to 30 minutes before meals can increase the comfort. The family is instructed to let the client eat at her own pace. Hurrying the client can result in an increased risk for aspiration, as well as make the experience less pleasant.

17. A, C, D, F

    As long as the stomach and lower GI system are functioning, clients can receive TEN to provide all or part of their nutritional needs regardless of their level of consciousness, if they are unable to meet these needs by eating (clients in

options C and F). The client with an intestinal blockage should be NPO and may require parenteral nutrition. The client who has no teeth or dentures can use liquids, semisolids, soft foods, and chopped or minced foods that require no chewing. The client with lung cancer and cachexia can receive TEN if he or she chooses to do so.

18. D

    If the position of the NG tube is in doubt or questionable, remove the tube. The fact that the client is continuously coughing is an indication that the tube may no longer be in the esophagus. Although a chest x-ray could establish tube placement, removal is warranted to prevent respiratory distress.

19. A, C, D, E

    Residual volume must be assessed at least every 6 hours to prevent reflux and aspiration, as well as other complications. Keeping the head of the bed elevated to at least 30 degrees also helps prevent reflux and aspiration. Clean technique is required to prevent GI infection, as is discarding any unused enteral products that have been open for 24 hours. The feeding bag and tubing are changed every 24 to 48 hours as needed and in accordance with agency policy. Warming of the enteral product is not required or recommended.

20. D

    Refeeding syndrome is a life-threatening complication of aggressive enteral feeding in a severely malnourished client that is caused by fluid and electrolyte shifts. This condition can lead to heart failure, muscle breakdown, seizures, and hemolysis. Main electrolyte imbalances are hypokalemia and hypophosphatemia. The hypokalemia causes shallow respiration, as does heart failure. Bleeding around the IV site can be caused by the accompanying hemolysis and poor clotting.

21. C

    The presence of insulin in the TPN solution activates the sodium-potassium ATPase pump on cell membranes and moves potassium from the extracellular fluid across the membranes into the cells, resulting in hypokalemia. Because the potassium is not present in the blood in high concentrations, any movement out of the blood can result in hypokalemia and serious physiologic changes.

22. B
The TPN infusion line cannot be capped and must remain patent. The nurse infuses a 10% glucose infusion to keep the line open and prevent changes in blood glucose levels.

23. C
Waist circumference (WC) is a strong predictor of coronary artery disease (CAD), and WC greater than 35 inches (89 cm) in women and greater than 40 inches (102 cm) in men indicates central obesity. A waist-to-hip ratio (WHR) of 0.95 or greater in men (0.8 or greater in women) indicates android obesity with excess fat at the waist and abdomen, which is also a strong predictor of CAD. Rheumatoid arthritis symptoms are made worse by obesity but are not caused by it. Type 2 diabetes is associated with obesity but type 1 is not. Chronic kidney disease is not directly related to obesity.

24. A
Orlistat inhibits lipase so that fats are only partially digested and absorbed. The nondigested fats and many fat-soluble nutrients are eliminated in the stool, potentially leading to vitamin deficiency.

25. B
Although all the listed assessments are important, airway management is the priority in the immediate postoperative period after bariatric surgery. Obese clients often have short, thick necks and compromised airways. These clients are more likely to need mechanical ventilation or other types of respiratory support to ensure adequate gas exchange.

26. D
These assessment findings strongly suggest an anastamotic leak, which is an emergency and can lead to peritonitis, sepsis, and death.

27. A, B, C, D, E
With the exception of maintaining the client on bedrest for 24 to 48 hours, all of the above actions are recommended as best practices to prevent the many potential complications associated with bariatric surgeries.

28. D
Dumping syndrome occurs when food enters the small intestine rather than the stomach after gastric bypass surgery, which results in increased blood flow to that site with decreased blood flow elsewhere. This causes hypotension and tachycardia from reduced central circulation and increased intestinal peristalsis with abdominal cramping and diarrhea from the stimulation caused by the sudden expansion of the intestinal lumen.

56
CHAPTER

Assessment of the Endocrine System

1. Which statements regarding endocrine function and hormones are correct? **Select all that apply**.
   A. All tissues and organs are affected by the endocrine system.
   B. Every hormone requires a receptor to modify the activities of its target tissue.
   C. Control over hormone secretion occurs through positive feedback mechanisms.
   D. Endocrine glands must be directly connected to their target tissues for efficient function.
   E. A tropic hormone from one endocrine gland has another endocrine gland as its target tissue.
   F. The body system that works most closely with the endocrine system to maintain homeostasis is the nervous system.

2. What is the expected **first** outcome of a hormone binding correctly to the receptor of its target tissue?
   A. Increased secretion of the hormone bound to the target tissue
   B. Decreased secretion of the hormone bound to the target tissue
   C. Increased specific function of the target tissue
   D. Decreased specific function of the target tissue

3. Which hormone levels will the nurse expect to be deficient in a client who has undergone removal of the posterior pituitary gland?
   A. Insulin and glucagon
   B. Oxytocin and vasopressin
   C. Estrogen and testosterone
   D. Growth hormone and somatomedins

4. Which change in appearance would the nurse expect to find in a client who has excessive production of melanocyte-stimulating hormone (MSH)?
   A. Acne
   B. Obesity
   C. Skin darkening
   D. Protruding eyes

5. Which hormone changes does the nurse expect when a client receives a continuous cortisol infusion for 24 hours when his or her endocrine feedback mechanisms are functioning normally?
   A. Lower than normal adrenocorticotropic hormone (ACTH) levels; lower than normal corticotropin-releasing hormone (CRH) levels
   B. Lower than normal adrenocorticotropic hormone (ACTH) levels; higher than normal corticotropin-releasing hormone (CRH) levels
   C. Higher than normal adrenocorticotropic hormone (ACTH) levels; lower than normal corticotropin-releasing hormone (CRH) levels
   D. Higher than normal adrenocorticotropic hormone (ACTH) levels; higher than normal corticotropin-releasing hormone (CRH) levels

6. Decreases of which hormone level does the nurse suspect may be responsible for a client's reduced catecholamine levels and decreased cardiac muscle excitability?
   A. Insulin
   B. Oxytocin
   C. Cortisol
   D. Glucagon

7. What effect on circulating levels of sodium and glucose does the nurse expect in a client who has been taking an oral cortisol preparation for 2 years because of a respiratory problem?
   A. Decreased sodium; decreased glucose
   B. Decreased sodium; increased glucose
   C. Increased sodium; decreased glucose
   D. Increased sodium; increased glucose

8. Which problems does the nurse expect in an older adult as a result of age-related changes in endocrine function? **Select all that apply**.
   A. Increased basal metabolic rate (BMR)
   B. Decreased core body temperature
   C. Dehydration
   D. Diarrhea
   E. Hyperglycemia
   F. Polyuria

9. Which client conditions will the nurse expect to stimulate the renin-angiotensin-aldosterone system (RAAS)? **Select all that apply**.
   A. Hypertension
   B. Hyperglycemia
   C. Hypokalemia
   D. Dehydration
   E. Hypoxemia
   F. Alkalemia

10. Which assessments are **most important** for the nurse to perform on an older client whose vasopressin levels are lower than normal?
    A. Vision and hearing
    B. Respiratory rate and depth
    C. Fasting blood glucose levels
    D. Skin turgor and urine output

11. Which client assessment finding indicates to the nurse the need to assess further for a possible endocrine problem?
    A. Has taken oral contraceptives for more than 2 years
    B. Has lost 15 lb in the last 6 weeks without dieting
    C. Now needs to wear corrective lenses
    D. Father has prostate cancer

12. Which food selections will the nurse, in collaboration with a registered dietitian nutritionist, teach a client who has a lower-than-normal level of thyroid hormones to increase in the diet? **Select all that apply**.
    A. Berries
    B. Cheese
    C. Protein
    D. Seafood
    E. Iodized salt
    F. Leafy green vegetables

13. Which serum electrolyte will the nurse need to monitor **most** closely after a client has surgery for total removal of the thyroid gland?
    A. Calcium
    B. Sodium
    C. Potassium
    D. Chloride

14. Which tissues or organs does the nurse expect will be evaluated in a male client who begins to have fluid secretion from the breast? **Select all that apply**.
    A. Testes
    B. Posterior pituitary
    C. Adrenal medulla
    D. Hypothalamus
    E. Parathyroid
    F. Anterior pituitary

15. Which actions will the nurse suggest to an older client to **prevent harm** as a result of decreased estrogen levels? **Select all that apply**.
    A. Use a skin moisturizer daily.
    B. Drink at least 2 L of water daily.
    C. Increase your intake of calcium and vitamin D.
    D. Walk a mile a day at least four times per week.
    E. Be sure to urinate immediately after sexual intercourse.
    F. Wear socks and gloves when going outside in cool weather.
    G. Weigh yourself daily at the same time and wearing the same amount of clothing.

16. What action does the nurse **avoid to prevent harm** when caring for a client with an enlarged thyroid gland who has indications of hyperthyroidism?
    A. Measuring blood pressure in either arm
    B. Urging the client to increase fluid intake
    C. Using excessive amounts of adhesive tape
    D. Touching or palpating the front of the neck

17. Which precaution or action is **most important** for the nurse to teach the client who is to collect a 24-hour urine specimen for endocrine testing?
    A. Eat a normal diet during the collection period.
    B. Wear gloves when you urinate to prevent contamination of the specimen.
    C. Urinate at the end of 24 hours and add that sample to the collection container.
    D. Avoid walking, running, dancing, or any vigorous exercise during the collection period.

18. For which suspected client condition will the nurse expect a needle biopsy of the thyroid gland to be performed in addition to imaging assessment?
    A. Hyperthyroidism
    B. Thyroid cancer
    C. Hypothermia
    D. Malnutrition

Chapter 56 Answer Key

1. A, B, E, F
   The endocrine system works closely with the nervous system for physiologic regulation to maintain homeostasis. Every tissue and organ is affected by the endocrine system and each hormone recognizes its specific target tissue(s) by the presence of a membrane or intracellular receptor. The target tissue of a tropic hormone is another endocrine gland.
   Endocrine glands are not directly connected to their target tissues; they are ductless with hormones being secreted into the blood.
   Control over hormone synthesis and release occurs through negative feedback mechanisms in which a change in function occurs to stimulate the release of a hormone that will cause an action that is opposite to the change.

2. C
   Correct binding of a hormone to its specific target tissue receptors first changes the activity of the target tissue by increasing its action. Over time, the increased target tissue activity indicates a decreased need for the hormone and will result in a decreased secretion of the hormone.

3. B
   The posterior pituitary gland secretes oxytocin and vasopressin. These hormone levels would be decreased in a client who no longer had a functioning posterior pituitary gland. Growth hormone is secreted by the anterior pituitary gland as are the tropic hormones that control the secretion of estrogen and testosterone. Insulin and glucagon are secreted by islet cells in the pancreas and are unaffected by loss of posterior pituitary function.

4. C
   MSH activates melanocytes to increase production of melanin, a pigment that darkens skin.

5. **A**
The release of CRH and ACTH is affected by the serum level of free cortisol acting through a negative feedback loop. The stimulus for release of CRH from the hypothalamus, which is responsible for stimulating the release of ACTH from the anterior pituitary gland, is a low blood level of cortisol. A continuous infusion of cortisol for 24 hours would be sensed by the hypothalamus as either adequate or elevated levels of cortisol, not low blood levels of cortisol. As a result, little if any CRH would be released from the hypothalamus and circulating levels would be lower than normal. With low levels of CRH, the anterior pituitary cells are not stimulated to release ACTH, thus circulating levels of this hormone would also be lower than normal. Adequate or elevated blood levels of cortisol *inhibit* the release of CRH and ACTH.

6. **C**
Cortisol must be present for catecholamine (epinephrine, norepinephrine [NE]) action and maintaining the normal excitability of the heart muscle cells. These are not the actions of insulin, oxytocin, or glucagon.

7. **D**
Cortisol is a glucocorticoid and has some mineralocorticoid activity that increases the reabsorption of sodium from the kidney tubules, which increases the serum sodium level. Cortisol also increases liver production of glucose (gluconeogenesis) and inhibits peripheral glucose uptake by the cells. Both these actions increase blood glucose levels.

8. **B, C, E, F**
The aging process generally causes a decline in the secretion of hormones from endocrine glands, especially those of the thyroid, pancreas, and adrenal glands. Decreased thyroid hormone secretion causes a decrease in overall metabolism and basal metabolic rate. The slower metabolism results in lower core body temperatures and constipation.

Decreased adrenal gland secretion limits the ability of the older adult to reabsorb water and sodium or to concentrate urine. This condition increases the risk for dehydration.

The decreased secretion of insulin from the pancreas and the decline in metabolism both result in hyperglycemia. When hyperglycemia is present, the osmolarity (osmolality) of the blood increases, causing the adult to have increased thirst and to move interstitial and intracellular fluids into the plasma volume, leading to polyuria.

9. **D, E**
Renin is produced by specialized cells of the kidney arterioles. Its release is triggered by a decrease in extracellular fluid volume from blood loss, sodium loss, or posture changes, and by hypoxemia. Renin converts renin substrate (angiotensinogen), a plasma protein, to angiotensin I. Angiotensin I is converted by an enzyme to form angiotensin II, the active form of angiotensin. In turn, angiotensin II stimulates the secretion of aldosterone. This system, although it cannot directly correct hypoxemia, causes the kidney to reabsorb sodium and water to bring the plasma volume and osmolarity back to normal and increase perfusion.

10. **D**
Vasopressin is antidiuretic hormone (ADH) and promotes reabsorption of water. Lower than normal levels of ADH result in increased urine output leading to dehydration.

11. **B**
An unintentional weight loss in excess of 5 lbs is significant. It may indicate an increase in metabolic rate or a problem with excessive fluid loss, either of which could be associated with an endocrine disorder.

12. **B, C, D, E**
Production of thyroid hormones requires a diet containing adequate amounts of protein (for the amino acid tyrosine) and iodide or iodine. Good food sources of protein include meat, fish, and dairy products. Dairy products and saltwater fish and seafood also contain iodine. Berries and leafy green vegetables contain very little protein or iodine/iodide.

13. A

The thyroid gland helps regulate serum calcium levels through the actions of thyrocalcitonin (TCT or calcitonin). Total removal of the thyroid gland disrupts this regulation. If the parathyroid glands are either damaged or removed along with the thyroid gland, parathyroid hormone production is also lost, resulting in even less regulation of serum calcium levels.

14. D, F

Breast fluid/milk production is induced by the presence of prolactin, secreted from the anterior pituitary gland. The hypothalamus regulates secretion of prolactin through the activity of prolactin-inhibiting hormone. A problem in either the hypothalamus or the anterior pituitary gland can cause lactation in men or women (without being pregnant or giving birth).

15. A, B, C, D, E

Decreased estrogen levels increase bone density loss, make skin drier and thinner, and increase the risk for cystitis. Weight-bearing activity and increasing intake of calcium and vitamin D can help slow this problem. Using skin moisturizer reduces dryness. Drinking at least 2 L of water daily and urinating immediately after intercourse help prevent cystitis.

Wearing socks and gloves in cool weather does not prevent harm associated with decreased estrogen levels and neither does obtaining daily weights.

16. D

If an enlarged thyroid gland is handled or palpated in a client with hyperthyroidism, large amounts of thyroid hormones could be released into the blood stream, leading to "thyroid storm" with exaggerated and severe symptoms of hyperthyroidism that are life-threatening. None of the other actions are likely to cause harm to a client with hyperthyroidism.

17. C

When a 24-hour urine specimen is started, the specimen should reflect all the urine produced during the specified time. The very first voiding is discarded because the urine has spent some time in the bladder and will not reflect what is happening during the actual 24 hours of the collection. The time of this discard is the beginning of the 24-hour collection period. The test requires that all urine voided after the start time be collected, including the specimen collected by emptying the bladder at end of the 24 hours, which marks the end of the test.

18. B

Needle biopsy of the thyroid (and many other glands) is performed after other types of assessment when the client is suspect to have cancer originating in that gland and surgery most likely will be needed.

Concepts of Care for Patients with Pituitary and Adrenal Gland Problems

1. Why is a deficiency in the production of the anterior pituitary hormone adrenocorticotropin hormone (ACTH) life threatening?
   A. Reduces sexual maturation leading to untreatable sterility
   B. Inhibits adrenal production of cortisol, which is necessary for life
   C. Reduces excretion of extracellular fluid leading to fluid overload and heart failure
   D. Lack of reabsorption of sodium and potassium leads to serious fluid and electrolyte imbalances

2. Which side effect will the nurse teach a male client receiving androgen therapy to expect?
   A. Increased testicular size
   B. Loss of body hair
   C. Gynecomastia
   D. Weight gain

3. Which statement made by a female client receiving hormone replacement therapy with estrogen and progesterone for anterior pituitary hypofunction indicates to the nurse correct understanding of the drug therapy?
   A. "I will switch to vaping instead of smoking cigarettes."
   B. "Reducing my use of hot showers and baths may help my dry skin."
   C. "If my breast sizes increase, I will report it to my primary health care provider."
   D. "I will report any leg pain or swelling immediately to my primary health care provider."

4. Which disorders will the nurse expect that a client with an abnormally functioning posterior pituitary gland could possibly have? **Select all that apply**.
   A. Hypothyroidism
   B. Bone density loss
   C. Growth retardation
   D. Diabetes insipidus (DI)
   E. Excessive virilization
   F. Syndrome of inappropriate antidiuretic hormone (SIADH)

5. What is the nurse's **best** response to a male client with a prolactinoma tumor of the anterior pituitary gland when he asks why he has not been able to achieve an erection?
   A. "The high levels of prolactin suppress release of your normal sex hormones."
   B. "You are probably embarrassed by the fact that fluid is coming from your nipples."
   C. "Don't worry. This problem is temporary and will most likely resolve after treatment."
   D. "Most men who are told they have a brain tumor experience psychological impotence."

6. Which assessment findings will the nurse expect to see in a 30-year-old client who has just been diagnosed with acromegaly? **Select all that apply**.
   A. Thickened lips
   B. Near-sightedness
   C. Hyperglycemia
   D. Hyponatremia
   E. Extremely long arms and legs
   F. Protruding lower jaw

7. A client who has been receiving bromocriptine therapy for 1 month to manage hyperpituitarism now has all of the following symptoms or changes. Which ones will the nurse report to the primary health care provider immediately to **prevent harm? Select all that apply**.
   A. Nausea
   B. Possible pregnancy
   C. Headaches
   D. Irregular heart beat
   E. Taste changes
   F. Watery nasal discharge

8. Which postoperative actions are appropriate for the nurse to take when caring for a client who is recovering from a transsphenoidal hypophysectomy? **Select all that apply**.
   A. Monitoring fluid and electrolyte balance closely
   B. Instructing the client how to perform incision care
   C. Performing neurologic checks hourly for first 24 hours
   D. Urging the client to cough vigorously every 2 hours while awake
   E. Encouraging the client to perform hourly deep-breathing exercises
   F. Instructing the client to use a soft-bristled toothbrush for oral hygiene

9. Which additional assessment is a **priority** for the nurse to perform on a client who develops a fever of 102°F (38.9°C) the day after a transsphenoidal hypophysectomy?
   A. Listening to breath sounds
   B. Checking pupillary responses
   C. Checking neck range of motion
   D. Asking about pain and burning on urination

10. Which hormone deficiency does the nurse associate with a client who has diabetes insipidus?
    A. Insulin
    B. Aldosterone
    C. Antidiuretic hormone
    D. Adrenocorticotropic hormone

11. Which assessment finding is **most important** for the nurse to report in a client with diabetes insipidus (DI)?
    A. Poor skin turgor
    B. Respirations of 26 beats/min
    C. Blood pressure of 130/80 mm Hg
    D. Potassium level of 4.8 mEq/L (mmol/L)

12. Which urine characteristics indicate to the nurse that a client being managed for diabetes insipidus requires another dose of desmopressin?
    A. Urine output volume increased; urine specific gravity increased
    B. Urine output volume increased; urine specific gravity decreased
    C. Urine output volume decreased; urine specific gravity increased
    D. Urine output volume decreased; urine specific gravity decreased

13. Which action will the nurse instruct assistive personnel (AP) to **avoid** when caring for a client with diabetes insipidus (DI) to **prevent harm**?
    A. Restricting fluids
    B. Taking blood pressures
    C. Urging the client to cough
    D. Allowing the client to sit with knees bent

14. Which client will the nurse recognize as being at increased risk for development of syndrome of inappropriate antidiuretic hormone (SIADH)?
    A. 27-year-old on high-dose steroids
    B. 47-year-old with acute renal failure
    C. 58-year-old with small cell lung cancer
    D. 60-year-old who had a myocardial infarction last year

15. Which changes in laboratory values will the nurse expect in a client who has untreated syndrome of inappropriate antidiuretic hormone (SIADH)? **Select all that apply**.
    A. Increased urine sodium
    B. Serum potassium 2.9 mEq/mL (mmol/L)
    C. Urine specific gravity 1.053
    D. Serum osmolarity 250 mOsm/L
    E. Increased hematocrit
    F. Serum sodium 119 mEq/mL (mmol/L)

16. Which change in laboratory values indicates to the nurse that the fluid restriction ordered for a client with syndrome of inappropriate antidiuretic hormone (SIADH) is having the desired effect?
    A. Decreased hematocrit
    B. Increased serum sodium
    C. Decreased serum osmolarity
    D. Increased urine specific gravity

17. Which action will the nurse take to **prevent harm** related to syndrome of inappropriate antidiuretic hormone (SIADH) when a client with the disorder is receiving feedings through a nasogatric (NG) tube?
    A. Turning off NG suction for an hour after feedings
    B. Using tape sparingly when anchoring the NG tube
    C. Removing the tube as soon as bowel sounds are present
    D. Using normal saline instead of water as the irrigation fluid

18. Which serum laboratory value in a client receiving conivaptin therapy for syndrome of inappropriate antidiuretic hormone (SIADH) will the nurse report **immediately** to the primary health care provider to **prevent harm**?
    A. Sodium 148 mEq/L (mmol/L)
    B. Potassium 3.2 mEq/L (mmol/L)
    C. Glucose 204 mg/mL (11.4 mmol/L)
    D. Arterial pH of 7.42

19. Which client will the nurse recognize as having a **high** risk for developing secondary adrenal insufficiency?
    A. 25-year-old using oral contraceptives
    B. 35-year-old with diabetes insipidus
    C. 45-year-old who suddenly stops taking high-dose corticosteroid therapy
    D. 55-year-old with an adrenal tumor causing excessive secretion of cortisol

20. Which action will the nurse instruct assistive personnel to perform to **prevent harm** for a client who has adrenal insufficiency?
    A. Padding the side rails of the client's bed
    B. Assisting the client to change positions slowly
    C. Using a lift sheet when repositioning the client
    D. Placing suctioning equipment at the client's bedside

21. Which change in a client's condition indicates to the nurse that corticosteroid therapy for the client in acute adrenal crisis is effective?
    A. Urine output is increased.
    B. Pitting edema has resolved.
    C. Client is alert and oriented.
    D. Blood glucose level is 60 mg/dL (3.3 mmol/L)

22. Which diuretic will the nurse expect to be prescribed by the primary health care provider to manage a client who has hyperaldosteronism?
    A. Mannitol
    B. Furosemide
    C. Spironolactone
    D. Ethacrynic acid

23. Which physical assessment findings will the nurse expect in a client with long-term Cushing disease? **Select all that apply**.
    A. "Moon-face"
    B. Body hair loss
    C. Truncal obesity
    D. Prominent lower jaw
    E. Thin, easily damaged skin
    F. Extremity muscle wasting

24. What is the nurse's **best** response when a client who is about to have a unilateral adrenalectomy for an adenoma that is causing hypercortisolism asks if she will have to continue the severe sodium restriction after surgery?
    A. "No, once the tumor has been removed and your cortisol levels have normalized, you will not retain excess sodium anymore."
    B. "No, after surgery you will have to take oral cortisol, which can easily be controlled so that your sodium levels do not rise."
    C. Yes, the fact that you are retaining sodium and have high blood pressure is related to your age and lifestyle, not the tumor."
    D. "Yes, sodium is very bad for people and everyone needs to eliminate sodium completely from their diets for the rest of their lives."

25. For which complications will the nurse assess, when planning prevention strategies with other interprofessional team members for client with hypercortisolism?
    A. Anorexia, constipation, hypotension
    B. Kidney stones, weight loss, cataracts
    C. Skin breakdown, infection, GI ulceration
    D. Diabetes insipidus, bradycardia, arthritis

26. Which action is **most appropriate** for the nurse to take in the preoperative holding area when a client who is scheduled to have an adrenalectomy for hypercortisolism is prescribed to receive cortisol by intravenous infusion?
    A. Requesting a "time-out" to determine whether this is a valid prescription
    B. Asking the client whether he or she usually takes prednisone
    C. Holding the dose because the client has a high cortisol level
    D. Administering the drug as prescribed

27. Which action taken by the nurse is **most likely** to reduce skin complications in a client who has hypercortisolism?
    A. Using roller gauze to anchor an IV
    B. Massaging the client's feet and calves
    C. Applying pressure after IM injections
    D. Applying dressings to areas with striae

28. Which precaution is **most important** for the nurse to teach to **prevent harm** in a client prescribed oral corticosteroids for hormone replacement therapy after a bilateral adrenalectomy?
    A. "Do not stop taking this drug without consulting your primary health care provider."
    B. "Avoid crowds and people who are ill."
    C. "Be sure to take this drug with food."
    D. "Reduce your salt intake."

29. What is the nurse's **best** response when a client who must continue to take a corticosteroid asks why an H_2 histamine blocker has been prescribed?
    A. "The drug therapy increases the development of allergies."
    B. "Corticosteroids are associated with an increased risk for gastric ulcers."
    C. "When taken together, the H_2 histamine blocker improves the absorption of the corticosteroid."
    D. "The H_2 histamine blocker counteracts the increased appetite stimulated by the corticosteroid."

Chapter 57 Answer Key

1. B
Deficiencies of adrenocorticotropic hormone (ACTH) or thyroid-stimulating hormone (TSH) are the most life threatening because they cause a decrease in the secretion of vital hormones from the adrenal and thyroid glands. Cortisol from the adrenal cortex is necessary for life by regulating the body's response to stress; carbohydrate, protein, and fat metabolism; emotional stability; immune function; sodium and water balance; and influencing other important body processes. For example, it must be present for epinephrine and norepinephrine action and maintaining the normal excitability of the heart muscle cells.

2. C
Side effects of androgen therapy include male breast development (gynecomastia), acne, baldness, and prostate enlargement. Although penile size increases with androgen therapy, testicular size usually decreases as a result of elevated blood androgen levels suppressing the release of gonadotropins from the hypothalamus because of negative feedback.

3. D
The use of exogenous estrogen and progesterone increases the risk for thrombus and emboli formation. This risk is even greater for women who use nicotine in any form (even vaping). Persistent leg pain and swelling without trauma are an indication of deep vein thrombosis in the extremity. Breast size increases are an expected side effect of this hormone replacement therapy. Exogenous estrogen and progesterone therapy are more likely to promote adequate skin oil production rather than dry skin.

4. D, F
The major hormone secreted on a daily basis by a normally functioning posterior pituitary gland is antidiuretic hormone (ADH, vasopressin). (Oxytocin secretion has less effects on day-to-day homeostasis.) Undersecretion of ADH results in DI. Oversecretion of ADH results in SIADH.

5. A
High levels of prolactin secreted by a prolactinoma suppress the release of gonadotropins. With reduced levels of gonadotropins, circulating levels of testosterone are too low to support normal sexual functioning. Although anxiety and embarrassment can lead to impotence, this does not really answer the client's question. Being told not to worry dismisses the client's valid concerns.

6. A, C, F
With acromegaly, the adult client has an over production of growth hormone (GH) that results in gradual enlargement of soft tissues and growth of desmoid bone, resulting in irreversible enlargement of the face, hands, feet, and protrusion of the lower jaw. Skeletal bones thicken but do not grow longer, and organs such as the liver and heart enlarge. The client also experiences breakdown of joint cartilage; and hypertrophy of ligaments, vocal cords, lips, and eustachian tubes are common. Hyperglycemia is common. Visual changes and electrolyte disturbances are not associated with acromegaly.

7. B, D, F
Bromocriptine can cause serious cardiac dysrhythmias, coronary artery spasms, and cerebrospinal fluid leakage. It is also contraindicated during pregnancy. Constipation, increased sleepiness, headaches, and nausea are possible side effects of the drug and their degree of discomfort to the client should always be considered; however, their presence does not constitute harm or require immediate attention. Change in taste sensation may or may not be related to bromocriptine therapy and is not considered a problem requiring further investigation.

8. A, C, E
A hypophysectomy removes all pituitary tissue and results in deficiency of all pituitary hormones, including antidiuretic hormone, which can lead to profound disturbances of fluid and electrolyte balance. Although limited in scope, a hypophysectomy can cause brain swelling

that leads to neurologic problems. This requires the performance of neurologic checks hourly for the first 24 hours. The client needs to avoid activity that could increase intracranial pressure, such as coughing, but still needs to prevent postoperative atelectasis by performing deep-breathing exercises hourly. With a transsphenoidal approach, the incision can be injured from inside the oral cavity. Thus, using any type of toothbrush is avoided until healing is complete.

9. C
Nuchal rigidity is a major indication of meningitis, a potential postoperative complication associated with this surgery. Meningitis is an infection and usually the client will also have a fever. Although a fever could indicate a respiratory or urinary tract infection and these must be ruled out, meningitis is more serious. Checking pupillary responses is not as critical as determining the presence or absence of nuchal rigidity and would not be performed first.

10. C
DI is caused by either the decreased production of antidiuretic hormone or the inability of the kidney tubules to respond to its presence. Deficiencies of insulin, aldosterone, and adrenocorticotropic hormone are not a cause of DI.

11. A
Clients with DI are at great risk for dehydration. Poor skin turgor is an indication of dehydration. Respiratory rate is slightly elevated, but is not a cause for concern. The blood pressure is at the upper limits of normal, but also is not a cause for concern. The potassium level is within normal limits.

12. B
Diabetes insipidus (DI) occurs with reduced or absent secretion of vasopressin (ADH). As a result, water is excessively excreted, causing a decrease in blood volume and an increase in urine volume. Blood is concentrated indicating dehydration and urine is very dilute, as measured by specific gravity, which is very low. When drug therapy with synthetic vasopressin

(desmopressin) is effective, the client increases water reabsorption so that urine output volume decreases at the same time that urine concentration increases, seen as an increased urine specific gravity. When urine volume increases and urine concentration decreases, another drug dose is needed to prevent hypovolemia and dehydration.

13. A
Restricting fluids in a client with DI greatly increases the risk for life-threatening dehydration. Clients are encouraged to take in as much fluid as they feel is necessary to satisfy thirst and prevent dehydration. Taking blood pressures, coughing, and sitting with the knees bent are not specifically harmful to the client with DI.

14. C
SIADH is more common among clients who have any type of continuing respiratory problem, especially lung cancer being managed with chemotherapy. None of the other health problems listed increase the risk for SIADH.

15. A, B, C, F
In SIADH, the kidney tubules reabsorb water and return it to the vascular volume leading to hypervolemia and dilution of all blood components. Urine output decreases and urine concentration increases, especially with sodium.

16. B
Increased serum sodium due to fluid restriction indicates effective therapy. Restricting fluid would result in increasing hematocrit levels as the fluid volume excess resolves. Plasma osmolality is decreased as a result of SIADH, so treatment would result in this level rising to near normal. Urine specific gravity is increased with SIADH and would decrease to near normal with treatment.

17. D
Preventing harm for a client with syndrome of inappropriate antidiuretic hormone (SIADH) involves avoiding care that could further dilute the electrolyte concentrations. By using normal

saline for NG irrigations instead of water, the risk for further dilution is reduced. The other actions relate to general NG issues.

18. A

The therapeutic effect of the vaptans, including conivaptan, is to induce water loss without an accompanying loss of sodium to bring the serum sodium level back to normal. A serum sodium level of 148 mEq/L (mmol/L) represents hypernatremia, which could have serious consequences and requires immediate action. The potassium is a little low but does not require immediate action. The pH is normal and the glucose level is high but not dangerously so.

19. C

The most common cause of secondary adrenal insufficiency is discontinuing higher dose corticosteroid therapy without an appropriate tapering down period to allow atrophied adrenal tissues to restart secretion of endogenous corticosteroids. None of the other conditions trigger adrenal insufficiency.

20. B

Adrenocortical insufficiency causes severe orthostatic (postural) hypotension, greatly increasing the client's risk for falls. Assisting the client to change positions slowly can help reduce the degree of blood pressure drop during position changes and reduce the risk for falls. The client has no need for padded side rails and does not have an increased risk for fractures. Although the client who has adrenal insufficiency may have a lower-than-normal serum sodium level, this level does not drop to the level that the client is at risk for seizure activity.

21. C

Clients with acute adrenal insufficiency are hypotensive and dehydrated with hypoglycemia, hyponatremia, and hyperkalemia. Their level of consciousness is altered to the point of lethargy and confusion. Edema is not present and urine output can be excessive. A major indication of drug therapy effectiveness is a return to an alert and oriented level of consciousness.

22. C

Aldosterone enhances the reabsorption of water and sodium, along with excretion of potassium. Clients with hyperaldosteronism have fluid overload, hyponatremia, and hypokalemia. Correction of these imbalances requires a diuretic, such as spironolactone, that increases sodium and water excretion and conserves potassium. Mannitol is an osmotic diuretic that promotes only water excretion. Furosemide and ethacrynic acid promote sodium and potassium loss along with water loss.

23. A, C, E, F

Common physical changes in a client who has had Cushing disease for more than a few months include fat redistribution that results in a moon-face and truncal obesity. The skin becomes thinner and more fragile. Skeletal muscles decrease in size and strength, especially in the extremities. Body hair is increased, not decreased and the jaw does not change thickness or position.

24. A

A tumor secreting excessive amounts of cortisol is this client's reason for needing to severely restrict her sodium. Once the tumor is removed, she will not have hypercortisolism but may have to take oral cortisol until the remaining adrenal gland begins to secrete sufficient cortisol. She will no longer experience severe sodium retention.

25. C

Under the influence of excessive amounts of cortisol, skin becomes thinner, prone to striations, and has decreased cell division. Although the white blood cell count may be high, the activity of the leukocytes (especially lymphocytes) is decreased and the client is immunosuppressed. The cortisol increases the risk for GI ulceration in many ways, including stimulating increased secretion of hydrochloric acid and thinning the protective mucus layer in the stomach.

26. D

Although the client has hypercortisolism, removal of the adrenal gland will stop the secretion of this important hormone that is essential for life. Further, the stress of surgery also increases the client's need for this hormone. Supplying the hormone throughout surgery prevents the complication (or at least reduces the risk) for acute adrenal crisis.

27. A

The client's skin is thin and easily injured. Once injured, the skin is slow to heal. When tape is needed, its use directly on the skin is minimized. Using roller gauze in place of tape helps to protect the client's skin. Massaging calves can promote embolization of a clot and is not recommended for any client. Applying pressure after IM injections can help reduce bleeding but does not prevent skin injury. Striae do not require dressings and their application can increase skin injury.

28. A

All of the choices are precautions that the nurse will teach the client taking an oral corticosteroid chronically. However, the most critical precaution is to not stop taking this drug because chronic corticosteroid use causes atrophy of the adrenal glands. With adrenal gland atrophy, the client no longer makes his or her own normal levels of corticosteroids, which are essential for life. Long-term steroid use is never suddenly stopped.

29. B

Corticosteroids increase the risk for gastric ulcer formation by stimulating increased production of stomach acids and thinning the stomach lining. H_2 histamine blockers reduce this risk by inhibiting the release of gastric acids. This drug category is not used for allergy prevention and does not suppress appetite. Combination therapy does not increase absorption of the corticosteroid.

58 CHAPTER

Concepts of Care for Patients with Problems of the Thyroid and Parathyroid Glands

1. Which statements regarding hypothyroidism are accurate? **Select all that apply**.
   A. Has a sudden onset of symptoms
   B. Can be diagnosed by the presence of a goiter
   C. Reduces cardiac and central nervous system function
   D. Often occurs weeks after a bacterial or viral infection
   E. Is much more common among women than among men
   F. Most common form has an autosomal dominant pattern of inheritance

2. Which history information provided by a client with hypothyroidism will the nurse consider as a possible cause of the disorder?
   A. Egg and peanut allergy
   B. Previous thyroid radiation
   C. Mother with Graves disease
   D. Has been pregnant three times in the past 4 years

3. Which symptoms will the nurse expect to find on assessment of a client with hypothyroidism? **Select all that apply**.
   A. Increased appetite
   B. Cold intolerance
   C. Constipation
   D. Hypotension
   E. Exophthalmia
   F. Palpitations
   G. Tremors
   H. Weight gain

4. Which laboratory values does the nurse specifically expect to find in a client who has primary hypothyroidism?
   A. Total serum T4 1 mcg/dL (22 nmol/L)
   B. Thyrotropin receptor antibodies (TRAbs) 0%
   C. Thyroid-stimulating hormone (TSH) 8 mU/mL
   D. White blood cell (WBC) count 6200/mm³ (6.2 × 10⁹/L)

5. Which precaution has the **highest priority** for the nurse to teach a client starting thyroid hormone replacement therapy (HRT) to **prevent harm**?
   A. "Take the drug at the same time every day."
   B. "Avoid caffeinated beverages and foods."
   C. "Take the drug exactly as prescribed."
   D. "Get plenty of sleep and rest."

6. Which condition does the nurse recognize as a life-threatening emergency and serious complication when a client's hypothyroidism is not treated or is undertreated?
   A. Exophthalmos
   B. Myxedema coma
   C. Toxic multinodular goiter
   D. Hashimoto thyroiditis

7. Which laboratory value in a client being managed for hypothyroidism will the nurse report to the primary health care provider **immediately**?
   A. Sodium 125 mEq/L (mmol/L)
   B. Potassium 3.0 mEq/L (mmol/L)
   C. Fasting blood glucose 68 mg/dL
   D. Platelet count of 220,000/mm³ (220 × 10⁹/L)

8. Which assessment findings in a client with myxedema coma indicate to the nurse that therapy is effective? **Select all that apply**.
   A. SpO$_2$ is 89%.
   B. Skin is cool and dry.
   C. Pulse is 62 beats/min.
   D. Blood pressure is 98/60.
   E. Urine output is greater about 10 mL/hr.
   F. Core body temperature is 98.6°F (36.8°C).

9. Which report from a client who has hypothyroidism and is taking synthetic thyroid hormone replacement therapy indicates to the nurse that more teaching is necessary?
   A. "I take the drug at the same time every day."
   B. "I always drink a full glass of water when I take the pill."
   C. "Even though the pill is small, I mix it with pudding to make it easier to swallow."
   D. "Most often, I take the drug as early in the morning as possible to prevent it from keeping me awake at night."

10. Which assessments have the **highest priority** for the nurse to perform on a 76-year-old client who began thyroid hormone replacement therapy (HRT) 2 weeks ago? **Select all that apply**.
    A. Checking for tremors
    B. Measuring blood pressure
    C. Checking oxygen saturation
    D. Asking about sleep patterns
    E. Asking about changes in appetite
    F. Determining the presence or absence of chest pain

11. What is the nurse's **best** response when a client with hypothyroidism asks how long hormone replacement therapy will be needed?
    A. "After your goiter is surgically removed, you should be able to stop HRT."
    B. "HRT will be needed for the rest of your life because hypothyroidism has no cure."
    C. "You will be able to stop HRT as soon as your blood levels of thyroid hormones rise to normal ranges."
    D. "Regardless of when your blood levels of thyroid hormones return to normal, HRT must be continued until all your symptoms subside."

12. The client who has been taking synthetic thyroid hormone replacement therapy (HRT) for 3 months reports all of the following conditions. Which condition indicates to the nurse that the drug dosage may need to be adjusted?
    A. Difficulty sleeping
    B. Increased urine output
    C. Decreased sense of smell
    D. Difficulty remembering to take the drug

13. Which client will the nurse consider to be at highest risk for development of Graves disease?
    A. 25-year-old who has been taking thyroid hormone replacement therapy for 9 years
    B. 35-year-old who has type 1 diabetes mellitus
    C. 45-year-old who eats a vegan diet that includes seaweed
    D. 55-year-old who lives near a uranium-processing plant

14. Which assessment findings that are unique to Graves disease will the nurse expect in a client who has hyperthyroidism?
    A. Goiter
    B. Fine tremors
    C. Protruding eyes
    D. Elevated body temperature
    E. Dry, waxy swelling on shins
    F. Multiple nodules in the thyroid gland

15. In collaboration with the registered dietitian nutritionist, which dietary modifications will the nurse suggest to a client with hyperthyroidism? **Select all that apply**.
    A. Increased salt water fish or seafood
    B. Increased overall calories
    C. Elimination of fatty food
    D. Increased carbohydrates
    E. Increased protein
    F. Fluid restriction

16. Which assessment technique will the nurse **avoid** during the examination of a client with hyperthyroidism to **prevent harm**?
    A. Using an oral thermometer for temperature assessment
    B. Checking hydration status by pinching up the skin
    C. Measuring blood pressure with an external cuff
    D. Palpating the thyroid gland

17. Which new-onset problem is **most important** for the nurse to instruct a client, starting on propylthiouracil as therapy for hyperthyroidism, to notify the primary health care provider immediately?
    A. Insomnia
    B. Ringing in the ears
    C. Heat intolerance
    D. Dark-colored urine

18. Which statement by a client undergoing radioactive iodine (RAI) therapy demonstrates to the nurse that the client has **correct understanding** of postprocedure precautions?
    A. "I will wear a wig until my hair grows back in."
    B. "I will be sure to use only one toilet and not let others use it for 2 weeks."
    C. "I will avoid crowds and people who are ill to reduce the risk for an infection."
    D. "I will avoid having a manicure or pedicure during the first month after treatment."

19. Which assessment finding of a client 10 hours after a subtotal thyroidectomy indicates to the nurse possible airway obstruction?
    A. Client is drooling.
    B. Oxygen saturation is 97%.
    C. Dressing has a moderate amount of serosanguinous drainage.
    D. Client responds to questions correctly but does not open the eyes while talking.

20. Which actions will the nurse take to help prevent strain on the suture line for a client who had a total thyroidectomy for thyroid cancer yesterday? **Select all that apply**.
    A. Keeping the client on total bedrest
    B. Placing a small pillow under the client's head
    C. Maintaining the head of the bed in the flat position
    D. Instructing the client to avoid deep-breathing exercises
    E. Applying an elastic wrap around the neck over the dressing
    F. Instructing the client to place both hands on the back of the neck while moving

21. Which complication does the nurse suspect when a client who had a thyroidectomy 1 day ago now has a weak voice and hoarseness?
    A. Impending hemorrhage
    B. Laryngeal nerve damage
    C. Partial airway obstruction
    D. Irritation from the endotracheal tube

22. Which client does the nurse consider to be at **highest** risk for a change in thyroid function from thyroiditis?
    A. 25-year-old woman who received a tetanus vaccination yesterday
    B. 38-year-old woman taking thyroid hormone replacement therapy
    C. 50-year-old man who sustained a neck injury in a car crash
    D. 61-year-old man who had influenza 3 weeks ago

23. Which laboratory value indicates to the nurse that a client who had a subtotal thyroidectomy for thyroid cancer several months ago may now have a recurrence of the disorder?
    A. Thyrotropin receptor antibody level of 0%
    B. Thyroglobulin level of 120 ng/mL (mcg/L)
    C. Serum calcium level of 10.0 mg/dL (2.37 mmol/L)
    D. Serum triiodothyronine (T3) 70 ng/dL (3.4 nmol/L)

24. For which laboratory value will the nurse immediately assess the reflexes of a client who has hypoparathyroidism?
    A. Sodium 131 mEq/L (mmol/L)
    B. Potassium 5.1 mEq/L (mmol/L)
    C. Calcium 7.8 mg/dL (1.76 mmol/L)
    D. pH 7.33

25. Which substances does the nurse expect to be prescribed for a client who has hypoparathyroidism to manage the symptoms? **Select all that apply**.
    A. Sodium supplement
    B. Calcium supplement
    C. Potassium supplement
    D. Phosphorus supplement
    E. Vitamin C
    F. Vitamin D

26. Which instruction will the nurse give to an assistive personnel (AP) who is providing morning care to a client with severe hypoparathyroidism to **prevent harm**?
    A. Apply a warming blanket.
    B. Offer oral fluids every 2 hours.
    C. Avoid using a firm-bristled toothbrush.
    D. Use a lift sheet when moving the client in bed.

27. With which client will the nurse be aware of an increased risk for hyperparathyroidism?
    A. 28-year-old woman with pregnancy-induced hypertension
    B. 45-year-old man receiving dialysis for end-stage kidney disease
    C. 55-year-old man with moderate heart failure after myocardial infarction
    D. 60-year-old woman on home oxygen therapy for chronic obstructive pulmonary disease

28. Which additional health problems will the nurse expect the client with chronic hyperparathyroidism to be at risk for if management is not effective? **Select all that apply**.
    A. Psychosis
    B. Kidney stones
    C. Thyroid cancer
    D. Bone deformities
    E. Chronic diarrhea
    F. Peptic ulcer disease

Chapter 58 Answer Key

1. C, D, E
   Hypothyroidism slows the metabolism and function of all systems, and the ones that are usually first noticed and can lead to life-threatening complications are the cardiac and central nervous systems. The most common form of the disorder is Hashimoto thyroiditis causing autoimmune destruction of thyroid cells starting several weeks after a bacterial or viral infection. All thyroid problems are five to ten times more common among women than men.

   The onset is slow and insidious. A goiter only indicates a thyroid problem and can occur with both hypothyroidism and hyperthyroidism. The disorder does not follow any particular genetic pattern of inheritance.

2. B
   One of the most common causes of hypothyroidism in North America is having thyroid radiation therapy for hyperthyroidism. Allergies and a family history of Graves disease do not increase hypothyroidism risk and neither does a history of close pregnancies.

3. B, C, D, H
   Hypothyroidism slows metabolism way below normal and weight gain is expected. Appetite is decreased, not increased.

   The client may not generate sufficient heat to maintain core body temperature. The GI system is slowed, resulting in constipation. Cardiac output decreases leading to hypotension.

Exophthalmia is a complication of the Graves form of hyperthyroidism. Palpitations and tremors occur when the central nervous system and the cardiovascular system are over stimulated by hypermetabolism. They are not associated with hypometabolism.

4. C

In primary hypothyroidism in which the thyroid gland cannot produce and secrete thyroid hormones, negative feedback first stimulates the hypothalamus to secrete more thyrotropin-releasing hormone (TRH) that, in turn, stimulates the anterior pituitary gland to secrete high levels of TSH. (The normal level of TSH is 0.3-5 mcg U/mL [0.35 mU/L]). This high level is trying to force unresponsive thyroid tissue cells to secrete thyroid hormones.

5. C

Although changes in dosages may eventually be prescribed, when starting HRT the client must take the drug exactly as prescribed. Taking a lower dose does not improve the hypothyroidism, which has serious consequences on body function. Increasing the dose can lead to dangerous cardiac and central nervous system toxicities.

6. B

General hypothyroidism is characterized by decreased metabolism in every tissue and organ. When poorly treated or untreated, the slow metabolism of hypothyroidism becomes profound with dangerously reduced cardiopulmonary and neurologic functioning, known as myxedema coma, although few affected adults become comatose. The heart muscle becomes flabby with increased chamber size causing decreased cardiac output with decreased perfusion and gas exchange in the brain and other vital organs.

7. A

All listed laboratory findings are low. The client with hypothyroidism is at risk for hypovolemic shock and reduced excitability of cardiac and nerve membranes. The low sodium level greatly increases the risk for shock and dysfunction of the cardiac and nervous systems.

8. C, D, F

An increasing core body temperature is a strong indication that the client's rate of metabolism is increasing in response to appropriate therapy. The SpO_2 is well below normal and an indication of ongoing poor perfusion and gas exchange. Cool dry skin is a characteristic of hypothyroidism, not an indication of improvement. Urine output is acceptable but still low and not a good indicator of therapy effectiveness. Both the pulse and blood pressure are in the lower normal ranges, which would indicate improvement during myxedema coma (both would have been much lower before the start of therapy).

9. C

Thyroid hormones should be taken on an empty stomach, at least 4 hours before or after a meal, because the dose is very small and almost any other substances interfere with its absorption. Drinking a full glass of water with the drug can help its absorption.

10. A, F

Although all the above-listed changes in client conditions can indicate whether HRT is effective, the most important parameters to assess are checking for tremors and chest pain because the therapy can induce a hyperthyroid state with cardiac and central nervous system toxicities, especially among older clients.

11. B

There is no cure for hypothyroidism and these hormones are critical for life. Therefore, the client must remain on HRT for the rest of his or her life.

12. A

If the dose of synthetic thyroid hormone is too high, manifestations of hyperthyroidism start appearing. Difficulty sleeping is a major manifestation of hyperthyroidism. This client's thyroid hormone levels need to be checked and the drug dosage possibly adjusted to a lower dose.

13. B

Graves disease is an autoimmune disorder that does not result from excessive intake of thyroid hormones (THs) or the substances needed to produce them (iodide/iodine present in seaweed). All autoimmune disorders have a strong genetic component and a person who has one autoimmune disorder is more likely to develop another. Exposure to any type of radiation can result in development of hypothyroidism, not any type of hyperthyroidism.

14. C, E

Hyperthyroidism is a hypermetabolic condition in which clients have fine tremors and elevated body temperature from central nervous system stimulation. Only the Graves disease form of hyperthyroidism results in exophthalmos and the buildup of mucinous tissue on the shins that presents as dry and waxy (pretibial edema). A goiter can be present in other forms of hyperthyroidism and is often also present in clients who have hypothyroidism. The goiter in Graves disease is a generalized swelling, and nodules are not present.

15. B, D, E

The client is hypermetabolic and has an increased need for calories, carbohydrates, and proteins. Proteins are especially important as the client is at risk for a negative nitrogen balance. Fatty foods do not need to be eliminated and fluids need to be increased to keep pace with the water loss from hypermetabolism and elevated body temperature. The client secretes too much thyroid hormones and does not need to increase his or her intake of iodine/iodide.

16. D

Manipulating or applying any pressure to the thyroid gland can release a bolus of thyroid hormones leading to the life-threatening complication of thyroid storm (crisis). Thus, palpation of the thyroid is **not** performed as part of the nurse's assessment.

17. D

Propylthiouracil can cause liver toxicity and must be stopped if this occurs. Persistently dark-colored urine is an indication of liver problems. Although this drug eventually suppresses thyroid hormone production, the client usually continues to have hyperthyroid symptoms (insomnia, heat intolerance) for some time after therapy is started. Even if ringing in the ears does occur (not a common side effect of therapy with this drug), its presence is not as urgent to report as any indications of liver toxicity.

18. B

The client's urine will contain small amounts of radioactive iodine that can pose a hazard to others, particularly if it is absorbed through mucous membranes. Until the client has completely cleared this material, he or she should use a separate toilet.

19. A

Drooling may be a normal response for some patients while sleeping; however, it is also a major indication of swelling in the neck that could result in airway obstruction. More assessment is needed to determine whether the client is in danger of losing his or her airway.

The oxygen saturation is within normal limits for a healthy adult. A moderate amount of drainage may be more than expected but is not an indication of obstruction.

After general anesthesia, most clients are sleepy. Not opening his or her eyes during a response to a question is not an indication of airway obstruction.

20. B, F

Strain or tension on the suture line after a thyroidectomy occurs whenever the client's neck is fully extended or hyperextended. This can be avoided by placing a small pillow under the head for neck flexion and by having the client support the neck when moving by placing both hands on the back of the neck.

Clients are placed in a semi-Fowler position rather than flat to prevent the effects of gravity from pulling on the incision during any movement. Deep-breathing exercises are encouraged. Elastic wraps are not applied to the neck because they could result in external airway obstruction.

21. B

Damage to the laryngeal nerve can occur during thyroid surgery, which reduces closure of the vocal cords and results in a weak, breathy voice that is hoarse-sounding. Partial airway obstruction would cause stridor and dyspnea. Irritation from the endotracheal tube causes a sore throat. Impending hemorrhage would not have vocal symptoms.

22. D

Thyroiditis that causes a decrease in thyroid function most often follows a bacterial or viral infection (such as influenza). The problem can occur at any age and with individuals of either gender. Mechanical trauma does not result in thyroiditis and neither does thyroid hormone replacement therapy. Although some people have flu-like symptoms with fever after any type of vaccination, a resulting change in thyroid function would require many days to weeks.

23. B

A hallmark of primary thyroid cancer or recurrence after surgery is an elevated serum thyroglobulin (Tg) level. The normal Tg level is 0.5 to 53.0 ng/mL (mcg/L) for men and 0.5 to 43.0 ng/mL (mcg/L) for women. All other laboratory values are within normal limits and are not associated with a recurrence of thyroid cancer.

24. C

All of the laboratory values are somewhat out of the normal range but do not reach critical values. Sodium is slightly decreased, potassium is slightly elevated, and pH is a little low. Only calcium is low enough to indicate severe problems and risk for seizure activity. Assessing the client for increased deep tendon reflexes can provide a reasonable determination of risk severity.

25. B, F

The client with hypoparathyroidism is calcium deficient and will need to take calcium supplements. Vitamin D helps increase GI absorption of calcium and also is prescribed. Phosphorus is avoided because it will make the calcium deficiency worse (calcium and phosphorus exist in the blood in a balanced reciprocal relationship, which means that an increase in one will result in a decrease in the other). None of the other minerals or vitamin C are prescribed as therapy for hypoparathyroidism.

26. D

A client with severe hypoparathyroidism may have very brittle bones that break easily. This client must be handled gently, including using a lift sheet for movement rather than grasping or pulling him or her.

27. B

Clients who have chronic renal failure do not completely activate vitamin D and poorly absorb calcium from the GI tract. They are chronically hypocalcemic, which triggers over stimulation of the parathyroid glands. None of the other disorders play a role in the development of hyperparathyroidism.

28. A, B, D, F

The constant leaching of calcium from bones leads to bone deformities in the extremities and back. High levels of PTH cause kidney stones. Calcium elevates serum gastrin levels, increasing the risk for peptic ulcer disease. Very high calcium levels increase the risk for psychosis with confusion.

Clients with hyperparathyroidism are usually constipated. The disorder is not associated with an increased risk for thyroid cancer.

59
CHAPTER

Concepts of Care for Patients with Diabetes Mellitus

1. Which physiologic actions result from normal insulin secretion? **Select all that apply**.
   A. Increased liver storage of glucose as glycogen
   B. Increased gluconeogenesis
   C. Increased cellular uptake of blood glucose
   D. Increased breakdown of lipids (fats) for fuel
   E. Increased production and release of epinephrine
   F. Decreased storage of free fatty acids in fat cells
   G. Decreased blood glucose levels
   H. Decreased blood cholesterol levels

2. What is the nurse's **best** response when a client who has type 1 diabetes asks why he shouldn't try to keep his blood glucose level as close to zero (0) as possible?
   A. "That would only frustrate you because there are many ways your body prevents your blood glucose level from going below 50 mg/L (2.8 mmol/L)."
   B. "You would have to eat absolutely no carbohydrates to accomplish this and just about all food contains some carbohydrates."
   C. "Glucose is an important nutrient, especially for your brain, and you cannot live if your blood glucose level gets too low."
   D. "Maintaining such a low glucose level would require a lot of very expensive drugs and not reduce the complications."

3. Which health problems that are complications of chronic hyperglycemia will the nurse reinforce to the client with diabetes could be *delayed or prevented* with long-term good glucose control? **Select all that apply**.
   A. Amputations
   B. Blindness
   C. Chronic kidney disease
   D. Heart attack
   E. Erectile dysfunction
   F. Stroke

4. Which assessment action is a **priority** for the nurse to perform **first** to **prevent harm** for a client with diabetes whose blood osmolarity is 345 mOsm/L?
   A. Checking skin turgor
   B. Measuring blood pressure
   C. Testing for ketones in the urine
   D. Checking the most recent serum electrolyte values

5. Which assessment finding will the nurse expect in a client with diabetes who has peripheral neuropathy of the *motor* neurons?
   A. Muscle weakness
   B. Orthostatic hypotension
   C. Absence of feeling in the feet
   D. Increased risk for myocardial infarction

6. Which assessment findings in a 33-year-old female client indicate to the nurse that she has an increased risk for type 2 diabetes? **Select all that apply**.
   A. A1C is 5.8%
   B. Weight is 25 lb (11.3 kg) above ideal
   C. Had a 10 lb (4.5 kg) baby 2 years ago
   D. Has irritable bowel syndrome with constipation
   E. Fasting blood glucose (FBG) level is 119 mg/dL (6.5 mmol/L)
   F. Mother, sister, and maternal grandmother all have type 2 diabetes

7. How will the nurse respond to the client newly diagnosed with type 2 diabetes who asks, "What does having metabolic syndrome and diabetes mean for me?"
   A. "Metabolic syndrome is helpful to anyone with diabetes because it increases the sensitivity of your cells to the presence of insulin."
   B. "People with diabetes and metabolic syndrome usually need to use insulin rather than oral antidiabetic drug to manage their blood glucose levels."
   C. "Metabolic syndrome is a problem in eliminating drugs from your body, so you will need to be on lower doses of your antidiabetic drugs to prevent severe side effects."
   D. "Your risk for having cardiovascular disease and a possible heart attack is higher and will require good control of your diabetes, blood pressure, and cholesterol to prevent them."

8. How will the nurse evaluate the level of glycemic control for a client with diabetes whose laboratory values include a fasting blood glucose level of 91 mg/dL (5.1 mmol/L) and an A1C of 8.2%?
   A. The client's glucose control for the past 24 hours has been good but the overall control is poor.
   B. The client's glucose control for the past 24 hours has been poor but the overall control is good.
   C. The values indicate that the client has poorly managed his or her disease.
   D. The values indicate that the client has managed his or her disease well.

9. Which action will the nurse recommend to a client with type 1 diabetes on insulin therapy who has been having a morning fasting blood glucose (FBG) level of 160 mg/dL (8.9 mmol/L) and is diagnosed with "Somogyi phenomenon" to achieve better control?
   A. "Avoid eating any carbohydrate with your evening meal."
   B. "Eat a bedtime snack containing equal amounts of protein and carbohydrates."
   C. "Inject the insulin into your arm rather than into the abdomen around the navel."
   D. "Take your evening insulin dose right before going to bed instead of at supper time."

10. Which client admitted to a surgical unit will the nurse recognize as having a higher risk for having type 2 diabetes?
    A. 30-year-old Hispanic female runner
    B. 36-year-old white female who has rheumatoid arthritis
    C. 40-year-old black male who is 10 lb (4.5 kg) underweight
    D. 48-year-old obese male American Indian

11. Which lifestyle changes will the nurse suggest to a 35-year-old client who has prediabetes to reduce the risk for developing type 2 diabetes? **Select all that apply**.
    A. Increasing fluid intake
    B. Increasing physical activity
    C. Quitting smoking and vaping
    D. Eliminating all dietary carbohydrates
    E. Reducing consumption of empty calories
    F. Keeping body weight at or slightly below ideal

12. Which precaution is a priority for the nurse to teach a client prescribed dulaglutide to **prevent harm**?
    A. Only take this drug once weekly.
    B. Do not drink alcohol when taking this drug.
    C. Take this drug right before or with the first bite of a meal.
    D. Report any genital itching to your diabetes health care provider immediately.

13. Which serum electrolyte level is **most important** for the nurse to monitor closely to **prevent harm** in a client who has hyperglycemia?
    A. Sodium
    B. Chloride
    C. Potassium
    D. Magnesium

14. Which issues regarding diabetes management will the nurse consider delaying to teach about to a client with newly diagnosed type 1 diabetes until after the initial phase? **Select all that apply**.
    A. Discussing exactly what causes type 1 diabetes
    B. Preparing and administering insulin
    C. Implementing sick-day management rules
    D. Recognizing indications of hypoglycemia and hyperglycemia
    E. Explaining the risk for passing on type 1 diabetes to one's children
    F. Monitoring urine ketone levels

15. With which classes of antidiabetic drugs will the nurse **most emphasize** to the client with diabetes how to recognize and manage hypoglycemia?
    A. Alpha-glucosidase inhibitors
    B. Biguanides
    C. Insulin
    D. Incretin mimetics
    E. Meglitinide analogs
    F. Second-generation sulfonylureas

16. Which assessment finding in a client with long-standing diabetes will the nurse interpret as an *early* sign of diabetic nephropathy?
    A. Positive urine red blood cells
    B. Microalbuminuria
    C. Positive urine glucose
    D. Positive urine white blood cells

17. With which signs and symptoms will the nurse teach a client to take action to **prevent harm** as indicators of *mild* hypoglycemia? **Select all that apply**.
    A. Headache
    B. Weakness
    C. Cold, clammy skin
    D. Irritability
    E. Pallor
    F. Tachycardia

18. For which client complication of diabetes will the nurse expect to administer glucagon intramuscularly?
    A. Diabetic retinopathy
    B. Severe hypoglycemia
    C. Diabetic ketoacidosis (DKA)
    D. Hyperglycemic-hyperosmolar state (HHS)

19. Which statement made by the client with type 1 diabetes during nutritional counseling indicates to the nurse that he or she correctly understands his or her nutritional needs?
    A. "If I completely eliminate carbohydrates from my diet, I will not need to take insulin."
    B. "I will make certain that I eat at least 130 g of carbohydrate each day regardless of my activity level."
    C. "My intake of protein in terms of grams and calories should be the same as my intake of carbohydrate."
    D. "My intake of unsaturated fats in terms of grams and calories should be the same as my intake of protein."

20. What is the **best** action for a nurse to take to **prevent harm** when a client with diabetes, who just received a premeal dose of regular insulin, is picked up by transportation to the radiation department for a scheduled x-ray before she has a chance to eat her lunch?
    A. Calling the radiation department and rescheduling the x-ray
    B. Sending the client's lunch with her to the radiation department
    C. Administering glucagon by the intramuscular route immediately
    D. Reminding the transporter that this client must be seen first in the radiation department

21. Which response on blood glucose level does the nurse expect to find in a client with diabetes who is now receiving corticosteroid therapy for an acute inflammation?
    A. Hypoglycemia
    B. Hyperglycemia
    C. Ketoacidosis
    D. No specific change

22. What is the nurse's **first** action on finding that the blood glucose level of a client with diabetes who is NPO for surgery in the next hour is 150 mg/dL (8.4 mmol/L)?
    A. Administer regular insulin IV.
    B. Administer a dose of glucagon.
    C. Notify the surgeon immediately.
    D. Document the finding as the only action.

23. For which client will the nurse question the diabetes health care provider's prescription for rosiglitazone?
    A. 22-year-old with new-onset asthma
    B. 40-year-old with hyperthyroidism
    C. 60-year-old with heart failure
    D. 65-year-old with kidney disease

24. Which situations or conditions will the nurse teach a client with diabetes are common causes of hypoglycemia? **Select all that apply**.
    A. Too much insulin taken compared with food intake
    B. Increased food intake especially after missed or delayed meals
    C. Insulin injected at the wrong time relative to food intake and physical activity
    D. Decreased insulin sensitivity as a result of regular exercise and weight loss
    E. Decreased insulin clearance from progressive kidney failure
    F. Decreased liver glucose production after alcohol ingestion

25. Which techniques will the nurse teach a client with diabetes about how to **prevent harm** from loss of insulin potency? **Select all that apply**.
    A. "Avoid exposing insulin to temperatures below 36°F (2.2°C) or above 86°F (30°C)."
    B. "Freeze bottles of insulin for long-term storage."
    C. "Always shake NPH insulin to assure it is evenly cloudy."
    D. "Avoid exposing insulin to heat or light."
    E. "Store unopened insulin bottles in a refrigerator."
    F. "A slight loss in potency may occur for bottles in use for more than 30 days but can still be used."

26. What problem does the nurse suspect when a client with well-controlled diabetes develops an unexpected increase in blood glucose level 2 days after surgery?
    A. Family bringing in food for client consumption
    B. Wound infection occurring before fever
    C. Response to interactions of newly prescribed drugs
    D. Progression of disease severity to type 1 diabetes

27. What is the **priority** action for the nurse and other members of the interprofessional health care team when caring for an older client admitted with hyperglycemic-hyperosmolar state (HHS)?
    A. Replacing potassium
    B. Preventing ketoacidosis
    C. Decreasing blood glucose levels
    D. Increasing circulating blood volume

28. Which condition will the nurse monitor closely for in a client with type 1 diabetes who has blood glucose level of 438 mg/dL (24.4 mmol/L)?
    A. Respiratory acidosis
    B. Metabolic alkalosis
    C. Respiratory alkalosis
    D. Metabolic acidosis

29. For which situations will the nurse teach a client to perform urine ketone testing?
    A. Anytime he or she is acutely ill or severely stressed
    B. When blood glucose levels are above 200 mg/dL (11.1 mmol/L)
    C. When symptoms of diabetic ketoacidosis (DKA) are present
    D. While participating in a weight-loss program
    E. Before engaging in strenuous exercise
    F. After eating citrus fruit or drinking alcohol

30. In collaboration with the registered dietitian nutritionists, what principle is **most important** for the nurse to reinforce to the client about changes in meal planning needed for management of type 1 diabetes?
    A. Eating at least five smaller meals per day plus a bedtime snack
    B. Taking extra insulin when planning to eat sweet foods
    C. Ensuring the inclusion of high-protein, low-carbohydrate, and low-fiber foods
    D. Considering the effects and peak action times of the prescribed insulin

31. Which class of antidiabetic drug will the nurse hold for a client after an imaging test using contrast medium until adequate kidney function is established?
    A. Alpha-glucosidase inhibitors
    B. Biguanides
    C. Meglitinides
    D. Second-generation sulfonylureas

32. What type of exercise will the nurse recommend for the client with diabetic retinopathy?
    A. Non-weight-bearing activities such as swimming
    B. Weight-bearing activities such as jogging
    C. Gradually increasing aerobic and resistance exercises
    D. Weight training and heavy lifting

33. Which action will the nurse teach a client with diabetes performing self-monitoring of blood glucose (SMBG) levels to **prevent harm** from bloodborne infections?
    A. Washing hands before beginning the test
    B. Not sharing the monitoring equipment with others
    C. Blotting away any excess blood from the strip
    D. Using gloves during monitoring

34. Which points will the nurse, in collaboration with a registered dietitian nutritionist, use to individualize a meal plan for a client with diabetes? **Select all that apply**.
    A. Maintaining blood glucose levels at or near the client's target range
    B. Allowing client food preferences whenever possible
    C. Permitting clients to eat as much as they desire
    D. Honoring the client's cultural preferences
    E. Limiting food choices to proteins and vegetables
    F. Suggesting the client avoid all forms of dietary fats

35. Which points are essential for the nurse to include in the teaching plan when instructing a client with diabetes how to select and wear appropriate shoes?
    A. "Have your shoes fitted by an experienced shoe fitter such as a podiatrist."
    B. "Make sure the shoes are 1 to 1.5 inches longer than your longest toe."
    C. "The heels of the shoes should be less than 2 inches high."
    D. "Avoid tight-fitting shoes that can damage your feet."
    E. "Rotate your shoes so you don't wear the same shoes 2 days in a row."
    F. "Get measured for shoes later in the day, when feet are normally larger."

36. How many grams of carbohydrate (CHO) will the nurse provide to a client who has symptoms of hypoglycemia with a blood glucose level between 69 mg/dL (3.9 mmol/L) and 50 mg/dL (2.8 mmol/L) to correct the problem and **prevent harm**?
    A. 5 g
    B. 10 g
    C. 15 g
    D. 30 g

37. What is the most appropriate action for the nurse to take when a client who has used insulin for diabetes control for 20 years now has a spongy swelling at the site used most frequently for insulin injection?
    A. Applying ice to this area
    B. Documenting the finding as the only action
    C. Assessing the client for other indications of cellulitis
    D. Instructing the client to use a different site for insulin injection

Chapter 59 Answer Key

1. A, C, G, H
   The main metabolic effects of insulin are to stimulate glucose uptake in skeletal muscle and heart muscle and to suppress liver production of glucose and very-low-density lipoprotein (VLDL). In the liver, insulin promotes the production and storage of glycogen (glycogenesis) at the same time that it inhibits glycogen breakdown into glucose (glycogenolysis). It increases protein and lipid (fat) synthesis and inhibits ketogenesis (conversion of fats to acids) and gluconeogenesis (conversion of proteins to glucose). In muscle, insulin promotes protein and glycogen synthesis. In fat cells, it promotes triglyceride storage. Overall, insulin keeps blood glucose levels from becoming too high and helps keep blood lipid levels in the normal range.

2. C
   Glucose is a critical nutrient for all cells and tissues. Although chronically high blood glucose levels cause many serious problems, low blood glucose levels can rapidly (within minutes) lead to neuron injury and death. Therefore, the desired outcome of diabetes management is to keep blood glucose levels in the range of 60 to 100 mg/dL (3.3 to 5.6 mmol/L) to support brain function and prevent death.

3. A, B, C, D, E, F
   All of these health problems are common complications of diabetes that develop as a result of chronic hyperglycemia. The hyperglycemia causes microvascular and macrovascular changes that reduce perfusion and gas exchange in these tissues resulting in hypoxia, anoxia,

ischemia, and buildup of toxic waste products that injure organs and lead to dysfunction. Long-term blood glucose delays or may even prevent these serious complications.

4. B

All the assessment actions are important for this client who is likely to be severely dehydrated. The priority assessment action is to measure blood pressure because the severe dehydration can cause profound hypotension with orthostatic hypotension leading to dangerously reduced organ perfusion and increasing the risk for falls.

5. A

Neuropathy of motor neurons leads to muscle weakness and increased risk for falls. Neuropathy of sensory neurons leads to loss of sensation in the feet and hands and can cause the client not to feel symptoms when MI occurs but does not increase the risk for having an MI. Cardiac autonomic neuropathy, not motor neuropathy, causes orthostatic hypotension.

6. A, B, C, E, F

Risk factors for type 2 diabetes include obesity, indications of gestational diabetes (first baby larger than 9 lb [4.1 kg]), and a family history of a parent or other first-degree relative with type 2 diabetes. In addition, although this client's A1C and FBG levels are not high enough for a diabetes diagnosis, they are consistent with prediabetes, a strong risk factor for development of type 2 diabetes. Irritable bowel syndrome is not a diabetes risk factor.

7. D

Metabolic syndrome is the simultaneous presence of metabolic factors that increase risk for developing type 2 DM and cardiovascular disease. Features include insulin resistance, higher blood lipid levels, abdominal obesity, and hypertension. The risk for atherosclerosis, along with heart disease and strokes is greatly increased. The two disorders together make blood glucose levels harder to control.

8. A

Fasting blood glucose levels provide an indication of the client's adherence to drug and nutrition therapy for DM for the previous 24 hours. This client's FBG is well within the normal range.

A1C provides an indication of general blood glucose control for the past several months because when glucose attaches to hemoglobin, the attachment is permanent for as long as those hemoglobin molecules are present within red blood cells. Normal red blood cell life span is about 120 days. This client's A1C level is outside the desirable range, indicating chronic hyperglycemia and poor long-term glucose control despite good short-term control.

9. B

The client with "Somogyi phenomenon," diagnosed by checking blood glucose levels during the night, has morning hyperglycemia caused by the counterregulatory response to nighttime hypoglycemia. Eating a bedtime snack to prevent nighttime hypoglycemia can result in suppression of counterregulatory hormone release.

A client with "dawn phenomenon," diagnosed by checking blood glucose levels during the night, has morning hyperglycemia that results from a nighttime release of adrenal hormones causing blood glucose elevations at about 5 to 6 a.m. It is managed by providing more insulin for the overnight period (e.g., giving the evening dose of intermediate-acting insulin at 10 p.m. instead of with the evening meal). Changing the injection site would not prevent morning hyperglycemia. Not eating any carbohydrate with a meal is more likely to cause severe hypoglycemia during the night and is dangerous.

10. D

The type 2 diabetes rate is about 13% among blacks and 12% in the Hispanic population, which is higher than that of non-Hispanic white Americans. At nearly 15.1%, American Indians and Alaska Indians have the highest age-adjusted prevalence of DM among U.S. racial and ethnic groups. The American-Indian client has an increased risk of obesity. The Hispanic female and black male have high activity levels or reduced weight, which decreases the risk.

11. B, E, F

    The two most important lifestyle changes to reduce the risk for development of type 2 diabetes are increasing activity and maintaining a healthy weight. Part of weight control is reducing consumption of surgery drinks and other sources of "empty" calories that increase overall weight and have minimal nutritional values. Increasing fluid intake and quitting smoking and vaping help prevent complications from diabetes but do not reduce the risk for developing the disorder. Eliminating all dietary carbohydrates is not part of a well-balanced diet, can cause other problems, and is not recommended for prevention of type 2 diabetes.

12. A

    This drug is an incretin mimetic (GLP1-agonist) that works with insulin to prevent hyperglycemia. It is taken as an injection only once per week. If taken more frequently, the client is at risk for an overdose. This drug is not associated with fasciitis of the perineum and does not require total abstinence from alcohol.

13. C

    Although all electrolytes can change as a result of hyperglycemia, potassium changes with either hyperkalemia or hypokalemia cause excitable membrane alterations that can be life threatening, especially in cardiac conduction and skeletal muscle contraction. The nurse must evaluate serum potassium levels most closely to prevent harm.

14. A, E, F

    Responses B, C, and D are "survival skills" and critically important for the client and family to know for safe management of this serious disorder. The other issues are less important for the client to know to prevent immediate harm.

15. C, D, E, F

    Insulin, incretin mimetics, meglitinide analogs, and sulfonylureas all increase blood insulin levels or insulin action and greatly increase the risk for hypoglycemia if the client does not match his or her food intake with peak drug action. Alpha-glucosidase inhibitors and biguanides have different mechanisms of action and do not increase the risk for hypoglycemia when taken alone.

16. B

    Microalbuminuria is the most common and reliable indicator of diabetic nephropathy. Red blood cells and white blood cells in the urine are indicators of urinary tract infection and not specific to nephropathy. Presence of glucose in the urine is more of an indication of hyperglycemia and not of the early stages of diabetic nephropathy.

17. A, B, D

    The earliest signs and symptoms of mild hypoglycemia are associated with changes in neurologic functioning including headache, sensation of hunger, irritability, and weakness. The other symptoms listed are present when hypoglycemia becomes more severe.

18. B

    Glucagon injections are administered to raise blood glucose levels when severe hypoglycemia is present. This drug breaks down liver glycogen stores into glycogen that is converted into glucose.

19. B

    Carbohydrates are the main fuel for human cells, especially neurons, and the substance most commonly used to make ATP. The dietary recommendations for clients who have diabetes is that, although the percentage of total calories needed is determined for each client, the diet should never contain less than 130 g of carbohydrate per day. Protein intake should range between 15% and 30% of total caloric intake per day.

20. A

    A client who receives premeal regular insulin and then does not eat the meal is at high risk for severe hypoglycemia. The best action is to not let the client go to the radiation department without eating. The nurse will reschedule the client's x-ray for a time after she has eaten. Sending the client's meal with her does not ensure sufficient intake to prevent hypoglycemia. The transporter has no responsibility in this matter. Giving glucagon is not a good option because the client's blood glucose level may not have decreased yet. Also, after glucagon is administered, the client requires close monitoring and would still not be able to have an x-ray at this time.

21. B
Corticosteroids increase blood glucose levels in a variety of ways, including increased release of liver glycogen and desensitizing the insulin receptor to insulin, which reduces cellular uptake of glucose from the blood.

22. D
The recommended blood glucose level for a client who has diabetes during surgery is between 140 mg/dL (7.8 mmol/L) and 180 mg/mL (10 mmol/L). This client's blood glucose is within the recommended range and no action regarding the level at this time is needed.

23. C
Rosiglitazone is a thiazolidinedione that has an increased risk for heart-related complications and deaths, bone fractures, and macular edema. Drugs from this class carry a black box warning to avoid their use in clients who have symptomatic heart failure.

24. A, C, E, F
The most common causes of hypoglycemia are: too much insulin compared with food intake and physical activity, insulin injected at the wrong time relative to food intake and physical activity, the wrong type of insulin injected at the wrong time, decreased food intake resulting from missed or delayed meals, delayed gastric emptying from gastroparesis, decreased liver glucose production after alcohol ingestion, and decreased insulin clearance due to progressive kidney failure.

25. A, D, E
To prevent loss of drug potency, clients are taught to avoid exposing insulin to temperatures below 36°F (2.2°C) or above 86°F (30°C), to avoid shaking bottles/vials, and to protect insulin from direct heat and light. Insulin is not to be frozen. Insulin potency decreases rapidly when bottles/vials have been opened and used for longer than 28 days and clients are instructed to discard open bottles after 28 days of use.

26. B
The most common cause of an elevated blood glucose level in a client who has maintained long-term good control is infection. Often the blood glucose level will rise before other indications of infection are present, including fever.

27. D
The client with HHS is severely dehydrated and at risk for death from decreased cardiac output. The first priority in management of HHS is replacing circulating fluid volume to ensure adequate perfusion. All other concerns, including decreasing blood glucose level, are secondary.

28. D
The client is severely hyperglycemic and is using fat for fuel, which increases the amount of ketone bodies released into the blood from fatty acid breakdown. This situation leads to diabetic ketoacidosis (DKA), a type of metabolic acidosis, with a low pH as hydrogen ion concentration increases. Although the client's compensatory efforts with breathing more rapidly and deeply can cause some respiratory alkalosis with a lower-than-normal carbon dioxide level, the acidosis is more likely to have serious consequences.

29. A, D, E
An acute illness or severe stress increases release of corticosteroids and results in high blood glucose levels that could increase the use of fatty acids for fuel and cause ketosis. Participation in a weight-loss program can result in insufficient intake of carbohydrates and result in increased breakdown of fatty acids, which causes formation of ketone bodies. Before heavy exercise, clients need to ensure a blood glucose level high enough to support the increased metabolism generated. When ketone bodies are present in the urine before exercise,

they indicate that a client does not have a sufficient glucose level to support exercise at this time. The client is taught to not exercise when ketone bodies are present and to test blood glucose levels. Ketones are rarely present when blood glucose levels are no higher than 200 mg/dL (11.1 mmol/L). The client who suspects DKA is present needs to go to the nearest emergency department and not waste time testing for ketone bodies. Citrus fruit does not increase acid production directly and alcohol causes hypoglycemia.

30. D
The guiding principle for meal planning for a client on insulin therapy (regardless of the specific insulin regimen) must take into consideration the effects and peak action times of all prescribed insulin. Meal times, composition, and sizes are based on these actions to promote euglycemia.

31. B
Metformin, the only drug in the biguanide class, can cause lactic acidosis in patients with kidney impairment and is not to be used by anyone with kidney disease. To prevent lactic acidosis and acute kidney injury, the drug is withheld before and after using contrast medium or any surgical procedure requiring anesthesia until adequate kidney function is established.

32. A
The client with retinopathy is at high risk for blindness as a result of increased bleeding inside the eye. These clients are taught to avoid any type of exercise that may increase damage to these blood vessels and cause vascular damage to many organs. Swimming is the only listed exercise that does not increase this risk.

33. B
Small particles of blood can adhere to the monitoring device and infection can be transported from one user to another. Therefore, the client is taught to not share his or her monitoring equipment with others. Washing hands

helps prevent general infection but not blood-borne infections.

34. A, B, D
The client is most likely to follow a diabetes diet plan when he or she is an active participant in plan development. Dietary habits of a lifetime are difficult to change. While maintaining blood glucose levels within the client's established target range is the desired outcome, this is more likely to be achieved when the plan includes some level of the client's specific food preferences and those that he or she considers part of their ethnic and cultural heritage. All food substances, including carbohydrates and fats, are included in a balanced diet, not just protein and vegetables, although the amount of the substances is more limited, as is the total caloric amount permitted daily.

35. A, C, D, E, F
All of the points are important for the client with diabetes to use when buying and wearing new shoes to prevent harm, with the exception of option B. Although the shoes should not be too tight, shoes that are too large can also injure the foot and cause the client to have a poor walking gait.

36. C
Current recommendations and guidelines for managing hypoglycemia in an alert client follow the 15-15 rule. With this rule, 15 g of CHO are given if the blood glucose level is less than 70 mg/dL (3.9 mmol/L) (or 30 g if less than 50 mg/dL [2.8 mmol/L]) or if the client is experiencing symptoms of hypoglycemia and can swallow safely. If the blood glucose recheck within 15 minutes is still low, the same treatment is given again.

37. D
The client has hypertrophic lipodystrophy as a result of repeated injections at the same site. Avoiding this site for an extended period of time allows the dystrophic changes to regress or at least not become worse.

60
CHAPTER

Assessment of the Renal/Urinary System

1. For which client does the nurse expect **increased** production of renin?
   A. 35-year-old who sustains significant blood loss
   B. 45-year-old diagnosed with hypertension
   C. 55-year-old who ingests an excessive amount of fluid
   D. 65-year-old who gets up two to three times nightly to void

2. Which substances will the nurse consider an abnormal finding in a client's routine urine sample? **Select all that apply.**
   A. Electrolytes
   B. Red blood cells
   C. Proteins
   D. Water
   E. Albumin
   F. Creatinine

3. Which blood pressure reading does the nurse expect will result in compromised kidney function for a client who sustained major injuries in an automobile accident?
   A. 160/80 mm Hg
   B. 140/100 mm Hg
   C. 80/60 mm Hg
   D. 68/40 mm Hg

4. What instructions would the nurse give an assistive personnel (AP) about the proper handling of a client's routine urinalysis specimen? **Select all that apply.**
   A. Leave the specimen in the bathroom.
   B. Ensure the container is tightly covered.
   C. Place the sample in a sterile container.
   D. Take the sample to the laboratory within 1 hour.
   E. Put the sample in a plastic sample bag.
   F. Refrigerate a sample that cannot be taken to the laboratory right away.

5. When a client's kidney hormonal function is not working properly, which condition does the nurse expect to occur?
   A. Leukemia
   B. Thrombocytopenia
   C. Anemia
   D. Neutropenia

6. Which client does the nurse expect is **most likely** to exceed the renal threshold when he or she is noncompliant with the prescribed therapeutic regimen?
   A. 45-year-old with biliary obstruction
   B. 55-year-old with type 2 diabetes mellitus
   C. 65-year-old with recurrent kidney stones
   D. 75-year-old with functional incontinence

7. Which nursing actions will the nurse take to provide safe care and **prevent harm** for an older client experiencing increased nocturia? **Select all that apply.**
   A. Ensure adequate lighting and a hazard-free environment.
   B. Use caution administering nephrotoxic drugs.
   C. Ensure the availability of a bedside toilet, bedpan, or urinal if needed.
   D. Encourage the client to use the toilet, bedpan, or urinal at least every 2 hours.
   E. Discourage excessive fluid intake for 2 to 4 hours before the client goes to bed.
   F. Respond as soon as possible to the client's indication of the need to void.

8. Which symptom will the nurse expect when caring for an older male client with an enlarged prostate?
   A. Passing a large amount of dilute urine
   B. Difficulty starting the urine stream
   C. Inability to sense the urge to urinate
   D. Burning sensation when voiding

9. Which topics will the nurse be sure to ask about when taking a history of a client with a change in urinary patterns? **Select all that apply.**
   A. History of chronic health problems such as diabetes and hypertension
   B. Status of financial resources for payment of treatments
   C. Likelihood of complying with treatment recommendations
   D. Occupational exposure to toxins and use of illicit substances
   E. Recent travel to geographic regions that pose infectious disease risk
   F. Previous kidney or urologic problems, including tumors, infections, stones

10. Which over-the-counter product will the nurse further explore with a client, for potential impact on kidney function?
    A. Mouthwash with alcohol
    B. Vitamin C
    C. Acetaminophen
    D. Fiber supplement

11. What is the **most common** symptom that prompts clients to seek medical attention for problems with the kidneys or urinary tract?

    A. Pain in flank or abdomen, or pain when urinating
    B. Change in the frequency or amount of urination
    C. Exposure to one or more nephrotoxic substances
    D. Change in color, clarity, or odor of the urine

12. Which problem or complication does the nurse suspect when a client with chronic kidney disease develops anorexia, nausea and vomiting, muscle cramping, and pruritus?
    A. Client has oliguria
    B. Client has anuria
    C. Client has uremia
    D. Client has azotemia

13. Which step will the nurse perform **first** on a client during assessment of the renal system?
    A. Listen for a bruit over each renal artery.
    B. Lightly palpate the abdomen in all four quadrants.
    C. Percuss from the lower abdomen toward the umbilicus.
    D. Observe the flank region for asymmetry or discoloration.

14. When the nurse provides care for a client with chronic kidney failure, what assessments will be made that support a finding of fluid overload? **Select all that apply.**
    A. Weigh the client and compare to baseline.
    B. Compare current blood pressure to baseline.
    C. Measure for residual urine with a bladder scanner.
    D. Auscultate the lung fields to determine if fluid is present.
    E. Check for pedal and periorbital swelling.
    F. Obtain a sterile urine specimen by catheterization.

15. What sound does the nurse expect to hear when listening over the renal artery of a client who has renal artery stenosis?
    A. Quiet, pulsating sound
    B. Swishing sound
    C. Occasional gurgling
    D. Faint wheezing

16. Which is the **best** technique for the nurse to use when assessing a client for bladder distention?
    A. Use one hand to gently depress the bladder as the client takes a deep breath, then percuss as the client slowly exhales.
    B. Place one hand under the client's back and palpate with the other hand over the bladder, percussing the lower abdomen until tympanic sounds are no longer heard.
    C. Gently palpate the outline of the bladder and percuss the lower abdomen toward the umbilicus until dull sounds are no longer produced.
    D. Locate the symphysis pubis, gently palpate for outline of the bladder, then auscultate for bowel sounds in the lower abdomen.

17. Which equipment and actions will the nurse use to assess a female client's urethra prior to inserting a urinary catheter? **Select all that apply.**
    A. Ensure a good light source is available.
    B. Record any discharge from the meatus.
    C. Assess for lesions or rashes and record.
    D. Remind the client to wipe from back to front.
    E. Ask about discomfort with urination.
    F. Wear well-fitting gloves during the assessment.

18. What question does the nurse ask to help interpret the result when a healthy adult client's urinalysis reveals a protein level of 0.9 mg/dL?
    A. "Have you ever been treated for a urinary tract infection?"
    B. "Are you sexually active and if so, do you use condoms?"
    C. "Do you have a family history of cardiac or biliary disease?"
    D. "Have you recently performed any strenuous exercise?"

19. Which laboratory values will the nurse monitor as **specific** indicators of a client's kidney function? **Select all that apply.**
    A. Creatinine
    B. Blood urea nitrogen (BUN)
    C. Cystatin-C
    D. Blood osmolarity
    E. BUN/creatinine ratio
    F. White blood cell count

20. Which questions will the nurse ask a client with a blood urea nitrogen (BUN) of 26 mg/dL to identify non-renal factors that may contribute to this laboratory result? **Select all that apply.**
    A. "Have you been trying to lose weight with severe calorie restrictions?"
    B. "Have you noticed any blood in your stool or vomited any blood?"
    C. "Have you been on a high-protein diet or been drinking high-protein drinks?"
    D. "Did you drink a lot of extra fluid before the blood sample was drawn?"
    E. "Are you taking or have you recently taken any steroid medications?"
    F. "Have you recently experienced any physical or emotional stress?"

21. Which assessment will the nurse complete before notifying the health care provider about an older client's blood osmolarity result of 313 mOsm/L?
    A. Checking lungs for respiratory status
    B. Assessing for any discomfort or pain
    C. Looking for signs of dehydration
    D. Smelling urine for odor and looking for particles

22. Which annual examinations to screen for kidney problems would the nurse recommend for an African-American client?
    A. Urinalysis, microalbuminuria, and serum creatinine
    B. Kidney ultrasound, blood urea nitrogen, and serum glucose
    C. Serum creatinine, blood urea nitrogen, and renal scan
    D. 24-hour urine collection, blood urea nitrogen, and urinalysis

23. Which client does the nurse expect is **most likely** to produce a urinalysis with a specific gravity (SG) of 1.004?
    A. Client with hypovolemia due to blood loss
    B. Client who has dehydration secondary to vomiting
    C. Client with syndrome of inappropriate antidiuretic hormone (SIADH)
    D. Client who is prescribed the diuretic medication furosemide every day

24. Which instruction will the nurse give the assistive personnel (AP) about when it is **best** to collect a client's urinalysis sample?
    A. In the evening before bedtime
    B. An hour after any meal
    C. With the first morning void
    D. After drinking two full glasses of water

25. Which actions will the nurse take to ensure that a client's 24-hour urine collection is completed appropriately? **Select all that apply.**
    A. Teach the client that a 24-hour collection of urine is necessary to quantify or calculate the rate of clearance of a particular substance.
    B. Check with the laboratory or procedure manual for proper technique to maintain the 24-hour collection.
    C. Do not remove urine from the collection container for other specimens during the 24-hour period.
    D. On initiation of the collection, ask the client to void, discard the urine, and note the time, then begin the collection.
    E. Twenty-four hours after initiation, ask the client to empty the bladder 24 hours after initiation and add that urine to the container.
    F. Place signs appropriately, then inform all personnel or family caregivers that the test is in progress.

26. Which action will the nurse include in postprocedural care for a client who has a renal scan?
    A. Administer captopril to increase renal blood flow.
    B. Encourage oral fluids to assist with excretion of the isotope.
    C. Insert a urinary catheter to measure urine output.
    D. Administer prescribed laxatives to cleanse the bowel.

27. What preprocedural instruction will the nurse provide for a client scheduled for an ultrasonography?
    A. "Empty your bladder just before the test begins."
    B. "Stop taking your routine medications 24 hours before the test."
    C. "You must have nothing to eat or drink after midnight before the test."
    D. "Drink 500 to 1000 mL of water 2 to 3 hours before the test."

28. Which actions will the nurse include in postprocedural care for a client who had a cystoscopy with general anesthesia? **Select all that apply.**
    A. Monitor for airway patency and breathing.
    B. Provide frequent vital sign checks including temperature.
    C. Record and monitor for any changes in urine output.
    D. Report pink-tinged urine to the urology care provider immediately.
    E. Irrigate the urinary catheter with sterile saline if prescribed.
    F. Encourage the client to take oral fluids to increase urine output.

29. What is the **priority** nursing assessment for a client who has undergone a kidney biopsy?
    A. Monitor for urinary retention.
    B. Assess for onset of hypertension.
    C. Perform frequent checks for hemorrhage.
    D. Observe for signs of nephrotoxicity.

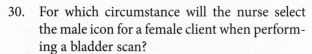

30. For which circumstance will the nurse select the male icon for a female client when performing a bladder scan?
    A. Female who self identifies as a male
    B. Woman with a history of hysterectomy
    C. Female who is 5 years postmenopausal
    D. Woman with a history of bladder cancer

31. Which **priority** teaching will the nurse provide to **prevent harm** for a client after a renal biopsy?
    A. Avoid lifting heavy objects for 1 to 2 weeks after the procedure.
    B. Do not go up or down stairs for at least 10 days.
    C. Avoid light house work including cooking and washing dishes.
    D. Stay out of the sun until after your follow-up appointment.

Chapter 60 Answer Key

1. A
   Renin assists in blood pressure control. It is formed and released when there is a decrease in blood flow, blood volume (e.g., blood loss), or blood pressure through the renal arterioles or when too little sodium is present in kidney blood.

2. B, C, E
   Large particles, such as blood cells, albumin, and other proteins, are too large to filter through the glomerular capillary walls. Therefore, these substances are **not** normally present in the excreted final urine.

3. D
   Glomerular filtration rate (GFR) is controlled by blood pressure and blood flow. The kidneys self-regulate their own blood pressure and blood flow, which keeps GFR constant. GFR is controlled by selectively constricting and dilating the afferent and efferent arterioles. When systolic pressure drops below 65 to 70 mm Hg, these self-regulation processes do **not** maintain GFR.

4. B, D, E, F
   The nurse teaches the AP that urine specimens become more alkaline when left standing unrefrigerated for more than 1 hour, when bacteria are present, or when a specimen is left uncovered. Alkaline urine increases cell breakdown. So, the presence of red blood cells may be missed on analysis. The AP ensures that urine specimens are covered and delivered to the laboratory promptly. A plastic bag protects against contact with urine that may be on the outside the cup. Urine specimen delayed 2 or more hours require refrigeration or other specific storage and transport precautions to ensure the integrity of the urine specimen. This is a routine urinalysis and does not need to be sterile. The sample should not be left in the bathroom.

5. C
   The kidneys produce the hormone erythropoietin for red blood cell (RBC) synthesis. When kidney function is poor, erythropoietin production decreases and anemia results.

6. B
   The point where the kidney is overwhelmed with glucose (e.g., diabetes mellitus) and can no longer reabsorb is called the renal threshold or transport maximum (tm) for glucose reabsorption. The renal threshold for glucose is greater than 180 mg/dL (10 mmol/L). When blood glucose levels are greater than 180 mg/dL (10 mmol/L), some glucose stays in the filtrate and is present in the urine.

7. A, C, E, F
   Actions A, C, E, and F are appropriate for preventing harm associated with falls related to frequent nocturia. Option B is an appropriate action for a client with decreased GFR. Option D is an appropriate action for a client with decreased bladder capacity. Option F is appropriate for decreased bladder capacity, but also appropriate for a client with nocturia to prevent falls.

8. **B**
    As male clients age, an enlarged prostate gland makes starting the urine stream difficult and may cause urinary retention.

9. **A, D, E, F**
    Options A, D, E, and F contribute important information to the client's history of urinary pattern changes. Finances and likelihood of compliance, although important, do not contribute to understanding the client's urinary pattern changes. Additional topics include the client's medical and surgical history, as well as previous kidney function laboratory values (e.g., proteinuria or albuminuria). See the section on taking a client history in your text for additional suggestions.

10. **C**
    The nurse asks for more information because high-dose or long-term use of NSAIDs or acetaminophen can seriously **reduce** kidney function.

11. **A**
    The onset of pain in the flank, in the lower abdomen or pelvic region, or in the perineal area causes concern and usually prompts the client to seek medical care. The nurse asks about the onset, intensity, and duration of the pain; its location; precipitating and relieving factors, and its association with any activity or event. Painful urination also leads clients to seek medical care.

12. **C**
    Uremia is the buildup of nitrogenous waste products in the blood from inadequate elimination as a result of kidney failure. Symptoms include anorexia, nausea and vomiting, muscle cramps, pruritus (itching), fatigue, and lethargy. Anuria is failure of kidneys to produce urine; oliguria is the production of abnormally small amounts of urine; and azotemia is the buildup of nitrogenous waste products in the blood.

13. **D**
    With assessment, inspection comes first. The nurse inspects the abdomen and the flank regions with the client in both supine and sitting positions. He or she observes for asymmetry (e.g., swelling) or discoloration (e.g., bruising or redness) in the flank region, especially in the area of the costovertebral angle (CVA). The CVA is located between the lower portion of the 12th rib and the vertebral column. Auscultation for bruits comes next. Auscultation is completed before percussion and palpation because these activities can alter bowel sounds and obscure abdominal vascular sounds. Palpation and percussion are usually completed by the health care provider or nurse practitioner.

14. **A, B, D, E**
    To assess for fluid overload, the nurse looks at the skin and tissues which may show edema associated with kidney disease, especially in the pedal (foot), pretibial (shin), and sacral tissues and around the eyes (periorbital). A stethoscope is used to listen to the lungs to determine whether fluid is present. The client is weighed and blood pressure measured as a baseline for later comparisons. A client with chronic kidney failure does not make much urine, thus checking for residual urine with a bladder scanner is not necessary. A sterile sample is not needed unless infection is suspected.

15. **B**
    A bruit is an audible swishing sound produced when the volume of blood or the diameter of the blood vessel changes. It often occurs with blood flow through a narrowed vessel, as in renal artery stenosis.

16. **C**
    A distended bladder sounds dull when percussed. After gently palpating to determine the outline of the distended bladder, the nurse begins percussion on the lower abdomen and continues in the direction of the umbilicus until dull sounds are no longer produced. If the nurse suspects bladder distention, a portable bladder scanner is used to determine the amount of retained urine.

17. **A, B, C, E, F**
    Using a good light source and wearing gloves, the nurse inspects the urethra by examining the

meatus and the tissues around it. Any unusual discharge such as blood, mucus, or pus is noted and recorded. The skin and mucous membranes of surrounding tissues are inspected. The nurse records the presence of lesions, rashes, or other abnormalities of the labia or vaginal opening. Urethral irritation is suspected when the client reports discomfort with urination. The nurse uses this opportunity to remind female clients to clean the perineum by wiping from **front to back** (**not** back to front). The client is taught that the front-to-back technique keeps organisms in stool from coming close to the urethra and decreases the risk for infection.

18. D

A random finding of **proteinuria** (usually albumin in the urine) followed by a series of negative (normal) findings does **not** imply kidney disease. Normal value for protein in the urine is 0-8 mg/dL. The nurse asks the client about recent strenuous exercise because urinary protein levels may be increased with exercise. Other causes of increased protein level include stress, infection, and glomerular disorders.

19. A, C, D, E

Serum creatinine is produced when muscle and other proteins are broken down. Because protein breakdown is usually constant, the serum creatinine level is a **good** indicator of kidney function. *Cystatin-C* measures glomerular filtration rate. Increased levels can be considered a predictor of chronic renal disease. Blood osmolarity is a measure of the overall concentration of particles in the blood and is a good indicator of hydration status. The kidneys excrete or reabsorb water to keep blood osmolarity in the range of 280 to 300 mOsm/kg (mmol/kg). When both the BUN and serum creatinine levels increase at the same rate, the BUN/creatinine ratio remains normal. However, elevations of *both* serum creatinine and BUN levels suggest kidney dysfunction. Blood urea nitrogen *(BUN)* measures the effectiveness of kidney excretion of urea nitrogen, a by-product of protein breakdown in the liver. Other factors influence the BUN level, and an

elevation does **not** always mean that kidney disease is present. WBC level provides more useful information about infection.

20. B, C, E, F

An increased BUN level may indicate liver or kidney disease, dehydration or decreased kidney perfusion, a high-protein diet, infection, stress, steroid use, Gl bleeding, or other situations in which blood is in body tissues. The nurse asks questions about these non-kidney factors that can cause increases in BUN.

21. C

The normal range for blood osmolarity is 280 to 300 mOsm/kg (mmol/kg). When blood osmolarity increases, vasopressin is released. Vasopressin increases the permeability of the distal tubules to water. The nurse assesses the client for signs of dehydration from water loss.

22. A

African-American clients are at **greater** risk for kidney failure than are white clients. The nurse recommends yearly health examinations including urinalysis, checking for the presence of microalbuminuria, and evaluating serum creatinine.

23. D

The normal urine SG is 1.005 to 1.030; usually 1.010 to 1.025. A client may have decreased SG in chronic kidney disease, diabetes insipidus, malignant hypertension, diuretic administration (e.g. furosemide, hydrochlorothiazide), and lithium toxicity.

24. C

Ideally, the urine specimen is collected at the morning's first voiding. Specimens obtained at other times may be too dilute.

25. A, B, C, D, E, F

All of these options are appropriate actions for the nurse to implement to ensure that a 24-hour urine collection is successfully completed. See Box 60.1 Collection of Urine Specimens in your text for additional information.

26. B

This imaging test is used to examine the perfusion, function, and structure of the kidneys by the IV administration of a radioisotope. The isotope is eliminated 6 to 24 hours after the procedure. The nurse encourages the client to drink fluids to aid in excretion of the isotope.

27. D

Ultrasonography usually requires a full bladder. The nurse asks the client to drink 500 to 1000 mL of water about 2 to 3 hours before the test to help fill the bladder. The nurse instructs the client **not** to void after drinking the water until the test is complete.

28. A, B, C, E, F

All of these actions are appropriate to the postprocedural care of a client after a cystoscopy with general anesthesia except option D. Pink-tinged urine is expected after this procedure. However, gross bleeding is not and should be reported immediately. Also, notify the urologist for obvious blood clots and a decrease or absence of urine output. Irrigate the Foley catheter with sterile saline, if prescribed by the urologist.

29. C

After a percutaneous kidney biopsy, the major risk is bleeding into the kidney or into the tissues external from the kidney at the biopsy site. For 24 hours after the biopsy, the nurse monitors the dressing site, vital signs (especially fluctuations in blood pressure), urine output, hemoglobin level, and hematocrit.

30. B

Before bladder scanning, the nurse selects the male or female icon on the bladder scanner. Using the female icon allows the scanner software to subtract the volume of the uterus from any measurement. Use the male icon on all men and on women who have undergone a hysterectomy.

31. A

If no bleeding occurs, the nurse teaches the client that he or she can resume general activities after 24 hours (e.g., light housework, such as cooking or washing dishes). The client is instructed to avoid lifting heavy objects, exercising, or performing other strenuous activities for 1 to 2 weeks after the biopsy procedure. Driving may also be restricted.

61 CHAPTER

Concepts of Care for Patients with Urinary Problems

1. What type of incontinence does the nurse recognize when a 45-year-old female client reports the loss of small amounts of urine during coughing, sneezing, jogging, or lifting?
   A. Urge incontinence
   B. Overflow incontinence
   C. Functional incontinence
   D. Stress incontinence

2. Which is the nurse's **best** action for an ambulatory obese older client with incontinence and dementia?
   A. Teach the client about strategies for weight reduction.
   B. Assist the client to apply estrogen cream.
   C. Provide the client assistance with toileting every 2 hours.
   D. Perform intermittent catheterization on the client.

3. When the nurse takes a history from an older adult, which drugs will he or she recognize as possible contributing factors to urinary incontinence? **Select all that apply.**
   A. Diuretics
   B. Opioid analgesics
   C. Beta$_3$ blockers
   D. Anticholinergic drugs
   E. Topical estrogen
   F. Tricyclic antidepressants

4. What is the nurse's **priority** concern for an older client with urinary incontinence, who is alert and oriented, but refuses to call for help and has fallen while trying to get to the bathroom alone?
   A. Managing incontinence
   B. Initiating fall precautions
   C. Managing noncompliance
   D. Accurately measuring urinary output

5. Which nonsurgical actions would the nurse include in the care of a middle-age female client with stress incontinence? **Select all that apply.**
   A. Suggest keeping a diary of urine leakage, activities, and foods eaten.
   B. Teach performance of pelvic floor (Kegel) exercise therapy.
   C. Encourage the client to take in adequate fluids, especially water.
   D. Instruct the client to consume a glass of cranberry juice every day.
   E. Refer to a registered dietitian nutritionist for diet or weight loss therapy.
   F. Prepare the client for a surgical sling or bladder suspension procedure.

6. Which outcome statement indicates to the nurse that the client's goal for pelvic floor (Kegel) exercises has been met?
   A. Client has no urinary leakage between voidings.
   B. Incontinence is still present, but frequency is decreased.
   C. Client is using fewer absorbent undergarments for protection.
   D. Reports of dysuria are no longer heard from the client.

7. Which questions will the nurse ask to provide effective screening for urinary incontinence by asking clients to respond "always," "sometimes," or "never"? **Select all that apply.**
   A. Do you ever leak urine after drinking two cups of coffee?
   B. Do you ever leak urine or water when you don't want to?
   C. Do you ever leak urine or water when you cough, sneeze, laugh, or exercise?
   D. Do you ever leak urine or water on the way to the toilet?
   E. Do you ever use pads, tissue, or cloth in your underwear to catch urine?
   F. Do you ever talk about leaking urine with your health care provider?

8. Which statement by a client to the nurse indicates that treatment for urge incontinence has been successful?
   A. "I have been using bladder compression and it works."
   B. "I lose a little urine when I sneeze, but I wear a thin pad."
   C. "I had a little trouble at first, but now I go to the toilet every 3 hours."
   D. "I'm doing the exercises, but I think that surgery is my best choice."

9. What is the nurse's **best** advice to a client with urge incontinence regarding fluid intake?
   A. Drink 120 mL every hour or 240 mL every 2 hours and limit fluid intake after dinner.
   B. Drink at least 2000 mL of water every day unless you have a heart problem.
   C. Drinking water is especially good for bladder health so drink as much as you can.
   D. Drink fluid freely in the morning hours but limit fluid intake after going to bed.

10. Which action associated with a habit training bladder program for an older client who is alert but mildly confused will the nurse delegate to the assistive personnel (AP)?
    A. Remind the client when it is time to use the bathroom and assist him or her on a regular schedule.
    B. Help the client record all incidents of incontinence that occur in a bladder diary.
    C. Change the client's incontinence pad or containment briefs every 4 hours.
    D. Gradually encourage the client's independence and increase the intervals between voidings.

11. Which action will the nurse **avoid** to **prevent harm** for a client with overflow incontinence?
    A. The Crede method to help initiating the emptying of the bladder
    B. The Valsalva maneuver when a client has heart disease
    C. Double voiding using a second attempt to empty the bladder
    D. Splinting to compress the bladder and move it into a better position

12. What **priority** information will the nurse teach a client and family about self-catheterization for the long-term problem of incomplete bladder emptying?
    A. Use sterile technique especially if the catheterization will be done by a family member.
    B. Use a large-lumen catheter with good lubrication for rapid emptying of the bladder.
    C. Catheterize yourself after you are incontinent or when your bladder feels distended.
    D. Perform careful handwashing and cleaning of the catheter to prevent risk for infection.

13. For which client prescription for urinary incontinence would the nurse be sure to question the health care provider?
    A. 74-year-old male client with bilateral glaucoma prescribed oxybutynin
    B. Older female client prescribed a thin application of estrogen vaginal cream daily
    C. Female client prescribed mirabegron whose blood pressure is 132/80 mm Hg
    D. Middle-aged male client prescribed imipramine who experiences slight morning dizziness

14. For which client is it appropriate for the nurse to teach intermittent self-catheterization?
    A. 18-year-old client with a severe head injury
    B. 25-year-old male client with paraplegia
    C. 48-year-old female client with stress incontinence
    D. 70-year-old client who wears absorbent briefs

15. In which situations will the nurse appropriately insert a urinary catheter into a client? **Select all that apply.**
    A. Acute urinary retention or bladder obstruction
    B. Accurate measurement of urine volume in critically ill clients
    C. To manage clients who are incontinent
    D. To assist in healing of open sacral wounds in incontinent clients
    E. To provide comfort at end of life
    F. Perioperatively for gynecological surgeries

16. Which actions will the nurse implement to minimize catheter-associated urinary tract infections (CAUTI) on a client care unit? **Select all that apply.**
    A. Leaving urinary catheters in place only as long as needed
    B. Using sterile equipment in the acute care setting when inserting a urinary catheter
    C. Maintaining a closed system by ensuring that catheter tubing connections are sealed securely
    D. Emptying the bag regularly, using a separate, clean container for each client
    E. Ensuring that the drainage spigot does not come into contact with nonsterile surfaces
    F. Securing the catheter to the client's thigh (women) or lower abdomen (men)

17. Which client does the nurse monitor carefully because of **high** risk for developing a complicated urinary tract infection (UTI)?
    A. 26-year-old male who is sexually active but consistently uses condoms
    B. 28-year-old male who has a neurogenic bladder due to a spinal cord injury
    C. 35-year-old woman who has had three full-term deliveries and one miscarriage
    D. 53-year-old woman who has some menstrual irregularities

18. What factors will the nurse recognize as contributors to a client diagnosis of complicated urinary tract infection (UTI)? **Select all that apply.**
    A. Pregnancy
    B. Obstruction
    C. Diabetes
    D. Pulmonary infection
    E. Chronic kidney disease
    F. Decreased immunity

19. Which circumstance is cause for the nurse's **greatest** concern when several clients in the long-term facility have developed urinary tract infections (UTIs)?
    A. Residents are not drinking enough fluids with meals and snacks.
    B. Assistive personnel (AP) are not assisting with toileting in a timely manner.
    C. A large percentage of residents have indwelling urinary catheters.
    D. Many residents have dementia and functional incontinence.

20. Which are the **most common** signs and symptoms of urinary tract infection that the nurse will recognize when assessing a client? **Select all that apply.**
    A. Nocturia
    B. Frequency
    C. Hematuria
    D. Urgency
    E. Suprapubic tenderness
    F. Dysuria

21. Which **priority** instructions will the nurse teach the client and family to **prevent harm** from urinary tract infections (UTIs) after discharge? **Select all that apply.**
    A. Drink fluids liberally, as much as 2 to 3 liters daily if not contraindicated by health problems.
    B. Be sure to get enough sleep, rest, and nutrition daily to maintain immunologic health.
    C. Do not routinely delay urination because the flow of urine can help remove bacteria that may be colonizing the urethra or bladder.
    D. For both men and women, gently wash the perineal area before intercourse.
    E. For women, be sure to douche before and after sexual intercourse.
    F. If spermicides are used, consider changing to another method of contraception.

22. What diagnostic test does the nurse expect the urologist to prescribe for a client with a urinary tract infection (UTI) who developed signs and symptoms of urosepsis (bacteremia)?
    A. Blood cultures
    B. Urine culture
    C. Culture of urinary meatus
    D. Repeat urinalysis

23. What problem will the nurse suspect when a client reports urgency, frequency, and bladder pain but the urinalysis shows a few white blood cells and red blood cells, but no bacteria and the urine culture results are negative?
    A. Interstitial cystitis
    B. Urethritis
    C. Kidney stones
    D. Incompletely treated bacterial cystitis

24. Which clients diagnosed with urinary tract infection (UTI) may need longer antibiotic treatment? **Select all that apply.**
    A. Postmenopausal woman
    B. Diabetic woman
    C. Immunosuppressed male
    D. Female client prescribed birth control
    E. Pregnant woman
    F. Older male with complicated UTI

25. Which intracollaborative therapy does the nurse expect the health care provider to prescribe for a postmenopausal client diagnosed with noninfectious urethritis?
    A. Antibiotic therapy
    B. Frequent sitz baths
    C. Estrogen vaginal cream
    D. Culture of drainage

26. Which circumstance does the nurse recognize as creating the **greatest** risk of recurrent urolithiasis when a client is admitted for an orthopedic procedure?
    A. Providing milk to the client with every meal tray or snack
    B. Insertion of an indwelling urinary catheter for the procedure
    C. Restricting foods and fluids for extended periods of time
    D. Administering an opioid narcotic drug for the severe pain

27. What is the nurse's **best** interpretation when a client is admitted with flank pain, and the urine report indicates turbidity, foul odor, rust color, presence of white and red blood cells as well as bacteria, and microscopic crystals?
    A. Staghorn calculus with infection
    B. Urolithiasis and infection
    C. Pyuria and cystitis
    D. Dysuria and urinary retention

28. What is the **priority** nursing concern when a client is admitted with a history of kidney stones and presents with severe flank pain, nausea and vomiting, pallor, and diaphoresis?
    A. Possible hemorrhage
    B. Urinary elimination blockage
    C. Impaired tissue perfusion
    D. Severe pain

29. Which **essential** nursing intervention will the nurse implement when a client returns from having shock wave lithotripsy?
    A. Strain the urine to monitor for the passage of stone fragments.
    B. Report bruising on the affected side immediately to the urologist.
    C. Apply a local anesthetic cream to the client's skin on the affected side.
    D. Continuously monitor the client's heart pattern for dysrhythmias.

30. Which information will the nurse include when teaching a client self-care measures after shock wave lithotripsy for kidney stones? **Select all that apply.**
    A. Finish the entire prescription of antibiotics to prevent infection.
    B. Pain in the region of the kidneys or bladder is to be expected.
    C. Balance regular exercise with adequate sleep and rest.
    D. Drink at the very least 3 liters of fluids every day.
    E. Your urine may appear bloody for a few days after the procedure.
    F. Watch for and immediately report any bruising to the urologist.

31. Which report or manifestation indicates to the nurse that a client's treatment for renal colic has been successful?
    A. Urine is pink tinged.
    B. Urine output is 50 mL per hour.
    C. Bladder scan shows no residual urine.
    D. Client reports that pain is relieved.

32. Which client would the nurse expect is at **highest** risk for development of bladder cancer?
    A. 25-year-old woman who has experienced three episodes of bacterial cystitis over the past year
    B. 27-year-old man with type 1 diabetes who is nonadherent with his therapeutic regimen
    C. 60-year-old woman with malnutrition secondary to chronic alcoholism and self-neglect
    D. 64-year-old man who smokes two packs of cigarettes a day and works in a chemical factory

33. Which urinary characteristic **most** concerns the nurse when assessing a client whose lifestyle choices and occupational exposure indicate a **high risk** for bladder cancer?
    A. Painless hematuria
    B. Occasional incontinence
    C. Increased nocturia
    D. Frequent voidings

34. Which home care instructions will the nurse provide the client who receives intravesical instillation of bacille Calmette-Guerin. At the outpatient clinic to prevent recurrence of superficial bladder cancer?
    A. "Your urine will be radioactive for 24 hours so avoid contact with children and pregnant women."
    B. "Drink a lot of extra fluid to flush your bladder but otherwise there are no special instructions."
    C. "For 24 hours others should not share your toilet and then you should clean it with 10% bleach before anyone else uses it."
    D. "Flush the toilet twice after every voiding and remind all family members to practice safe hand hygiene."

Chapter 61 Answer Key

1. D
   The most common type of incontinence in younger women is stress incontinence. Its main feature is the inability to retain urine when laughing, coughing, sneezing, jogging, or lifting. Clients with stress incontinence cannot tighten the urethra enough to overcome the increased bladder pressure caused by contraction of the detrusor muscle.

2. C
   The client has dementia and is cognitively impaired, which leads to functional incontinence. Habit training (scheduled toileting) is a type of bladder training that is successful in reducing incontinence in cognitively impaired clients. To use habit training, caregivers help the client void at specific times (e.g., every 2 hours on the even hours). The goal is to get the client to the toilet before incontinence occurs. The nurse could assign this assistance to an LPN/LVN or delegate it to the assistive personnel (AP).

3. A, B, D
   Diuretics cause frequent urination, often in large amounts. Opioid analgesics decrease a client's level of consciousness and awareness of the need to void. Anticholinergic drugs affect the ability to urinate as well as cognition. Beta$_3$ blockers, estrogen cream, and tricyclic antidepressants are used to treat incontinence.

4. B
   A common cause of falls in health care facilities is related to client efforts to get out of bed unassisted to use the toilet. The nurse collaborates with all staff members, including assistive personnel (AP), to consistently implement a toileting schedule and prevent incontinence.

5. A, B, C, E
   Options A, B, C, and E are appropriate nonsurgical stress incontinence management strategies. Option D, the use of cranberry juice may be recommended to prevent urinary tract infections, but does not affect incontinence. Surgical sling or bladder suspension procedures are both surgical management options for treatment of stress incontinence.

6. A
   With appropriate therapy, the client with altered urinary elimination due to incontinence is expected to develop continence of urine elimination. For stress urinary incontinence, the best indicator is no urine leakage between voidings and no urine leakage with increased abdominal pressure (e.g., sneezing, laughing, lifting).

7. B, C, D, E
   Incontinence may be underreported because health care professionals do not ask clients

about urine loss. Many clients are hesitant to initiate the subject. Effective screening includes asking clients to respond "always," "sometimes," or "never" to these questions:

- Do you ever leak urine or water when you don't want to?
- Do you ever leak urine or water when you cough, sneeze, laugh, or exercise?
- Do you ever leak urine or water on the way to the toilet?
- Do you ever use pads, tissue, or cloth in your underwear to catch urine?

8. C
For urge urinary incontinence, the best outcome is that the client responds to the urge in a timely manner, gets to toilet between urge and passage of urine, and avoids substances that stimulate the bladder (e.g., caffeine, alcohol).

9. A
For urge urinary incontinence, the nurse teaches the client to avoid foods that irritate the bladder such as caffeine and alcohol. Spacing fluids at regular intervals throughout the day (e.g., 120 mL every hour or 240 mL every 2 hours) and limiting fluids after the dinner hour (e.g., only 120 mL at bedtime) help avoid fluid overload on the bladder and allow urine to collect at a steady pace.

10. A
The nurse collaborates with all staff members, including assistive personnel (AP), to consistently implement the toileting schedule for habit training. The scope of practice for an AP includes assisting clients with toileting and reminding them when it is time to use the bathroom. Habit training is undermined when absorbent briefs are used in place of timed toileting. Do not tell clients to "just wet the bed."

11. B
The Valsalva maneuver is contraindicated in clients who have some cardiac problems because it can trigger a vagal response and cause bradycardia.

12. D
The nurse focuses on these important points when teaching the intermittent self-catheterization technique: proper handwashing and cleaning of the catheter to reduce the risk for infection; a small lumen and good lubrication of the catheter prevent urethral trauma; and a regular schedule for bladder emptying prevents distention and mucosal trauma. Clients must be able to understand instructions and have the manual dexterity to manipulate the catheter. Caregivers or family members in the home can also be taught to perform intermittent catheterization using clean (rather than sterile) technique with good outcomes.

13. A
Oyxbutynin is an anticholinergic drug. The nurse asks whether the client has glaucoma before starting any drugs from this class because anticholinergics can increase intraocular pressure and make glaucoma worse.

14. B
Clients for whom intermittent catheterization or other alternatives to indwelling catheters are considered include those with spinal cord injuries or conditions. The client who performs this procedure must be able and willing to learn, as well as have the dexterity to complete it safely.

15. A, B, D, E, F
All of these situations are appropriate for insertion of a urinary catheter except for option C, the management of incontinence. There are many other strategies and interventions that can be used successfully to treat incontinence. Remember that the longer a urinary catheter is in place, the more risk for the client to develop a urinary tract infection (UTI).

16. A, B, C, D, E, F
All of these options are appropriate actions for the nurse to implement to prevent the occurrence of CAUTIs. For additional suggestions, see Best Practice for Patient Safety & Quality Care **QSEN** Minimizing Catheter-Associated Urinary Tract Infections (CAUTI) in your text.

17. B
Neurogenic bladder is among the factors that contribute to a diagnosis of complicated UTI.

18. A, B, C, E, F
Some factors and conditions that contribute to a diagnosis of complicated UTI are pregnancy, male gender, obstruction, diabetes, neurogenic bladder, chronic kidney disease, and reduced immunity. Pulmonary infection does not contribute to complicated UTI diagnosis.

19. C
The major concern is that many clients in the facility have indwelling urinary catheters. Ensuring that urinary catheters are used appropriately and discontinued as early as possible is essential. Catheters must not be left in place for staff convenience. Indwelling catheters are a major factor for the number of catheter-associated urinary tract infections (CAUTI).

20. B, D, F
Frequency, urgency, and dysuria are the most common symptoms of a urinary tract infection (UTI), but other symptoms may be present. See Key Features of UTI in your text for additional symptoms that may also be noted when a client has a UTI.

21. A, B, C, D, F
The nurse teaches all of these options to prevent a UTI, except option E. Women must be taught to **avoid** using irritating substances such as douches, scented lubricants for intercourse, bubble bath, tight-fitting underwear, and scented toilet tissue.

22. A
The spread of the infection from the urinary tract to the bloodstream is termed bacteremia or urosepsis. Catheter-associated urinary tract infections are the leading cause of urosepsis. To determine which organism is in the bloodstream, blood culture samples are ordered.

23. A
Cystoscopy is needed to accurately diagnose interstitial (noninfectious) cystitis. A urinalysis usually shows WBCs and RBCs but no bacteria.

24. B, C, E, F
Longer antibiotic treatment (7 to 21 days) is required for hospitalized clients and those with complicated UTIs (e.g., men, pregnant women, and clients with anatomic, functional or metabolic derangements that affect the urinary tract). Men in general need longer antibiotic treatment. Postmenopausal women or women taking birth control pills do not require longer treatment.

25. C
Noninfectious urethritis symptoms usually resolve spontaneously over time, regardless of treatment. Postmenopausal women often have improvement in urethral symptoms with the use of estrogen vaginal cream. Estrogen cream applied in a thin layer locally to the vagina increases the amount of estrogen in the urethra as well, reducing irritating symptoms.

26. C
The nurse urges clients to drink enough fluids to maintain dilute urine throughout the day and night unless fluid restriction is needed for another health problem. Some urologists recommend sufficient fluid intake to result in at least 1.5 L of urine output or 7 to 12 voidings daily. Food can provide 20% or more of fluid intake, particularly the intake of fruits and vegetables. Insufficient fluid intake can lead to recurrent urolithiasis (the presence of *calculi* [stones] in the urinary tract). A history of calculi in the urinary tract is also a risk factor for recurrence.

27. B
Hematuria during renal colic is common, and blood may make the urine appear smoky or rusty. RBCs are usually caused by stone-induced trauma to the lining of the ureter, bladder, or urethra. WBCs and bacteria may be present as a result of urinary stasis. Increased turbidity (cloudiness) and odor indicate that infection may also be present. Thus, the nurse's best interpretation of these results is urolithiasis with infection.

28. D
The major symptom of stones is severe pain, commonly called renal colic. Drug therapy is needed in the first 24 to 36 hours when pain is most severe. Opioid analgesics are used to

control the severe pain caused by stones in the urinary tract and may be given IV for rapid pain relief.

29. A

After lithotripsy, the nurse implements straining the urine to monitor the passage of stone fragments. Bruising on the affected side is expected after this procedure. Anesthetic cream is not needed after the procedure, nor is cardiac monitoring.

30. A, C, D, E

Options A, C, D, and E include important content for the nurse to teach a client for self-management after lithotripsy. See Patient and Family Education: Preparing for Self-Management Urinary Calculi in your text for additional content to teach a client after lithotripsy.

31. D

Renal colic is the severe pain that occurs with the presence of kidney stones. When the treatment is successful, the client's pain is relieved.

32. D

Exposure to toxins such as gasoline and diesel fuel, as well as to chemicals used in hair dyes and in the rubber, paint, electric cable, and textile industries, increases the risk for bladder cancer. The **greatest risk** factor for bladder cancer is tobacco use.

33. A

The nurse's highest concern is blood in the urine because it is often the **first** indication of bladder cancer. It may be gross or microscopic and is usually painless and intermittent.

34. C

Prophylactic immunotherapy with intravesical instillation of bacille Calmette-Guérin (BCG), a live virus compound, is used to prevent tumor recurrence of superficial cancers. Usually the agent is instilled in an outpatient cancer clinic and allowed to dwell in the bladder for a specified length of time. When the client urinates, live virus is excreted with the urine. The nurse teaches clients receiving this treatment to prevent contact of the live virus with other members of the household by **not** sharing a toilet with others for at least 24 hours after instillation. Instruct men to urinate while sitting down to avoid splashing the urine. After 24 hours, the toilet should be completely cleaned using a solution of 10% liquid bleach.

62 CHAPTER

Concepts of Care for Patients with Kidney Disorders

1. Which findings will the nurse assess when a client is experiencing problems with urinary elimination caused by acute pyelonephritis? **Select all that apply.**
   A. Hypertension
   B. Pain and burning with urination
   C. Client reports back, flank, or loin pain
   D. Urine is cloudy and has a foul odor
   E. Client produces large amounts of dilute urine
   F. Urine sample is dark or smoky colored

2. What **priority** question will the nurse be sure to ask a client at risk for acute pyelonephritis?
   A. "Have you recently been treated for a urinary tract infection?"
   B. "Are you taking birth control pills as contraception?"
   C. "Do your have a family history of stroke or myocardial infarction?"
   D. "Have you ever leaked urine when laughing, jogging, or coughing?"

3. Which laboratory tests would the nurse expect the health care provider to order when a client has acute pyelonephritis? **Select all that apply.**
   A. Urine culture for specific infective organism to be treated
   B. Complete blood count with differential to monitor for increased WBCs
   C. Urinalysis for bacteria, leucocyte esterase, nitrate, and RBCs
   D. C-reactive protein and erythrocyte sedimentation rate (ESR) to determine immune response and inflammation
   E. Blood urea nitrogen (BUN) and serum creatinine levels to monitor for elevation
   F. Test to determine whether a woman is pregnant

4. Which client will the nurse monitor carefully for **highest** risk of developing acute pyelonephritis?
   A. 32-year-old man with diabetes insipidus
   B. 34-year-old woman with diabetes mellitus in the second trimester of pregnancy
   C. 75-year-old man who drinks four beers each day
   D. 78-year-old woman prescribed diuretics for mild heart failure

5. Which client findings cause the nurse to suspect the possibility of chronic pyelonephritis? **Select all that apply.**
   A. Sudden onset of massive proteinuria
   B. Inability to conserve sodium
   C. Decreased urine-concentrating ability and nocturia
   D. Abscess formation
   E. Hypertension
   F. Hyperkalemia and acidosis

6. Which condition **best** indicates to the nurse that a client's fluid intake is sufficient to manage acute pyelonephritis?
   A. Client estimates an intake of 1.5 liters of water per day.
   B. Client reports no burning or pain with urination.
   C. Urine output is clear yellow and dilute.
   D. Antibiotic treatment was completed exactly as prescribed.

7. Which information is **most important** for the nurse to include when teaching a client and family about home care for acute pyelonephritis? **Select all that apply.**
   A. Role of nutrition and adequate fluid intake
   B. Need for a balance between rest and activity
   C. Signs and symptoms of disease recurrence
   D. Use of successful coping mechanisms
   E. Care of a permanent indwelling catheter
   F. Drug regimen (purpose, timing, frequency, duration, and possible side effects)

8. What **priority** finding will the nurse assess for when inspecting the hands, face, and eyelids of a client with possible acute glomerulonephritis (GN)?
   A. Redness
   B. Rash
   C. Dryness
   D. Edema

9. What is the nurse's **next** action after assessing a client with glomerulonephritis (GN) who reports mild shortness of breath and finding crackles in all lung fields, distended neck veins?
   A. Obtaining a urine sample to check for proteinuria
   B. Checking for costovertebral angle tenderness or flank pain
   C. Assessing carefully for additional signs of fluid overload
   D. Alerting the health care provider about the respiratory symptoms

10. What results will the nurse expect from a 24-hour urine test for total protein when a client is diagnosed with glomerulonephritis (GN)?
    A. Protein excretion rate may be increased from 500 mg/24 hr to 3 g/24 hr.
    B. Protein excretion rate may be decreased from 500 mg/24 hr to 250 mg/24 hr.
    C. Protein excretion rate will be within normal limits for the client.
    D. Protein excretion rate will vary from normal to slightly increased.

11. Which interventions will the nurse expect to implement for management of infection as the cause for glomerulonephritis (GN)? **Select all that apply.**
    A. Corticosteroids
    B. Antibiotics
    C. Cytotoxic drugs
    D. Personal hygiene
    E. Fluid restriction
    F. Handwashing

12. When a client with glomerulonephritis has a urine output over the past 24 hours of 1050 mL, how much fluid will the nurse allow the client during the next 24-hour period?
    A. 1050 to 1150 mL
    B. 1250 to 1350 mL
    C. 1450 to 1550 mL
    D. 1550 to 1650 mL

13. Which symptoms will the nurse expect to find on assessment when a client with chronic glomerulonephritis (GN) develops uremia? **Select all that apply.**
    A. Ataxia
    B. Slurred speech
    C. Neck vein distention
    D. Asterixis
    E. Crackles in lung bases
    F. Itching

14. When the nurse reviews laboratory values for a client with chronic glomerulonephritis, and the serum phosphorus level is 5.3 mg/dL, which other change does the nurse expect to see?
    A. Serum calcium level is low normal or slightly below normal
    B. Serum potassium level below the normal range
    C. Elevated serum sodium levels related to dehydration
    D. Elevated chloride levels related to elevated sodium

15. Which actions will the nurse delegate to the assistive personnel (AP) for appropriate care of a client with acute glomerulonephritis?
    A. Teaching how to collect a 24-hour urine specimen
    B. Weighing the client every morning with the same scale
    C. Assessing for changes in the urine sample
    D. Evaluating the client's ability to safely get to the bathroom

16. Which health problem does the nurse suspect when a client with decreased kidney function has increased proteinuria, decreased serum albumin, lipids in blood and urine, increased aPTT and INR, facial edema, and hypertension?
    A. Glomerulonephritis
    B. Pyelonephritis
    C. Nephrotic syndrome
    D. Chronic kidney failure

17. Which nursing and collaborative actions are implemented by the nurse when caring for a client with nephrotic syndrome (NS)? **Select all that apply.**
    A. Administration of mild diuretics
    B. Fluid restrictions
    C. Frequent assessment of hydration status
    D. Administration of angiotensin-converting enzyme inhibitors
    E. Collection of urine sample for culture
    F. Assessment for periorbital swelling

18. What is the **priority** action the nurse will take for a client admitted with nephrotic syndrome (NS) who has proteinuria, hypertension, lipidemia, and facial edema?
    A. Monitoring client's fluid volume and hydration status
    B. Consulting with registered dietician nutritionist about adequate intake
    C. Using clean and sterile techniques to prevent infections
    D. Teaching the client about and preparing for a renal biopsy

19. Which factors promote long-term adherence to the prescribed antihypertensive drug therapy for a client diagnosed with nephrosclerosis? **Select all that apply.**
    A. Monthly reminders
    B. Once-a-day dosing
    C. Written drug information
    D. Low cost
    E. Minimal side effects
    F. Eliminating diet restrictions

20. Which questions will the nurse ask a client suspected of having polycystic kidney disease (PKD)? **Select all that apply.**
    A. "Do you have a family history of PKD or kidney disease?"
    B. "Have you ever had any problems with muscle aches or joint pains?"
    C. "Do you have any problems with headaches?"
    D. "Have you had any difficulty with constipation or abdominal discomfort?"
    E. "Do you have a history of any sexually transmitted infections?"
    F. "Have you noticed any changes in the color or frequency of urine?"

21. What **early** sign would the nurse expect when a client is suspected of autosomal dominant polycystic kidney disease (ADPKD)?
    A. Headache
    B. Nocturia
    C. Pruritus
    D. Facial edema

22. Which self-care management techniques will the nurse teach a client with polycystic kidney disease (PKD) to prevent constipation? **Select all that apply.**
    A. Consume adequate fluid intake of 2 to 3 liters daily.
    B. Use stool softeners daily.
    C. Take NSAIDs for discomfort.
    D. Avoid aspirin-containing drugs.
    E. Maintain your fiber intake and exercise regularly.
    F. Increase your dietary protein intake with meals.

23. For which minimal risk diagnostic test will the nurse prepare the client with polycystic kidney disease to have as initial screening?
    A. Kidney-ureter-bladder (KUB) x-rays
    B. Computed tomography with angiography
    C. Renal ultrasonography
    D. Renal needle biopsy

24. For which symptoms or changes will the nurse instruct a client with polycystic kidney disease (PKD) to contact the health care provider immediately? **Select all that apply.**
    A. Presence of a foul urine odor
    B. Going more than 1 day between bowel movements
    C. Development of a headache that does not go away
    D. Getting up twice nightly to urinate
    E. Experiencing a sudden weight gain
    F. Consuming some small salty pretzels

25. What is the nurse's **priority** concern when caring for clients with hydronephrosis or hydroureter?
    A. Dilute urine
    B. Dehydration
    C. Pain with urination
    D. Obstruction

26. What does the nurse suspect when assessment reveals a distended bladder and the client reports passing very small amounts of urine today despite a normal fluid intake and feeling the urge to urinate?
    A. Urethral stricture
    B. Polycystic kidney disease
    C. Hydroureter
    D. Hydronephrosis

27. Which finding will the nurse associate with an obstruction in the urinary system **specifically** associated with hydronephrosis?
    A. Chills and fever
    B. Flank asymmetry
    C. Urge incontinence
    D. Bladder distention

28. Which client signs and symptoms cause the nurse to suspect the possibility of renovascular disease? **Select all that apply.**
    A. Sudden onset of hypertension
    B. Distended bladder on palpation
    C. Difficult to control hypertension
    D. Sustained hyperglycemia
    E. Elevated serum creatinine
    F. Decreased glomerular filtration rate

29. What is the nurse's **best** response when a client with renovascular disease asks why the endovascular procedure, stent placement, is preferable to surgery to correct his or her condition?
    A. "The procedure will make a bypass route for blood to enter your kidney and does not leave a scar."
    B. "Stent placement is less risky and requires less time for recovery than does renal artery bypass surgery."
    C. "A synthetic blood vessel graft is inserted to redirect blood flow from the abdominal aorta into the renal artery."
    D. "An endovascular procedure is more cost-effective and does not need to be repeated."

30. Which postoperative action will the nurse take for a client who had a nephrostomy and a nephrostomy tube is now in place?
    A. Monitor the amount of drainage in the collection bag.
    B. Keep the client NPO for at least 6 to 8 hours.
    C. Irrigate the tube until the return drainage is clear.
    D. Instruct the client to sleep with the operative side down.

31. What is the nurse's **best** response when a client with kidney cancer, who had a nephrectomy, asks if the remaining kidney can take over kidney function immediately?
    A. "Your remaining kidney isn't able to provide adequate function, so other therapies will be necessary."
    B. "That's a good question. We'll ask your health care provider about it during next rounds."
    C. "The kidney you have left will provide adequate function, but it may take a few days or weeks."
    D. "It varies from person to person, but you can expect normal kidney function to return the same day."

32. Which therapy does the nurse expect after a client's nephrectomy to prevent an adrenal complication?
    A. Administration of a potassium supplement
    B. Prescription for steroid supplement
    C. Addition of extra calcium to diet
    D. Estrogen supplements for postmenopausal women

33. Which assessment findings will the nurse expect to see documented when a client is first admitted with renal cell carcinoma?
    A. Gross hematuria, hypertension, diabetes, and oliguria
    B. Flank pain, blood in the urine, palpable renal mass, and renal bruit
    C. Nocturia and urinary retention with difficulty initiating the urine stream
    D. Dysuria, polyuria, dehydration, and palpable kidney mass

34. What will the nurse teach a client and family about prevention of kidney and genitourinary trauma? **Select all that apply.**
    A. Wear a seat belt.
    B. Practice safe walking habits.
    C. Use caution when riding bicycles and motorcycles.
    D. Wear appropriate protective clothing when participating in contact sports.
    E. Avoid all contact sports and high-risk activities if you have only one kidney.
    F. Penetrating trauma is responsible for most kidney injuries.

Chapter 62 Answer Key

1. B, C, D, F
   Options B, C, D, and F are manifestations of acute pyelonephritis. See Key features of Acute Pyelonephritis in your text for additional signs and symptoms. Hypertension occurs with chronic pyelonephritis. Urine will be decreased and have characteristics of infections (e.g., turbidity, foul odor), not dilute.

2. A
   Acute pyelonephritis is an active bacterial infection, which results from bacterial infection, with or without obstruction or reflux. An important feature is recent cystitis or treatment for urinary tract infection (UTI).

3. A, B, C, D, E, F
   The nurse expects that all of these laboratory tests will be ordered to determine the presence of acute pyelonephritis.

4. B
   The woman in option B has two risk factors for pyelonephritis: diabetes and pregnancy. Pyelonephritis from an ascending infection may follow manipulation of the urinary tract (e.g., placement of a urinary catheter), particularly in clients who have reduced immunity or diabetes. Hormonal changes as well as obstruction caused by the fetus during pregnancy make acute pyelonephritis more common during the second trimester and beginning of the third trimester.

5. B, C, E, F
   The nurse recognizes manifestations that define chronic pyelonephritis from acute by the following characteristics: hypertension; inability to conserve sodium; decreased urine-concentrating ability, resulting in nocturia; and a tendency to develop hyperkalemia and acidosis.

6. C
Fluid intake is recommended at 2 L/day, sufficient to result in dilute (pale yellow) urine, unless another health problem requires fluid restriction.

7. A, B, C, D, F
All of these options are taught by the nurse to the client and family before discharge except option E. Clients are rarely discharged with a urinary catheter in place, and chronic urinary catheter care is only taught if necessary.

8. D
The nurse assesses a client's face, eyelids, hands, as well as other areas for edema because this is present in most clients with acute GN.

9. C
The nurse assesses for fluid overload and pulmonary edema that may result from fluid and sodium retention occurring with acute GN. He or she asks about any difficulty breathing or shortness of breath. Assessment for crackles in the lung fields, an S_3 heart sound (gallop rhythm), and neck vein distention would also be completed. With this information, the nurse would then notify the health care provider of the findings.

10. A
When a 24-hour urine collection for total protein is obtained, the nurse expects the protein excretion rate for clients with acute GN to be increased from 500 mg/24 hr to 3 g/24 hr.

11. B, D, F
Managing infection as a cause of acute GN begins with appropriate antibiotic therapy. Penicillin, erythromycin, or azithromycin is prescribed for GN caused by streptococcal infection. The nurse stresses personal hygiene and basic infection control principles (e.g., handwashing) to prevent spread of the organism. Clients are taught the importance of completing the entire course of the prescribed antibiotic.
Corticosteroids and cytotoxic drugs are used for GN that is **not** caused by infection. Fluid

restriction may be used with the complication of fluid overload.

12. D
For clients with fluid overload, hypertension, and edema, diuretics and sodium and water restrictions are prescribed. The usual fluid allowance is equal to the previous 24-hour urine output plus 500 to 600 mL. In this case the client would be allowed 1050 mL plus 500 to 600 mL which equals 1550 to 1650 mL for the next 24 hours.

13. A, B, D, F
Uremic symptoms include slurred speech, ataxia, tremors, or asterixis (flapping tremor of the fingers or the inability to maintain a fixed posture with the arms extended and wrists hyperextended). Skin symptoms of uremia include a yellowish color, texture changes, bruises, rashes, or eruptions. Itching and areas of dryness or excoriation from scratching are often present.

14. A
The client's phosphorus level is elevated, so the nurse expects the client's calcium level to below normal, or slightly below normal. This occurs because calcium and phosphorus exist in the blood in a balanced reciprocal relationship. Whenever one electrolyte is elevated, the other is decreased.

15. B
The scope of practice for an AP includes assisting with activities of daily living, weighing the client, assisting to the bathroom and other ambulation. The nurse instructs the AP to weigh the client every morning at the same time, wearing the same amount of clothes, and using the same scale. Teaching, assessing, and evaluating are higher level skills performed by the professional RN.

16. C
Signs and symptoms of nephrotic syndrome (NS) include sudden onset of: massive proteinuria; hypoalbuminemia; edema (especially facial and periorbital); lipiduria; hyperlipidemia;

delayed clotting or increased bleeding with higher-than-normal values for serum activated partial thromboplastin time (aPTT) coagulation or international normalized ratio for prothrombin (INR, PT); and reduced kidney function with elevated blood urea nitrogen (BUN) and serum creatinine and decreased glomerular filtration rate (GFR).

17. A, C, D, F
Angiotensin-converting enzyme inhibitors (ACEIs) can decrease protein loss in the urine and lower blood pressure for clients with NS. Mild diuretics and sodium restriction may be needed to control edema (facial and periorbital) and hypertension. The nurse assesses the client's hydration status because vascular dehydration is common.

18. A
The nurse's priority action is to assess the client's fluid volume and hydration status. Assessing the client's hydration status is essential because vascular dehydration is common. If plasma volume is depleted, kidney problems worsen.

19. B, D, E
Although many antihypertensive drugs may lower blood pressure, the client's response is important in ensuring long-term adherence to the prescribed therapy. Factors that promote adherence include once-a-day dosing, low cost, and minimal side effects.

20. A, C, D, F
The nurse gathers essential information when taking a client's history. Explore the family history of a client with suspected or actual PKD and ask whether either parent was known to have PKD or whether there is any family history of kidney disease. Important information to obtain includes the age at which the problem was diagnosed in the parent and any related complications. Ask about pain, abdominal discomfort, constipation, changes in urine color or frequency, hypertension, headaches, and a family history of stroke or sudden death.

21. B
Nocturia (the need to urinate excessively at night) is an early symptom and occurs because of decreased urine-concentrating ability when a client develops PKD.

22. A, B, E
The nurse teaches the client who has adequate urine output to prevent constipation by maintaining adequate fluid intake (generally 2 to 3 liters daily in food and beverages), maintaining dietary fiber intake, and exercising regularly. The client is advised about the use of stool softeners and bulk agents, including careful use of laxatives, to prevent chronic constipation. Aspirin-containing drugs are avoided to decrease the risk of bleeding, not constipation. NSAIDs are used cautiously because they can reduce kidney blood flow, but do not cause constipation. Protein intake may be limited to slow the development of end-stage kidney disease (ESKD), but is not an action that will reduce constipation.

23. C
Ultrasound is the primary method for diagnosing PKD. The size of the kidney is measured by ultrasound as well as cysts within the kidney.

24. A, C, E
The nurse teaches a client and family to notify the primary health care provider for sudden weight gain, headache that does not go away, and for changes in urine such as a foul odor and new-onset blood in the urine. Missing a bowel movement for 1 day is not enough to establish constipation. Nocturia is characteristic of PKD. Consuming salty foods is a concern because of sodium restrictions, but eating a few small pretzels does not require notification of the primary health care provider.

25. D
Hydronephrosis and hydroureter are problems of urinary elimination with outflow **obstruction**. Urethral strictures obstruct urine outflow and may contribute to bladder distention, hydroureter, and hydronephrosis. Prompt recognition and treatment are crucial to preventing permanent kidney damage.

26. A

Urethral strictures obstruct urine outflow and may contribute to development of bladder distention, hydroureter, and hydronephrosis.

27. B

In hydronephrosis, the kidney enlarges as urine collects in the renal pelvis and kidney tissue. Because the capacity of the renal pelvis is normally 5 to 8 mL, obstruction in the renal pelvis or at the point where the ureter joins the renal pelvis quickly distends the renal pelvis. Since this condition usually affects only one kidney, flank asymmetry is often present due to the enlarged kidney.

28. A, C, D, E, F

All of these options suggest a diagnosis of renovascular disease except option B, distended bladder. Renovascular disease includes processes affecting the renal arteries that may severely **narrow** the lumens and greatly reduce blood flow to the kidney tissues.

29. B

Endovascular techniques are nonsurgical approaches to repair renal artery stenosis. Stent placement with or without balloon angioplasty is an example of an endovascular intervention. These techniques are less risky and require less time for recovery than does renal artery bypass surgery. The procedure does not create a bypass route. Depending on other client factors, the procedure may need to be repeated.

30. A

The nurse monitors the nephrostomy site for leaking urine or blood as well as amount of drainage. Urine drainage may be bloody for the first 12 to 24 hours after the procedure but should gradually clear. If prescribed, the nephrostomy tube can be irrigated with 5 mL sterile saline to check patency and dislodge clots. However, the volume used for this purpose is not intended to irrigate the nephrostomy until urine drainage is clear. Diuresis can occur once the tube is in place.

31. C

Although overall kidney function decreases after a nephrectomy, the remaining kidney tissue usually works well enough for a healthy life. It may take a few days or weeks for the remaining kidney to assume all kidney functions.

32. B

Adrenal insufficiency is possible as a complication when a kidney and adrenal gland are removed. Although only one adrenal gland may be affected, the remaining gland may not be able to secrete sufficient glucocorticoids immediately after surgery and steroid replacements may be needed.

33. B

Clients with renal cell carcinoma (RCC) have flank pain, obvious blood in the urine, and a kidney mass that can be palpated. The abdominal mass may be felt with *gentle* palpation and a renal bruit may be heard on auscultation.

34. A, B, C, D, E

All of these options are appropriate for the nurse to teach a client and family for prevention of traumatic kidney or genitourinary injuries except option F. The main cause of kidney trauma is blunt injuries.

63

CHAPTER

Concepts of Care for Patients with Acute Kidney Injury and Chronic Kidney Disease

1. Which criteria does the nurse understand are included in the current definition of acute kidney injury (AKI)? **Select all that apply.**
   A. Signs and symptoms of fluid overload such as peripheral edema and crackles in the lungs
   B. Urine volume of less than 0.5 mL/kg/hr for 6 hours
   C. Presence of polyuria, nocturia, and very dilute pale yellow urine
   D. Increase in serum creatinine by 0.3 mg/dL (26.2 µmol/L) or more within 48 hours
   E. Hypotension and tachycardia with progressively decreased amounts of urine
   F. Increase in serum creatinine to 1.5 times or more from baseline in the previous 7 days

2. For which causes will the nurse monitor clients for development of intrarenal (intrinsic) acute kidney injury (AKI)? **Select all that apply.**
   A. Glomerulonephritis
   B. Bladder cancer
   C. Exposure to nephrotoxins
   D. Embolism in renal blood vessels
   E. Severe dehydration
   F. Kidney stones

3. When prerenal and postrenal causes of acute kidney injury occur, how does the nurse expect a client's kidneys to compensate? **Select all that apply.**
   A. Constricting of blood vessels in the kidneys
   B. Restricting of secretion of glucocorticoids
   C. Releasing antidiuretic hormone (ADH)
   D. Crushing then passing fragments of kidney stones
   E. Dilating of peripheral arteries throughout the body
   F. Activating the renin-angiotensin-aldosterone pathway

4. Which health promotion teaching will the nurse stress to healthy adults to **prevent harm** from acute kidney injury (AKI)?
   A. Check your blood pressure every day.
   B. Find out if you have a family history of diabetes.
   C. Avoid dehydration by drinking 2 to 3 liters of water daily.
   D. Have annual testing for blood urea nitrogen (BUN), creatinine, protein, and glucose.

5. Which condition will the nurse recognize increases the risk for a client with benign prostatic hyperplasia (BPH) to develop?
   A. Perfusion reduction (prerenal failure)
   B. Intrinsic or intrarenal failure
   C. Urine flow obstruction (postrenal failure)
   D. End-stage kidney disease

6. Which assessment questions are **most appropriate** for the nurse to ask a client at risk for acute kidney injury (AKI)? **Select all that apply.**
   A. "Have you noticed any changes in your urine's appearance, frequency, or volume?"
   B. "Have you experienced any leakage of urine when coughing or laughing?"
   C. "Do you weigh yourself and have you noticed any unexpected weight loss?"
   D. "Do you have a history of diabetes, hypertension, or peripheral vascular disease?"
   E. "Do you use any nonsteroidal anti-inflammatory drugs regularly?"
   F. "Have you had and recent surgeries, traumas, or transfusions?"

7. Which laboratory results will the nurse monitor when a client is receiving IV gentamicin? **Select all that apply.**
   A. Platelet count
   B. Hemoglobin and hematocrit
   C. Blood urea nitrogen (BUN)
   D. Prothrombin time
   E. Creatinine
   F. Gentamicin peak and trough levels

8. Based on the Kidney Disease: Improving Global Outcomes classification (KDIGO), how will the nurse interpret this client data (serum creatinine increases 1.5 times over baseline with urine output of less than 0.5 mL/kg/hr for 6 hours or longer)?
   A. Stage 1
   B. Stage 2
   C. Stage 3
   D. End-stage kidney disease

9. When a client is in the diuretic phase of acute kidney injury (AKI), what **priority** action will the nurse take?
   A. Assessing for hypertension and fluid overload
   B. Monitoring for hypovolemia and electrolyte loss
   C. Adjusting the dosage of diuretic medications
   D. Balancing diuretic therapy with intake and output

10. Which are the goals of nutritional support for a client with acute kidney injury (AKI) when the nurse collaborates with the registered dietitian nutritionist (RDN)? **Select all that apply.**
    A. Maintaining or improving nutritional status
    B. Creating a program for weight loss
    C. Preserving lean body mass
    D. Restoring or maintaining fluid balance
    E. Preserving kidney function
    F. Preventing end-state kidney disease

11. Which client does the nurse understand has the **greatest** risk of developing acute kidney injury (AKI)?
    A. 23-year-old female who was recently treated for a urinary tract infection
    B. 32-year-old female who is pregnant and has gestational diabetes
    C. 49-year-old male who is obese and has a history of skin cancer
    D. 73-year-old male who has hypertension and peripheral vascular disease

12. For a client diagnosed with acute kidney injury (AKI), the nurse considers questions an order for which diagnostic test?
    A. Ultrasonography
    B. Kidney-ureter-bladder x-ray (KUB)
    C. Computed tomography with contrast
    D. Kidney biopsy

13. Which type of medication does the nurse expect the health care provider to prescribe for a client with acute kidney injury to improve blood flow to the kidneys?
    A. Loop diuretics
    B. Phosphate binders
    C. Calcium channel blockers
    D. Erythropoietin-stimulating agents

14. What is the nurse's **priority** action when the health care provider orders IV fluids at a rate of 1 mL/kg/hr for 12 hours prior to a CT scan with contrast media for a client who weighs 152 lbs?
    A. Set the IV pump to deliver fluid at 69 mL/hr.
    B. Set the IV pump to deliver fluid at 152 mL/hr.
    C. Call the health care provider for clarification of the order.
    D. Ask the radiologist for clarification of the order.

15. Which outcome statement indicates to the nurse that the goal of giving a client IV therapy after a diagnostic imaging test with contrast media has been met?
    A. Lung sounds are clear and there are no signs or symptoms of fluid overload.
    B. The client has no signs or symptoms of contrast-induced immune response.
    C. Urine output is 150 mL/hr for 6 hours after the use of the contrast agent.
    D. Urine output is 0.5mL/kg/hr for 6 hours and the client remains euvolemic.

16. Which electrolyte imbalance does the nurse expect when a client is in the early phase of chronic kidney disease (CKD)?
    A. Hyperkalemia
    B. Hyponatremia
    C. Hypercalcemia
    D. Hypokalemia

17. When the nurse reviews the laboratory results and finds that a client with chronic kidney disease (CKD) has a serum potassium level of 8 mEq/L (mmol/L), which assessment will be completed before notifying the health care provider?
    A. Cardiac rhythm
    B. Respiratory rate and depth
    C. Tremors of the hands
    D. Change in urine appearance

18. For which condition does the nurse suspect a client with chronic kidney disease (CKD) is attempting to compensate for when respirations increase in rate and depth?
    A. Hypoxia
    B. Alkalosis
    C. Acidosis
    D. Hypoxemia

19. Which instruction will the nurse give an assistive personnel (AP) to **prevent harm** when providing care to a client who has osteodystrophy?
    A. Assist the client with feeding for all meals.
    B. Gently wash the client's skin with a mild soap and rinse well.
    C. Assist the client with ambulation to the toilet every 2 hours.
    D. Use a lift sheet when moving or lifting the client.

20. For which emergency procedure does the nurse prepare when a client with chronic kidney disease develops chest pain, tachycardia, low-grade fever, friction rub, and muffled heart tones?
    A. Hemodialysis
    B. Removal of pericardial fluid
    C. Cardioversion
    D. Endotracheal intubation

21. What urinalysis findings does the nurse expect when a client is in the **early** stage of chronic kidney disease? **Select all that apply.**
    A. Proteinuria
    B. Increased specific gravity
    C. Red blood cells (RBCs)
    D. Increased urine osmolarity
    E. White blood cells (WBCs)
    F. Glucosuria

22. Which laboratory result will the nurse expect when a client with chronic kidney disease reports fatigue, lethargy with weakness, and mild shortness of breath with dizziness when rising to a standing position?
    A. Low blood glucose
    B. Low white blood cell count
    C. Low blood urea nitrogen (BUN)
    D. Low hemoglobin/hematocrit

23. The nurse collaborates with the registered dietician nutritionist (RDN) to teach a client about which recommendations for management of chronic kidney disease? **Select all that apply.**
    A. Reducing calories
    B. Controlling protein intake
    C. Limiting fluid intake
    D. Restricting potassium
    E. Increasing sodium
    F. Restricting phosphorus

24. To **avoid harm** and prevent osteodystrophy, which intracollaborative action does the nurse implement?
    A. Encouraging high-quality protein foods
    B. Administering iron supplements twice a day
    C. Encouraging extra milk with meals and snacks
    D. Administering phosphate binders with each meal

25. Which nutritional supplements does the nurse expect the health care provider will prescribe for a client with chronic kidney disease? **Select all that apply.**
    A. Water-soluble vitamins
    B. Calcium
    C. Iron
    D. Magnesium
    E. Vitamin D
    F. Phosphorus

26. What is the nurse's **first** action when a client with chronic kidney disease (CKD) develops restlessness, anxiousness, shortness of breath, a rapid heart rate, frothy sputum, and crackles in the bases of the lungs?
    A. Facilitating transfer to the intensive care unit for aggressive treatment
    B. Placing the client's head of bed in the high-Fowler position
    C. Monitoring vital signs and assessing the lungs every 15 minutes
    D. Administering an IV loop diuretic such as furosemide

27. Which drug will the nurse **avoid** administering to a client with chronic kidney disease (CKD) to **prevent harm**?
    A. Opioids
    B. Antibiotics
    C. Oral antihyperglycemics
    D. Magnesium antacids

28. Which client will the nurse consider **most likely** to be a candidate for continuous kidney replacement therapy (CKRT) using venovenous hemofiltration?
    A. 65-year-old with fluid volume overload
    B. 55-year-old who needs long-term management
    C. 45-year-old who is critically ill and unstable
    D. 35-year-old with a peritoneal infection

29. For which client conditions does the nurse expect the possibility of emergent hemodialysis (HD)? **Select all that apply.**
    A. Severe uncontrollable hypertension
    B. Pericarditis
    C. Symptomatic hyperkalemia with ECG changes
    D. Myocardial infarction
    E. Pulmonary edema
    F. Some drug overdoses

30. What are the criteria used for selection of clients for hemodialysis (HD)? **Select all that apply.**
    A. Client values and preferences
    B. Client's family member or partner who is willing to learn about HD
    C. Irreversible kidney failure when other therapies are unacceptable or ineffective
    D. No disorders that would seriously complicate HD
    E. Expected ability to continue or resume roles at home, work, or school
    F. Insurance plan will cover costs of procedures

31. Which gastrointestinal changes does the nurse expect to find when assessing a client with uremia?
    A. Increased salivation
    B. Halitosis
    C. Stomatitis
    D. Anorexia
    E. Nausea and vomiting
    F. Hiccups

32. What is the nurse's **best** response when a client asks how often and for how long he or she will have to go for hemodialysis (HD)?
    A. "It varies and you will need to discuss this with your nephrology health care provider for specific instructions."
    B. "Most clients require about 12 hours per week, which is usually divided into three 4-hour treatments."
    C. "If you follow the diet and fluid therapies you will spend less time in dialysis, about 8 hours each week."
    D. "Many clients prefer to have home treatment dialysis that occurs every night while sleeping."

33. How does the nurse **best** interpret a condition when a client is undergoing hemodialysis (HD) and develops symptoms including headache, nausea, vomiting, and fatigue?
    A. Mild dialysis disequilibrium syndrome
    B. Adverse reaction to the dialysate solution
    C. Transient symptoms in a client new to hemodialysis
    D. Expected manifestations of end-stage kidney disease

34. What instructions will the nurse give to the assistive personnel (AP) regarding care of a client with an arteriovenous fistula?
    A. Assess for bleeding at the needle insertion sites every 2 hours.
    B. Monitor the client's distal pulses and capillary refill for circulation.
    C. Palpate the dialysis site for thrills and auscultate for a bruit every 4 hours.
    D. Avoid taking blood pressure readings on the client's arm with the arteriovenous fistula.

35. What does the nurse expect when comparing a client's posthemodialysis weight and blood pressure with predialysis data?
    A. Blood pressure is increased and weight is decreased
    B. Blood pressure and weight are slightly increased
    C. Blood pressure and weight are the same
    D. Blood pressure and weight are decreased

36. Which **priority** teaching will the nurse provide to the client receiving peritoneal dialysis (PD) when the effluent becomes cloudy?
    A. The change means that more waste products are being removed from the blood.
    B. The presence of cloudiness is an early sign of an infection called peritonitis and is very serious.
    C. Effluent cloudiness is the result of eating foods that contain too much protein and electrolytes.
    D. The effluent is expected to be cloudy because it has spent time (dwelled) in the abdomen, in close contact with the intestines.

37. Which actions will the nurse take to check the peritoneal dialysis system of a client when the dialysate outflow is slow? **Select all that apply.**
    A. Ensuring that the drainage bag is elevated above the client's abdomen
    B. Inspecting the tubing to ensure there is no kinking or twisting
    C. Making sure that clamps are open and unclamped
    D. Repositioning the client to the other side and ensuring good body alignment
    E. Instructing the client to stand up at the bedside and cough
    F. Placing the client in a supine low-Fowler position

38. What is the **best** method for the nurse to monitor the weight of a client who is receiving peritoneal dialysis (PD)?
    A. Calculating the client's dry weight by comparing daily weights to baseline weights
    B. Determining dry weight by comparing the client's weight to a standard weight chart
    C. Checking the weight after a drain and before the next fill to monitor the dry weight
    D. Weighing the client daily and subtracting dialysate volume to determine dry weight

39. What is the nurse's **best** action when a client receiving PD has slightly less outflow than inflow?
    A. Placing the client on an oral fluid intake restriction
    B. Notifying the nephrology health care provider
    C. Recording the difference as intake on the flow sheet
    D. Instructing the client to stand and walk then measuring the next outflow

40. Which client conditions will the nurse recognize as absolute contraindications to receiving a kidney transplant? **Select all that apply.**
    A. Breast cancer and metastasis to the lungs
    B. Type 2 diabetes controlled with diet and exercise
    C. Urinary tract infection
    D. Active treatment for peptic ulcer disease
    E. Chemical dependency
    F. Living related donor

41. For how many hours will the nurse instruct the assistive personnel (AP) to check the hourly urine output of a postoperative client who had a kidney transplant?
    A. 8 hours
    B. 12 hours
    C. 24 hours
    D. 48 hours

42. Why will the nurse **immediately** notify the nephrology health care provider if a client develops hypotension and diuresis postoperatively after a kidney transplant?
    A. These problems place the client at risk for hypervolemia and dehydration.
    B. Dehydration with hypotension reduces perfusion and oxygen to the new kidney.
    C. These assessment findings are indicators of a possible serious acute infection.
    D. Increased work by the kidney for diuresis results in excessive buildup of cellular toxins that damage the new kidney's tubules.

43. What does the nurse expect the nephrology health care provider to prescribe when a post kidney transplant client develops oliguria, elevated temperature of 100° F (37.8° C), increased blood pressure, and signs of fluid retention 9 days after the surgery?
    A. Immediate removal of the transplanted kidney
    B. Increased doses of immunosuppressive drugs
    C. Immediate return to either hemodialysis or peritoneal dialysis
    D. Antibiotic therapy until infection symptoms are resolved

Chapter 63 Answer Key

1. B, D, F
   The most current definition of AKI is an increase in serum creatinine by 0.3 mg/dL (26.2 μmol/L) or more within 48 hours; or an increase in serum creatinine to 1.5 times or more from baseline, which is known or presumed to have occurred in the previous 7 days; or a urine volume of less than 0.5 mL/kg/hr for 6 hours.

2. A, C, D
   Examples of disorders causing intrinsic renal AKI include allergic disorders, embolism or thrombosis of the renal vessels, and nephrotoxic agents. Severe dehydration causes prerenal failure. Bladder cancer and kidney stones cause postrenal failure. For additional causes, see Table 63.4 Diseases and Conditions That Contribute to Acute Kidney Injury in your text.

3. A, C, F
   When prerenal or postrenal causes of AKI occur, the kidneys compensate by three responses: constricting kidney blood vessels, activating the renin-angiotensin-aldosterone pathway, and releasing antidiuretic hormone (ADH).

4. C
   Dehydration (severe blood volume depletion) reduces perfusion and can lead to AKI even in adults who have no known kidney problems. The nurse urges all healthy adults to avoid dehydration by drinking 2 to 3 liters of water daily.

5. C
   BPH (enlarged prostate gland) increases the client's risk for urine flow obstruction leading to postrenal failure because the prostate gland surrounds and puts pressure on the urethra.

6. A, D, E, F
   The nurse asks about any noted changes in urine, as well as any exposure to nephrotoxic substances or drugs. Other important information from the client's medical history includes surgeries, trauma, transfusions, and chronic conditions such as diabetes, hypertension, and peripheral vascular disease. For additional essential topic, see the History section on AKI in your text.

7. C, E, F
   If a client is receiving a known nephrotoxic drug, the nurse will closely monitor laboratory values, including BUN, creatinine, and drug (gentamicin) peak and trough levels, for indications of reduced kidney function.

8. A
   Based on the Kidney Disease: Improving Global Outcomes classification (KDIGO), a value of serum creatinine increases 1.5 times over baseline with urine output of less than 0.5 mL/kg/hr for 6 hours or longer indicates stage 1. See Table 63.2 in your text for information on the other stages for this system.

9. B
   For the client in the diuretic phase of AKI, the nurse plans care that focuses on fluid and electrolyte replacement and monitoring. Onset of polyuria can signal the start of recovery from AKI.

10. A, C, D, E
    Nutrition support goals in AKI are to provide sufficient nutrients to maintain or improve nutrition status, preserve lean body mass, restore or maintain fluid balance, and preserve kidney function.

11. D
    Risk factors for AKI include shock, cardiac surgery, hypotension, prolonged mechanical ventilation, and sepsis. Older adults or adults with diabetes, hypertension, peripheral vascular disease, liver disease, or CKD are at higher risk of AKI if hospitalized. The client in option D is an older adult with two important risk factors. Thus, he is at highest risk of AKI development.

12. C
    The client's diagnosis is AKI. To complete the CT with contrast, the client will be injected with a contrast dye, which is nephrotoxic, therefore the nurse considers questioning that diagnostic test.

13. C

Calcium channel blockers can improve the GFR and blood flow within the kidney. They also help to control blood pressure.

14. A

The nurse calculates the client's weight in kilograms (152 lb divided by 2.2 = 69 kg). Then the nurse sets the IV pump to run at 69 mL/hr.

15. C

A common desired outcome for clients undergoing a procedure with contrast medium is a urine output of 150 mL/hr for the first 6 hours after administration of the contrast agent.

16. B

Early in CKD, the nurse expects the client's laboratory values to reveal hyponatremia (sodium depletion) because there are fewer healthy kidney nephrons to reabsorb sodium.

17. A

Normal potassium level is within 3.5 to 5 mEq/L (mmol/L). With CKD, high potassium (K+) levels can develop quickly, reaching 7 to 8 mEq/L (mmol/L) or greater. Life-threatening changes in cardiac rate and rhythm result from K+ elevation because of abnormal depolarization and repolarization.

18. C

As CKD worsens and acid retention increases, increased respiratory action is needed to keep the blood pH normal. The respiratory system adjusts or compensates for the increased blood hydrogen ion levels (acidosis or decreased pH) by increasing the rate and depth of breathing to excrete carbon dioxide through the lungs. This breathing pattern, called Kussmaul respiration, increases with worsening kidney disease.

19. D

Clients with osteodystrophy have thin, fragile bones that are at risk for fractures with even slight trauma. When lifting or moving a client with fragile bones, the AP is instructed to use a lift sheet rather than pulling the client.

20. B

The client's signs and symptoms suggest pericarditis which often occurs in CKD and can cause tamponade. Treatment of tamponade, which is a medical emergency, requires immediate removal of pericardial fluid (pericardiocentesis) by placement of a needle, catheter, or drainage tube into the pericardium.

21. A, C, E, F

In the early stages of CKD, the nurse expects the urinalysis may show protein, glucose, red blood cells (RBCs) and white blood cells (WBCs), and decreased or fixed specific gravity. Urine osmolarity is usually decreased. As CKD progresses, urine output decreases dramatically, and osmolarity then increases.

22. D

The client's symptoms suggest anemia which is common in clients in the later stages of CKD and makes symptoms worse. The causes of anemia include a decreased production of erythropoietin by the kidneys which causes reduced red blood cell (RBC) production and low hemoglobin and hematocrit levels.

23. B, C, D, F

The nurse collaborates with the RDN to teach the client about diet changes that are needed as a result of CKD. Common changes include control of protein intake; fluid intake limitation; restriction of potassium, sodium, and phosphorus intake; taking vitamin and mineral supplements; and consuming enough calories to meet metabolic need.

24. D

Phosphorus restriction for control of phosphorus levels is started early in CKD to avoid renal osteodystrophy. The nurse administers phosphate binders at mealtime to increase their effectiveness in slowing or preventing the absorption of dietary phosphorus.

25. A, B, C, E

The nurse expects the health care provider to prescribe daily vitamin and mineral supplements for most clients with CKD. Low-protein diets are also low in vitamins, and water-soluble vitamins are removed from the blood during dialysis. Anemia also is a problem in clients with CKD because of the limited iron content of low-protein diets and decreased kidney production of erythropoietin. Thus, supplemental iron is needed. Calcium and vitamin D supplements may be needed, depending on the client's serum calcium levels and bone status.

26. B
The nurse recognizes this client's symptoms as indicators of pulmonary edema. First, the client is placed in a high-Fowler position and given oxygen to improve gas exchange. Then health care provider or Rapid Response Team is notified for treatment and management of pulmonary edema.

27. D
The nurse questions a prescription for magnesium-containing antacids for clients with CKD because they cannot excrete magnesium and need to avoid any additional intake and buildup of magnesium. To avoid hypermagnesemia, the nurse teaches clients with kidney disease to avoid antacids containing magnesium.

28. C
Clients who need continuous kidney replacement therapy (CKRT) are hospitalized and are too unstable to tolerate the changes in blood pressure that occur with intermittent conventional hemodialysis. This treatment occurs in an intensive care unit and is continuous over 24 hours.

29. A, B, C, E, F
Some indications for emergent dialysis include: pulmonary edema; severe uncontrollable hypertension; symptomatic hyperkalemia with ECG changes; other severe electrolyte or acid-base disturbances; some drug overdoses; and pericarditis.

30. A, C, D, E
Selection criteria for HD include: irreversible kidney failure when other therapies are unacceptable or ineffective; no disorders that would seriously complicate HD; client values and preferences; and expected ability to continue or resume roles at home, work, or school.

31. B, C, D, E, F
Uremia affects the entire GI system. The flora of the mouth change with uremia. The mouth contains the enzyme urease, which breaks down urea into ammonia. The ammonia generated remains and then causes halitosis (uremic fetor) and stomatitis (mouth inflammation). Anorexia, nausea, vomiting, and hiccups are common in clients with uremia. For more information about uremic changes in the body, see chart 63.2 Key Features of Uremia.

32. B
The best answer the nurse can provide this client is the most common treatment. Most clients receive three 4-hour treatments over the course of a week. The nurse provides additional information for some clients with ongoing urine production, who may need only two 5- to 6-hour treatments a week. If a client gains large amounts of fluid, a longer HD treatment time may be needed to remove the fluid without hypotension or other severe side effects.

33. A
Dialysis disequilibrium syndrome may develop during HD or after HD has been completed. It is characterized by mental status changes and can include seizures or coma, although this severity of disequilibrium syndrome is rare with today's HD practice. A **mild form** of disequilibrium syndrome includes symptoms of nausea, vomiting, headaches, fatigue, and restlessness. It is thought to be the result of a rapid reduction in electrolytes and other particles.

34. D
The AP's scope of practice includes taking and recording vital signs. For a hemodialysis client, checking blood pressure includes **not** taking blood pressure readings using the extremity in which the vascular access is placed. Assessment, monitoring, palpation, and auscultation are more advanced skills performed by the professional registered nurse. For more information

on care of a client's arteriovenous fistula, see Best Practice for Patient Safety & Quality Care QSEN Caring for the Patient With an Arteriovenous Fistula or Arteriovenous Graft in your text.

35.   D
Posthemodialysis, the nurse obtains vital signs and weight for comparison with predialysis measurements. After dialysis, the nurse expects blood pressure and weight to be reduced as a result of fluid removal.

36.   B.
The nurse teaches the client to recognize indications of peritonitis (e.g., cloudy dialysate outflow [effluent], fever, abdominal tenderness, abdominal pain, general malaise, nausea, and vomiting). Cloudy or opaque effluent is the **earliest** indication of peritonitis. The client is taught to examine all effluent for color and clarity to detect peritonitis early and to report indications of peritonitis immediately to the nephrology health care provider.

37.   B, C, D, F
When PD outflow drainage is slow, actions that can help improve flow include: ensuring that the drainage bag is lower than the client's abdomen to enhance gravity drainage; inspecting the connection tubing and PD system for kinking or twisting; and ensuring that clamps are open. If outflow drainage is still inadequate, reposition the client to stimulate outflow. Turning the client to the other side or ensuring that he or she is in good body alignment may help. Having the client in a supine low-Fowler position reduces abdominal pressure. Increased abdominal pressure from sitting or standing or from coughing contributes to leakage at the PD catheter site.

38.   C
The client's actual weight is his or her "dry weight". For a client receiving PD, dry weight is checked after a drain and before the next fill.

The client is always weighed on the same scale, with the same amount of clothes.

39.   C
When outflow is less than inflow, the difference is retained by the client during dialysis and it is counted as fluid intake.

40.   A, C, E
Absolute contraindications to kidney transplant include active cancer, current infection, active psychiatric illness, active substance abuse, and nonadherence with dialysis or medical regimen.

41.   D
A postoperative client who had a kidney transplant has a urinary catheter in place for accurate measurements of urine output and decompression of the bladder. Decompression prevents stretch on sutures and ureter attachment sites on the bladder. The nurse and AP check urine output at least hourly during the first 48 hours. This includes examining the urine for color.

42.   B
If hypotension or excessive diuresis (e.g., unanticipated urine output 500 to 1000 mL greater than intake over 12 to 24 hours or other goal for intake and output) is present, respond by notifying the nephrology health care provider because hypotension reduces perfusion and oxygen to the new kidney, threatening the kidney's survival.

43.   B
These symptoms within the time frame of a week or more indicate that the client may be having an acute rejection. The treatment for acute rejection is increased dosages of immunosuppressive drugs. Immunosuppressive drugs protect the transplanted organ. These drugs include corticosteroids, inhibitors of T-cell proliferation and activity (azathioprine, mycophenolic acid, cyclosporine, and tacrolimus), mTOR inhibitors (to disrupt stimulatory T-cell signals), and monoclonal antibodies.

64

CHAPTER

Assessment of the Reproductive System

1. When the normal vaginal flora is disrupted, what condition does the nurse expect that a female client is **most likely** to experience?
   A. Vaginal infection
   B. Vaginal dryness
   C. Irregular menstrual cycles
   D. Infertility

2. When the nurse takes a history from a male client and finds that he had mumps with orchitis, which **common** potential complication is possible?
   A. Decreased libido
   B. Prostate hypertrophy
   C. Testicular atrophy
   D. Impotence

3. Which factors will the nurse assess in a male client who reports decreased libido? **Select all that apply.**
   A. Timing of exercise program
   B. Use of tobacco
   C. Occupation
   D. Consumption of alcohol
   E. Weight gain or loss
   F. Illicit substance use

4. Which condition does the nurse expect when a female client reports altered nutritional intake resulting in changes in metabolism?
   A. Excessive bleeding
   B. Pelvic inflammatory disease
   C. Endometriosis
   D. Amenorrhea

5. Which **priority** action will the nurse implement when an older male client reports difficulty starting the urine stream?
   A. Teach the importance of testicular self-exam (TSE).
   B. Discuss exercises to strengthen pelvic floor muscles.
   C. Teach signs of urethral obstruction and importance of prostate cancer screening.
   D. Provide information on testosterone functions and supplements.

6. Which reproductive physiologic changes will the nurse expect in an older female client? **Select all that apply.**
   A. Drying, smoothing, and thinning of the vaginal walls
   B. Increased size of the uterus
   C. Loss of tone and elasticity of the pelvic ligaments and connective tissue
   D. Hypertrophy of the endometrium
   E. Increased flabbiness and fibrosis of the breasts
   F. Decreased size of the labia majora and clitoris

7. Which health and lifestyle habits does the nurse assess when taking a history from a client with a reproductive health problem? **Select all that apply.**
   A. Socioeconomic status
   B. Dietary intake
   C. Exercise pattern
   D. Sleep pattern
   E. Sexual practices
   F. Occupational status

8. Which **priority** question will the nurse ask to evaluate the current condition of a 40-year-old client who is experiencing heavy vaginal bleeding?
   A. "Are you sexually active and do you use oral contraceptives?"
   B. "Are you feeling weak, dizzy, or light-headed?"
   C. "Is the bleeding related to your menstrual cycle or intercourse?"
   D. "Are you having any sensations of pain or cramping?"

9. What finding does the nurse expect when reviewing a male client's laboratory results and finding a testosterone level of 200 ng/dL?
   A. Increased muscle mass and weight
   B. Increase in urinary output
   C. Testicular pain with nausea
   D. Changes in sexual performance

10. What does the nurse expect that a 30-year-old female client is **most likely** to experience when she reports a history of blockages in her fallopian tubes?
   A. Difficulty conceiving
   B. Vaginal discharge
   C. Difficulty controlling weight
   D. Irregular menses

11. Which findings will the nurse expect to see when assessing the scrotum of a client? **Select all that apply.**
   A. Contracts with exposure to cold
   B. Suspended below the pubic bone
   C. Skin of scrotum is lightly pigmented
   D. Sparse hair follicles
   E. Pouch skin is thin walled
   F. Warm compared to surrounding tissues

12. Which instruction will the nurse give the client **immediately** before a pelvic exam and Pap test?
   A. Clean your genitals with warm water.
   B. Empty your bladder in the bathroom.
   C. Relax and the test will be less painful.
   D. Lie flat on the table until the test is over.

13. Which client does the nurse prioritize as **most** in need of a pelvic examination?
   A. 25-year-old with possible urinary tract infection (UTI)
   B. 53-year-old who reports decreased libido and fatigue
   C. 62-year-old who reports resumption of menses
   D. 74-year-old with 25-lb intentional weight loss

14. What does the nurse tell an African-American client whose prostate-specific antigen (PSA) level is less than 2.5 ng/mL?
   A. African-American men typically have lower-than-normal PSA levels.
   B. This level indicates the need for follow-up for possible prostate cancer.
   C. The test should be repeated on an annual basis to monitor for abnormalities.
   D. A PSA level of less than 2.5 ng/mL is generally considered a normal value.

15. When the nurse explains to a group of women that annual screening mammograms are not recommended for women under 40 years of age, what is the underlying rationale for this decision?
   A. Breast tumors are uncommon among women under the age of 40 years.
   B. The amount of radiation exposure outweighs the benefit for women of child-bearing age.
   C. In younger women there is little difference in the density of normal tissue and malignant tumors.
   D. In younger women the tumors are likely too small to be detected by mammography.

16. For which client is the nurse **most likely** to administer an iron supplement?
    A. 23-year-old who has pelvic inflammatory disease
    B. 32-year-old with heavy menstrual bleeding and an intrauterine device
    C. 53-year-old who is entering menopause and has a breast mass
    D. 70-year-old who is diagnosed with benign prostatic hyperplasia

17. For which conditions are a pelvic examination and Pap test indicated to assess for? **Select all that apply.**
    A. Menstrual irregularities
    B. Rape trauma or other pelvic injury
    C. Unexplained abdominal or vaginal pain
    D. Vaginal discharge, itching, sores, or infection
    E. Physical changes in the vagina, cervix, and uterus
    F. Pregnancy and infertility

18. Which actions will the nurse include in the postoperative care of a client who had a laparoscopy? **Select all that apply.**
    A. Administering oral analgesics for incisional pain
    B. Notifying the health care provider for postoperative shoulder pain
    C. Instructing the client to change the small adhesive bandage as needed
    D. Reassuring the client that most painful sensations disappear within 1 to 2 weeks
    E. Teaching the client to observe the incision for signs of infection or hematoma
    F. Reminding the client to avoid strenuous activity for 3 to 4 weeks after the procedure

19. Which actions will the nurse instruct the client to **avoid** to **prevent harm** after having a colposcopy procedure?
    A. Do not douche, use tampons, and have sexual intercourse for 1 week after the procedure.
    B. Wear a perineal pad and expect bleeding with small clots for the first 24 hours.
    C. Do not drive or operate heavy machinery while taking the prescribed pain medication.
    D. Perform breast self-examination every month and report changes to the health care provider.

20. Which postprocedural findings will the nurse instruct a client who had a prostate biopsy to expect?
    A. Swelling of the biopsy area and difficulty urinating are expected during the first week.
    B. A low-grade fever and bright red penile discharge are normal for several days.
    C. Slight soreness and light rectal bleeding that is bright red are expected for a few days.
    D. Seminal fluid will appear normal within a day after the procedure.

21. Which preprocedural instructions will the nurse give a client before a mammogram?
    A. Do not eat or drink anything 2 to 3 hours before the procedure.
    B. Abstain from sexual relations for 24 hours prior to the procedure.
    C. Do not use lotions, creams, or powder on your breasts before the study.
    D. Wear a supportive bra and bring a breast pad for use after testing.

Chapter 64 Answer Key

1. A
   The normal vaginal bacteria (flora) interact with the secretions to produce lactic acid and maintain an acidic pH (3.5 to 5.0) in the vagina. This acidity helps prevent infection in the vagina. Thus, the nurse expects the client to develop a vaginal infection.

2. C

A history of mumps in men may cause orchitis (painful inflammation and swelling of the testes), which can lead to testicular atrophy.

3. B, D, F

Assess for alcohol, tobacco, and illicit drug use. In males, libido (sex drive), sperm production, and the ability to have or sustain an erection can be affected by these substances.

4. D

Disorders that affect a woman's metabolism or nutrition can depress ovarian function and cause amenorrhea.

5. C

When an older man has difficulty initiating his urine stream, it is most likely related to an enlarged prostate gland which may lead to obstruction. The nurse teaches the client about signs of urethral obstruction and importance of prostate cancer screening.

6. A, C, E, F

Options A, C, E, and F are expected changes in the reproductive system as women age. Option B is not correct because the uterus decreases in size with age (unless another problem is present). Option D is not correct because the endometrium atrophies with age.

7. B, C, D, E

The nurse assesses general health habits such as sleep, exercise, diet, and sexual practices. Occupation and socioeconomic status are important, but may not contribute to knowledge about reproductive problems.

8. B

Option B assesses the effects of the bleeding on the condition of the client which is of immediate concern. These signs can indicate significant bleeding. The nurse will pass this information on to the health care provider.

9. D

Testosterone production is fairly constant in the adult male. Only a slight and gradual reduction of testosterone production occurs in the older adult male until he is in his 80s. This client's testosterone level is low (normal is 280 to 1080 ng/dL). Low testosterone levels decrease muscle mass, reduce skin elasticity, and lead to changes in sexual performance.

10. A

The fallopian tubes insert into the fundus of the uterus and extend laterally close to the ovaries. They provide a duct between the ovaries and the uterus for the passage of ova and sperm. When there is blockage in the fallopian tubes, there is no passage for the ova and sperm, thus, conception is difficult if not impossible.

11. A, B, D, E

The scrotum is a thin-walled, fibromuscular pouch that is behind the penis and suspended below the pubic bone. This pouch protects the testes, epididymis, and vas deferens in a space that is slightly cooler than inside the abdominal cavity. The scrotal skin is darkly pigmented and contains sweat glands, sebaceous glands, and few hair follicles. It contracts with cold, exercise, tactile stimulation, and sexual excitement.

12. B

Immediately before the pelvic examination and pap test, the nurse asks the client to empty her bladder and undress completely before draping and positioning her in the lithotomy position for the procedure.

13. C

Resumption of menses after menopause is never a normal event. This client is most in need of a pelvic examination with workup and testing to determine why she is experiencing bleeding again.

14. D

Although elevated PSA levels may be associated with prostate cancer, there is variance among health care providers in interpretation of results. Levels less than 2.5-4.0 ng/mL are generally considered normal.

15. C

In young women's breasts, there is little difference in the density between normal glandular tissue and malignant tumors, which makes the mammogram less useful for evaluation of breast masses in these clients. For this reason, annual screening mammograms are not recommended for women younger than 40 years.

16. B
Women have special nutrition needs. Heavy menstrual bleeding, particularly in women who have intrauterine devices, may require iron supplements.

17. A, B, C, D, E, F
All of these options are conditions for which a pelvic examination and Pap test are helpful assessment tools.

18. A, C, E
The client is usually discharged on the day of the laparoscopy procedure. Incisional pain is managed by oral analgesics. The greatest discomfort is usually caused by referred shoulder pain from positioning during the procedure. Most of these sensations disappear within 48 hours depending on the extent of the procedure. The nurse instructs the client to change the small adhesive bandage as needed and to observe the incision for signs of infection or hematoma.
The client is also reminded to avoid strenuous activity for the first week after the procedure.

19. A
The client should be instructed to refrain from douching, using tampons, and having sexual intercourse for 1 week (or as instructed by the health care provider).

20. C
After prostate biopsy, the nurse reminds the client that he may experience slight soreness, light rectal bleeding that is bright red for a few days, and moderate hematuria which should resolve in a few days. Tell the client that his seminal fluid may be discolored red or rust for several weeks.

21. C
Remind the client not to use creams, lotions, powders, or deodorant on the breasts or underarms before the study because these products may be visible on the mammogram and contribute to misdiagnosis.

65 CHAPTER

Concepts of Care for Patients with Breast Disorders

1. Which condition is **most likely** when the nurse admits a 25-year-old female client, with a self-detected mass in the right breast that is oval-shaped, freely mobile, and rubbery?
   A. Fibroadenoma
   B. Ductal ectasia
   C. Macrocyst
   D. Papilloma

2. Which are characteristics that the nurse expects to find in clients with a history of fibrocystic changes (FCC) in the breast? **Select all that apply.**
   A. Breast pain
   B. Tender breast lumps
   C. Oval shape
   D. Breast swelling
   E. Symptom relief after menstruation
   F. Gynecomastia

3. What will the nurse teach about self-care management to a client with mild discomfort from a fibrocystic breast condition? **Select all that apply.**
   A. Use analgesics such as acetaminophen for discomfort.
   B. Avoid dietary caffeine and other stimulants.
   C. Wear a supportive bra, even when in bed.
   D. Limit salt intake before menses.
   E. Local ice or heat application may help control pain.
   F. Diuretics may help decrease premenstrual breast engorgement.

4. Which male client does the nurse understand has the **greatest** risk of developing gynecomastia?
   A. 25-year-old injured in a touch football game
   B. 38-year-old with stable angina
   C. 49-year-old prescribed spironolactone
   D. 61-year-old with hypothyroidism

5. For which conditions would the nurse prepare and teach a client about breast biopsy? **Select all that apply.**
   A. Fluid was not aspirated during fine needle aspiration.
   B. Hormonal replacement therapy is prescribed.
   C. Mammogram shows suspicious findings.
   D. Fluid buildup recurs after aspiration.
   E. Mass remains palpable after aspiration.
   F. Aspirated fluid reveals cancer cells.

6. Which action does the nurse teach a client to **prevent harm** after breast augmentation surgery?
   A. Begin exercising by twisting at the waist the day after surgery.
   B. Walk every few hours to prevent venous thromboembolism (VTE).
   C. Wait a week or more after surgery before resumption of smoking.
   D. Have someone stay with you during the first 6 hours after discharge.

7. What normal findings will the nurse expect when assessing the breasts of an older woman?
   A. Gentle palpation may cause discomfort or mild pain.
   B. Nipples are retracted and there may be a discharge.
   C. Tissue is difficult to palpate because of fat deposits.
   D. Breasts are atrophied, flattened, and elongated.

8. What does the nurse suspect when a client reports identification of a hard breast mass with irregular borders, redness, swelling, nipple discharge, and enlarged axillary nodes?
   A. Intraductal papilloma
   B. Ductal ectasia
   C. Fibroadenoma
   D. Fibrocystic changes

9. In addition to routine assessment, what **specific** assessment will the nurse perform on a client with very large breasts?
   A. Careful examination of the size and shape of nipples
   B. Ask if client has considered breast reduction mammoplasty
   C. Observe for fungal infection underneath the breasts
   D. Assess for pain in the bones and joints

10. During a breast examination, the nurse practitioner palpates a small mass in the client's right breast. What are the **most important** items to include when documenting this finding? **Select all that apply.**
    A. "Face of the clock" location of the mass
    B. Amount of pressure required to detect the mass
    C. Size and shape of the mass
    D. Method used to examine the breast
    E. Whether the mass is fixed or moveable
    F. Skin changes around the mass such as dimpling

11. What advice will the nurse give to a postmenopausal client about when to perform breast self-examination (BSE)?
    A. Perform breast self-examination on the 15th day of each month.
    B. The last day of the month is the best day for breast self-examination.
    C. After menopause, breast self-examination will not detect a mass.
    D. Choose any day of the month but follow a consistent schedule.

12. What will the nurse teach a client who had breast reconstruction about the Jackson-Pratt drain left in place? **Select all that apply.**
    A. The drain will be emptied every hour and the amount recorded.
    B. A drain is usually left in place 1 to 3 weeks after surgery.
    C. There should be less than 30 mL over 24 hours before the drain is removed.
    D. Contact the health care provider for excessive drainage.
    E. Record the color and amount of drainage when the drain is emptied.
    F. Drainage tubes collect any fluid that accumulates under the surgical area.

13. What teaching about the affected arm will the nurse provide for a client who had a partial mastectomy (lumpectomy)?
    A. Do not start any arm or hand exercises until the drains are removed from the incision.
    B. Do push-ups and arm circles on a routine basis for a full recovery.
    C. Avoid using the affected arm for having blood pressure measured, receiving injections, or having blood drawn for 2 weeks after surgery.
    D. Elevate the head of the bed at least 30 degrees, with the affected arm elevated on a pillow while awake.

14. Which exercise will the nurse teach a client to perform on the first day after mastectomy surgery?
    A. Squeezing the affected hand around a soft, round object
    B. Hand wall climbing
    C. Shoulder blade squeezing
    D. Rope turning

15. What question does the nurse ask a client, who reported a breast mass 6 months ago, related to possible metastases of breast cancer?
    A. "Have you had any exposure to radiation or toxic chemicals?"
    B. "Has your mother or sister ever been diagnosed with breast cancer?"
    C. "Have you noticed any joint or bone pain or other changes in your body?"
    D. "Have you developed a cough, shortness of breath, or difficulty sleeping?"

16. Which sign or symptom detected by the nurse practitioner during clinical breast examination of a client suggests advanced breast cancer?
    A. Thin, milky discharge from nipple
    B. Edematous thickening and pitting of breast skin called peau d'orange
    C. Oval-shaped, mobile, rubbery mass
    D. Replacement of normal cells with connective tissue and collagen

17. What is the nurse's **best** action when an anxious, upset client has just been diagnosed with breast cancer and informed that surgery is likely the best treatment option?
    A. Provide education about treatment options.
    B. Assist with making independent decisions.
    C. Provide reassurance about long-term outcomes.
    D. Listen and allow open discussion about feelings.

18. When will the nurse expect a client with breast cancer to receive neoadjuvant therapy?
    A. After surgery to ensure that all cancer cells have been destroyed
    B. Before surgery to shrink the tumor and make it easier to remove
    C. With radiation therapy to treat any metastasis that may occur
    D. During surgery to make sure that all of the tumor cells are removed

19. What **priority** teaching will the nurse provide to a client after mastectomy surgery?
    A. Begin exercises 3 to 4 days after the surgery.
    B. A regular diet can be started the first day after surgery.
    C. Check the surgical site for signs of infection or bleeding.
    D. Start ambulating the day after surgery.

20. Which advice will the nurse provide for a client who is prescribed tamoxifen to decrease the chance of breast cancer recurrence, with regard to the side effects of the drug?
    A. Ginger ale with the drug will decrease the nausea.
    B. Have a handrail installed around the bathtub to prevent falls.
    C. Check your weight and report weight gain to the health care provider.
    D. Use a soft-bristled toothbrush to prevent bleeding.

21. What symptoms will the nurse expect a client who had a prophylactic oophorectomy to report? **Select all that apply.**
    A. Night sweats
    B. Mood changes
    C. Hot flashes
    D. Weight gain
    E. Difficulty sleeping
    F. Chills

22. What advantage does the nurse discuss with a client who is prescribed trastuzumab for treatment of breast cancer?
    A. The drug will shrink the tumor.
    B. It is less likely to harm normal cells.
    C. Nausea and vomiting are rare side effects.
    D. Cardiac side effects are not a concern.

23. Which factors will the nurse question a male client about to assess risk for breast cancer? **Select all that apply.**
    A. Family history
    B. *BRCA1* and/or *BRCA2* mutation
    C. Respiratory disease
    D. Testicular disorders
    E. Obesity
    F. Hyperthyroidism

Chapter 65 Answer Key

1. A
   A fibroadenoma is a well-defined solid mass of connective tissue that is unattached to the surrounding breast tissue and is usually discovered by the woman herself, or during mammography. On clinical assessment, fibroadenomas are oval, freely mobile, rubbery, and variable in size.

2. A, B, D, E
   Typical symptoms of FCC include breast pain, and firm, hard, tender lumps or swelling in the breasts, particularly before a woman's menstrual period. Symptoms usually resolve after menstruation and then recur before the next menstrual period in a cyclic fashion.

3. A, B, C, D, E
   The nurse teaches a client with a fibrocystic breast condition about all of these options. Options A, B, C, D, and E are more appropriate for a mild condition. Option F is incorrect because diuretics are added for the treatment of more severe FCC.

4. C
   Drugs such as spironolactone can cause gynecomastia. The first line of treatment is to discontinue any drugs that may contribute to this condition. If a medical condition such as hyperthyroidism or hypogonadism contributes to the condition, treatment of the underlying issue often helps to resolve gynecomastia.

5. A, C, E, F
   A needle biopsy or surgical biopsy may be ordered after fine needle aspiration. Biopsy may

be indicated in these situations: no fluid is aspirated; mammogram shows suspicious findings; mass remains palpable after aspiration; and aspirated fluid reveals cancer cells.

6. B
   The nurse teaches the client to walk every few hours to prevent venous thromboembolism (VTE). The client must avoid strenuous activity or twisting above the waist. Smoking cessation is important for healing and should not be resumed. The client is usually discharged on the day of surgery and someone must be with her for the first 24 hours.

7. D
   As women age, the breast tissue becomes flattened and elongated, and is suspended loosely from the chest wall. On palpation, the breast tissue of the older woman has a finer, more granular feel than the lobular feel in a younger woman. Breast examination in older adults may be easier because of tissue atrophy and relaxation of the suspensory ligaments.

8. B
   Ductal ectasia is described as a hard, irregular mass or masses with nipple discharge, enlarged axillary nodes, redness, and edema. It can be difficult to distinguish from cancer without a biopsy.

9. C
   A woman with large breasts may develop a recurrent fungal infection under the breasts, especially in hot weather, because it is difficult to keep this area dry and exposed to air.

10. A, C, E, F

See the box, Best Practice for Patient Safety & Quality Care **QSEN** Assessing a Breast Mass, in your text. Important documentation includes: identifying the location of the mass by using the "face of the clock" method; describing the shape, size, and consistency of the mass; assessing whether the mass is fixed or movable; noting any skin changes around the mass, such as dimpling of the skin, increased vascularity, nipple retraction, nipple inversion, or skin ulceration; assessing the adjacent lymph nodes, both axillary and supraclavicular nodes; and asking clients if they experience pain or soreness in the area around the mass.

11. D

The nurse teaches women whose breast tissue is no longer influenced by hormonal fluctuations, such as after a total hysterectomy or menopause, to pick a day each month to do BSE and consistently perform BSE on the same day each month.

12. B, C, D, E, F

All of these options are correct topics for the nurse to teach the client except option A. In the immediate postoperative period, measurement of drainage is more frequent than in the later postoperative period, when the nurse checks the amount and color of drainage and the wound site when vital signs are checked (e.g., every 2, 4 or 6 hours).

13. D

The client should have the head of the bed elevated at least 30 degrees, with the affected arm elevated on a pillow while awake. Keeping the affected arm elevated promotes lymphatic fluid return after removal of lymph nodes and channels during the surgery.

14. A

After mastectomy, beginning exercises must not stress the incision and can usually be started on the first day after surgery. These exercises include squeezing the affected hand around a soft, round object (e.g., a ball or rolled washcloth) and flexion/extension of the elbow.

15. C

The nurse asks the client about joint or bone pain because the most common sites for metastases of breast cancer include bones, brain, liver, and lung; however, breast cancer can spread to any organ.

16. B.

A sign that sometimes indicates a client has late-stage breast cancer is an edematous thickening and pitting of breast skin called peau d'orange (orange peel skin).

17. D

A client with breast cancer may have difficulty coping and experience anxiety related to their disease and treatment. The nurse assesses the client's perceptions of the situation, then listens carefully and allows her to express these feelings.

18. B

Before surgery, a large tumor is sometimes treated with chemotherapy, called neoadjuvant therapy, to shrink the tumor before it is surgically removed. An advantage of this therapy is that cancer then can be removed by lumpectomy rather than mastectomy.

19. C

To decrease the chance of surgical site infection, priority teaching by the nurse includes the need to carefully observe the surgical wound for signs of swelling and infection throughout recovery. The client looks at the incision and flap for signs of bleeding, infection, and poor tissue perfusion, then reports any abnormalities to the health care provider.

20. C

Tamoxifen is a selective estrogen receptor modulator (SERM) drug. Common side effects of SERMs include hot flashes and weight gain. Rare but serious side effects of these drugs include endometrial cancer and thromboembolic events. The nurse would recommend the client check weight frequently and report weight gain to the health care provider.

21. A, B, C, D, E, F
The nurse expects a woman who undergoes an oophorectomy to have menopausal symptoms which includes all of these options.

22. B
The monoclonal antibody trastuzumab is a targeted cancer therapy. These drugs target specific characteristics of cancer cells, such as a protein, an enzyme, or the formation of new blood vessels. The advantage of targeted therapy over traditional chemotherapy is that targeted therapy is less likely to harm normal, healthy cells and therefore it has fewer side effects.

23. A, B, D, E
Risk factors for male breast cancer include previous radiation, a family history of breast cancer (male or female), *BRCA1* and/or *BRCA2* mutation, diabetes, alcohol and liver disease, testicular disorders, and obesity.

66 CHAPTER

Concepts of Care for Patients with Gynecologic Problems

1. About which factors will the nurse ask a client who is suspected of having uterine leiomyomas? **Select all that apply.**
   A. Hypertension
   B. Type 2 diabetes
   C. Early menarche
   D. Alcohol use
   E. Postmenopausal
   F. Heavy consumption of red meat

2. What does the nurse expect was documented as the presenting symptom for a female client admitted with uterine leiomyomas?
   A. Foul-smelling vaginal discharge
   B. Intermittent abdominal pain
   C. Heavy vaginal bleeding
   D. Urinary stress incontinence

3. What are the nurse's **best** actions when a client with uterine leiomyomas reports pelvic pressure, constipation, and urinary retention? **Select all that apply.**
   A. Check the lower extremities for fluid retention.
   B. Assess the abdomen for distention or enlargement.
   C. Measure fluid intake and urinary output.
   D. Ask the client if her pants fit tighter now.
   E. Measure residual urine using a urinary catheter.
   F. Measure the abdomen as a baseline for comparison.

4. For which complications will the nurse monitor in a client after hysteroscopic surgery for uterine leiomyomas? **Select all that apply.**
   A. Embolism
   B. Fluid overload
   C. Pneumonia
   D. Hemorrhage
   E. Persistent increased menstrual bleeding
   F. Cardiac dysrhythmias such as atrial fibrillation

5. In addition to the pelvic examination, for which diagnostic test will the nurse **most likely** prepare a client suspected to have uterine leiomyomas?
   A. Transvaginal ultrasound
   B. Laparoscopy
   C. Hysteroscopy
   D. Endometrial biopsy

6. Which client does the nurse understand is **most suitable** to undergo a uterine artery embolization procedure for leiomyomas?
   A. 18-year-old who is unmarried
   B. 25-year-old who is engaged to be married
   C. 35-year-old who is married and wants a child
   D. 46-year-old who is divorced with four children

7. Which activity restrictions will the nurse teach a client to follow after vaginal hysterectomy? **Select all that apply.**
   A. Limit stair climbing to less than five times a day.
   B. Do not lift anything heavier than 5 to 10 lb.
   C. Gradually increase walking as exercise.
   D. Do not cross your legs at the knees.
   E. Avoid sitting for extended periods of time.
   F. Do not drive until the surgeon tells you it's permitted.

8. Which condition is the client **most likely** to report to the nurse after uterine prolapse?
   A. "I have to use the bathroom much more often than I used to."
   B. "It feels like something is falling out down there."
   C. "I leak urine whenever I laugh, cough, or sneeze."
   D. "I've had two urinary tract infections in the last 3 months."

9. Which nonsurgical treatments for pelvic organ prolapse would the nurse teach a client about? **Select all that apply.**
   A. Pelvic floor muscle (Kegel) exercises
   B. Space-filling vaginal pessaries
   C. Bladder training program
   D. Low-fiber diet
   E. Stool softeners
   F. Laxatives

10. Which statement by a client to the nurse indicates that her anterior colporrhaphy has achieved the desired therapeutic outcome?
    A. "That constipated feeling has resolved."
    B. "The abdominal pain is almost gone."
    C. "I have good control over my urination."
    D. "My vaginal bleeding has completely stopped."

11. Which client does the nurse understand has the **greatest** need for evaluation of possible endometrial cancer?
    A. 63-year-old having bleeding after menopause
    B. 51-year-old having irregular menses for 6 months
    C. 35-year-old with report of multiple sexual partners
    D. 23-year-old with no menstrual period for 3 months

12. Which body parts does the nurse teach a client are removed during surgery for endometrial cancer? **Select all that apply.**
    A. Uterus
    B. Vagina
    C. Fallopian tubes
    D. Rectum
    E. Ovaries
    F. Bladder

13. Which care action will the nurse assign to the assistive personnel (AP) for a client receiving external radiation therapy for treatment of endometrial cancer?
    A. Gently washing the markings outlining the treatment site
    B. Monitoring for skin breakdown in the perineal area
    C. Assisting the client to ambulate to the bathroom if she feels fatigued
    D. Assessing the urinary catheter and urine output for color and odor

14. What **primary** factor does the nurse understand is the reason for low survival rates in clients with ovarian cancer?
    A. Ovarian cancer develops in clients with underlying immunosuppression and poor health.
    B. There are no specific diagnostic tests that can confirm or rule out ovarian cancer.
    C. Ovarian cancer does not respond well to conventional radiation or chemotherapy treatments.
    D. Symptoms are mild and vague, so the cancer is often not detected until in its late stage.

15. Which action will the nurse expect to take when a client diagnosed and treated for ovarian cancer has a recurrence?
    A. Arranging discussions with others who have recurring cancer
    B. Assessing readiness to explore palliative care and hospice
    C. Assisting to identify complementary therapies that may be helpful for palliation
    D. Teaching about radical hysterectomy followed by brachytherapy

16. What information will the nurse include when providing discharge teaching to a client who had a local cervical ablation? **Select all that apply.**
    A. Do not use tampons or douche.
    B. Take tub baths instead of showers.
    C. Refrain from sexual activity.
    D. Avoid lifting heavy objects.
    E. Expect to run a fever for the first week to 10 days.
    F. Report heavy bleeding or foul-smelling drainage.

17. When teaching a client about the loop electro-surgical excision procedure (LEEP) for cervical cancer, what does the nurse instruct the client is expected after the surgery?
    A. Spotting with slight pain
    B. Menses-like vaginal bleeding
    C. Cramps lasting during the first 48 hours
    D. Watery discharge during the first week

18. Which instruction will the nurse provide to the client who is currently receiving brachytherapy for gynecologic cancer?
    A. Call for help when getting out of bed.
    B. Stay in bed during the treatment session.
    C. Use a separate bathroom when you go home.
    D. Avoid being near children when you are home.

19. Which common **nonsexually** transmitted causes will the nurse ask a client about to determine possible causes of vulvovaginitis? **Select all that apply.**
    A. Yeast infection
    B. Herpes simplex
    C. Feminine hygiene sprays
    D. Pediculosis pubis
    E. Tight-fitting clothes
    F. Vaginal sponges

20. What self-management strategy will the nurse recommend to a client to prevent vulvovaginitis?
    A. Wear lightweight nylon underwear.
    B. Apply antiseptic cream to the perineal area daily.
    C. Cleanse the inner labial mucosa with antiseptic soap.
    D. Choose breathable fabrics to wear such as cotton.

21. Which question does the nurse ask when a 22-year-old female client is being evaluated for possible toxic shock syndrome (TSS)?
    A. "How many pads do you use on heavy flow days?"
    B. "Have you every used intravaginal estrogen therapy?"
    C. "Do you have a history of multiple sexual partners?"
    D. "Do you use an insertable contraceptive device?"

22. Which clinical signs and symptoms will the nurse assess for when a client is admitted with a diagnosis of toxic shock syndrome (TSS)? **Select all that apply.**
    A. Itching
    B. Fever
    C. Macular rash
    D. Hypertension
    E. Myalgias
    F. Vaginal lesions

23. Which preventive measure will the nurse include when teaching a group of female clients about prevention of toxic shock syndrome?
    A. "Use sanitary napkins on heavy flow days."
    B. "Use superabsorbent tampons only at night."
    C. "Change the tampon every 3 to 6 hours."
    D. "Void before and immediately after intercourse."

Chapter 66 Answer Key

1. A, C, D, F
   Known risk factors that are associated with development of leiomyomas that the nurse would be familiar with include early menarche, significant consumption of red meats, use of alcohol, and hypertension.

2. C
   The nurse expects that a woman admitted with uterine leiomyomas most likely presented with heavy vaginal bleeding. Many women with leiomyomas report painful menstruation, often with heavy flow and the presence of clots, which cause them to seek medical care.

3. B, D, F
   When a client reports feeling of pelvic pressure and altered elimination patterns, including constipation and urinary frequency or retention, these symptoms are the result of the enlarged fibroid pressing on other organs. The client may notice that her abdomen has increased in size. Assess the woman's abdomen for distention or enlargement and measure for a baseline comparison. Ask if her clothes are fitting tighter or it's difficult to zip or button her pants.

4. A, B, D, E
   The nurse monitors for rare but potential complications of hysteroscopic surgery, which include: fluid overload (fluid used to distend the uterine cavity can be absorbed); embolism; hemorrhage; perforation of the uterus, bowel, or bladder and ureter injury; persistent increased menstrual bleeding; and incomplete suppression of menstruation. Severe pain or heavy bleeding are reported immediately to the surgeon or Rapid Response Team.

5. A
   To diagnose uterine leiomyomas, transvaginal ultrasound (US), a procedure in which the ultrasound probe is placed into the vagina for visualization, is the diagnostic study of choice.

6. D
   An alternative to surgery for a woman who does not desire pregnancy is uterine artery embolization (also called uterine fibroid embolization) which is performed under local anesthesia, or with sedation if the client requests. The interventional radiologist uses a percutaneous catheter inserted through the femoral artery to inject polyvinyl alcohol and gelatin-like pellets into the uterine artery. The uterine artery then carries these materials into the blood vessels that feed the leiomyoma. The resulting blockage starves the tumor of circulation, allowing it to shrink and may lead to infertility.

7. A, B, C, D, E, F
   The nurse would teach a client all of these activity restrictions after a vaginal hysterectomy. For more information on teaching clients after hysterectomy, see the box in your text titled, Patient and Family Education: Preparing for Self-Management Care After a Total Vaginal or Abdominal Hysterectomy.

8. B
   Clients with suspected uterine prolapse may report a feeling of "something falling out," dyspareunia (painful intercourse), backache,

and/or heaviness or pressure in the pelvis. Options A, C, and D are signs of cystocele or bladder prolapse.

9. A, B, C, E, F
Nonsurgical management of pelvic organ prolapse includes teaching women to improve pelvic support and tone by doing pelvic floor muscle exercises (PFMEs, or Kegel exercises). Space-filling devices such as a vaginal pessary can be worn to elevate the uterine prolapse. Women with bladder symptoms may benefit from bladder training and attention to complete emptying. The primary health care provider usually prescribes a **high**-fiber diet, stool softeners, and laxatives.

10. C
An anterior colporrhaphy (anterior repair) tightens the pelvic muscles for better bladder support, and is usually only performed after the client has unsuccessfully tried conservative management and continues to have bothersome symptoms. The desired outcome is that the client will have better control of urine output.

11. A
The main symptom of endometrial cancer is abnormal uterine bleeding [AUB], especially postmenopausal. The 51-year-old is likely going through menopause, and the 23-year-old may be pregnant. Having multiple sexual partners is not a risk factor for endometrial cancer.

12. A, C, E
The most common surgical procedure to address endometrial cancer involves the removal of the uterus, fallopian tubes, and ovaries (total hysterectomy and bilateral salpingo-oophorectomy [BSO]).

13. C
An AP's scope of practice includes aspects of client care such as bathing, feeding, ambulating, and checking and recording vital signs. The nurse is familiar with this scope of practice and appropriately assigns client care tasks to the AP. The AP is instructed not to wash the radiation therapy markings. The nurse monitors and assesses clients.

14. D
The survival rates for ovarian cancer are low because many women do not seek care early. They associate common early symptoms (e.g., bloating, urinary urgency or frequency, difficulty eating or feeling full, and pelvic pain) and other vague symptoms (weight gain, constipation, bloating) with menopause. Survival rates are low because this cancer is often not detected until in its late stages.

15. B
Ovarian cancer has a high recurrence rate. After recurrence, the cancer is treatable but no longer curable. When this occurs, the client may deny symptoms at first or express feelings of anger and grief. The client and family are often fearful of the outcome. The nurse provides encouragement and support during this difficult time and references to grief counseling, spiritual leaders (if desired), and community support groups. For clients with advanced metastatic disease, the nurse collaborates with members of the interprofessional team for possible referral to palliative care and hospice.

16. A, C, D, F
Discharge teaching for a client who had a local cervical ablation includes: refraining from sexual intercourse; not using tampons; not douching; taking showers rather than tub baths; avoiding lifting heavy objects; and reporting any heavy vaginal bleeding, foul-smelling drainage, or fever.

17. A
LEEP is both a diagnostic procedure and a treatment because it provides a specimen that can be examined by a pathologist to ensure that the lesion was completely removed. Spotting (very scant bleeding) and slight pain after the procedure is common.

18. B
While the radioactive implant is in place for brachytherapy, radiation is emitted that can affect other people, so others will not be in the room. Inform the client that she is restricted to bedrest during the treatment session (10 to 20 minutes) to prevent dislodgment of the

radioactive source. At the completion of treatment, the client may go home the same day. There are no restrictions for the client to stay away from her family or the public between treatments.

19. A, C, E, F
The most common nonsexual causes of vulvovaginitis include: yeast infections and chemicals such as spermicides, vaginal sponges, feminine hygiene sprays, bubble baths and soaps, and new or different laundry detergent. Other causes include wearing tight-fitting clothing and wiping from back to front, introducing bacteria from the stool into the vagina. Herpes simplex and pediculosis pubis are sexually transmitted.

20. D
The nurse recommends that the client wear breathable fabrics such as cotton to prevent development of vulvovaginitis. See Patient and Family Education: Preparing for Self-Management Prevention of Vulvovaginitis in

your text for additional prevention strategies for prevention of vulvovaginitis.

21. D
Toxic shock syndrome (TSS) can result from leaving a tampon, contraceptive sponge, or diaphragm in the vagina.

22. B, C, E
Common signs and symptoms of TSS include fever (which remains elevated despite treatment), diffuse macular rash, myalgias, and hypotension. The rash associated with TSS often looks like a sunburn, and clients can develop broken capillaries in the eyes and skin.

23. C
To prevent TSS, the nurse would advise clients to change tampons every 3 to 6 hours. See Patient and Family Education: Preparing for Self-Management Prevention of Toxic Shock Syndrome in your text for additional preventive strategies for TSS.

Concepts of Care for Patients with Male Reproductive Problems

1. Which symptom does the nurse **most likely** expect when admitting a client diagnosed with benign prostatic hyperplasia (BPH)?
   A. Erectile dysfunction
   B. Pain in the scrotum
   C. Difficulty passing urine
   D. Constipation

2. Which technique is **best** when the nurse assesses an obese client who reports symptoms associated with benign prostatic hyperplasia?
   A. Instructing the client to urinate, then using the bedside ultrasound bladder scanner
   B. Applying gentle pressure to the bladder to elicit urgency, then instructing the client to void
   C. Having the client drink several large glasses of water, then percussing the bladder
   D. Instructing the client to undress from the waist down, then inspecting and palpating the bladder

3. Which questions will the nurse ask a client to determine the presence of signs and symptoms of benign prostatic hyperplasia (BPH)? **Select all that apply.**
   A. "Have you noticed a sensation of incomplete bladder emptying?"
   B. "Have you recently experienced a testicular or bladder infection?"
   C. "Have you noticed dribbling or leaking after you finish urination?"
   D. "How many times do you have to get up during the night to urinate?"
   E. "Have you noticed blood at the start or at the end of urination?"
   F. "Have you noticed increased force or size of your urine stream?"

4. What action will the advanced practice nurse take after performing a digital rectal examination on a client with benign prostatic hyperplasia (BPH)?
   A. Instruct the client to remain in a supine position with knees bent.
   B. Massage the prostate to obtain a fluid sample for possible prostatitis.
   C. Use a sterile cotton-tipped applicator for a sample from the penis for possible infection.
   D. Administer pain medication to relieve the discomfort from the examination.

5. Which behavioral modification instructions will the nurse teach a client with benign prostatic hyperplasia (BPH)? **Select all that apply.**
   A. Take diuretics to increase urine output.
   B. Limit alcohol intake.
   C. Avoid caffeine containing beverages.
   D. Do not consume large amounts of fluid in a short time.
   E. Avoid sexual intercourse.
   F. Avoid taking antihistamine drugs.

6. Which laboratory tests does the nurse expect to be ordered to screen for prostate cancer in a client with benign prostatic hyperplasia (BPH)? **Select all that apply.**
   A. Urinalysis and urine culture
   B. Complete blood count (CBC)
   C. Prostate-specific antigen (PSA)
   D. Blood urea nitrogen (BUN)
   E. Serum acid phosphatase
   F. Serum creatinine

7. Which question will the nurse ask a client to determine whether the drug tamsulosin is achieving the desired therapeutic effect?
   A. "Do you have a green or yellow discharge from your penis?"
   B. "Are you having any problems achieving an erection?"
   C. "Does your urine have a strong odor or appear cloudy?"
   D. "Are you continuing to have difficulty passing urine?"

8. Which diagnostic procedure does the nurse expect the health care provider to order to test a client with an enlarged bladder, for bladder outlet obstruction?
   A. Bladder ultrasound scan
   B. Urodynamic pressure-flow study
   C. Computed tomography scan
   D. Transrectal ultrasound

9. Which action does the nurse teach a client with BPH to perform that can help relieve obstructive symptoms?
   A. Urinate before going to bed and immediately upon waking.
   B. Consume fluids regularly throughout the day.
   C. Increase the frequency of sexual intercourse.
   D. Urinate forcefully after drinking a large glass of water.

10. Which criteria will the nurse assess in a client with benign prostatic hyperplasia that indicate the need for a surgical treatment? **Select all that apply.**
    A. Hydronephrosis
    B. Acute urinary tract infection unresponsive to first-line antibiotics
    C. Hematuria
    D. Chronic urinary tract infection secondary to residual urine in bladder
    E. Recurrent kidney stones
    F. Acute urinary retention due to obstruction

11. What does the nurse teach an older client with prostate cancer who is scheduled to have a digital rectal examination (DRE) and a prostate-specific antigen (PSA) test?
    A. The PSA laboratory test is drawn before the DRE.
    B. The DRE is completed 2 weeks before the PSA.
    C. The PSA is reviewed first because DRE may not be necessary.
    D. Both tests can be completed at the client's convenience.

12. Which nursing actions are included in the care of a client who had a transurethral resection of the prostate (TURP)? **Select all that apply.**
    A. Helping the client out of the bed to the chair as soon as permitted to prevent complications of immobility
    B. Using normal saline solution for the intermittent bladder irrigant unless otherwise prescribed
    C. Monitoring and documenting the color, consistency, and amount of urine output
    D. Providing a safe environment for the client because of temporary changes in mental status
    E. Assessing the client for reports of severe bladder spasms with decreased urinary output
    F. Checking the drainage tubing frequently for external obstructions such as kinks, and internal obstructions such as blood clots

13. Which client does the nurse recognize has the **highest** risk for development of prostate cancer?
    A. 45-year-old Asian American with a history of benign prostatic hyperplasia
    B. 55-year-old Hispanic American who practices poor dietary intake
    C. 65-year-old Caucasian American with two cousins who developed prostate cancer
    D. 75-year-old African American whose father and brother developed prostate cancer

14. Which laboratory test suggests to the nurse that a client with prostate cancer has metastasis to the bone?
    A. Decreased alpha-fetoprotein
    B. Increased blood urea nitrogen (BUN)
    C. Elevated serum alkaline phosphatase
    D. Decreased serum creatinine

15. To which common sites does the nurse expect metastasis when a client has prostate cancer? **Select all that apply.**
    A. Liver
    B. Pancreas
    C. Lungs
    D. Lumbar spine
    E. Kidneys
    F. Bones of the pelvis

16. After a transrectal ultrasound with biopsy for prostate cancer, what instructions will the nurse provide the client? **Select all that apply.**
    A. Report fever, chills, bloody urine, and any difficulty voiding.
    B. The biopsy will diagnose if you have prostate cancer.
    C. Drink plenty of fluids during the first 24 hours.
    D. Expect to see bright red bleeding at first.
    E. Report any pink color in the urine to the health care provider.
    F. Avoid strenuous physical activity.

17. What is the nurse's **best** action when assessing a client after open radical prostatectomy and finding scrotal and penile swelling?
    A. Notify the health care provider and monitor for inability to urinate.
    B. Elevate the scrotum and penis, then apply ice to the area intermittently.
    C. Assist the client to increase mobility by using early ambulation.
    D. Observe the urethral meatus for redness, discharge, and abnormal output.

18. Which common serum tumor markers does the nurse expect will be ordered to confirm a client's suspected diagnosis of testicular cancer? **Select all that apply.**
    A. Early prostate cancer antigen (EPCA-2)
    B. Lactate dehydrogenase (LDH)
    C. Alpha-fetoprotein (AFP)
    D. Beta human chorionic gonadotropin (hCG)
    E. BRCA1 mutation
    F. Glutathione S-transferase (GST P1)

19. What does the nurse practitioner suspect when performing an examination on a young male client and finding a testicular lump that is hard and painless?
    A. Prostate cancer
    B. Epididymitis
    C. Testicular cancer
    D. Erectile dysfunction

20. Which instructions will the nurse teach a client after an open retroperitoneal lymph node dissection (RPLND) for testicular cancer? **Select all that apply.**
    A. Do not lift anything that weighs over 15 lbs.
    B. Limit intake of fluids to 1000 to 1200 mL per day.
    C. Do not drive a car until the health care provider allows it.
    D. Perform monthly testicular self-examination on the remaining testicle.
    E. Report fever, drainage, or increasing tenderness around the incision.
    F. Avoid climbing stairs during the first week after surgery.

21. Which **priority** information will the nurse gather from a client who is seeking a prescription for sildenafil for erectile dysfunction?
    A. Medication prescription for nitrate drugs
    B. Presence of nocturnal or morning erections
    C. Use of any illicit drugs or substances
    D. Dietary consumption of proteins each day

22. Which potential causes of organic erectile dysfunction does the nurse assess for in a client? **Select all that apply.**
    A. Kidney disease
    B. Diverticulitis
    C. Thyroid disorders
    D. Obesity
    E. Diabetes mellitus
    F. Penile trauma

23. Which instruction will the nurse provide to a client who is taking a phosphodiesterase-5 (PDE5) inhibitor drug for erectile dysfunction?
    A. If one pill does not work, wait an hour and take a second pill.
    B. Use relaxation techniques before and after taking this drug.
    C. Abstain from alcohol use before sexual intercourse.
    D. Do not perform heavy lifting while using this medication.

24. What is the nurse's **best** response when a client who had a vasectomy asks when sexual intercourse can be safely resumed?
    A. "Your surgeon will discuss the timing and will tell you when it is safe to have sex again."
    B. "It depends on how much swelling, pain, and bruising you experience after the surgery."
    C. "Just to be safe, you should probably wait at least 6 months or more before having sex."
    D. "Sexual intercourse should be avoided for at least 1 week after your surgery."

Chapter 67 Answer Key

1. C
   As the client's prostate gland enlarges, it extends upward into the bladder and inward, causing bladder outlet obstruction. Because of this, the nurse expects the symptom of difficulty in starting and continuing urination.

2. A
   Clients with obesity are best assessed with percussion by the health care provider, or bedside ultrasound bladder scanner by the nurse, rather than by inspection or palpation. Instruct the client to urinate before the examination.

3. A, C, D, E
   The nurse asks the client about the number of times he awakens during the night to void (nocturia). Other important topics to question a client about include: difficulty in starting (hesitancy) and continuing urination; reduced force and size of the urinary stream ("weak" stream); sensation of incomplete bladder emptying; straining to begin urination; postvoid (after voiding) dribbling or leaking; and hematuria (blood in the urine) when starting the urine stream or at the end of urination.

4. B
   After palpating the prostate gland through a digital rectal examination (DRE), the nurse practitioner may massage the prostate to obtain a fluid sample for examination to rule out prostatitis (inflammation and possible infection of the prostate), a common problem that can occur with BPH.

5. B, C, D, F
   Behavioral modifications that the nurse teaches a client with BPH include avoidance of drinking large amounts of fluid in a short period of time, especially before going out or at bedtime; limiting caffeine and alcohol consumption, as these have a diuretic effect; and avoiding drugs that can cause urinary retention, especially anticholinergics, antihistamines, antipsychotics, and muscle relaxants.

6. C, E
   Laboratory tests for cancer screening include PSA (most commonly used to test for early prostate cancer), and serum acid phosphatase (to screen for metastatic prostate cancer). Creatinine and BUN evaluate renal function. CBC

looks for evidence of systemic infection or anemia. A urinalysis and urine culture evaluate for systemic infection and if there is blood in the urine, for anemia.

7. D
Tamsulosin is an alpha^1 adrenergic antagonist drug. These drugs act to relax smooth muscle in the bladder neck, which will help make urination less difficult.

8. B
The health care provider orders a urodynamic pressure-flow study to help in determining if there is urine blockage or weakness of the detrusor muscle.

9. C
The nurse teaches the client that frequent sexual intercourse can reduce obstructive symptoms because it causes the release of prostatic fluid. This approach is helpful for a client whose obstructive symptoms result from an enlarged prostate with a large amount of retained prostatic fluid.

10. A, C, D, F
For a client with BPH, some or all of these criteria indicate the need for surgery: acute urinary retention due to obstruction; chronic urinary tract infections secondary to residual urine in the bladder; hematuria; hydronephrosis; and persistent pain with decrease in urine flow.

11. A
The PSA laboratory test should be drawn before the DRE because this examination can cause an increase in PSA due to prostate irritation.

12. A, B, C, D, E, F
All of these options are appropriate nursing actions when caring for a client after a TURP. See Best Practice for Patient Safety & Quality Care **QSEN** Care of the Patient After Transurethral Resection of the Prostate in your text for additional appropriate nursing care actions to take after a client has a TURP.

13. D
The risk of prostate cancer increases for men who have a first-degree relative (father, brother, son) with the disease, and for African-American men.

14. C
The laboratory test result that suggests metastasis of prostate cancer to the bones is elevated serum alkaline phosphatase levels. These clients also have severe pain.

15. A, C, D, F
Common sites of metastasis from prostate cancer are the nearby lymph nodes and bones, although it can also metastasize to the lungs or liver. The bones of the pelvis, sacrum, and lumbar spine are most often affected.

16. A, B, C, F
After a transrectal ultrasound with biopsy, the nurse teaches a client to report fever, chills, bloody urine, and any difficulty voiding. He is advised to avoid strenuous physical activity and to drink plenty of fluids, especially in the first 24 hours after the procedure. The nurse teaches that a small amount of bleeding turning the urine pink is expected during this time. Bright red bleeding should be reported to the health care provider immediately. The biopsy provides an accurate diagnosis for prostate cancer.

17. B
After open radical prostatectomy, when the nurse assesses and finds swelling of the scrotum and penis, the best action is to elevate the scrotum and penis and apply ice to the area intermittently for the first 24 to 48 hours. The cause of this swelling is from the disrupted pelvic lymph flow.

18. B, C, D
Common serum tumor markers that are used when formulating a diagnosis of testicular cancer are: alpha-fetoprotein (AFP), beta human chorionic gonadotropin (hCG), and lactate dehydrogenase (LDH). Early prostate cancer antigen (EPCA-2) may be a serum marker for prostate cancer. Glutathione S-transferase

(GST P1) mutation increases the risk for prostate cancer. BRCA1 mutation increases a woman's risk for breast cancer.

19. C
The most common finding in a client with testicular cancer is a painless, hard swelling or enlargement of the testicle. A health care provider palpates the testes for lumps and swelling that are often not visible.

20. A, C, D, E
The nurse teaches the client the following instructions after RPLND: do not lift anything over 15 lb (6.8 kg), avoid stair climbing, and do not drive a car for several weeks. Notify the surgeon immediately if chills, fever, vomiting, increasing incisional pain, drainage, or dehiscence of the incision occurs. Perform monthly testicular self-examination (TSE) on the remaining testis. The client should **not** limit fluid intake to 1000 to 1200 mL per day.

21. A
The nurse asks the client whether he takes nitrates. Men who are prescribed nitrates must avoid PDE5 inhibitors (e.g., sildenafil) because the vasodilation effects can cause a profound hypotension and reduce blood flow to vital organs.

22. A, C, E, F
Potential causes of organic erectile dysfunction include: vascular endocrine, or neurologic diseases; chronic diseases (e.g., diabetes mellitus, renal failure); penile disease or trauma; and surgery or pharmaceutical therapies.

23. C
The nurse teaches a client taking PDE5 inhibitors to abstain from alcohol before sexual intercourse because it may impair the ability to have an erection.

24. D
Heavy lifting, sports, and sexual intercourse should be avoided for at least 1 week. Teach the client and partner to use an alternate form of contraception until a 3-month follow-up. At that time, a semen analysis will be performed to determine if the procedure was effective.

Concepts of Care for Transgender Patients

CHAPTER 68

1. Which statement made to the nurse by a client **most accurately** describes self-identification as transgender?
   A. "Since childhood I have always felt like I was born in the wrong body."
   B. "I have always been attracted to other women and they are attracted to me."
   C. "I think women are more amazing and influential and I prefer to be viewed as a woman."
   D. "I enjoy wearing women's clothes because they are pretty and feel so nice."

2. What question will the nurse ask **first** when a client's medical record states that he has gender dysphoria?
   A. "Do you think of yourself as male or female?"
   B. "Are you seeking interventions for sex reassignment?"
   C. "How do you prefer to be addressed?"
   D. "What issues of sexuality would you like to talk about?"

3. When the nurse interviews a transgender client, which statement is of **greatest** concern for failure to cope with major life stressors?
   A. "I smoke two to three packs of cigarettes every day."
   B. "I've tried to commit suicide four times in my life."
   C. "When I feel really down, I drink and use marijuana."
   D. "Last night I went to a bar and picked up a stranger for sex."

4. From the acronym LGBTQ, which terms will the nurse understand refer to the sexual orientation of a client? **Select all that apply.**
   A. Questioning
   B. Queer
   C. Transgender
   D. Bisexual
   E. Gay
   F. Lesbian

5. Which recommendations will nurses follow to create a safe, welcoming environment for LGBTQ client care? **Select all that apply.**
   A. Designating unisex or single-stall restrooms
   B. Making waiting rooms inclusive of LGBTQ clients and families
   C. Not limiting gender options on medical forms to "male" and "female"
   D. Ensuring that visitation policies are equitable for families of LGBTQ clients
   E. Reflecting the client's choice of terminology in communication and documentation
   F. Including gender-neutral language on all medical forms and documents

6. In which circumstance will the nurse make a clinical judgment to forgo extensive questioning about a client's gender identity?
   A. The client is dressed like a man and wants information about hormones that feminize the body.
   B. The client has recurrent urinary tract infections despite compliance with the medication treatment regime.
   C. The client appears to be male but requests a pelvic examination by a female health care provider.
   D. The client requires treatment for a severely sprained ankle sustained during a soccer game.

7. What will the nurse do **first** when a natal male client who appears to be female has an order for placement of a urinary indwelling catheter for hourly urine output measurement?
   A. Introduce himself or herself, ask how the client prefers to be addressed, verify the client's identity by checking the name band, and explain the procedure.
   B. Respectfully address the client by the name on the chart and armband, then perform catheter insertion for a male client.
   C. Inspect the genitalia and adapt the catheter insertion as appropriate while avoiding the use of gender-specific language.
   D. Politely leave and obtain advice from the charge nurse about whether to treat the client as male or female.

8. What is the nurse's **best** action after inadvertently making an error when addressing a transgender client by not using their preferred name or pronoun?
   A. Apologize and explain that working with transgender clients is a new experience.
   B. Assume that the client is used to this type of error and continue providing care.
   C. Self-correct and continue providing care rather than making a prolonged apology.
   D. Observe the client's nonverbal behavior to determine whether the error was noticed.

9. Which **increased** health risks will the nurse monitor for when a transgender client is prescribed estrogen therapy? **Select all that apply.**
   A. Elevated blood glucose
   B. Fluid retention
   C. Hypotension
   D. Estrogen-dependent cancer
   E. Kidney disease
   F. Venous thromboembolism

10. What physical changes will the nurse teach a client to expect when undergoing estrogen therapy for male-to-female (MtF) transition? **Select all that apply.**
    A. Decreased testicular size
    B. Increased libido (sex drive)
    C. Reduced muscle mass
    D. Increased erectile function
    E. Softening of skin
    F. Increased body hair growth

11. Based on the guidelines from the World Professional Association for Transgender Health (WPATH), which clients meet the criteria for gender-affirming hormonal therapy? **Select all that apply.**
    A. 16-year-old who has experienced gender dysphoria since early childhood
    B. 30-year-old with gender dysphoria and no physical or mental health problems
    C. 40-year-old who would like to temporarily try being a member of the opposite sex
    D. 45-year-old with gender dysphoria since grade school and well-controlled hypertension
    E. 62-year-old with known history of gender dysphoria and symptoms of dementia
    F. 65-year-old lesbian with history of multiple suicide attempts

12. Which laboratory result will the nurse monitor to **prevent harm** when a client on estrogen therapy is also prescribed spironolactone?
    A. Blood glucose level
    B. Platelet count
    C. White blood cell count
    D. Serum potassium level

13. Which finding does the nurse assess to determine that a female-to-male (FtM) client prescribed testosterone is having the desired effect?
    A. Client reports breast tenderness.
    B. Nurse observes increased body hair.
    C. Client reports decreased sex drive.
    D. Nurse observes average sized male penis.

14. Which nursing actions are included in the preoperative care of a male-to-female (MtF) client who will undergo a vaginoplasty? **Select all that apply.**
    A. Give nothing by mouth for 24 hours prior to surgery.
    B. Administer an enema and laxatives as prescribed.
    C. Instruct the client to ambulate because positioning for surgery will be prolonged.
    D. Monitor for and report hematocrit and hemoglobin level results.
    E. Administer preoperative antimicrobials to minimize infection.
    F. Monitor and record the drainage from the Jackson-Pratt drain.

15. Which client report indicates to the nurse that one of the **most serious** complications of vaginoplasty has occurred?
    A. Burning sensation during urination
    B. Urinary incontinence when sneezing
    C. Leakage of stool from the vagina
    D. Tenderness and bruising of the labia

16. Which information will the nurse include when teaching a client who had a vaginoplasty about self-care management? **Select all that apply.**
    A. Do not take baths (submerged in water) for 8 months after surgery.
    B. Avoid tobacco or smoking for at least a month after surgery to promote healing.
    C. Carefully follow the prescribed individualized dilator protocol.
    D. Do not have sexual intercourse until at least 3 months after surgery.
    E. Avoid swimming or bike riding for 3 weeks.
    F. Take acetaminophen as prescribed for pain control at home.

Chapter 68 Answer Key

1. A
   A client who identifies self as transgender does not view this as a choice or lifestyle but, rather, an inner sense of being born in the wrong body.

2. C
   A client with gender dysphoria experiences emotional or psychological distress caused by an incongruence between one's natal (birth) sex and gender identity. The most appropriate question for the nurse to ask is how the client prefers to be addressed.

3. B
   For transgender clients, major life stressors, emotional distress, and lack of resources can lead to suicidal ideation or suicide attempts when all other methods of coping have failed. This client requires follow-up with regard to suicide ideation. The health care provider must be notified and a mental health assessment with counselling and follow-up may be needed.

4. D, E, F
   L (lesbian), G (gay), and B (bisexual) refer to specific sexual orientation. However, transgender is nonspecific for sexual orientation and clients may identify as heterosexual, homosexual, both, or neither. Q refers to clients who are queer or questioning (people who do not feel they belong in any other subgroup).

5. A, B, C, D, E, F
   All of these options will help make waiting rooms safer and more welcoming for LBGTQ clients. See the box titled Best Practice for Patient Safety & Quality Care **QSEN** The Joint Commission Recommendations for Creating a Safe, Welcoming Environment for LGBTQ Patients in your text for additional suggestions.

6. D

The treatment of the injury for the client in option D does not require sexual assessment, so there is no need to ask extensive questions about sexual identity. The clients in options A, B, and C have problems that will likely require questioning about sexual identity.

7. A

As with any client, introduce yourself, and ask how he or she prefers to be addressed. Verify his or her identity, then explain the procedure and answer any questions before performing the catheter insertion.

8. C

Occasionally nurses recognize the cues and know their client's preferred name or pronoun, but accidentally say the wrong one. Transgender clients encounter this situation often and typically anticipate an occasional error. When this error occurs, simply self-correct and continue with care rather than make a prolonged apology. Focusing too much on the error may make the client more uncomfortable because more attention has been drawn to the situation.

9. A, B, D, F

Estrogen therapy can cause increased health risks such as increased blood clotting leading to venous thromboembolism (VTE), elevated blood glucose, hypertension, estrogen-dependent cancers, and fluid retention.

10. A, C, E

The nurse providing care for a client undergoing a MtF transition would teach about these changes: breast tissue development, reduced or absent sperm count and ejaculatory fluid, reduced muscle mass, change in emotions, change in sweat and odor patterns, decreased testicular size, reduced erectile function, decreased libido (sex drive), decreased body hair growth, and softening of skin.

11. B, D

According to WPATH's most recent Standards of Care (2011), the criteria for gender-affirming hormonal therapy include continuing and well-documented gender dysphoria, client ability to make a fully informed decision and give consent to treatment, client older than 18 years, and well-controlled existing medical or mental health problems.

12. D

Spironolactone is used as an androgen blocker. It is a low-cost potassium-sparing diuretic that also inhibits testosterone secretion and androgen binding to androgen receptors. Periodic laboratory tests to assess for hyperkalemia may be needed especially for clients with renal insufficiency.

13. B

Expected changes when a FtM client is taking testosterone therapy include voice deepening, body hair growth (hirsutism) with possibly hairline recession and male pattern baldness, increased muscle mass, increased libido, increased aggression, vaginal dryness, clitoral growth, redistribution of fat, and cessation of menses.

14. B, D, E

Preoperative care for a MtF client having a vaginoplasty includes a bowel preparation which may be started 24 hours before surgery, and may include a clear liquid diet, laxatives, and sodium phosphate/saline enemas. Increased fluids are recommended until the client goes to bed the night before surgery because the bowel preparation can be very dehydrating. Antimicrobials are typically given on the day of surgery to minimize the risk for infection. Adequate hemoglobin and hematocrit (H&H) levels are especially important because some blood is lost during surgery. Jackson-Pratt drainage is monitored postoperatively.

15. C

One of the worst complications is a vaginal-rectal fistula, which is caused by rectal perforation during surgery. The nurse teaches a client to report any leakage of stool into the vagina immediately to their surgeon.

16. B, C, D, F
    See the box titled Best Practice for Patient Safety & Quality Care Postoperative Teaching for Clients Who Have a Vaginoplasty in your text for a list of postoperative teaching that the nurse must include for a client who has a vaginoplasty. Option A is not correct because the client should not take a bath for 8 weeks postoperatively, and option E is not correct because swimming and bike riding should be avoided for 3 months.

CHAPTER 69

Concepts of Care for Patients with Sexually Transmitted Infections

1. Which client situations will the nurse understand have the **greatest** risk of acquiring a sexually transmitted infection (STI)? **Select all that apply.**
   A. Having more than one sexual partner
   B. Engaging in anal, rectal, or vaginal sex without a condom
   C. Having sex while using drugs or alcohol
   D. Engaging in sex with a partner who was successfully treated for an STI in the past
   E. Having sex with a partner who uses intravenous drugs
   F. Having engaged in sexual activities with more than one partner in the past

2. Which safer sex practices will the nurse teach clients to prevent sexually transmitted infections (STIs)? **Select all that apply.**
   A. Wearing gloves for finger or hand contact with the vagina or rectum
   B. Using a latex or polyurethane condom for genital and anal intercourse
   C. Practicing serial monogamy
   D. Wash hands immediately after contact with vagina or rectum
   E. Using a condom or latex barrier during oral-genital or oral-anal sexual contact
   F. Practicing abstinence

3. What is the nurse's **best** advice when a client reports contracting genital herpes (GH) several years ago and asks about recurrences?
   A. "If you haven't had any further episodes, the GH is inactive and you are not contagious."
   B. "If you don't have any open sores or notice any drainage, the GH is not contagious."
   C. "GH can recur and not show symptoms but infection is still possible, so you should always use a condom."
   D. "The majority of adults have already been exposed to GH, so you don't have to worry about passing it on."

4. What **priority** teaching will the nurse provide to a young female client with a severe case of genital herpes (GH) regarding long-term consequences of the infection?
   A. Provide instructions about an increased risk for central nervous system complications.
   B. Teach about the increased risk for neonatal transmission and acquiring HIV infection.
   C. Discuss the increased risk for multiple types of reproductive cancer in young women.
   D. Tell the client about the increased risk for scarring and adhesions of the fallopian tubes.

5. Which interprofessional treatments will the nurse discuss with a client with genital herpes (GH)? **Select all that apply.**
   A. Administering sitz baths three or four times a day
   B. Encouraging genital hygiene by keeping the skin clean and dry
   C. Never using a urinary catheter because of increased risk for infection
   D. Encouraging frequent urination while pouring water over the genitalia
   E. Washing hands thoroughly after contact with lesions
   F. Applying local anesthetic sprays or ointments as prescribed

6. What does the nurse suspect when a client reports itching and tingling for 2 days followed by a blister on the penis that ruptured spontaneously and is painful?
   A. Syphilis
   B. Genital warts
   C. Gonorrhea
   D. Genital herpes

7. What information does the nurse include when teaching a young male client about the use of condoms to prevent sexually transmitted infections (STIs)? **Select all that apply.**
   A. Use spermicide (nonoxynol-9) with condoms.
   B. Put condoms on before any genital contact.
   C. Assure that a lubricant, if used, is oil-based.
   D. Never use a condom more than once.
   E. Keep condoms in a cool, dry place.
   F. Always handle a condom with care to avoid damaging it.

8. What **first** symptom(s) will the nurse assess for when a client has been exposed to syphilis?
   A. A small painless sore called a chancre
   B. Urinary frequency and burning with incontinence
   C. Malaise, low-grade fever, and headache
   D. Rash that appears on the palm, soles, and trunk

9. What is the nurse's **best** advice for a client who was exposed to syphilis about 3 weeks ago and reports being asymptomatic and abstinent since the incident?
   A. "Continue abstinence for up to 6 months and report any painless sores that appear on your genitals."
   B. "The first symptoms can appear anytime between 12 days and 12 weeks after exposure, so you should come in and be tested."
   C. "If you are still asymptomatic at 3 weeks after exposure, it is unlikely that you have contracted this sexually transmitted infection."
   D. "It's recommended that you check with your partner or partners to make sure that they have the disease and may have passed it on to you."

10. What instruction will the nurse provide the assistive personnel (AP) when a client is admitted to the emergency department (ED) with a pustular rash related to secondary syphilis?
    A. Gloves should always be worn when caring for or touching the client.
    B. If the skin is open and draining fluid, use gloves only during client care.
    C. The lesions are highly contagious so let the client perform his or her own hygiene care.
    D. No instructions are given because the client's privacy and confidentiality are essential.

11. Which interprofessional collaborative care action and teaching does the nurse expect to complete when a client is diagnosed with primary syphilis?
    A. Administering benzathine penicillin G given intramuscularly for 7 days and teaching about follow-up evaluations at 3, 6, and 12 months
    B. Administering ceftriaxone intramuscularly in a single dose plus azithromycin 1 g orally in a single dose, and teaching about follow-up evaluations at 3, 6, and 12 months
    C. Administering metronidazole orally twice daily for 14 days and instructing the client about follow-up evaluations at 6, 12, and 24 months
    D. Administering benzathine penicillin G given intramuscularly as a single high dose, and instructing the client about follow-up evaluations at 6, 12, and 24 months

12. What is the nurse's **priority** action after a client has received an intramuscular injection of benzathine penicillin G?
    A. Ask the client for contact information on all sexual partners.
    B. Observe the client for at least 30 minutes to detect an allergic reaction.
    C. Instruct the client to go home and rest for at least 2 to 4 hours.
    D. Observe the injection site for redness, fever, and any signs of infection.

13. Which actions does the nurse anticipate when a client develops a Jarisch-Herxheimer reaction after antibiotic treatment for syphilis? **Select all that apply.**
    A. Administering oxygen
    B. Starting IV resuscitation fluids
    C. Giving analgesics
    D. Injecting IV epinephrine
    E. Administering antipyretics
    F. Placing a nasogastric tube

14. What does the nurse practitioner suspect when assessing a client and finding multiple large cauliflower-like growths on the genitalia?
    A. Gonorrhea
    B. Genital herpes
    C. Salpingitis
    D. Genital warts

15. What **priority** teaching will the nurse provide for a client with condylomata acuminata (genital warts) who will continue treatment at home after discharge?
    A. Proper application of imiquimod cream
    B. Use of trichloroacetic acid or bichloracetic acid
    C. Implementation of cryotherapy with liquid nitrogen
    D. Administration of podophyllin resin in tincture of benzoin

16. Which sexually transmitted infections (STIs) in clients will the nurse report to local health authorities? **Select all that apply.**
    A. Chlamydia
    B. Genital herpes
    C. Gonorrhea
    D. Syphilis
    E. Human immune deficiency virus
    F. Salpingitis

17. Which specific **priority** action will the nurse teach a client to prevent genital warts infection?
    A. Decrease the number of sexual partners.
    B. Always use a condom for any sexual encounter.
    C. Get a vaccination against human papilloma virus (HPV).
    D. Remain mutually monogamous in a sexual relationship.

18. Which information will the nurse teach a client who is diagnosed with chlamydia trachomatis? **Select all that apply.**
    A. Antibiotic therapy with azithromycin 1 g orally is given in a single dose.
    B. Abstaining from sexual encounters for 7 days from the start of treatment is necessary.
    C. Rescreening for reinfection with women should occur at 2 to 3 years after treatment.
    D. Complications of untreated chlamydia include infertility and ectopic pregnancy.
    E. Most recurrences are reinfections from a new or untreated partner.
    F. The incubation period for chlamydia ranges from 6 to 8 weeks.

19. Which symptoms would the nurse expect when a male client reports that his female partner was diagnosed and treated for gonorrhea?
    A. A small painless lump on the penis that spontaneously disappeared
    B. Dysuria and a profuse yellowish green or scant clear penile discharge
    C. Numerous small, painless papillary growths in the genital region
    D. Painful intercourse with scrotal swelling and epididymitis

20. For which client would the nurse expect a test-of-cure to be recommended after treatment is completed?
    A. Client treated with azithromycin for chlamydia infection
    B. Client treated with cefixime for gonorrheal infection
    C. Client treated with benzathine penicillin for syphilis
    D. Client treated with ceftriaxone for gonorrheal infection

21. Which client circumstance does the nurse understand is **most appropriate** for expedited partner treatment?
    A. Partner is afraid to come to the health care facility.
    B. Partners are clients of a commercial sex worker.
    C. Client and partner are both HIV positive.
    D. Client and partner both have multiple other partners.

22. For which condition does the nurse understand that women with pelvic inflammatory disease (PID) are at **increased** risk?
    A. Cardiovascular disease
    B. Amenorrhea
    C. Infertility
    D. Ovarian cancer

23. Which instruction will the nurse provide an assistive personnel (AP) when caring for a client with pelvic inflammatory disease (PID)?
    A. Place the client in a semi-Fowler position.
    B. Restrict the client to complete bedrest.
    C. Allow the client only clear liquids.
    D. Reposition the client every 2 hours.

24. Which factors will the nurse monitor for that will increase a female client's risk for pelvic inflammatory disease? **Select all that apply.**
    A. Caffeine use
    B. Smoking cigarettes
    C. Consistent use of condoms
    D. Multiple sex partners
    E. Vaginal douching
    F. History of sexually transmitted infections (STIs)

25. Which actions will the nurse take to relieve the pain of a client with pelvic inflammatory disease (PID)? **Select all that apply.**
    A. Administer antibiotic therapy as prescribed.
    B. Apply heat to the lower abdomen or back.
    C. Give opioid pain relievers.
    D. Place client in semi-Fowler position.
    E. Administer mild analgesics.
    F. Massage lower extremities.

26. Which actions will the nurse teach a client with pelvic inflammatory disease (PID) who is being treated on an ambulatory care basis?
    A. Check your blood pressure twice a day.
    B. Take your opioid pain drug as soon as you feel pain starting.
    C. Weigh yourself every morning and report a weight gain or loss.
    D. Avoid sexual intercourse for the full course of antibiotic treatment.

Chapter 69 Answer Key

1. A, B, C, E, F
   Individuals at greatest risk for acquiring an STI include: those who have more than one sexual partner (especially anonymous partners); have had more than one sexual partner in the past; engage in sexual activity with someone who has an STI; have a history of having an STI; use intravenous drugs; have or had a partner who uses (used) intravenous drugs; engage in anal, vaginal, or oral sex without a condom; and have sex while using drugs or alcohol. A partner who was successfully treated for an STI in the past and is no longer infectious does not increase the risk for STIs.

2. A, B, E, F
   Safer sex practices that a nurse teaches clients include: using a latex or polyurethane condom for genital and anal intercourse, using a condom or latex barrier (dental dam) over the genitals or anus during oral-genital or oral-anal sexual contact, wearing gloves for finger or hand contact with the vagina or rectum, practicing abstinence, practicing mutual (not serial) monogamy, and decreasing the number of sexual partners.

3. C
   Many people do not have symptoms during the primary outbreak. After the primary outbreak, the virus is dormant and recurs periodically, even if the client is asymptomatic. Recurrences are not caused by reinfection; they are related to viral shedding, and the client is infectious. Thus, the client should be advised to always use a condom. The nurse reminds the client that antiviral drugs are used to treat GH. The drugs decrease the severity, promote healing, and decrease the frequency of recurrent outbreaks, but do **not** cure the infection.

4. B
   The nurse teaches this client about the long-term complications of GH, which include the risk for neonatal transmission and an increased risk for acquiring HIV infection.

5. A, B, D, E, F
   See the box titled Best Practice for Patient Safety & Quality Care: Care of or Self-Management for the Patient with Genital Herpes in your text for additional suggestions for client self-management when a client has GH. Option C is not correct because insertion of a urinary catheter may be ordered by the health care provider.

6. D
   When a client experiences GH, symptoms include an itching or a tingling sensation in the skin 1 to 2 days before the outbreak, known as the prodrome. These sensations are usually followed by the appearance of vesicles (blisters) in a cluster on the vulva, vagina, cervix, scrotum, penis, or perianal region at the site of inoculation. The blisters rupture spontaneously in 1 to 2 days and leave ulcerations that can become extensive and cause pain.

7. B, D, E, F
   The nurse teaches the client about how to properly use condoms. See the box titled Patient and Family Education: Preparing for Self-Management: Use of Condoms in your

text for additional suggestions for correct use of condoms. Option A is not correct because use of spermicides with condoms has **not** been proven to be more or less effective against STIs than use without spermicide. Option C is not correct because if a lubricant is used with a condom, it should be water-based to be easily washed away with water.

8. A
The first visible sign of syphilis is a small, painless sore, called a "chancre", which may appear from 12 days to 12 weeks after exposure. Chancres may be found on any area of the skin or mucous membranes but occur most often on the genitalia. They begin as small papules, approximately 1 to 2 cm in diameter with a raised margin.

9. B
Because it may take up to 12 weeks for a client to develop symptoms of syphilis, the best advice is to have the client come in for testing, then treatment if the test is positive because untreated syphilis can lead to organ damage and death.

10. A
When a client has lesions related to secondary syphilis, they are highly contagious and should not be touched without gloves. The nurse instructs the AP to wear gloves whenever providing care or touching this client.

11. D
Interprofessional collaborative care includes drug therapy and health teaching to resolve the infection and prevent transmission to others. The nurse expects to administer benzathine penicillin G given IM as a single high dose as the evidence-based treatment for primary, secondary, and early latent syphilis. Additionally, the CDC recommends follow-up evaluation, including blood tests at 6, 12, and 24 months. Repeat treatment may be needed if the client does not respond to the initial antibiotic.

12. B
Allergic reactions to benzathine penicillin G can occur. Monitor the client for allergic signs and symptoms (e.g., rash, edema, shortness of breath, chest tightness, anxiety). Keep all clients at the health care agency for at least 30 minutes after they have received the antibiotic, so signs and symptoms of an allergic reaction can be detected and treated. The most severe reaction is anaphylaxis. Treatment must be available and implemented immediately if symptoms occur.

13. C, E
A Jarisch-Herxheimer reaction may follow antibiotic therapy for syphilis. This reaction is caused by the rapid release of products from the disruption of the cells of the organism. Symptoms include fever, generalized aches, rigors, vasodilation, diaphoresis, hypotension, and worsening of any rash that was present. These symptoms are usually benign and begin within 24 hours after therapy, and are treated symptomatically with analgesics and antipyretics.

14. D
The diagnosis of condylomata acuminata (genital warts) is made by examination of the lesions. They are initially small, papillary growths that are white or resemble the color of the client's skin that may grow into large cauliflower-like masses. Multiple warts usually occur in the same area.

15. A
Imiquimod topical cream is an immune-mediated therapy that can be self-applied to treat genital warts. The nurse teaches the client to wash their hands, then wash the area where the cream is to be applied. The cream is applied in a thin layer and left in place. The client must wash hands carefully after applying the cream. After the cream has been left in place for the prescribed amount of time, the area can be washed with mild soap and water and hands carefully washed again.

16. A, C, D, E
Chlamydia infection, gonorrhea, syphilis, chancroid, and human immune deficiency virus (HIV) infection (through HIV Stage III - AIDS)

are notifiable to local health authorities in every state.

17. C
All of these actions are important to prevent HPV, but vaccination is specific to the protection of clients against HPV, which causes genital warts. It is one of the **most important** interventions available, especially for men having sex with men (MSM) and immunocompromised young adults. The nurse teaches clients about the various vaccinations available (see Table 69.3 in your text) and encourages them to be immunized.

18. A, B, D, E
The nurse teaches the client about chlamydia infection including: the sexual mode of transmission; the incubation period (1 to 3 weeks); the high possibility of asymptomatic infections and the usual symptoms, if present; the need for antibiotic treatment of infection and the need to complete all medications, even if feeling better; the need for abstinence from sexual intercourse until the client and partner(s) have all completed treatment (7 days from the start of treatment, including a single-dose regimen); that women should be rescreened for reinfection 3 to 12 months after treatment because of the high risk for pelvic inflammatory disease (PID); also, that there is less evidence of the need for rescreening of treated men, but it should be considered; the need to return for evaluation if symptoms recur or new symptoms develop (most recurrences are re-infections from a new or untreated partner); and that complications of untreated or inadequately treated infection may include PID, infertility, ectopic pregnancy, or newborn complications.

19. B
With gonorrhea, if symptoms are present, men usually notice dysuria and a penile discharge that can be either profuse, yellowish-green fluid or scant, clear fluid.

20. B
Because of the potential for resistance of gonorrhea to cefixime, a test-of-cure is recommended after treatment is completed. A test-of-cure is performed 3 to 4 weeks after treatment and is only done if concern exists regarding persistence of infection despite treatment, if symptoms of infection persist, or if lack of adherence to the treatment regimen is suspected.

21. A.
Expedited partner therapy (EPT) involves treating sexual partners of clients diagnosed with chlamydia infection or gonorrhea by providing prescriptions or medication to the client, which they can take to their partner(s), without the partner(s) having to be examined by a provider of care. Evidence shows that when the client gives the drug to their partner(s), rates of infection **decrease**, and more partners report receiving treatment.

22. C
Complications of PID include chronic pelvic pain, **infertility**, risk for ectopic pregnancy, and tubo-ovarian abscess (TOA), a serious short-term condition requiring hospitalization in which an inflammatory mass arises on the fallopian tube, ovary, and/or other pelvic organs.

23. A
Teach the AP to have the client rest in a semi-Fowler position and encourage limited ambulation to promote gravity drainage of the infection that may help relieve **pain**. The client does not need to be limited to clear liquids, kept on bedrest, or to be repositioned every 2 hours.

24. B, D, E, F
Factors that increase a sexually active woman's risk of developing PID include: being younger than 26 years old; having a new sexual partner, or having multiple sexual partners; having a sexual partner who has other concurrent sexual partners; practicing inconsistent use of condoms; having a history of PID; having a concurrent chlamydial or gonococcal infection, or having bacterial vaginosis; practicing vaginal douching; having a history of sexually transmitted infections (STIs); and having had an intrauterine device (IUD) placed within the previous 3 weeks (this is noted as a small risk).

25.   A, B, D, E
Antibiotic therapy relieves pain by destroying the pathogens and decreasing the inflammation caused by infection. Other measures to treat pain include administering mild analgesics and applying heat to the lower abdomen or back. Teach the client to rest in semi-Fowler position and encourage limited ambulation to promote gravity drainage of the infection that may help relieve pain.

26.   D
The nurse instructs women who are being treated for PID on an ambulatory care basis to avoid sexual intercourse for the full course of antibiotic treatment and until their symptoms have resolved. They are also taught to check their temperature twice daily, and to report an increase in temperature to their health care provider.

Next Generation NCLEX®
Examination Unfolding
Case Studies

NGN Unfolding Case Study #1: Musculoskeletal Trauma (Concepts of Mobility and Perfusion)

1-A. A 25-year-old male client riding his motorcycle was struck by a speeding truck while passing him on a narrow rural road. As a result of the accident, the client was thrown into a ditch with the motorcycle landing on his right leg. His riding helmet remained intact during the accident. After lifting the motorcycle from the client's entrapped right leg, first responders at the scene found him to be alert and oriented × 3, and able to move both arms and his left leg. The only visible injury was severe bone and soft-tissue damage of his right leg. The client states that his pain was a 10/10 on a 0 to 10 pain intensity scale. Vital signs: pulse = 90 beats/min, respirations = 24 breaths/min, and blood pressure = 130/78 mm Hg. The client was immobilized and transported to the emergency department (ED). Upon admission to the ED, the nurse reviews the prehospital documentation. **Indicate which client assessment finding requires immediate follow-up by the ED nurse at this time.**

Assessment Finding	Assessment Finding that Requires Immediate Follow-Up
Alert and oriented × 3	
Unable to move his right leg	
Pulse = 90 beats/min	
Respirations = 24 breaths/min	
Blood pressure = 130/78 mm Hg	
10/10 right leg pain	
Severe right leg bone and soft-tissue damage	

1-B. A 25-year-old male client riding his motorcycle was struck by a speeding truck while passing him on a narrow rural road. As a result of the accident, the client's right leg was severely damaged by the motorcycle and he was transported to the hospital by ambulance. After evaluation by the interprofessional health care team in the ED and multiple x-ray examinations, the client was found to have several closed fractures of the femur, tibia, and fibula. Large portions of skin and soft tissues were damaged, but most of the skeletal muscle on the right leg remained intact. The client was sedated for fracture reduction and immobilization with a fiberglass splint. After this procedure, he was admitted to the acute care orthopedic unit with an IV infusion and client-controlled analgesia. **Use an X to indicate which potential issues listed in the left column may place this client at risk while in the hospital.**

Potential Issues	Risk to Client
Constipation	
Neurovascular compromise	
Atelectasis	
GI bleeding	
Pressure injury	
Venous thromboembolism	

1-C. A 25-year-old male client experienced severe right leg trauma due to a motorcycle accident. After reduction and immobilization of several right leg fractures, the client was admitted to the acute care orthopedic unit with an IV infusion and client-controlled analgesia. The surgeon told the client that he would have an open reduction internal fixation after swelling in the right leg decreases. The admitting nurse is planning care for the client. **Choose the**

most likely **options for the information missing from the statements below by selecting from the lists of options provided.**

Based on the client's condition, the client's priority need will be to prevent _____**1**_____.
In addition, he will need interventions to prevent potentially life-threatening complications of immobility, especially _____**2**_____ and _____**2**_____.

Options for 1	Options for 2
Pressure injury	Venous thromboembolism
GI bleeding	Stress ulcer
Neurovascular compromise	Stroke
Stroke	Pressure injury
Pneumonia	Atelectasis

1-D. A 25-year-old male client experienced severe right leg trauma due to a motorcycle accident. After reduction and immobilization of several right leg fractures, the client was admitted yesterday to the acute care orthopedic unit with an IV infusion and client-controlled analgesia. This morning, the client's IV was converted to a saline lock because the client was eating and drinking adequate fluids. His pain level this morning was a 3/10 with PCA morphine, but the PCA is scheduled to be discontinued by 8 p.m. this evening. The night nurse discontinued the PCA per surgeon's order and assured the client that he could still have morphine when needed.

At 4 a.m., the nurse gave the client the prescribed dose of morphine for his report of 9/10 pain. At 5 a.m., the client reported that the pain was now "more like a 12 out of 10" and he feels painful tingling in his right foot. He states that the morphine he received an hour ago "did not touch" his pain. **Use an X for the nursing actions listed below that are Indicated (appropriate or necessary),** Contra-indicated **(could be harmful), or** Non-Essential **(makes no difference or not necessary) for the client's care at this time.**

Nursing Action	Indicated	Contraindicated	Non-Essential
Perform a neurovascular assessment of the client's lower extremities.			
Place the client's right leg on 2 pillows to decrease swelling.			
If possible, loosen the leg splint but keep the leg immobilized.			
Administer additional morphine to alleviate pain.			
Collaborate with the physical therapist.			
Prepare the client for possible fasciotomy.			
Contact the primary health care provider immediately.			

1-E. A 25-year-old male client experienced severe right leg trauma due to a motorcycle accident 5 days ago and was admitted to the acute care orthopedic unit. Since that time, he has had two surgeries, including a fasciotomy due to compartment syndrome, and open reduction internal fixation (ORIF) of the tibia. His fasciotomy wound is open but healing well with new granular tissue at the base of the wound. The ORIF incision is well-approximated and beginning to heal. The client has a new leg splint that begins above his knee and ends under his foot for support during the healing process. What nursing actions are appropriate for the client at this time? **Select all that apply.**

A. Manage the client's pain to achieve a 2/10 to 3/10 on a 0 to10 pain intensity scale.
B. Perform frequent lower extremity neurovascular assessments ("circ checks").
C. Collaborate with the case manager to plan for hospital discharge planning.
D. Reinforce teaching about crutch-walking using a three-point gait.
E. Remind assistive personnel to assist the client in changing positions every 1-2 hours.
F. Encourage client to select high-fiber foods to help prevent constipation.
G. Reinforce leg exercises and ankle "pumps" to prevent deep vein thrombosis.
H. Remind the client to use his incentive spirometer at least every 2 hours.
I. Ask the client to report any burning or pressure sensation of the right heel.

1-F. A 25-year-old male client experienced severe right leg trauma due to a motorcycle accident. After 10 days in the hospital for ORIF of the tibia, skin grafts of the lower leg, and a fasciotomy for relief of compartmental pressure, the client spent 2 weeks in a rehabilitation unit. Today the client sees his orthopedic surgeon for a follow-up visit 6 weeks after his initial injury. The nurse performs a brief health assessment prior to the client's visit with the surgeon. **For each client finding, use an X to indicate whether the interventions for the client were <u>Effective</u> (helped to meet expected outcomes), <u>Ineffective</u> (did not help to meet expected outcomes), or <u>Unrelated</u> (not related to the expected outcomes).**

Client Finding	Effective	Ineffective	Unrelated
Able to ambulate independently with crutches			
Needs oral opioid medication every 4 hours to control pain			
Feels very anxious and sometimes depressed			
Has no drainage or redness of ORIF incision			
Reports having signs and symptoms of seasonal allergies			
Continuing regular exercises at home as prescribed by the physical therapist			

NGN Unfolding Case Study #2: Venous Thromboembolism (Concepts of Clotting and Perfusion)

2-A. A 79-year-old female client was diagnosed as having a mesenteric thrombosis for which she had a colon resection to remove the ischemic bowel via a traditional laparotomy 2 days ago. The client's medical history includes hypertension, diabetes mellitus type 2, peripheral arterial disease, rheumatoid arthritis, and osteoarthritis. Prior to her hospitalization, the client lived independently in a senior apartment complex. The client is alert and oriented, and her incisional pain has been well managed. Vital signs for over 24 hours have been stable. Today the nurse is planning to begin discharge teaching for follow-up care at home with her daughter. When the nurse enters the room, the client tells the nurse that her left leg is "hurting a lot" and seems larger than her right leg. Upon inspection, the nurse notes that the client's left leg calf is swollen and reddened. The nurse instructs the client to remain in bed.

Highlight the client findings that are of *immediate* concern to the nurse.

2-B. A 79-year-old female client was diagnosed as having a mesenteric thrombosis for which she had a colon resection to remove the ischemic bowel via a traditional laparotomy 2 days ago. The client's medical history includes hypertension, diabetes mellitus type 2, peripheral arterial disease, rheumatoid arthritis, and osteoarthritis. When the nurse enters the room, the client tells the nurse that her left leg is "hurting a lot" and seems larger than her right leg. Upon inspection, the nurse notes that the client's left leg calf is swollen and reddened. The nurse instructs the client to remain in bed. **Choose the *most likely* options for the information missing from the statement below by selecting from the list of options provided.**

The nurse recognizes that based on the client's history and current assessment findings, she is currently at risk for complications from surgery and decreased mobility, especially _____, _____, and _____.

Options
Infection
Osteoporosis
Cholelithiasis
Venous thromboembolism (VTE)
Pancreatitis
Pressure injury
Bowel obstruction

2-C. A 79-year-old female client was diagnosed as having a mesenteric thrombosis for which she had a colon resection to remove the ischemic bowel via a traditional laparotomy 2 days ago. The client's medical history includes hypertension, diabetes mellitus type 2, peripheral arterial disease, rheumatoid arthritis, and osteoarthritis. When the nurse enters the room, the client tells the nurse that her left leg is "hurting a lot" and seems larger than her right leg. Upon inspection, the nurse notes that the client's left leg calf is swollen and reddened. The nurse instructs the client to remain in bed. **Choose the *most likely* options for the information missing from the statements below by selecting from the lists of options provided.**

The nurse recognizes that based on the client's new onset of signs and symptoms, she *most likely* has a _____1_____. The **priority** for her care will be to prevent the life-threatening complications of this health problem, especially _____2_____.

Options for 1	Options for 2
Peripheral arterial occlusion	Myocardial infarction
Deep vein thrombosis	Arterial wall rupture
Venous valvular disease	Atrial fibrillation
Arterial aneurysm	Pulmonary embolism
Cellulitis	Sepsis

2-D. A 79-year-old female client was diagnosed as having a mesenteric thrombosis for which she had a colon resection to remove the ischemic bowel via a traditional laparotomy 2 days ago. The client's medical history includes hypertension, diabetes mellitus type 2, peripheral arterial disease, rheumatoid arthritis, and osteoarthritis. When the nurse enters the room, the client tells the nurse that her left leg is "hurting a lot" and seems larger than her right leg. Upon inspection, the nurse notes that the client's left leg calf is swollen and reddened. The nurse instructs the client to remain in bed and notifies the primary health care provider. The nurse anticipates primary health care provider orders. **For each provider order, select whether it is Anticipated (expected and necessary), Contraindicated (could be harmful), or Non-Essential (makes no difference or not necessary).**

Provider Order	Anticipated	Contraindicated	Non-Essential
Initiate vascular access.			
Obtain a 12-lead electrocardiogram (ECG).			
Lower the client's legs to below the heart.			
Begin administration of anticoagulant therapy.			
Draw blood for laboratory testing, including coagulation studies, CBC, and platelets.			
Administer supplemental oxygen.			
Check urine and stool for occult blood.			

2-E. A 79-year-old female client was diagnosed as having a mesenteric thrombosis for which she had a colon resection to remove the ischemic bowel via a traditional laparotomy 2 days ago. Based on this morning's nursing assessment, the client was diagnosed as having a calf deep vein thrombosis in her left leg. The nurse initiated IV unfractionated heparin therapy 1200 units per hour as ordered after health care team review of laboratory test results. What actions would the nurse take related to heparin administration? **Select all that apply.**

a. Use a programmable infusion pump for heparin administration.

b. If any aPTT level is greater than 70 seconds, stop the infusion immediately.

c. Ensure that vitamin K as the drug antidote is available if needed for bleeding.

d. Monitor for any symptoms of bleeding, including bruising, epistaxis, and blood in the urine or stool.

e. Frequently check the client's platelet count and report any value less than 350,000/mL.

f. Remind assistive personnel to avoid massaging the client's legs.

g. Call the Rapid Response Team if the client experiences chest pain and dyspnea.

2-F. A 79-year-old female client was diagnosed as having a mesenteric thrombosis for which she had a colon resection to remove the ischemic bowel via a traditional laparotomy 2 days ago. She was treated for venous thromboembolism and then went home to stay at her daughter's house. Since her discharge, she has been on rivaroxaban therapy. Today she is scheduled for a 4-week follow-up visit with her primary health care provider. The nurse takes a brief history and physical assessment prior to her examination with the provider.

For each client finding, use an X to indicate whether the interventions for the client were Effective (helped to meet expected outcomes), Ineffective (did not help to meet expected outcomes), or Unrelated (not related to the expected outcomes).

Client Finding	Effective	Ineffective	Unrelated
Abdominal incision healed without infection			
Has had no bleeding or unusual bleeding while on the anticoagulant			
States that she knows to call 911 if she has any shortness of breath and/or chest pain			
Needs help with ADLs and is not ready to go back to her apartment from her daughter's house			
States that she is having her annual cardiology appointment next week			
Left leg calf is not red and only slightly swollen			

NGN Unfolding Case Study #3: Chronic Obstructive Pulmonary Disease (Concepts of Gas Exchange and Infection)

3-A. A 68-year-old male client with a history of stable chronic obstructive pulmonary disease (COPD) is accompanied by his wife to the emergency department this morning. He has a history of controlled hypertension, mild heart failure, and atrial fibrillation. Today he reports muscle aches, increased fatigue, and shortness of breath that has been getting progressively worse; he states "I can't seem to catch my breath." The client also reports chills and a fever ranging from 100.8°F (38.2°C) up to 102.6°F (38.7°C) over the past 3 days and coughing up large amounts of rust-colored mucus. He is being admitted to the hospital with a diagnosis of possible influenza and pneumonia. On arrival to the acute care unit, the nurse notes that the client is using his portable oxygen via nasal cannula (NC) at 2 L/min. He is sitting in the wheelchair in a forward bending position with his arms resting on his knees, and is having difficulty breathing when talking. His wife states that he has been unable to perform activities of daily living at his usual level. She tells the nurse that he becomes extremely fatigued and short of breath even when brushing his teeth. He always sleeps in a semi-sitting position but has been sleeping poorly now because of his cough. **Use an X to indicate which client assessment findings require immediate follow-up by the nurse at this time.**

Assessment Finding	Assessment Finding that Requires Immediate Follow-Up
Sleeps in a semi-sitting position	
Using oxygen at 2 L/min via NC	
Sitting in a forward bending position with the arms resting on his knees	
Has increased fatigue and shortness of breath	
Expectorating rust-colored mucus	
Has chills and fever	

3-B. A 68-year-old male client with a history of stable chronic obstructive pulmonary disease (COPD) is admitted to the acute care hospital unit for possible influenza and pneumonia. On admission assessment, the nurse notes that the client is thin and pale, with a loss of muscle mass in his extremities. His skin is warm, moist, and intact. Vital signs: temperature = 102.8°F (39.3°C), heart rate = 88 beats/min with regular rhythm, respirations = 24 breaths/min and shallow, oxygen saturation = 89%, and blood pressure = 138/92 mm Hg. Using the Visual Analog Dyspnea Scale (VADS), the nurse determines that the client has moderate dyspnea. He has a barrel chest with decreased breath sounds in both lower lobes and wheezing heard bilaterally. Coarse crackles are present on inspiration and expiration in the right middle lobe. No cyanosis; finger clubbing present; 1+ edema bilaterally in feet and ankles. Pain level at 7/10 on the right side when coughing; 3/10 on inspiration and expiration. **Use an X to indicate which assessment findings are commonly associated with each client condition.** *Note that all assessment findings should be used. Each assessment finding may be used only.*

Assessment Finding	COPD	Pneumonia
Temperature = 102.8°F (39.3°C)		
Barrel chest		
Thin, pale, loss of muscle mass in extremities		
Coarse crackles on inspiration and expiration in middle right lobe		
Finger clubbing		
Pain level = 7/10 on right side when coughing		

3-C. A 68-year-old male client with a history of stable chronic obstructive pulmonary disease (COPD) was admitted to the acute care hospital unit for possible influenza and pneumonia. The collaborative plan of care includes the following:
- Vital signs every 4 hours
- Fall Precautions
- Droplet Precautions
- Continue with oxygen at 2 L/min via NC
- Continuous pulse oximetry
- Start IV of 0.9% normal saline at 30 mL/hr
- Influenza A/B and RSV assay
- Sputum culture
- Blood cultures
- CBC, BMP, CRP, ABGs
- ECG and chest x-ray
- Acetaminophen 650 mg orally every 4 hours PRN for fever or discomfort
- Ceftriaxone 1g IV every 24 hours
- Consults: respiratory, nutritional, occupational and physical therapy.

Choose the *most likely* options for the information missing from the statement below by selecting from the lists of options provided. The nurse recognizes that the client's *priority* need for care is to _____1_____ followed by _____2_____.

Options for 1	Options for 2
Administer ceftriaxone	Obtaining a chest x-ray
Collect sputum and blood cultures	Contacting the respiratory therapist
Obtain an ECG	Asking the dietary department to bring a meal
Initiate Droplet Precautions	Starting the IV infusion

3-D. A 68-year-old male client with a history of stable chronic obstructive pulmonary disease (COPD) was admitted to the acute care hospital unit for possible influenza and pneumonia. Shortly after admission, his wife reports that the client is having a harder time breathing. The nurse quickly assesses the client and notes that respirations are 32 breaths/min and labored, and observes chest retractions and use of accessory muscles for breathing. He is coughing and expectorating large amounts of rust-colored sputum; he is gasping as he tries to talk. His color is pale. **Use an X to indicate which nursing actions listed below are <u>Indicated</u> (appropriate or necessary), <u>Contraindicated</u> (could be harmful), or <u>Non-Essential</u> (make no difference or not necessary) for the client's care at this time.**

Nursing Action	Indicated	Contraindicated	Non-Essential
Increase the flow of the IV rate to 125 mL/hr.			
Check the pulse oximetry reading.			
Increase the flow of oxygen to 6 L/min.			
Check the client's temperature.			
Check the client's heart rate.			
Monitor the client's respiratory rate.			
Check elevation of the head of the bed.			
Auscultate lung sounds.			
Contact respiratory therapy immediately.			

3-E. A 68-year-old male client with a history of stable chronic obstructive pulmonary disease (COPD) was admitted to the acute care hospital unit for possible influenza and pneumonia. Shortly after admission, his wife reported that the client was having a hard time breathing. Interventions were immediately implemented and effective in alleviating the respiratory distress. The prescribed plan of care was then resumed. The client had an uneventful evening and slept comfortably through the night. The primary health care provider examined the client the next morning and prescribed a repeat chest x-ray for later in the day. The plan is to discharge the client tomorrow with an oral antibiotic for home if he continues to improve and the chest x-ray shows beginning pneumonia resolution. The nurse creates and begins to implement a discharge teaching plan for the client and his wife. Which instructions would the nurse include in the teaching? **Select all that apply.**
a. How to safely use a dehumidifier
b. The regimen for taking the oral antibiotics
c. The technique for performing effective coughing
d. The procedure for performing diaphragmatic breathing
e. The need to maintain hydration up to at least 3.5 L intake daily
f. The technique for performing pursed-lip breathing techniques
g. How to increase the oxygen flow when breathing difficulty occurs

3-F. A 68-year-old male client with a history of stable chronic obstructive pulmonary disease (COPD) was admitted to the acute care hospital unit for possible influenza and pneumonia. Shortly after admission, his wife reported that the client was having a hard time breathing. Interventions were immediately implemented and effective in alleviating the respiratory distress. The prescribed plan of care was then resumed and the nurse began to plan for the client's discharge teaching. **For each underlined teaching area, use an X to indicate whether the behavior or statement listed seems to be <u>Understood</u> by the client or <u>Requires Further Teaching</u>.**

Client Behavior or Statement	Understood	Requires Further Teaching
Pursed-lip breathing Purses the lips and breathes in slowly through the mouth and out slowly through the nose.		
Antibiotic administration States "I will take antibiotics until they are gone."		
Coughing technique Sits on the side of the bed with feet placed firmly on the floor. Turns the shoulders inward and bends the head slightly downward, hugging a pillow against the stomach. Takes a few breaths, attempting to exhale more fully. After the third to fifth breath, a deeper breath is taken and he bends forward slowly while coughing 2-3 times.		
Exercise States "If I get short of breath when walking, I will stop and wait until the next day to try again."		
Oxygen use States "I know it's safe to use burning candles when I am using my oxygen as long as the candles are 4 feet away from the oxygen tank."		
Diaphragmatic breathing Performs diaphragmatic breathing by sitting in a chair, placing hands on the abdomen, breathing from the abdomen while keeping the chest still.		

NGN Unfolding Case Study #4: Spinal Cord Injury (Concepts of Mobility and Perfusion)

4-A. A 45-year-old male client sustained a spinal cord injury at T6 as a result of a gunshot wound. Surgery was performed 4 days ago to remove the bullet. Today the client is transferred to the neurosurgical unit from critical care. During hand-off report, the nurse is told that the client is a high-level paraplegic. The client is currently alert and oriented and able to describe how his injury occurred. Psychosocial assessment reveals anxiety and fear about his prognosis. He states, "I can't feel or move anything below my waist and I'm worried about what this means. I'm still single and only 45 years old and don't have any kids yet." Additional assessment findings include:
- Temperature = 98.8°F (37.1°C)
- Pulse = 82 beats/min
- Respirations = 20 breaths/min
- Oxygen saturation = 93% (on room air)
- Blood pressure = 122/82 mm Hg
- Pain level = 0/10 (states: "I can't feel my legs")
- Skin integrity intact
- Breath sounds = fine crackles in the right lower lobe
- Abdomen is distended and firm
- Bowel sounds present × 4

The client states he is not sure when he had his last bowel movement (BM) and there is no documentation of a BM postoperatively. He has an indwelling urinary catheter that is draining clear, yellow urine. **Use an X to indicate which client assessment findings require immediate follow-up by the nurse at this time.**

Assessment Finding	Assessment Finding that Requires Follow-Up
Client was able to describe how his injury occurred when asked	
Client states "I'm single and only 45 years old and don't have any kids yet."	
Breath sounds reveal fine crackles in the right lower lobe	
Bowel sounds heard in all 4 quadrants	
No documentation of a BM since surgery 4 days ago	
Indwelling urinary catheter draining clear, yellow urine	
Vital signs: T = 98.8°F (37.1°C), P = 82 beats/min, R = 20 breaths/min, oxygen saturation = 93%, BP = 122/82 mm Hg	

4-B. A 45-year-old male client sustained a spinal cord injury at T6 as a result of a gunshot wound which was surgically treated 4 days ago. He was transferred from the critical care unit to the neurosurgical unit this morning. He has an indwelling urinary catheter draining clear, yellow urine, but has not yet had a postoperative bowel movement (BM). The nurse enters the client's room to set up lunch and notes that the client's face is very flushed. He reports having a "terrible throbbing headache" at a 10/10 on a 0 to 10 pain intensity scale and nasal congestion. The nurse quickly checks the client's vital signs and documents: T = 99.0°F (37.2°C), P = 58 beats/min, R = 20 breaths/min oxygen saturation = 90% (on room air [RA]), and BP = 210/120 mm Hg. Breath sounds reveal fine crackles in the right lower lobe.

For each client assessment finding, use an X to indicate whether it is associated with pneumonia or autonomic dysreflexia. *All assessment findings should be used, and each finding should be used only once.*

Assessment Finding	Pneumonia	Autonomic Dysreflexia
Facial flushing		
T = 99.0°F (37.2°C)		
P = 58 beats/min		
Oxygen saturation = 90% (on RA)		
Headache		
BP = 210/120 mm Hg		
Fine crackles in the right lower lobe		

4-C. A 45-year-old male client sustained a spinal cord injury at T6 as a result of a gunshot wound which was surgically treated 4 days ago. He has an indwelling urinary catheter draining clear, yellow urine, but has not yet had a postoperative bowel movement (BM). The nurse enters the client's room to set up lunch and notes that the client's face is very flushed. He reports having a "terrible throbbing headache" at a 10/10 and nasal congestion. The nurse quickly checks the client's vital signs and documents: T = 99.0°F (37.2°C), P = 58 beats/min, R = 20 breaths/min, oxygen saturation = 90% (on RA), BP = 210/120 mm Hg. Breath sounds reveal fine crackles in the right lower lobe.

Which client assessment findings are a **priority** concern for the nurse? **Select all that apply.**
a. Pulse rate
b. Flushed face
c. Body temperature
d. Oxygen saturation
e. Blood pressure
f. Fine crackles in the right lower lobe
g. Lack of a postoperative bowel movement
h. Report of a headache and nasal congestion
i. Clear, yellow urine draining from catheter

4-D. A 45-year-old male client sustained a spinal cord injury at T6 as a result of a gunshot wound which was surgically treated 4 days ago. He has an indwelling urinary catheter draining clear, yellow urine, but has not yet had a postoperative bowel movement (BM). The nurse enters the client's room to set up lunch and notes that the client's face is very flushed. He reports having a "terrible throbbing headache" at a 10/10 and nasal congestion. The nurse quickly checks the client's vital signs and documents: T = 99.0°F (37.2°C), P = 58 beats/min. R = 20 breaths/min, oxygen saturation = 90% (on RA), BP = 210/120 mm Hg. Breath sounds reveal fine crackles in the right lower lobe.

Use an X for the nursing actions listed below that are <u>Indicated</u> (appropriate or necessary), <u>Contraindicated</u> (could be harmful), or <u>Non-Essential</u> (makes no difference or not necessary) for the client's care at this time.

Nursing Action	Indicated	Contraindicated	Non-Essential
Raise the head of the bed.			
Clamp the urinary catheter.			
Monitor the client's temperature.			
Check for a fecal impaction and disimpact if needed.			
Administer nifidepine.			
Monitor breath sounds.			
Monitor deep tendon reflexes.			

4-E. A 45-year-old male client sustained a spinal cord injury at T6 as a result of a gunshot wound which was surgically treated 4 days ago. He has an indwelling urinary catheter draining clear, yellow urine, but has not yet had a postoperative bowel movement (BM). The nurse enters the client's room to set up lunch and notes that the client's face is very flushed. He reports having a "terrible throbbing headache" at a 10/10 and nasal congestion. The nurse quickly checks the client's vital signs and documents: T = 99.0°F (37.2°C), P = 58 beats/min, R = 20 breaths/min, oxygen saturation = 90% (on RA), BP = 210/120 mm Hg. Breath sounds reveal fine crackles in the right lower lobe. The nurse suspects that the client is experiencing autonomic dysreflexia. **Choose the** *most likely* **options for the information missing from the statement below by selecting from the lists of options provided.**

The **first** action that the nurse would take is to _____ 1 _____ to _____ 2 _____.

Options for 1	Options for 2
Check for fecal impaction	Reduce the blood pressure
Administer nifidipine	Increase urinary flow
Raise the head of the bed	Increase oxygen saturation
Start supplemental oxygen	Identify the cause
Obtain a 12-lead ECG	Prevent myocardial infarction

4-F. A 45-year-old male client sustained a spinal cord injury at T6 as a result of a gunshot wound which was surgically treated 4 days ago. Shortly after his transfer from the critical care unit to the neurosurgical unit, he experienced autonomic dysreflexia due to a fecal impaction. After implementing appropriate interventions, the nurse reassesses the client. Which of the following client assessment findings indicate that this complication has been adequately managed? **Select all that apply.**

a. Vision is clear
b. Pulse = 70 beats/min
c. BP = 130/88 mm Hg
d. Oxygen saturation = 92% (on RA)
e. Headache is 2/10
f. Breath sounds = fine crackles
g. Temperature = 99.2°F (37.1°C)
h. Facial color pink
i. Skin warm and dry

NGN Unfolding Case Study #5: Chronic Kidney Disease (Concepts of Elimination and Infection)

5-A. A 42-year-old female client is admitted to the renal unit of the hospital from the emergency department (ED) with a long-term history of polycystic kidney disease and diabetes mellitus (DM) type 1. Over the past few years her kidneys have slowly and progressively failed. Three years ago, the client was diagnosed with chronic kidney disease (CKD) and started peritoneal dialysis (PD). She has a peritoneal catheter and performs automated peritoneal dialysis procedure every night using a continuous cycling machine. The client states that she has been unusually tired, "been running fevers" on and off for the last few weeks, and had difficulty controlling her blood glucose levels. She has abdominal discomfort and "bloating," for which she has been taking ibuprofen 200 mg every 6 hours. The client states that she came to the ED today because her temperature was elevated to 101.8°F (38.8°C) this morning after ending her dialysis treatment. She had chills alternating with sweating consistently last night. She reports that her blood glucose reading before breakfast was 325 mg/dL (18.1 mmol/L). When asked about fluid intake and output, the client reports that her fluid intake is approximately 32 oz (1 L) daily depending on her dialysis output and weight, and that she urinates approximately 20 mL a day. The client also reports that the effluent (outflow) from the catheter this morning contained some "white flecks." She was hospitalized due to a diagnosis of catheter-related peritonitis. The nurse reviews the ED notes and diagnostic results, and performs a head-to-toe admission assessment. The following data are documented.

Nursing Assessment:

- Pain in the abdomen that worsens with touch; 5/10 on a 0 to 10 pain intensity scale
- Abdominal bloating and distention
- Poor appetite
- Nausea, but denies vomiting
- Thirst
- Fatigue
- Fever and chills
- Dry dressing covering the catheter exit site
- Vital signs: temperature = 101.6°F (38.6°C), pulse = 72 beats/min, respirations = 22 breaths/min, blood pressure = 160/92 mm Hg, oxygen saturation = 93%
- Breath sounds clear bilaterally
- Last bowel movement yesterday was soft and formed

- Weight = 158 lb (71.7 kg) (states no change from yesterday morning)
- Finger stick blood glucose (FSBG) = 345 mg/dL (19.2 mmol/L)

Laboratory and Diagnostic Results:

- White blood cell count = 17,500 mm³ (17.5 × 10⁹/L)
- Glomerular filtration rate = 20 mL/min
- Hemoglobin =12 g/dL (120 mmol/L)
- Hematocrit = 37% (0.37)

- Blood urea nitrogen = 42 mg/dL (15.12 mmol/L)
- Creatinine = 3.9 mg/dL (343 μmol/L)
- Sodium = 145 mg/dL (145 mmol/L)
- Potassium = 4.9 mg/dL (4.9 mmol/L)
- Abdominal computed tomography (CT) of the abdomen shows irregular peritoneal thickening and fluid collection.

Indicate which client assessment findings require immediate follow-up by the nurse at this time.

Assessment Finding	Assessment Finding that Requires Follow-Up
Weight = 158 lb (71.7 kg)	
Urinary output approximately 20 mL/day	
Dry dressing covering the catheter exit site	
Temperature = 101.6°F (38.6°C)	
Finger stick blood glucose (FSBG) = 345 mg/dL (19.2 mmol/L)	
White blood cell count = 17,500/mm³ (17.5 × 10⁹/L)	
Last bowel movement yesterday	
Abdominal discomfort and bloating	
Pulse = 72 beats/min	
Blood pressure (BP) =160/92 mm Hg	
White flecks in PD effluent	

5-B. A 42-year-old female client is admitted to the renal unit of the hospital from the emergency department (ED) with a long-term history of polycystic kidney disease and diabetes mellitus (DM) type 1. Over the past few years her kidneys have slowly and progressively failed. Three years ago, the client was diagnosed with chronic kidney disease (CKD) and started peritoneal dialysis (PD). She has a peritoneal catheter and performs automated peritoneal dialysis procedure every night using a peritoneal continuous cycling machine. The client states that she has been unusually tired, "been running fevers" on and off for the last few weeks, and had difficulty controlling her blood glucose levels. She has abdominal discomfort and "bloating," for which she has been taking ibuprofen 200 mg every 6 hours. The client states that she came to the ED today because her temperature was elevated to 101.8°F (38.8°C) this morning after ending her dialysis treatment. She had chills alternating with sweating consistently last night. She reports that her blood glucose reading this morning was 325 mg/dL (18.1 mmol/L). When asked about fluid intake and output, the client reports that her fluid intake is approximately 32 oz (1 L) daily depending on her dialysis output and weight, and that she urinates approximately 20 mL a day. The client also reports that the effluent (outflow) from the catheter this morning contained some "white flecks." She was hospitalized due to a diagnosis of catheter-related peritonitis. **Indicate which assessment finding is associated with each of the client's health problems.** *All assessment findings must be used. Any assessment finding may be used more than once.*

Assessment Finding	Peritonitis	Chronic Kidney Disease	DM Type 1
Abdominal discomfort and bloating			
FSBG = 345 mg/dL(19.2 mmol/L)			
Drinks 32 oz (1 L) of fluids daily			
Fatigue			
Temperature = 101.6°F (38.6°C)			
Chills			
BP = 160/92 mm Hg			
White flecks in peritoneal output			
White blood cell count = 17,500 mm³ (17.5 × 10⁹/L)			
Glomerular filtration rate = 20 mL/min			
Blood urea nitrogen = 42 mg/dL (15.12 mmol/L)			
Creatinine = 3.9 mg/dL (343 μmol/L)			
Abdominal pain = 5/10 on a 0 to 10 scale			

5-C. A 42-year-old female client is admitted to the renal unit of the hospital from the emergency department (ED) with a long-term history of polycystic kidney disease and diabetes mellitus (DM) type 1. Over the past few years her kidneys have slowly and progressively failed. Three years ago, the client was diagnosed with chronic kidney disease (CKD) and started peritoneal dialysis (PD). The client was hospitalized due to a diagnosis of catheter-related peritonitis. The nurse contacts the nephrologist to report admission assessment findings and to obtain admission orders. The client's assessment data include:

Nursing Assessment:

- Pain in the abdomen that worsens with touch; 5/10 on a 0 to 10 pain intensity scale
- Abdominal bloating and distention
- Poor appetite
- Nausea, but denies vomiting
- Thirst
- Fatigue
- Fever and chills
- Dry dressing covering the catheter exit site
- Vital signs: temperature = 101.6°F (38.6°C), pulse = 72 beats/min, respirations = 22 breaths/min, blood pressure = 160/92 mm Hg, oxygen saturation = 93%

- Breath sounds clear bilaterally
- Last bowel movement yesterday was soft and formed
- Weight = 158 lb (71.7 kg) (states no change from yesterday morning)
- Finger stick blood glucose (FSBG) = 345 mg/dL (19.2 mmol/L)

Laboratory and Diagnostic Results:

- White blood cell count = 17,500 mm³ (17.5 × 10⁹/L)
- Glomerular filtration rate = 20 mL/min
- Hemoglobin =12 g/dL (120 mmol/L)
- Hematocrit = 37% (0.37)
- Blood urea nitrogen = 42 mg/dL (15.12 mmol/L)
- Creatinine = 3.9 mg/dL (343 μmol/L)
- Sodium = 145 mg/dL (145 mmol/L)
- Potassium = 4.9 mg/dL (4.9 mmol/L)
- Abdominal computed tomography (CT) of the abdomen shows irregular peritoneal thickening and fluid collection

Based on the client's assessment findings, what are the **priority** concerns for the nurse? **Select all that apply.**

a. Pain
b. Fatigue
c. Infection

d.   Hyperpnea
e.   Hypertension
f.   Hyperthermia
g.   Hyperglycemia

5-D. A 42-year-old female client is admitted to the renal unit of the hospital from the emergency department (ED) with a long-term history of polycystic kidney disease and diabetes mellitus (DM) type 1. Over the past few years her kidneys have slowly and progressively failed. Three years ago, the

client was diagnosed with chronic kidney disease (CKD) and started peritoneal dialysis (PD). The client was hospitalized due to a diagnosis of catheter-related peritonitis.

For each provider order, select whether it is Anticipated (expected and necessary), Contraindicated (could be harmful), or Non-Essential (makes no difference or not necessary) for the client at this time.

Provider Order	Anticipated	Contraindicated	Non-Essential
Obtain a specimen of dialysis effluent.			
Remove the peritoneal catheter immediately.			
Obtain a blood culture.			
Administer the prescribed insulin infusion.			
Administer the prescribed IV antibiotic.			
Continue with nightly peritoneal dialysis.			
Administer ibuprofen for pain as needed.			
Flush the dialysis catheter per agency protocol.			

5-E. A 42-year-old female client is admitted to the renal unit of the hospital from the emergency department (ED) with a long-term history of polycystic kidney disease and diabetes mellitus (DM) type 1. Over the past few years her kidneys have slowly and progressively failed. Three years ago, the client was diagnosed with chronic kidney disease (CKD) and started peritoneal dialysis (PD). The client was hospitalized due to a diagnosis of catheter-related

peritonitis. The nurse reviews the nephrologist's orders. **Choose the *most likely* options for the information missing from the statement below by selecting from the lists of options provided.**

The **priority** action that the nurse would take is to _____1_____ to _____2_____ followed by _____3_____ to _____4_____.

Options for 1	Options for 2	Options for 3	Options for 4
Obtain a blood culture and dialysis effluent specimen	Achieve normal glucose levels	Obtaining blood cultures and dialysis outflow specimen	Improve the GFR
Remove the dialysis catheter	Determine the organism causing infection	Removing the dialysis catheter	Achieve normal glucose levels
Initiate an IV insulin infusion	Improve the GFR	Initiating an IV insulin infusion	Resolve infection
Administer prescribed antibiotics	Resolve infection	Administering antibiotics	Determine the organism causing infection

5-F. A 42-year-old female client is admitted to the renal unit of the hospital from the emergency department (ED) with a long-term history of polycystic kidney disease and diabetes mellitus (DM) type 1. Over the past few years her kidneys have slowly and progressively failed. Three years ago, the client was diagnosed with chronic kidney disease (CKD) and started peritoneal dialysis (PD). The client was hospitalized due to a diagnosis of catheter-related peritonitis. The nurse reviews and implements the nephrologist's admitting orders. When the nurse obtains the dialysis effluent specimen to send to the laboratory, white stringy material is noted in a cloudy fluid. The nurse initiates IV antibiotics (IV vancomycin and ceftazidime) as prescribed.

Three days later, the nurse performs a client assessment and documents the following findings:

- Pain in the abdomen; 1 on a 0-10 pain intensity scale
- Abdomen soft with minimal distention
- Denies nausea or vomiting
- Ate 90% breakfast this morning
- Dialysis effluent from the overnight treatment clear with no sediment
- Dry dressing covering the catheter exit site
- Vital signs: temperature = 98.9.°F (37.1°C), pulse = 68 beats/min, respirations = 18 breaths/min, blood pressure = 142/80 mm Hg, oxygen saturation = 94% (on room air[RA])
- Breath sounds clear bilaterally
- Weight = 156 lb (70.8 kg)
- Fasting serum glucose = 148 mg/dL (8.24 mmol/L)

Hospital discharge is planned for the following day if the client's condition continues to improve. The nurse begins to implement a discharge teaching plan for the client. **Use an X to indicate which client statement indicates that the home care instruction is either <u>Understood</u> or <u>Requires Further Teaching</u>.**

Client Statement	Understood	Requires Further Teaching
"I need to alter my diet and eat foods high in fiber."		
"It's important not to limit my fluid intake to prevent those white specks and threads that were in my dialysis output."		
"I should anchor my catheter to my skin with tape."		
"I should check my temperature at least once a day."		
"It is okay to skip one treatment a week if I have a social commitment that I want to participate."		
"I need to be sure to eat some more protein foods like meat, milk, and eggs, and decrease the intake of foods like beans, nuts, and chocolate."		
"I need to watch my blood glucose closely because of my diabetes, but the dialysis procedure should not affect my glucose level."		

NGN Unfolding Case Study #6: Traumatic Brain Injury (Concepts of Cognition and Perfusion)

6-A. A 51-year-old male client who sustained a closed head injury was brought to the emergency department (ED) this morning by emergency medical services (EMS). The client was accompanied by his wife who reported that he fell from a ladder while trying to clean the gutters on their house. On arrival to the hospital, the client was alert and responding appropriately to questions wearing a neck collar that was applied by first responders for neck stabilization. Vital signs: temperature = 98.7°F (37°C), apical heart rate = 78 beats/min and regular, respirations = 18 breaths/min, blood pressure (BP) = 126/78 mm Hg.

Oxygen saturation is 95% (on room air [RA]). The client reported a mild headache of 3/10 on a 0 to 10 pain intensity scale. Cardiac monitor reading revealed normal sinus rhythm. The client denied nausea or vomiting. Glasgow Coma Scale score = 15 ; PERRLA. In addition to routine lab work, a computed tomography (CT) scan of the brain, and cervical and spinal x-rays were performed. The CT scan of the brain showed regions of hypodensity. Two hours later, the client was transferred to the acute neurological unit. The unit admission assessment was the same as the baseline assessment in the ED. The client was placed on bedrest with the head of the bed elevated, and a lunch tray was requested.

Highlight the client findings <u>below</u> that are of *immediate* concern to the nurse.

The nurse performs a neurological check on the client about an hour after lunch. Vital signs: temperature = 98.8°F (37.1°C), apical heart rate = 60 beats/min and regular, respirations = 16 breaths/min blood pressure (BP) = 142/68 mm Hg. Oxygen saturation is 92% (on RA). The client reports a headache of 5/10 on a 0 to 10 pain intensity scale and has a new onset of nausea. Glasgow Coma Scale score = 12. The client seems sleepy and confused as to where he is, but he

responds to localized painful stimuli and opens his eyes in response to sound. Slight pupil dilation is noted in the right eye.

6-B. A 51-year-old male client who sustained a closed head injury was admitted from the ED to the neurological unit today around noon. After lunch, the nurse performed a neurological check on the client about an hour after lunch. Vital signs: temperature = 98.8°F (37.1°C), apical heart rate = 60 beats/min and regular, respirations = 16 breaths/min, blood pressure (BP) = 142/68 mm Hg. Oxygen saturation is 92% (on RA). The client reported a headache of 5/10 on a 0 to 10 pain intensity scale and had a new onset of nausea. Glasgow Coma Scale score = 12. The client seemed sleepy and confused as to where he was, but he responded to localized painful stimuli and opened his eyes in response to sound. Slight pupil dilation was noted in the right eye. **Choose the *most likely* options for the information missing from the statement below by selecting from the lists of options provided.**

The nurse recognizes that the client's decline in neurological status is likely the result of _____**1**_____ caused by _____**2**_____.

Options for 1	Options for 2
Dehydration	Hospitalization
Increasing intracranial pressure	Low oxygen saturation
Sensory deprivation	Intracranial bleeding
Hypoxia	Hypertension
Increasing headache pain	Inadequate fluid intake

6-C. A 51-year-old male client who sustained a closed head injury was admitted from the ED to the neurological unit today around noon. After lunch, the nurse performed a neurological check on the client about an hour after lunch. Vital signs: temperature = 98.8°F (37.1°C), apical heart rate = 58 beats/min and regular, respirations = 16 breaths/min, blood pressure (BP) = 142/68 mm Hg. Oxygen saturation is 92% (on RA). The client reported a headache of 5/10 on a 0 to 10 pain intensity scale and had a new onset of nausea. Glasgow Coma Scale score = 12. The client seemed sleepy and confused as to where he was, but he responded to localized painful stimuli

and opened his eyes in response to sound. Slight pupil dilation was noted in the right eye. Based on the neurological assessment, what changes would the nurse identify as the **priority** for the client? **Select all that apply.**

a. Increased headache pain
b. New-onset confusion
c. Bradycardia
d. Pupillary dilation
e. Decreased level of consciousness
f. Increased blood pressure
g. Decreased respiratory rate

6-D. A 51-year-old male client who sustained a closed head injury was admitted from the ED to the neurological unit today around noon. After lunch, the nurse performed a neurological check on the client about an hour after lunch. Vital signs: temperature = 98.8°F (37.1°C), apical heart rate = 58 beats/min; and regular, respirations =16 breaths/min, blood pressure (BP) = 142/68 mm Hg. Oxygen saturation is 92% (on RA). The client reported a headache of 5/10 on a 0 to 10 pain intensity scale and had a new onset of nausea. Glasgow Coma Scale score was 12 points. The client seemed sleepy and confused as to where he was, but he responded to localized painful stimuli and opened his eyes in response to sound. Slight pupil dilation was noted in the right eye. The neurosurgeon examines the client and determines that he is experiencing increased intracranial pressure due to an epidural hematoma. A plan of care is developed.

For each provider order, select whether it is Anticipated (expected and necessary), Non-Essential (makes no difference or not necessary), or Contraindicated (could be harmful) for the client at this time.

Provider Order	Anticipated	Non-Essential	Contraindicated
Discontinue IV infusion.			
Administer osmotic diuretic.			
Place the client on a hypothermia blanket.			
Check skin integrity.			
Assess bowel sounds.			
Elevate the head of the bed to 30 degrees.			
Prepare for evacuation of the hematoma.			

6-E. A 51-year-old male client who sustained a closed head injury was admitted from the ED to the neurological unit today around noon. After lunch, the nurse performed a neurological check on the client about an hour after lunch. Vital signs: temperature = 98.8°F (37.1°C), apical heart rate = 58 beats/min and regular, respirations = 16 breaths/min, blood pressure (BP) = 142/68 mm Hg. Oxygen saturation is 92% (on RA). The client reported a headache of 5/10 on a 0 to10 pain intensity scale and had a new onset of nausea. Glasgow Coma Scale score was 12 points. The client seemed sleepy and confused as to where he was, but he responded to localized painful stimuli and opened his eyes in response to sound. Slight pupil dilation was noted in the right eye. The neurosurgeon examines the client and determines that he is experiencing increased intracranial pressure due to an epidural hematoma. A plan of care is developed.

Choose the *most likely* options for the information missing from the statement below by selecting from the lists of options provided.

The **first** action that the nurse would take for the client is to _____1_____ to _____2_____, followed by _____3_____ to _____4_____.

Options for 1	Options for 2	Options for 3	Options for 4
Ensure the head of the bed is at 30 degrees	Minimize bleeding	Ensuring the head of the bed is at 30 degrees	Minimize bleeding
Prepare for evacuation of the hematoma	Reduce intracranial pressure	Preparing for evacuation of the hematoma	Reduce intracranial pressure
Administer osmotic diuretic	Provide adequate cerebral perfusion	Administering osmotic diuretic	Provide adequate cerebral perfusion

6-F. A 51-year-old male client who sustained a closed head injury was admitted from the ED to the neurological unit today around noon. About 2 hours later, the nurse noted a decline in the client's neurological status which was determined to be caused by an epidural hematoma. The client returns from PACU after undergoing a burr hole procedure to remove the accumulated blood from the epidural space. The dura and scalp were closed and there is no drain in place. The nurse assesses the client and documents the following data. Vital signs: temperature = 99.2°F (37.3°C), apical heart rate = 72 beats/min and regular, respirations = 16 breaths/min, blood pressure (BP) = 132/70 mm Hg. Oxygen saturation is 95% (on 2 L oxygen via nasal cannula). The client is sleepy but arousable. Pain is reported as 4/10 on a 0 to 10 pain intensity scale. Glasgow Coma Scale score = 15.

Highlight the findings below that indicate the client is _not_ progressing as expected and exhibiting symptoms of potential complications.

Two hours later, the nurse re-assesses the client and finds that his airway remains patent. A quarter-sized amount of clear wetness is noted on the head dressing. Oxygen saturation is 94% (on 2 L oxygen via nasal cannula). The client is awake and states his name, but is unsure where he is, what happened to him, and what day it is. Glasgow Coma Scale score = 10. Vital signs: temperature = 99.2°F (37.3°C), apical heart rate = 70 beats/min and regular, respirations = 18 breaths/min, BP = 155/60 mm Hg. The client reports his headache is now 8/10 on a 0 to 10 pain intensity scale. He opens his eyes in response to pain. Pupils equal and react to light slowly.

NGN Unfolding Case Study #7: ST Elevation Myocardial Infarction (STEMI) (Concept of Perfusion)

7-A. The wife of a 64-year-old male client calls 911 to report that her husband was raking leaves in the yard, clutched his chest, and is having severe crushing chest pain (10/10 on a 0 to 10 pain intensity scale). The client is quickly attached to the cardiac monitor, which reveals ST elevation and a 12-lead ECG is transmitted to the emergency department (ED) for further evaluation. EMS obtains a rapid health assessment and determines that the client has no history of cardiac disease or hypertension and has no allergies. The ECG reveals that he currently has ST elevations. Vital signs: temperature = 99.2°F (37.3°C) apical heart rate = 88 beats/min and regular, respirations = 24 breaths/min, blood pressure (BP) = 178/98 mm Hg. Oxygen saturation is 89% (on room air [RA]). Oxygen at 3 L/min is applied to the client and an IV catheter is inserted. Aspirin 325 mg is administered with nitroglycerin 0.4 mg sublingually. The client arrives at the ED and the nurse assesses the client and notes the following:

- Chest pain is a pressure-like feeling at 8/10 on a 0 to 10 pain intensity scale

- Temperature = 99.2°F (37.3°C)
- Apical heart rate = 98 beats/min and irregular
- Respirations = 24 breaths/min
- Blood pressure (BP) = 154/84 mm Hg
- Oxygen saturation = 93% (on 3 L/min oxygen via NC)

IV morphine sulfate is administered as prescribed. The nurse maintains oxygen therapy at 3 L/min, obtains another 12-lead ECG, and places the client on a continuous cardiac monitor. Laboratory and diagnostic studies are prescribed including complete metabolic profile (CMP), cardiac troponin I and troponin T. Reperfusion (antithrombotic) therapy is initiated. An echocardiography imaging, and coronary angiography with possible percutaneous coronary intervention is prescribed.

Use an X to indicate which client assessment findings require immediate follow-up by the nurse at this time.

Assessment Finding	Assessment Finding that Requires Immediate Follow-Up
Pain level = 8/10	
Temperature = 99.2°F (37.3°C)	
Apical heart rate = 98 beats/min and irregular	
Respirations = 20 breaths/min	
Blood pressure (BP) = 154/84 mm Hg	
Oxygen saturation = 93% (on 3 L/min)	
ST elevations on initial ECG	

7-B. A 64-year-old male client arrives at the ED with his wife via ambulance with the following admission assessment:

- Chest pain is a pressure-like feeling at 8/10 on a 0 to 10 pain intensity scale
- Temperature = 99.2°F (37.3°C)
- Apical heart rate = 98 beats/min and irregular
- Respirations = 24 breaths/min
- Blood pressure (BP) = 154/84 mm Hg
- Oxygen saturation = 93% (on 3 L/min oxygen via NC)
- ST elevations on initial ECG

Based on the assessment data, the nurse recognizes that the client is at risk for which potential complications? **Select all that apply.**

a. Sepsis
b. Pneumonia
c. Heart failure
d. Atrial fibrillation
e. Sinus bradycardia
f. Hypovolemic shock
g. Ventricular fibrillation
h. Ventricular tachycardia

7-C. A 64-year-old male client arrives at the ED with his wife via ambulance with the following admission assessment:

- Chest pain is a pressure-like feeling at 8/10 on a 0 to 10 pain intensity scale
- Temperature = 99.2°F (37.3°C)
- Apical heart rate = 98 beats/min and irregular
- Respirations = 24 breaths/min
- Blood pressure (BP) = 154/84 mm Hg
- Oxygen saturation = 93% (on 3 L/min oxygen via NC)
- ST elevations on initial ECG

Choose the *most likely* options for the information missing from the statements below by selecting from the lists of options provided.

Based on the nurse's assessment findings, the nurse determines that the client's temperature reading _____1_____ and the client's BP reading _____2_____. The ST elevation noted on the initial ECG most likely _____3_____.

Options for 1	Options for 2	Options for 3
Is an expected finding	Is too high	Indicates acute myocardial infarction
Indicates infection	Is decreased due to medication	Indicates a normal finding
Indicates the need for respiratory precautions	Requires immediate intervention	Occurs if a client is having chest pain

7-D. A 64-year-old male client arrives at the ED with his wife via ambulance with the following admission assessment:

- Chest pain is a pressure-like feeling at 8/10 on a 0 to 10 pain intensity scale
- Temperature = 99.2°F (37.3°C)
- Apical heart rate = 98 beats/min and irregular
- Respirations = 24 breaths/min
- Blood pressure (BP) = 154/84 mm Hg
- Oxygen saturation = 93% (on 3 L/min oxygen via NC)
- ST elevations on initial ECG

The nurse is monitoring the client closely while awaiting transfer from the ED to the cardiac catheterization department. The client reports that his pain level is 5/10 now but is feeling really weak and dizzy as though he might "pass out." He is having some trouble breathing and feeling palpitations. The nurse notes this cardiac rhythm:

Based on the cardiac rhythm strip, use an X for the nursing actions listed below that are <u>Indicated</u> **(appropriate or necessary),** <u>Contraindicated</u> **(could be harmful), or** <u>Non-Essential</u> **(makes no difference or not necessary) for the client's care at this time.**

Nursing Action	Indicated	Contraindicated	Non-Essential
Begin cardiopulmonary resuscitation (CPR).			
Check vital signs.			
Be sure the client is in a semi-Fowler position.			
Obtain a 12-lead ECG.			
Stop the reperfusion therapy.			
Obtain a chest x-ray.			
Prepare to administer IV diltiazem.			
Prepare to administer IV amiodarone.			
Prepare to administer IV digoxin.			

7-E. A 64-year-old male client arrives at the ED with his wife via ambulance with the following admission assessment:

- Chest pain is a pressure-like feeling at 8/10 on a 0 to 10 pain intensity scale
- Temperature = 99.2°F (37.3°C)
- Apical heart rate = 98 beats/min and irregular
- Respirations = 24 breaths/min
- Blood pressure (BP) = 154/84 mm Hg
- Oxygen saturation = 93% (on 3 L/min oxygen via NC)
- ST elevations on initial ECG

The nurse is monitoring the client closely while awaiting transfer from the ED to the cardiac catheterization department. The client reports that his pain level is 5/10 now but is feeling really weak and dizzy as though he might "pass out." He is having some trouble breathing and feeling palpitations. The nurse notes that the client has atrial fibrillation on the cardiac monitor.

Choose the _most likely_ options for the information missing from the statements below by selecting from the lists of options provided.

The _immediate_ action that the nurse would take is to _____1_____ to _____2_____ followed by _____3_____ to _____4_____.

Options for 1	Options for 2	Options for 3	Options for 4
Prepare to administer IV digoxin	Control the heart rate	Preparing to administer IV digoxin	Control the heart rate
Check vital signs	Provide oxygen and circulation to all body tissues	Checking vital signs	Provide oxygen and circulation to all body tissues
Place the client in a semi-Fowler position	Determine a baseline status and specific plan for treatment	Placing the client in a semi-Fowler position	Determine a baseline status and specific plan for treatment

7-F. A 64-year-old male client is admitted to the ED with an ST elevation myocardial infarction (STEMI). While awaiting transfer from the ED to the cardiac catheterization department, the client had an episode of atrial fibrillation (AF). Following immediate treatment of the AF, the cardiac catheterization department calls the ED and indicates that the department is prepared to perform the procedure. Before transferring the client and providing a hand-off report, a cardiac rhythm strip from the heart monitor is obtained, which reveals normal sinus rhythm. The nurse obtains additional assessment data to evaluate the effectiveness of interventions to treat the dysrhythmia. **For each client finding, use an X to indicate whether the interventions for the client were <u>Effective</u> (helped to meet expected outcomes), <u>Ineffective</u> (did not help to meet expected outcomes), or <u>Unrelated</u> (not related to the expected outcomes).**

Client Finding	Effective	Ineffective	Unrelated
Temperature = 99.2°F (37.3°C)			
Apical heart rate = 80 beats/min and regular			
Respirations = 20 breaths/min			
Oxygen saturation = 90% (on 3 L/min oxygen)			
Blood pressure (BP) = 130/72 mm Hg			
Cardiac rhythm = Normal sinus rhythm			
Dyspnea			
Chest pain 5/10 on 0 to 10 pain intensity scale			

NGN Unfolding Case Study #8: Diabetes Mellitus Type 2 (Concepts of Metabolism and Fluid and Electrolyte Balance)

8-A. An 85-year-old female client was brought to the emergency department this morning by her daughter because of confusion and lethargy. The daughter reports that her mother lives with her, and over the past few weeks she has become increasingly tired, weak, and very thirsty. The daughter tells the nurse that her mother has a history of diabetes mellitus type 2 and heart failure. Home medications include metformin 500 mg in the morning with breakfast and again at dinner, 10 mg furosemide every other morning, lisinopril 2.5 mg daily, and carvedilol 3.125 mg twice daily. This morning the daughter reports that she had to help her mother to the bathroom because of her weakness. She noticed a "funny smell" to her mother's urine and thought it looked concentrated. After laboratory and diagnostic testing were completed, the client was diagnosed with hyperglycemic hyperosmolar syndrome (HHS) and urinary tract infection (UTI).

The client arrives to the medical unit and has an IV solution of 0.45% normal saline infusing at 100 mL/hr via an infusion device. The admission nurse in the medical unit reviews the notes from the ED and notes that the client received 5 units regular insulin by IV bolus and has a continuous

IV insulin solution infusing at a rate of 5 units/hr. Ciprofloxacin 400 mg IV every 8 hours is prescribed. The nurse performs an admission assessment and documents the findings. **Highlight the client findings <u>below</u> that require immediate follow-up by the nurse.**

Vital signs: temperature = 101°F (38.3°C), apical heart rate = 96 beats/min and regular, respirations = 20 breaths/min, oxygen saturation = 92% on room air (RA), blood pressure = 104/68 mm Hg. Skin dry with decreased turgor. Finger stick blood glucose (FSBG) = 450 mg/dL (25 mmol/L). Client reports thirst and tolerating oral fluids without nausea. Weight = 112 lb (50.8 kg) which is a weight loss of 8 lb (3.6 kg) since 2 weeks ago. Fine crackles noted bilaterally in the lungs. Denies shortness of breath. No cyanosis; capillary refill 3 seconds. Pedal pulses 2+ bilaterally; 2+ edema bilaterally in feet and ankles; neck vein distention noted. Abdomen soft, bowel sounds present × 4, states last bowel movement yesterday (soft, brown, moderate amount). Has low abdominal discomfort on palpation; 3/10 on a 0 to 10 pain intensity scale. States she is urinating every 3 to 4 hours with no burning. Moves all extremities but is weak and needs assistance with standing and ambulating. Is alert and oriented. States no numbness or tingling in extremities; PERRLA.

8-B. An 85-year-old female client was admitted from home this morning with hyperglycemic hyperosmolar syndrome (HHS) and urinary tract infection (UTI). The daughter reported that her mother lives with her, and over the past few weeks she has become increasingly tired, confused, and very thirsty. The client has a history of diabetes mellitus type 2 and heart failure. Home medications include metformin 500 mg in the morning with breakfast and again at dinner, 10 mg furosemide every other morning, lisinopril 2.5 mg daily, and carvedilol 3.125 mg twice daily. The admission nurse in the medical unit reviews the notes from the ED and notes that the client received 5 units regular insulin by IV bolus and has a continuous IV insulin solution infusing at a rate of 5 units/hr. Ciprofloxacin 400 mg IV every 8 hours is prescribed. The nurse performs an admission assessment and documents the findings, including the following:

Vital signs: temperature = 101°F (38.3°C), apical heart rate = 96 beats/min and regular, respirations = 20 breaths/min, oxygen saturation = 92% on RA, blood pressure = 104/68 mm Hg. Skin dry with decreased turgor. Finger stick blood glucose (FSBG) = 450 mg/dL (25 mmol/L). Client reports thirst and tolerating oral fluids without nausea. Weight = 112 lb (50.8 kg) which is a weight loss of 8 lb (3.6 kg) since 2 weeks ago. Fine crackles noted bilaterally in lung bases. Pedal pulses 2+ bilaterally; 2+ edema bilaterally in feet and ankles; neck vein distention noted.

Use an X to indicate which assessment finding is associated with each of the client's health problems. *All assessment findings must be used. Each assessment finding can be used more than once.*

Assessment Finding	Heart Failure	HHS	UTI
Confusion and lethargy			
States she is thirsty			
Temperature = 101°F (38.3°C)			
Fine crackles bilaterally in lung bases			
FSBG = 450 mg/dL (25 mmol/L)			
2+ edema bilaterally in feet and ankles			
Weight loss			
Neck vein distention			

8-C. An 85-year-old female client was admitted from home this morning with hyperglycemic hyperosmolar syndrome (HHS) and urinary tract infection (UTI). The daughter reported that her mother lives with her, and over the past few weeks she has become increasingly tired, confused, and very thirsty. The client has a history of diabetes mellitus type 2 and heart failure. Home medications include metformin

500 mg in the morning with breakfast and again at dinner, 10 mg furosemide every other morning, lisinopril 2.5 mg daily, and carvedilol 3.125 mg twice daily. The admission nurse in the medical unit reviews the notes from the ED and notes that the client received 5 units regular insulin by IV bolus and has a continuous IV insulin solution infusing at a rate of 5 units/hr. Ciprofloxacin 400 mg IV every 8 hours is prescribed. The nurse performs an admission assessment and documents the findings, including the following:

Vital signs: temperature = 101°F (38.3°C), apical heart rate = 96 beats/min and regular, respirations = 20 breaths/min, oxygen saturation = 92% on RA, blood pressure = 104/68 mm Hg. Skin dry with decreased turgor. Finger stick blood glucose (FSBG) = 450 mg/dL (25 mmol/L). Client reports thirst and tolerating oral fluids without nausea. Weight = 112 lb (50.8 kg) which is a weight loss of 8 lb (3.6 kg) since 2 weeks ago. Fine crackles noted bilaterally in lung bases. Pedal pulses 2+ bilaterally; 2+ edema bilaterally in feet and ankles; neck vein distention noted. Based on the admission assessment, what findings would the nurse identify as the **priority** when planning the client's care? **Select all that apply.**

a. Weight loss
b. Adventitious breath sounds
c. Dehydration
d. Ankle and foot edema
e. Hyperglycemia
f. Urinary tract infection
g. Confusion
h. Fever
i. Hypotension

8-D. An 85-year-old female client was admitted from home this morning with hyperglycemic hyperosmolar syndrome (HHS) and urinary tract infection (UTI). The daughter reported that her mother lives with her, and over the past few weeks she has become increasingly tired, confused, and very thirsty. The client has a history of diabetes mellitus type 2 and heart failure. The admission nurse in the medical unit reviews the notes from the ED and notes that the client received 5 units regular insulin by IV bolus and has a continuous IV insulin solution infusing at a rate of 5 units/hr. Ciprofloxacin 400 mg IV every 8 hours is prescribed. The nurse prepares a plan of care for the client.

Use an X to indicate the nursing actions listed below that are <u>Indicated</u> (appropriate or necessary), <u>Contraindicated</u> (could be harmful), or <u>Non-Essential</u> (makes no difference or not necessary) for the client's care at this time.

Nursing Action	Indicated	Contraindicated	Non-Essential
Monitor intake and output carefully.			
Maintain continuous bedrest.			
Maintain the client in a flat position.			
Place the client on a continuous cardiac monitor.			
Monitor vital signs frequently.			
Perform frequent FSBGs.			
Limit fluids to 240 mL every 8 hours.			
Send urine for urinalysis daily.			
Monitor lung sounds every shift.			

8-E. An 85-year-old female client was admitted from home this morning with hyperglycemic hyperosmolar syndrome (HHS) and urinary tract infection (UTI). The daughter reported that her mother lives with her, and over the past few weeks she has become increasingly tired, confused, and very thirsty. The client has a history of diabetes mellitus type 2 and heart failure. The admission nurse in the medical unit reviews the notes from the ED and notes that the client received 5 units regular insulin by IV bolus and has a continuous IV insulin solution infusing at a rate of 5 units/hr. Ciprofloxacin 400 mg IV every 8 hours is prescribed. Several hours after unit admission, the nurse reassesses the client and notes that she is increasingly confused and very lethargic. Vital signs: temperature = 101.8°F (38.8°C), apical heart rate = 72 breaths/min, respirations = 20 breaths/min, BP = 172/60 mm Hg, and oxygen saturation = 92%. The client complains of a headache and feels nauseated. **Choose the *most likely* options for the information missing from the statement below by selecting from the lists of options provided.**

The *immediate* action that the nurse would take is to _____1_____ to _____2_____ followed by _____3_____ to _____4_____.

Options for 1	Options for 2	Options for 3	Options for 4
Elevate the head of the bed to 30 to 40 degrees	Prevent an allergic reaction	Administering an antiemetic	Determine the change in status
Contact the primary health care provider	Report the findings	Checking the blood glucose level	Relieve the nausea
Stop the IV infusion of ciprofloxacin	Decrease intracranial pressure	Increasing the IV flow of the normal saline	Prevent further dehydration

8-F. An 85-year-old female client was admitted from home this morning with Hyperglycemic hyperglycemic hyperosmolar syndrome (HHS) and urinary tract infection (UTI). The daughter reported that her mother lives with her, and over the past few weeks she has become increasingly tired, confused, and very thirsty. The client has a history of diabetes mellitus type 2 and heart failure. The admission nurse in the medical unit reviews the notes from the ED and notes that the client received 5 units regular insulin by IV bolus and has a continuous IV insulin solution infusing at a rate of 5 units/hr. Ciprofloxacin 400 mg IV every 8 hours is prescribed.

As part of the night shift assessment, the nurse notes that the client's FSBG is 275 mg/dL (15.3 mmol/L). The primary health care provider prescribes the following: acetaminophen 650 mg orally or rectally by suppository, change IV infusion to 0.9% normal saline, and discontinue IV insulin infusion. A CMP and blood osmolarity test is ordered. The nurse evaluates the effectiveness of interventions.

For each assessment finding, use an X to indicate whether interventions were Effective (helped to meet expected outcomes), Ineffective (did not help to meet expected outcomes), or Unrelated (not related to the expected outcomes).

Assessment Finding	Effective	Ineffective	Unrelated
BP = 140/70 mm Hg			
FSBG = 275 mg/dL (15.3 mmol/L)			
Urine output = 20 mL/hr			
Sodium = 145 mg/dL (145 mmol/L)			
Potassium = 5.5 mEq/L (5.5 mmol/L)			
Blood osmolarity = 350 mOsm/kg (0.28 mmol/kg)			
Oxygen saturation = 93%			
Fine crackles noted bilaterally in lung bases			
2+ edema bilaterally in feet and ankles			

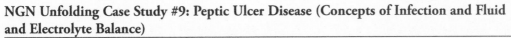

NGN Unfolding Case Study #9: Peptic Ulcer Disease (Concepts of Infection and Fluid and Electrolyte Balance)

9-A. A 50-year-old male client arrives to the emergency department and states that he vomited a small amount of bright red blood this morning. A nursing assessment reveals the following data:

The client has epigastric pain after meals and describes it like heartburn or gnawing. He reports that he has some difficulty swallowing and feels full after eating. He has been slowly losing weight and easily gets constipated. His abdomen is soft and tender on palpation with no guarding; abdominal pain is 3/10 on a 0 to 10 pain intensity scale. Bowel sounds are heard × 4 and his last bowel movement was yesterday – hard, black, and tarry stool. The client reports no previous history of gastrointestinal health problems. When asked about *Helicobacter pylori* infection, he denies ever being told that he had an infection. Skin color is pale and client reports feeling tired lately. Vital signs are within normal limits except B/P = 98/60 mm Hg.

The client has a 5-year history of coronary artery disease (CAD) and reports that it is well controlled with medication. Medication history includes metoprolol 50 mg twice daily, aspirin 325 mg daily, lisinopril 2.5 mg daily, and simvastatin 20 mg daily, but he has not taken any medication today. He states that he drinks alcohol on weekends and stopped smoking when he was told he had heart disease. He has a 30–pack-year smoking history.

The ED physician assistant prescribes laboratory and diagnostic studies including a hemoglobin and hematocrit (H&H), electrolytes, liver enzymes, blood urea nitrogen (BUN) and creatinine (Cr), coagulation studies, an ECG, and cardiac enzymes. Type and crossmatch are also prescribed. The client is NPO and oxygen via nasal cannula at 2 L/min is started. Two large-bore peripheral IV lines are inserted and lactated Ringer's solution is infused at 125 mL/hr.

Use an X to indicate which client findings require immediate follow-up by the nurse at this time.

Client Finding	Client Finding that Requires Immediate Follow-Up
Has some difficulty swallowing and feels full after meals	
Abdomen is soft and tender on palpation with no guarding	
Stools are black and tarry	
Skin color is pale	
History of coronary artery disease	
Drinks alcohol on the weekends	
Has lost weight	
Takes aspirin daily	
B/P = 98/60 mm Hg	
Vomited red blood this morning	

9-B. A 50-year-old male client arrives to the emergency department and states that he vomited a small amount of bright red blood this morning. A nursing assessment reveals the following data:

The client has epigastric pain after meals and describes it like heartburn or gnawing. He reports that he has some difficulty swallowing and feels full after eating. He has been slowly losing weight and easily gets constipated. His abdomen is soft and tender on palpation with no guarding; abdominal pain is 3/10 on a 0 to 10 pain intensity scale. Bowel sounds are heard × 4 and his last bowel movement was yesterday – hard, black, and tarry stool. The client reports no previous history of gastrointestinal health problems, but has a history of CAD. When asked about *Helicobacter pylori* infection, he denies ever being told that he had an infection. Skin color is pale and client reports feeling tired lately. Vital signs are within normal limits except B/P = 98/60 mm Hg.

Use an X to indicate which assessment finding is *most likely* **associated with each of the client's health problems.** *All assessment findings should be used. Any assessment finding may be used more than once.*

Assessment Finding	Peptic Ulcer Disease	GI Bleeding	Coronary Artery Disease
Heartburn or a gnawing or burning feeling			
Abdominal pain = 3/10			
Black and tarry stool			
Skin color is pale			
Feeling tired			
Apical heart rate = 96 beats/min			
Blood pressure (BP) = 98/60 mm Hg			
Oxygen saturation = 89%			

9-C. A 50-year-old male client arrives to the emergency department and states that he vomited a small amount of bright red blood this morning. A nursing assessment reveals the following data:

The client has epigastric pain after meals and describes it like heartburn or gnawing. He reports that he has some difficulty swallowing and feels full after eating. He has been slowly losing weight and easily gets constipated. His abdomen is soft and tender on palpation with no guarding; abdominal pain is 3/10 on a 0 to 10 pain intensity scale. Bowel sounds are heard × 4 and his last bowel movement was yesterday – hard, black, and tarry stool. The client reports no previous history of gastrointestinal health problems, but has a history of CAD. When asked about *Helicobacter pylori* infection, he denies ever being told that he had an infection. Skin color is pale and client reports feeling tired lately. Vital signs are within normal limits except B/P = 98/60 mm Hg. The nurse reviews the laboratory results and the ECG report. All laboratory results were within normal limits except for hemoglobin (Hgb) = 9 g/dL (90 mmol/L) and hematocrit (Hct) = 38.3% (0.383). The ECG confirmed sinus tachycardia.

Based on the client findings, the nurse begins to plan the client's care. What does the nurse recognize as the **priority** problems for the client?
a. Bleeding
b. Dysphagia

c. Weight loss
d. Hypotension
e. Anemia
f. Constipation
g. Epigastric pain

9-D. A 50-year-old male client arrives to the emergency department and states that he vomited a small amount of bright red blood this morning. A nursing assessment reveals the following data:

The client has epigastric pain after meals and describes it like heartburn or gnawing. He reports that he has some difficulty swallowing and feels full after eating. He has been slowly losing weight and easily gets constipated. His abdomen is soft and tender on palpation with no guarding; abdominal pain is 3/10 on a 0 to 10 pain intensity scale. Bowel sounds are heard × 4 and his last bowel movement was yesterday – hard, black, and tarry stool. The client reports no previous history of gastrointestinal health problems, but has a history of CAD. When asked about *Helicobacter pylori* infection, he denies ever being told that he had an infection. Skin color is pale and client reports feeling tired lately. Vital signs are within normal limits except B/P = 98/60 mm Hg. The nurse reviews the laboratory results and the ECG report. All laboratory results were within normal limits except for hemoglobin (Hgb) = 9 g/dL (90 mmol/L) and hematocrit (Hct) = 38.3% (0.383). The ECG confirmed sinus tachycardia.

A gastroenterologist is consulted and the nurse awaits new orders. **For each provider order, select whether it is __Anticipated__ (expected and necessary),** __Non-Essential__ **(makes no difference or not necessary), or __Contraindicated__ (could be harmful) for the client at this time.**

Provider Order	Anticipated	Contraindicated	Non-Essential
Insertion of a nasogastric tube			
Preparation for endoscopy			
Cardiologist consult			
Administration of a proton pump inhibitor and prokinetic agent			
Administration of a blood transfusion			
Administration of IV morphine			
Administration of IV ondansetron			

9-E. A 50-year-old male client arrives to the emergency department and states that he vomited a small amount of bright red blood this morning. The gastroenterologist schedules the client for an immediate endoscopy to determine the cause of the bleeding and explains the procedure to the client. The nurse immediately prepares the client. **Choose the *most likely* options for the information missing from the statement below by selecting from the lists of options provided.**

The ***priority*** action that the nurse would take is _____1_____ to _____2_____ followed by _____3_____ to _____4_____.

Options for 1	Options for 2	Options for 3	Options for 4
Check vital signs	Obtain approval for endoscopy	Checking vital signs	Obtain approval for endoscopy
Administer a proton pump inhibitor and prokinetic agent	Alleviate nausea and vomiting	Administering a proton pump inhibitor and prokinetic agent	Alleviate nausea and vomiting
Call for a cardiologist consult	Determine any changes	Requesting a cardiologist consult	Determine any cardiac changes
Administer IV ondansetron	Improve stomach visualization and suppress acid secretion	Administering IV ondansetron	Improve stomach visualization and suppress acid secretion
Perform gastric lavage	Clear the stomach of blood or sediment	Performing gastric lavage	Clear the stomach of blood or sediment

9-F. A 50-year-old male client admitted to the ED with GI bleeding has an endoscopy to determine the cause of the bleeding. Results reveal that the client has a gastric ulcer that was treated with therapeutic hemostasis intervention. Stomach tissue biopsies were obtained to assess for *Helicobacter pylori* infection. An H&H, coagulation studies, and ECG have been prescribed 1 hour postprocedure. After 4 hours of postprocedure observation and stable vital signs, laboratory results, and ECG, the client can be discharged to home. Home medications will include a proton pump inhibitor (esomeprazole) and cytoprotective agent (sucralfate). The nurse begins to implement a discharge teaching plan for the client. **Use an X to indicate which client statement indicates that the home care instruction is either __Understood__ or __Requires Further Teaching__.**

Client Statement	Understood	Requires Further Teaching
"I will cut my daily aspirin dose in half."		
"It may be a good idea to eat some foods with probiotics such as yogurt."		
"I can continue to drink alcohol as long as it is only on the weekends."		
"I should avoid any foods that contain vitamin C."		
"I may have to take some more medications if my biopsies are positive for infection."		
"It is a good thing that I stopped smoking a while back because smoking can increase the acid in my stomach."		
"I can't skip any doses of my prescribed medications because they are needed to protect my stomach and help my ulcer heal."		
"I may have another black and tarry bowel movement next time I go but if I continue to see these kind of bowel movements or see any blood, I need to notify my doctor."		
"If I should feel lightheaded, dizzy, and week, it is probably from the new medication and I don't need to worry about that."		

NGN Unfolding Case Study #10: Bowel Obstruction (Concepts of Elimination and Fluid and Electrolyte Balance)

10-A. A 69-year-old male client with a history of colorectal cancer arrives at the ED and reports that he has abdominal pain of 5/10 on a 0 to 10 pain intensity scale. The client reports a history of benign premature ventricular contractions (PVCs) and is taking metoprolol 50 mg twice daily for control. He tells the nurse that he recently completed his chemotherapy treatments and since then has had extreme fatigue, loss of appetite, sores in his mouth, and diarrhea. He is wondering if his symptoms are due to the effects of chemotherapy. He reports no allergies.

Nursing assessment findings include:

- Vital signs: temperature = 99.2°F (37.3°C), apical heart rate = 90 beats/min and irregular with an occasional skipped beat, respirations = 24 breaths/min, blood pressure (BP) = 168/90 mm Hg, oxygen saturation = 93% (on RA), abdominal pain level = 5/10 on a 0 to 10 pain intensity scale
- Reports loss of appetite, vomiting, constipation with diarrhea containing blood streaks, abdominal distention and tenderness; mass in mid-abdomen palpated, bowel sounds are high-pitched tinkling sounds; last bowel movement was during the night; weight is 145 lb (65.8 kg); reports a loss of 10 lb (4.5 kg) in the last month
- Breath sounds are clear bilaterally and client denies dyspnea or chest pain
- Skin is intact, dry, with poor turgor; sore white patches on mucous membranes in the mouth
- Reports urine output has decreased over the past week; denies burning or difficulty
- Moves all extremities and is able to ambulate independently; reports general fatigue and weakness
- Alert and oriented, coherent and responds appropriately; denies forgetfulness or memory loss; reports numbness and tingling in the ankles and feet bilaterally

Highlight the client findings that require immediate follow-up by the nurse.

10-B. A 69-year-old male client with a history of colorectal cancer arrives at the ED and reports that he has abdominal pain of 5/10 on a 0 to 10 pain intensity scale. The client reports a history of benign premature ventricular contractions (PVCs) and is taking metoprolol 50 mg twice daily for control. He tells the nurse that he recently completed his chemotherapy treatments and since then has had extreme fatigue, loss of appetite, sores in his mouth, numbness and tingling in the ankles and feet bilaterally, and diarrhea. He is wondering if his symptoms are due to the effects of chemotherapy.

Nursing assessment findings include:

- Vital signs: temperature = 99.2°F (37.3°C), apical heart rate = 90 beats/min and irregular with an occasional skipped beat, respirations = 24 breaths/min, blood pressure (BP) = 168/90 mm Hg, oxygen saturation = 93% (on RA), abdominal pain level = 5/10 on a 0 to 10 pain intensity scale
- Reports loss of appetite, vomiting, constipation with diarrhea containing blood streaks, abdominal distention and tenderness; mass in mid-abdomen palpated, bowel sounds are high-pitched tinkling sounds; last bowel movement was during the night; weight is 145 lb (65.8 kg); reports a loss of 10 lb (4.5 kg) in the last month

Use an X to indicate which assessment finding is associated with each of the client's health problems. *All assessment findings should be used. Each assessment finding may be used more than once.*

Assessment Finding	Bowel Obstruction	Chemotherapy
Sore white patches on mucous membranes of the mouth		
Abdominal pain of 5/10 on a 0 to 10 pain intensity scale		
Loss of appetite and weight loss		
Numbness and tingling in the ankles and feet bilaterally		
High-pitched tinkling bowel sounds		
Apical heart rate = 90 beats/min		
BP = 168/90 mm Hg		

10-C. A 69-year-old male client with a history of colorectal cancer arrives at the ED and reports that he has abdominal pain of 5/10 on a 0 to 10 pain intensity scale. He tells the nurse that he recently completed his chemotherapy treatments and since then has had extreme fatigue, loss of appetite, sores in his mouth, numbness and tingling in the ankles and feet bilaterally, and diarrhea.

Nursing assessment findings include:

- Vital signs: temperature = 99.2°F (37.3°C), apical heart rate = 90 beats/min and irregular with an occasional skipped beat, respirations = 24 breaths/min, blood pressure (BP) = 168/90 mm Hg, oxygen saturation = 93%, abdominal pain level = 5/10 on a 0 to 10 pain intensity scale
- Reports loss of appetite, vomiting, constipation with diarrhea containing blood streaks, abdominal distention and tenderness; mass in mid-abdomen palpated, bowel sounds are high-pitched tinkling sounds; last bowel movement was during the night; weight is 145 lb (65.8 kg); reports a loss of 10 lb (4.5 kg) in the last month

Laboratory and diagnostic tests results include:

- White blood cell count = 4,500 mm³ (4.5 × 10⁹/L)
- Hemoglobin = 11 g/dL (110 mmol/L)
- Hematocrit = 37% (0.37)
- Blood urea nitrogen = 25 mg/dL (9 mmol/L)
- Creatinine = 2.0 mg/dL (176 μmol/L)
- Sodium = 149 mg/dL (149 mmol/L)
- Potassium = 3.2 mg/dL (3.2 mmol/L)
- X-ray: A blockage in the large intestine is suspected; gas and liquid bowel contents above the area of the blockage appear to be present. Follow-up with CT scan is recommended.

- CT scan: A partial obstruction is seen in the large intestine. Gas and liquid bowel contents are seen both above and below the area of the blockage.
- ECG: normal sinus rhythm with occasional PVCs

Based on the client findings, the nurse begins to plan the client's care. What does the nurse recognize as the **priority** problems for the client? **Select all that apply.**
a. Abdominal pain
b. Dehydration
c. Acute kidney injury
d. Abnormal ECG
e. Tachycardia
f. Weight loss
g. Intestinal perforation
h. Electrolyte imbalance
i. High blood pressure

10-D. A 69-year-old male client with a history of colorectal cancer arrives at the ED and reports that he has abdominal pain of 5/10 on a 0 to 10 pain intensity scale. He tells the nurse that he recently completed his chemotherapy treatments and since then has had extreme fatigue, loss of appetite, sores in his mouth, numbness and tingling in the ankles and feet bilaterally, and diarrhea.

Nursing assessment findings include:

- Vital signs: temperature = 99.2°F (37.3°C), apical heart rate = 90 beats/min and irregular with an occasional skipped beat, respirations = 24 breaths/min, blood pressure (BP) = 168/90 mm Hg, oxygen saturation = 93% (on RA),

abdominal pain level = 5/10 on a 0 to 10 pain intensity scale
- Reports loss of appetite, vomiting, constipation with diarrhea containing blood streaks, abdominal distention and tenderness; mass in mid-abdomen palpated, bowel sounds are high-pitched tinkling sounds; last bowel movement was during the night; weight is 145 lb (65.8 kg); reports a loss of 10 lb (4.5 kg) in the last month

Laboratory and diagnostic tests results include:

- White blood cell count = 4,500 mm^3 (4.5 × 10^9/L)
- Hemoglobin = 11 g/dL (110 mmol/L)
- Hematocrit = 37% (0.37)
- Blood urea nitrogen = 25 mg/dL (9 mmol/L)
- Creatinine = 2.0 mg/dL (176 μmol/L)
- Sodium = 149 mg/dL (149 mmol/L)
- Potassium = 3.2 mg/dL (3.2 mmol/L)
- X-ray: A blockage in the large intestine is suspected; gas and liquid bowel contents above the area of the blockage appear to be present. Follow-up with CT scan is recommended.
- CT scan: A partial obstruction is seen in the large intestine. Gas and liquid bowel contents are seen both above and below the area of the blockage.
- ECG: normal sinus rhythm with occasional PVCs

Place an X to indicate the nursing actions listed below that are <u>Indicated</u> (appropriate or necessary), <u>Contraindicated</u> (could be harmful), or <u>Non-Essential</u> (makes no difference or not necessary) for the client's care at this time.

Nursing Action	Anticipated	Contraindicated	Non-Essential
Sips of clear liquids only			
Administration of a laxative			
Bowel rest			
IV potassium replacement			
Vital signs every 30 minutes			
Prepare for surgery			
Antibiotic administration			
Insertion of a nasogastric tube			
Increase the IV flow rate to 100 mL/hr			

10-E. A 69-year old male client with a history of colorectal cancer arrives at the ED and reports that he has abdominal pain of 5/10 on a 0 to 10 pain intensity scale.

Nursing assessment findings include:

- Vital signs: temperature = 99.2°F (37.3°C), apical heart rate = 90 beats/min and irregular with an occasional skipped beat, respirations = 24 breaths/min, blood pressure (BP) = 168/90 mm Hg, oxygen saturation = 93% (on RA), abdominal pain level = 5/10 on a 0 to 10 pain intensity scale
- Reports loss of appetite, vomiting, constipation with diarrhea containing blood streaks, abdominal distention and tenderness; mass in mid-abdomen palpated, bowel sounds are high-pitched tinkling sounds; last bowel movement was during the night; weight is 145 lb (65.8 kg); reports a loss of 10 lb (4.5 kg) in the last month

Laboratory and diagnostic tests results include:

- White blood cell count = 4,500 mm^3 (4.5 × 10^9/L)
- Hemoglobin = 11 g/dL (110 mmol/L)
- Hematocrit = 37% (0.37)

- Blood urea nitrogen = 25 mg/dL (9 mmol/L)
- Creatinine = 2.0 mg/dL (176 μmol/L)
- Sodium = 149 mg/dL (149 mmol/L)
- Potassium = 3.2 mg/dL (3.2 mmol/L)
- X-ray: A blockage in the large intestine is suspected; gas and liquid bowel contents above the area of the blockage appear to be present. Follow-up with CT scan is recommended.
- CT scan: A partial obstruction is seen in the large intestine. Gas and liquid bowel contents are seen both above and below the area of the blockage.
- ECG: normal sinus rhythm with occasional PVCs

Choose the _most likely_ options for the information missing from the statement below by selecting from the lists of options provided.

The nurse is prioritizing actions. The nurse would first _____ **1** _____, and then would _____ **2** _____ followed by _____ **3** _____ .

Options for 1	Options for 2	Options for 3
Increase the flow rate of the IV to 100 mL/hr and administer IV potassium	Increase the flow rate of the IV to 100 mL/hr and administer IV potassium	Increasing the flow rate of the IV to 100 mL/hr and administer IV potassium
Insert a nasogastric tube	Insert a nasogastric tube	Inserting a nasogastric tube
Prepare for surgery	Prepare for surgery	Preparing the client for surgery

10-F. A 69-year-old male client with a history of colorectal cancer arrives at the ED and reports that he has abdominal pain of 5/10 on a 0 to 10 pain intensity scale client due to a partial intestinal obstruction. Based on diagnostic test results, he was scheduled for a bowel resection. The tumor and a small portion of the intestine was removed and the remaining intestine was anastomosed. A colostomy was not required.

The client had an uneventful night and is progressing postoperatively as expected. An IV solution of lactated Ringers is infusing at 100 mL/hr and a client-controlled analgesic (PCA) pump is providing pain control. The surgeon visits the client this morning and plans to start a liquid diet with slow progression to soft foods. The surgeon informs the client that discharge will be in 2-3 days if the client progresses as expected. The nurse prepares a home care teaching plan for the client and begins to implement the teaching. **Use an X to indicate which client statement indicates that the home care instruction is either <u>Understood</u> or <u>Requires Further Teaching</u>.**

Client Statement	Understood	Requires Further Teaching
"I should eat small amounts of food every day rather than 3 large meals."		
"It is okay to take a mild laxative if I don't have a bowel movement in 4 days."		
"I need to contact my surgeon if I see any oozing of clear yellow drainage coming from my incision or if the incision edges seem to be separating."		
"The pain medication that I take may make it difficult to have a bowel movement."		
"I would like to plan some walks outside because the weather is so beautiful right now, but I know that I have to limit my activity."		
"I need to check my temperature every day. If it is ever 101°F (38.3°C) or higher, I need to call my surgeon."		

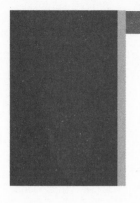

Answers and Rationales for Next Generation NCLEX® Examination Unfolding Case Studies

NGN Unfolding Case Study #1: Musculoskeletal Trauma (Concepts of Mobility and Perfusion)

1-A.

Answers:

Assessment Finding	Assessment Finding that Requires Immediate Follow-Up
Alert and oriented × 3	
Unable to move his right leg	X
Pulse = 90 beats/min	
Respirations = 24 breaths/min	
Blood pressure = 130/78 mm Hg	
10/10 right leg pain	X
Severe right leg bone and soft-tissue damage	X

Rationales: The client's major injury seems to be severe right leg damage from the motorcycle accident. He is unable to move his leg and is in severe excruciating pain. Changes in his vital signs are likely due to a sympathetic response to the trauma and the intense pain he is experiencing. Therefore, these values do not require follow-up by the nurse at this time.

Clinical Judgment Cognitive Skill: Recognize Cues

Reference: Ignatavicius, et al., 2021, Chapter 47

1-B.

Answers:

Potential Issues	Risk to Client
Constipation	X
Neurovascular compromise	X
Atelectasis	X
GI bleeding	
Pressure injury	X
Venous thromboembolism	X

Rationales: The client will have impaired mobility during his recovery and therefore is at risk for complications of immobility such as constipation, atelectasis, pressure injury, and venous thromboembolism. Due to his severe leg injury affecting both bone and soft tissue, he is at risk for swelling and neurovascular compromise. Although he could experience a stress ulcer, he will likely not have GI bleeding as a result.

Clinical Judgment Cognitive Skill: Analyze Cues

Reference: Ignatavicius, et al., 2021, Chapter 47

1-C.

Answers:

Based on the client's condition, the client's priority need will be to prevent **neurovascular compromise.** In addition, he will need interventions to

prevent potentially life-threatening complications of immobility, especially **atelectasis** and **venous thromboembolism**.

Rationales: Because the client is young and he can move except for his right leg, his priority need is to maintain arterial perfusion to his right leg and foot. Due to massive bone and soft-tissue trauma, he is at high risk for neurovascular compromise which could lead to compartment syndrome. Additionally, he will need interventions to prevent complications of immobility, especially those that could be life-threatening like pulmonary complications, venous thromboembolism (e.g., a pulmonary embolus), or fat embolism syndrome (FES).

Clinical Judgment Cognitive Skill: Prioritize Hypotheses

Reference: Ignatavicius, et al., 2021, Chapter 47

1-D.

Answers:

Nursing Action	Indicated	Contraindicated	Non-Essential
Perform a neurovascular assessment of the client's lower extremities.	X		
Place the client's right leg on 2 pillows to decrease swelling.		X	
If possible, loosen the leg splint but keep the leg immobilized.	X		
Administer additional morphine to alleviate pain.	X		
Collaborate with the physical therapist.			X
Prepare the client for possible fasciotomy.	X		
Contact the surgeon immediately.	X		

Rationales: The client is most likely experiencing compartment syndrome which may require a fasciotomy to relieve the pressure and restore adequate perfusion. The nurse would perform a complete neurovascular assessment of the lower extremities to compare peripheral circulation of each foot and leg before contacting the orthopedic surgeon. The client's injured leg would not be elevated because that position would slow arterial flow to the foot. Loosening the splint, if possible, would reduce lower leg

pressure and may help prevent the client from needing the fasciotomy.

Clinical Judgment Cognitive Skill: Generate Solutions

Reference: Ignatavicius, et al., 2021, Chapter 47

1-E.

Answers: A, B, C, E, F, G, H

Rationales: The client remains at risk for neurovascular compromise and complications of impaired mobility. Therefore, the nurse would plan care to prevent and assess for those health problems. The client would learn to ambulate with crutches, but a three-point gait would require partial weight bearing on the affected leg and he would not be allowed to bear any weight while the bones are healing, which is expected to take at least 6 weeks. The nurse would want to know if the client experiences burning or pressure sensations on his right heel due to the splint to prevent a major pressure injury.

Clinical Judgment Cognitive Skill: Take Action

Reference: Ignatavicius, et al., 2021, Chapters 33 and 47

1-F.

Answers:

Client Finding	Effective	Ineffective	Unrelated
Able to ambulate independently with crutches	X		
Needs oral opioid medication every 4 hours to control pain		X	
Feels very anxious and sometimes depressed		X	
Has no drainage or redness of leg wounds	X		
Reports having symptoms of seasonal allergies			X
Continuing regular exercises at home as prescribed by the physical therapist	X		

Rationales: The client's injury was 6 weeks ago and he should be weaning off of opioids such that he takes them only when needed instead of taking them every 4 hours. He is anxious and depressed, and needs treatment for these mental health disorders. Having allergy symptoms is not related to his injury.

The plan of care was effective for the client because his wounds are healed and he is ambulating independently with crutches.

Clinical Judgment Cognitive Skill: Evaluate Outcomes

Reference: Ignatavicius, et al., 2021, Chapter 47

NGN Unfolding Case Study #2: Venous Thromboembolism (Concepts of Clotting and Perfusion)

2-A.

Answers:

A 79-year-old female client was diagnosed as having a mesenteric artery thrombosis for which she had a colon resection to remove the ischemic bowel via a traditional laparotomy 2 days ago. The client's medical history includes hypertension, diabetes mellitus type 2, peripheral arterial disease, rheumatoid arthritis, and osteoarthritis. Prior to her hospitalization, the client lived independently in a senior apartment complex. The client is alert and oriented, and her incisional pain has been well managed. Vital signs for over 24 hours have been stable. Today the nurse is planning to begin discharge teaching for follow-up care at home with her daughter. When the nurse enters the room, the client tells the nurse that her left leg is "hurting a lot" and seems larger than her right leg. Upon inspection, the nurse notes that the client's left leg calf is swollen and reddened. The nurse instructs the client to remain in bed.

Rationales: The client was apparently recovering well from her surgery until she had a new onset of symptoms in her left leg that included pain, redness, and swelling. The nurse recognizes that a postoperative client is at risk for deep vein thrombosis, especially because her surgery was due to a mesenteric arterial clot.

Clinical Judgment Cognitive Skill: Recognize Cues

Reference: Ignatavicius, et al., 2021, Chapter 33

2-B.

Answers:

The nurse recognizes that based on the client's history and current assessment findings, she is currently at risk for complications from surgery and decreased mobility, especially **infection**, **pressure injury**, and **venous thromboembolism (VTE)**.

Rationales: The client is at risk for VTE and pressure injury due to her surgery, decreased mobility, and advanced age. Having had a major abdominal surgery, she is also at risk for infection.

Clinical Judgment Cognitive Skill: Analyze Cues

Reference: Ignatavicius, et al., 2021, Chapter 33

2-C.

Answers:

The nurse recognizes that based on the client's new onset of signs and symptoms, she *most likely* has a **deep vein thrombosis.** The **priority** for her care will be to prevent the life-threatening complication of this health problem, that is **pulmonary embolism.**

Rationales: The client has the classic signs and symptoms of peripheral deep vein thrombosis (DVT). The major concern for a client with a DVT is her risk that a piece of the clot dislodges and travels to the lungs causing the potentially life-threatening complication of pulmonary embolism.

Clinical Judgment Cognitive Skill: Prioritize Hypotheses

Reference: Ignatavicius, et al., 2021, Chapter 33

2-D.

Answers:

Provider Order	Anticipated	Contraindicated	Non-Essential
Initiate vascular access.	X		
Obtain a 12-lead ECG.			X
Lower the client's legs to below the heart.		X	
Begin administration of anticoagulant therapy.	X		
Draw blood for laboratory testing, including coagulation studies, CBC, and platelets.	X		
Administer supplemental oxygen.			X
Check urine and stool for occult blood.	X		

Rationales: The client diagnosed with a DVT is usually started on an anticoagulant, often as an infusion requiring vascular access. Before beginning a heparin infusion, laboratory tests are performed to have a baseline for coagulation studies, CBC, and platelets. Urine and stool occult blood testing may also be done. The client's legs should be elevated on several pillows to facilitate venous flow and decrease swelling. Supplemental oxygen and an ECG are not required unless there are other signs and symptoms indicating breathing or central circulation problems.

Clinical Judgment Cognitive Skill: Generate Solutions

Reference: Ignatavicius, et al., 2021, Chapter 33

2-E.

Answers: A, B, D, F, G

Rationales: All of these nursing actions are appropriate except that vitamin K is not the antidote for heparin. Protamine sulfate is the antidote for heparin; vitamin K is the antidote for warfarin. If the platelet count falls below 150,000/mL, the nurse would stop the heparin infusion and notify the primary health care provider.

Clinical Judgment Cognitive Skill: Take Action

Reference: Ignatavicius, et al., 2021, Chapter 33

2-F.

Answers:

Client Finding	Effective	Ineffective	Unrelated
Abdominal incision healed without infection	X		
Has had no bleeding or unusual bleeding while on the anticoagulant	X		
States that she knows to call 911 if she has any shortness of breath and/or chest pain	X		
Needs help with ADLs and is not ready to go back to her apartment from her daughter's house		X	
States she is having her annual cardiology appointment next week			X
Left leg calf is not red and only slightly swollen	X		

Rationales: All of the client findings show that the client is recovering well, but she still needs help with ADLs perhaps due to weakness or anxiety. The nurse would explore the client's concerns further. Having an annual cardiology evaluation is unrelated to her abdominal surgery and postoperative complication of venous thromboembolism.

Clinical Judgment Cognitive Skill: Evaluate Outcomes

Reference: Ignatavicius, et al., 2021, Chapter 33

NGN Unfolding Case Study #3: Chronic Obstructive Pulmonary Disease (Concepts of Gas Exchange and Infection)

3-A.

Answers:

Assessment Finding	Assessment Finding that Requires Immediate Follow-Up
Sleeps in a semi-sitting position	
Using oxygen at 2 L/min via NC	
Sitting in a forward bending position with the arms resting on his knees	
Has increased fatigue and shortness of breath	X
Expectorating rust-colored mucus	X
Has chills and fever	X

Rationales: Respiratory infection risk increases in COPD because of the increased mucus and poor gas exchange. Chills and fever, increased fatigue and shortness of breath, and expectoration of rust-colored mucus are manifestations of pneumonia and are concerns requiring immediate follow-up. It is common for COPD clients to sleep in a semi-sitting position because breathlessness is worse when lying down (orthopnea). It is also common for the client with COPD to require use of home oxygen, and to sit in a forward bending position with the arms held forward (this position helps reduce dyspnea because it allows maximum expansion of the chest).

Clinical Judgment Cognitive Skill: Recognize Cues

Reference: Ignatavicius, et al., 2021, Chapter 27

3-B.

Answers:

Assessment Finding	COPD	Pneumonia
Temperature = 102.8°F (39.3°C)		X
Barrel chest	X	
Thin, pale, loss of muscle mass in extremities	X	
Coarse crackles on inspiration and expiration in middle right lobe		X
Finger clubbing	X	
Pain level = 7/10 on right side when coughing		X

Rationales: The client with COPD may have a "barrel chest;" this is caused by air trapping. The client with progressive COPD is thin, with loss of muscle mass in the extremities. Finger clubbing is characteristic and indicates chronically decreased arterial oxygen levels. Manifestations of pneumonia, a common complication of COPD, include chills and fever, increased fatigue and shortness of breath, and expectoration of rust-colored mucus. Coarse crackles or low-pitched crackles are characteristic of pneumonia. Infection and infiltrates that occur in pneumonia can cause pain when breathing or coughing.

Clinical Judgment Cognitive Skill: Analyze Cues

Reference: Ignatavicius, et al., 2021, Chapter 24 & 27

3-C.

Answers:

The nurse recognizes that the client's *priority* need for care is to **collect sputum and blood cultures** followed by **obtaining a chest x-ray**.

Rationales: The client is suspected of having an infection so this is the priority. Sputum and blood cultures will provide information about the specific organism, if present, that is causing the infection. It is a priority to obtain these specimens before administering the antibiotic because the antibiotic can affect culture growth, resulting in inaccurate results. Since infection and potential pneumonia are the concerns, the next action is to obtain the chest x-ray to assist in confirming the client's diagnosis. There are no data that indicate that the client is experiencing cardiac complications, so it is not a priority to do an ECG. Although a respiratory consult is necessary, it is not the next action considering the data provided.

Clinical Judgment Cognitive Skill: Prioritize Hypotheses

Reference: Ignatavicius, et al., 2021, Chapter 24 & 27

3-D.

Answers:

Nursing Action	Indicated	Contraindicated	Non-Essential
Increase the flow of the IV rate to 125 mL/hr.		X	
Check the pulse oximetry reading.	X		
Increase the flow of oxygen to 6 L/min.		X	
Check the client's temperature.			X
Check the client's heart rate.	X		
Monitor the client's respiratory rate.	X		
Check elevation of the head of the bed.	X		
Auscultate lung sounds.	X		
Contact respiratory therapy immediately.	X		

Rationales: The nurse would check for head elevation to assist with breathing and then would quickly assess the client's respiratory status. The respiratory rate is noted as 32 breaths/min and should be monitored. The heart rate, pulse oximetry, and lung sounds need to be checked to assist in determining client status and potential problem. Checking the client's temperature is nonessential at this time; it is not going to provide significant data about the client's current status. Respiratory therapy would be contacted because a respiratory treatment may be necessary for bronchodilation. Considering the client's history of heart failure, increasing the IV flow rate to 125 ml/hr is contraindicated because of the risk of fluid overload and exacerbation of the heart failure. The need for oxygen therapy and its effectiveness can be determined by ABG values and oxygen saturation. The client with COPD may need an oxygen flow of 2 to 4 L/min via nasal cannula or up to 40% via Venturi mask. The nurse would not increase the oxygen flow rate in a client with COPD without a specific prescription to do so.

Clinical Judgment Cognitive Skill: Generate Solutions

Reference: Ignatavicius, et al., 2021, Chapter 24 & 27

3-E.

Answers: B, C, D, F

Rationales: Humidifiers may be useful to help keep secretions thin in the client who lives in a dry climate or uses dry heat during the winter. A dehumidifier would dry the environmental air and could also dry secretions; this could be harmful because it would cause thickening of secretions. Antibiotics need to be taken for the full course of the prescribed therapy to prevent recurrence of the infection. Diaphragmatic or abdominal and pursed-lip breathing may be helpful for managing dyspneic episodes. Coughing effectively can improve gas exchange by helping increase airflow in the larger airways and removing excess mucus. Maintaining hydration may thin the thick, tenacious (sticky) secretions, making them easier to remove by coughing. Unless hydration needs to be avoided for other health problems, the client with COPD should be taught to drink at least 2 L/day of fluid. Since the client has a history of mild heart failure, 3.5 L of fluid per day may be an excessive amount and the nurse should consult with the primary health care provider. The nurse needs to teach the client the safety measures for oxygen use such as ensuring that there are no open flames in rooms in which oxygen is in use. The client should know how to operate the oxygen equipment but must be taught that the oxygen flow should not be increased unless specifically prescribed. If the client feels as though he or she needs more oxygen or is having a difficult time breathing, the PHCP should be contacted immediately.

Clinical Judgment Cognitive Skill: Take Action

Reference: Ignatavicius, et al., 2021, Chapter 27

3-F.

Answers:

Client Behavior or Statement	Understood	Requires Further Teaching
Pursed-lip breathing Purses the lips and breathes in slowly through the mouth and out slowly through the nose.		X
Antibiotic administration States "I will take antibiotics until they are gone."	X	
Coughing technique Sits on the side of the bed with feet placed firmly on the floor. Turns the shoulders inward and bends the head slightly downward, hugging a pillow against the stomach. Takes a few breaths, attempting to exhale more fully. After the third to fifth breath, a deeper breath is taken and he bends forward slowly while coughing 2-3 times.	X	
Exercise States "If I get short of breath when walking, I will stop and wait until the next day to try again."		X
Oxygen use States "I know it's safe to use burning candles when I am using my oxygen as long as the candles are 4 feet away from the oxygen tank."		X
Diaphragmatic breathing Performs diaphragmatic breathing by sitting in a chair, placing hands on the abdomen, breathing from the abdomen while keeping the chest still.	X	

Rationales: The client states the correct procedure for antibiotic administration. The client is performing correct coughing technique and diaphragmatic breathing technique. The client is performing pursed-lip breathing incorrectly. The client needs to close the mouth and breathe in through the nose, purse the lips as if to whistle, and breathe out slowly through the mouth. The simplest exercise plan is having the client walk (indoors or outdoors) daily at a self-paced rate until symptoms limit further walking; this is followed by a rest period, and then walking is continued until 20 minutes of actual walking has been accomplished. Therefore, the client's statement that he will stop the exercise if shortness of breath occurs and wait until the next day to try again is incorrect. The client's statement about oxygen therapy is incorrect. The oxygen container needs to be away from open flames such as candles, fireplaces, gas stoves, or water heaters. "No smoking" signs should be posted in the window of the client's home as well.

Clinical Judgment Cognitive Skill: Evaluate Outcomes

Reference: Ignatavicius, et al., 2021, Chapter 27

NGN Unfolding Case Study #4: Spinal Cord Injury (Concepts of Mobility and Perfusion)

4-A.

Answers:

Assessment Finding	Assessment Finding that Requires Follow-Up
Client was able to describe how his injury occurred when asked.	
Client states "I'm single and only 45 years old and don't have any kids yet."	X
Breath sounds reveal fine crackles in the right lower lobe.	X
Bowel sounds heard in all 4 quadrants	
No documentation of a BM since surgery 4 days ago	X
Indwelling urinary catheter draining clear, yellow urine	
Vital signs: T = 98.8°F (37.1°C), P = 82 beats/min, R = 20 breaths/min, oxygen saturation = 93%, BP = 122/82 mm Hg	

Rationales: Clients with SCI are at a high risk for complications that result from prolonged impaired mobility, including pressure injuries, venous thromboembolism (VTE), and pneumonia. Other complications include autonomic dysreflexia, cognition problems, and psychosocial concerns. They may have significant behavior and emotional reactions as a result of changes in functional ability, body image, role performance, and self-concept.

Clinical Judgment Cognitive Skill: Recognize Cues

Reference: Ignatavicius, et al., 2021, Chapter 40

4-B.

Answers:

Assessment Finding	Pneumonia	Autonomic Dysreflexia
Facial flushing		X
T = 99.0°F (37.2°C)	X	
P = 58 beats/min		X
Oxygen saturation = 90% (on RA)	X	
Headache		X
BP = 210/120 mm Hg		X
Fine crackles in the right lower lobe	X	

Rationales: Autonomic dysreflexia (AD) is a potentially life-threatening condition in which noxious visceral or cutaneous stimuli cause a sudden, massive, uninhibited reflex sympathetic discharge in people with high-level SCI. The manifestations are a sudden, significant rise in blood pressure accompanied by bradycardia, severe throbbing headache, nasal congestion, blurred vision, profuse sweating above the level of the lesion, goose bumps above or possibly below the level of the lesion, flushing of the skin above the level of the lesion—especially in the face, neck, and shoulders, and a feeling of apprehension. Pneumonia occurs as a result of immobility and airway compromise from ineffective breathing patterns. Some indications include elevated temperature, adventitious breath sounds, and signs of compromise such as lowered pulse oximetry reading.

Clinical Judgment Cognitive Skill: Analyze Cues

Reference: Ignatavicius, et al., 2021, Chapter 27 & 40

4-D.

Answers:

Nursing Action	Indicated	Contraindicated	Non-Essential
Raise the head of the bed.	X		
Clamp the urinary catheter.		X	
Monitor the client's temperature.			X
Check for a fecal impaction and disimpact if needed.	X		
Administer nifidepine.	X		
Monitor breath sounds.			X
Monitor deep tendon reflexes.			X

Rationales: The nurse needs to analyze all assessment data to determine that the client is experiencing AD. Next, the nurse needs to have knowledge of how this emergency is treated. The nurse would place the client in a sitting position to help lower the BP. The cause needs to be quickly determined and managed. Causes include catheter blockage so clamping the urinary catheter is contraindicated. Constipation is a cause of AD, so it is essential that the nurse check for fecal impaction and disimpact if needed. Monitoring the temperature and breath sounds is non-essential at this time and is unrelated to treatment for AD. The BP would be monitored every 10 to 15 minutes. Nifedipine or nitrate may be prescribed to lower blood pressure as needed.

Clinical Judgment Cognitive Skill: Generate Solutions

Reference: Ignatavicius, et al., 2021, Chapter 40

4-C.

Answers: A, B, E, G, H

Rationales: AD is a potentially life-threatening condition that needs to be treated immediately to prevent a stroke. Some manifestations are sudden, significant rise in systolic and diastolic blood pressure accompanied by bradycardia, severe throbbing headache, nasal congestion, and flushing of the skin above the level of the lesion. Some specific risk factors are bladder distention and bowel distention or impaction from constipation. Although the temperature reading, pulse oximetry reading, and breath sounds need to be addressed, these are not the immediate critical concerns. Absent deep tendon reflexes, mobility, and sensory perception are expected manifestations in SCI.

Clinical Judgment Cognitive Skill: Prioritize Hypotheses

Reference: Ignatavicius, et al., 2021, Chapter 27 & 40

4-E.

Answers:

The **first** action that the nurse would take is **raise the head of the bed** to **reduce the blood pressure.**

Rationales: If the patient experiences AD, the head of the bed is raised immediately to help reduce the blood pressure; this is the first action. The Rapid Response Team or primary health care provider is notified for drug therapy to quickly reduce blood pressure. The nurse needs to quickly determine the cause of AD and manage it promptly to resolve the condition.

Clinical Judgment Cognitive Skill: Take Action

Reference: Ignatavicius, et al., 2021, Chapter 40

4-F.

Answers: A, B, C, E, H, I

Rationales: The signs and symptoms of AD are sudden, significant rise in systolic and diastolic blood pressure accompanied by bradycardia, severe throbbing headache, nasal congestion, blurred vision, profuse sweating above the level of lesion, goose bumps above or possibly below the level of the lesion, and flushing of the skin above the level of the lesion. Therefore, resolution of these manifestations determine effectiveness of interventions.

Clinical Judgment Cognitive Skill: Evaluate Outcomes

Reference: Ignatavicius, et al., 2021, Chapter 40

NGN Unfolding Case Study #5: Chronic Kidney Disease (Concepts of Elimination and Infection)

5-A.

Answers:

Assessment Finding	Assessment Finding that Requires Follow-Up
Weight = 158 lb (71.7 kg)	
Urinary output approximately 20 mL/day	
Dry dressing covering the catheter exit site	
Temperature = 101.6°F (38.6°C)	X
Finger stick blood glucose (FSBG) = 345 mg/dL (19.2 mmol/L)	X
White blood cell count = 17,500 mm^3 (17.5 × 10^9/L)	X
Last bowel movement yesterday	
Abdominal discomfort and bloating	X
Pulse = 72 beats/min	
Blood pressure (BP) =160/92 mm Hg	
White flecks in PD effluent	X

Rationales: Peritonitis is inflammation of the peritoneum that is usually due to a bacterial or fungal infection. It is a complication of peritoneal dialysis and can be life threatening if not treated promptly. Signs and symptoms include fever, chills, abdominal pain and tenderness, abdominal distension, loss of appetite, thirst, nausea and vomiting, fatigue, cloudy dialysis output, white flecks or strands or clumps in the dialysis output, or an unusual odor to the output.

These findings require immediate follow-up. A finger stick blood glucose (point of care) reading of 345 mg/dL (19.2 mmol/L) is an elevated level requiring intervention; this indicates uncontrolled diabetes in addition to the presence of infection. A white blood cell (WBC) count of 17,500/mm^3 (17.5 × 10^9/L) is elevated indicating infection. Normal WBC count is 5000-10,000/mm^3 (5-10 × 10^9/L). Weight of 158 lb is unchanged from the previous measurement and is not a concern. A urine output of 20 mL/day is an expected finding in chronic kidney disease. A dry dressing covering the catheter site indicates no signs of a concern, such as leakage around the catheter. Having a bowel movement a day ago is a positive finding as peritonitis can cause difficulty with passing stool or flatus. A pulse of 72 beats/min is within the normal range. A BP of 160/92 mm Hg is above the normal range, but it is not a cause for immediate follow-up because an elevated BP is an expected finding in chronic kidney disease.

<u>Clinical Judgment Cognitive Skill:</u> Recognize Cues

<u>Reference:</u> Ignatavicius et al., 2021, Chapter 63

5-B.

Answers:

Assessment Finding	Peritonitis	Chronic Kidney Disease	DM Type 1
Abdominal discomfort and bloating	X		
FSBG = 345 mg/dL(19.2 mmol/L)			X
Drinks 32 oz (1 L) of fluids daily		X	
Fatigue	X	X	
Temperature = 101.6°F (38.6°C)	X		
Chills	X		
BP = 160/92 mm Hg		X	
White flecks in peritoneal output	X		
White blood cell count = 17,500 mm³ (17.5 × 10⁹/L)	X		
Glomerular filtration rate = 20 mL/min		X	
Blood urea nitrogen = 42 mg/dL (15.12 mmol/L)		X	
Creatinine = 3.9 mg/dL (343 μmol/L)		X	
Abdominal pain = 5/10 on a 0-10 scale	X		

<u>Rationales:</u> Signs and symptoms of peritonitis include fever, chills, abdominal pain and tenderness, abdominal distension, loss of appetite, thirst, nausea and vomiting, fatigue, cloudy dialysis output, white flecks or strands or clumps in the dialysis output, or an unusual odor to the output. An elevated glucose reading occurs in infection. Thirst and an elevated glucose reading are also findings noted in uncontrolled diabetes in hyperglycemia. An elevated WBC count of 17,500/mm³ (17.5 × 10⁹/L) indicates infection. In chronic kidney disease, the kidneys have lost their ability to eliminate excess fluid and wastes from the body so wastes and fluids build up. Water and electrolyte imbalance occur, which leads to thirst and the need for fluid restriction. Some other manifestations of chronic kidney disease include malaise, fatigue, elevated blood pressure, and loss of appetite. The blood urea nitrogen and creatinine levels elevate as the kidneys lose their filtering ability. As chronic kidney disease progresses, the glomerular filtration rate decreases.

<u>Clinical Judgment Cognitive Skill:</u> Analyze Cues

<u>Reference:</u> Ignatavicius et al., 2021, Chapter 59 & 63.

5-C.

<u>Answers:</u> A, C, F, G

<u>Rationales:</u> Primary immediate concerns need to focus on the manifestations that indicate life-threatening conditions or are abnormal manifestations requiring intervention. Pain is an immediate concern and needs to be addressed to provide comfort.

Hyperthermia is a sign of infection, therefore both hyperthermia and infection are a concern; infection can be life threatening for this patient. For the patient with type 1 diabetes mellitus, hyperglycemia is also an immediate concern and intervention is necessary. If the blood glucose continues to rise, diabetic ketoacidosis can occur. Fatigue is a manifestation of chronic kidney disease and although nursing interventions need to focus on reducing the fatigue, it is not an immediate concern. The respiratory rate

is slightly above normal range; this could be due to pain and will likely return to normal once the pain is controlled. Although the blood pressure is elevated above normal, this is expected in chronic kidney disease. In addition, pain could be a factor in its elevation.

Clinical Judgment Cognitive Skill: Prioritize Hypotheses

Reference: Ignatavicius et al., 2021, Chapter 63

5-D.

Answers:

Provider Order	Anticipated	Contraindicated	Non-Essential
Obtain a specimen of dialysis effluent.	X		
Remove the peritoneal catheter immediately.		X	
Obtain a blood culture.	X		
Administer the prescribed insulin infusion.			X
Administer the prescribed IV antibiotic.	X		
Continue with nightly peritoneal dialysis.	X		
Administer ibuprofen for pain as needed.		X	
Flush the dialysis catheter per agency protocol.		X	

Rationales: When peritonitis is suspected, it needs to be confirmed. A specimen of the dialysate outflow needs to be obtained for culture and sensitivity study, Gram stain, and cell count to identify the infecting organism. Antibiotics are needed to treat peritonitis; thus, these laboratory studies are necessary to determine the most effective antibiotic treatment. Because the patient has chronic kidney disease, continuation of the peritoneal dialysis is necessary to rid the body of wastes and excess fluid. Blood cultures are necessary to ensure the absence of bacteria in the blood and to rule out septicemia. Intravenous insulin administration is unnecessary and is used when the patient is experiencing a dangerously high blood glucose, such as in diabetic ketoacidosis. Immediate catheter removal is contraindicated; the catheter is needed for dialysis and the condition is initially treated with antibiotic therapy. Nonsteroidal anti-inflammatory drugs (NSAIDs) such as ibuprofen can cause progressive kidney damage. These drugs block prostaglandins, which result in decreased blood flow to

the kidneys. Dialysis catheter flushes are not a part of care for peritoneal dialysis and are contraindicated. In addition, flushing infected fluid into the body will worsen infection.

Clinical Judgment Cognitive Skill: Generate Solutions

Reference: Ignatavicius et al., 2021, Chapter 63

5-E.

Answers:

The **priority** action that the nurse would take is to **obtain blood cultures and a dialysis effluent specimen** to **determine the organism causing infection,** followed by **administering antibiotics** to **resolve infection.**

Rationales: Blood cultures and culture and sensitivity study, Gram stain, and cell count studies need to be completed before any antibiotic therapy is initiated. These tests will determine the organism causing infection and this is critical to know so that effective treatment is administered. Administering an antibiotic prior to obtaining and testing specimens can alter the results of the tests. Following specimen collection, antibiotics are started. Intravenous insulin administration is unnecessary and is used when the client is experiencing a dangerously high blood glucose, such as in diabetic ketoacidosis. Catheter removal is contraindicated and is needed for the dialysis treatment; the condition is initially treated with antibiotic therapy.

Clinical Judgment Cognitive Skill: Take Action

Reference: Ignatavicius et al., 2021, Chapter 63

5-F.

Answers:

Client Statement	Understood	Requires Further Teaching
"I need to alter my diet and eat foods high in fiber."	X	
"It's important not to limit my fluid intake to prevent those white specks and threads that were in my dialysis output."		X
"I should anchor my catheter to my skin with tape."	X	
"I should check my temperature at least once a day."	X	
"It is okay to skip one treatment a week if I have a social commitment that I want to participate."		X
"I need to be sure to eat some more protein foods like meat, milk, chicken, fish, and eggs, and decrease my intake of foods like beans, liver, nuts, and chocolate."	X	
"I need to watch my blood glucose closely because of my diabetes but the dialysis procedure should not affect my glucose at all."		X

Rationale: To avoid constipation, the nephrologist may prescribe a diet that is high in fiber, as well as a stool softener or laxative. These interventions will prevent constipation, which can cause abdominal discomfort and straining. People who use peritoneal dialysis lose protein with every exchange so they need an increased amount of protein in the diet. Protein is found in meat, milk, chicken, fish, and eggs; lower-quality protein is found in some vegetables and grains. Other changes in diet may include reducing the amount of phosphorus foods. Phosphorus is found in dairy products, cheese, dried beans, liver, nuts, and chocolate. A fluid restriction will be prescribed. Fluid intake and dialysis output needs to be monitored. When dialysis outflow is less than dialysis inflow, the difference is retained by the client during dialysis and is counted as fluid intake. The client is also instructed to weigh herself daily to monitor fluid status. The dialysate contains a high concentration of dextrose and will affect the blood glucose level because the body absorbs the glucose. The client needs to continue with the dialysis treatment as done before hospitalization and not skip treatments unless the nephrologist prescribes an alternate treatment. The client is taught to check her temperature daily to monitor for signs of infection.

Clinical Judgment Cognitive Skill: Evaluate Outcomes

Reference: Ignatavicius et al., 2021, Chapter 63

NGN Unfolding Case Study #6: Traumatic Brain Injury (Concepts of Cognition and Perfusion)

6-A.

Answers:

The nurse performs a neurological check on the client about an hour after lunch. Vital signs: temperature = 98.8°F (37.1°C), apical heart rate = 60 beats/min and regular, respirations = 16 breaths/min, blood pressure (BP) = 142/68 mm Hg. Oxygen saturation is 92% (on RA). The client reports a headache of 5/10 on a 0 to 10 pain intensity rating scale and has a new onset of nausea. Glasgow Coma Scale score = 12. The client seems sleepy and confused as to where he is, but he responds to localized painful stimuli and opens his eyes in response to sound. Slight pupil dilation is noted in the right eye.

Rationales: The client with a head injury should always be monitored for signs of increased intracranial pressure (ICP). Signs include elevated temperature, slowing of the pulse rate, rise in blood pressure with a widening pulse pressure, headache, nausea and vomiting, pupil changes, and signs of neurological deterioration. The client's temperature increased by only 0.1 degrees and this is insignificant. The apical heart rate has dropped from 78 to 60 beats/min and this is significant. Cardiac status reveals normal sinus rhythm and this is not significant. The client's headache has worsened, and neurological status is deteriorating as noted by the drop in the Glasgow Coma Scale score. Unilateral pupil dilation can be a sign of cranial nerve III compression.

Clinical Judgment Cognitive Skill: Recognize Cues

Reference: Ignatavicius et al., 2021, Ch. 40.

6-B.

Answers:

The nurse recognizes that the client's decline in neurological status is likely the result of **increasing intracranial pressure** caused by **intracranial bleeding.**

Rationale: The client sustained a closed head injury. Whenever an injury occurs, edema results. The brain is a closed space and does not have room for a build-up of fluid or blood from edema. When this occurs, pressure is placed on the structures in the brain resulting in increased ICP and neurological alterations. The client is not vomiting or exhibiting signs of dehydration. Likewise, no data indicate sensory deprivation.

Clinical Judgment Cognitive Skill: Analyze Cues

Reference: Ignatavicius et al., 2021, Chapter 40

6-C.

Answers: A, D, E, F

Rationales: The primary concern when caring for a client with a head injury is increased intracranial pressure (ICP). Since the client's headache has worsened from 3/10 to 5/10, this is a concern. Unilateral pupil dilation can be a sign of cranial nerve III compression from increased ICP and is a concern. The blood pressure reading has changed from 126/78 to 142/68 mm Hg showing an increase and widened pulse pressure, an indication of increased ICP. Although hyperthermia and abnormal respirations are a sign of increased ICP, the client is not exhibiting these manifestations. A decrease in the Glasgow Coma Scale score and neurological changes are also an indication of increased ICP.

Clinical Judgment Cognitive Skill: Prioritize Hypotheses

Reference: Ignatavicius et al., 2021, Chapter 40

6-D.

Answers:

Provider Order	Anticipated	Non-Essential	Contraindicated
Discontinue IV infusion.			X
Administer osmotic diuretic.	X		
Place the client on a hypothermia blanket.			X
Check skin integrity.		X	
Assess bowel sounds.		X	
Elevate the head of the bed to 30 degrees.	X		
Prepare for evacuation of the hematoma.	X		

Rationales: If the client is exhibiting signs of increased ICP, the head of the bed should be elevated to assist in the drainage of fluid from the cranium. Osmotic diuretics, such as mannitol or hypertonic saline, may be used to diminish intracranial pressure. These agents reverse the pressure gradient across the blood-brain barrier, reducing intracranial pressure. Surgical evacuation of the hematoma is usually required in this condition. Checking skin integrity and bowel sounds may be a part of the assessment but they are nonessential actions at this time and are unrelated to the client's condition. IV fluids are not discontinued and are needed to maintain euvolemia and to provide adequate cerebral perfusion pressure. There is no data to indicate that the client needs a hypothermia blanket and its use could be harmful.

Clinical Judgment Cognitive Skill: Generate Solutions

Reference: Ignatavicius et al., 2021, Chapter 40

6-E.

Answers:

The **first** action that the nurse would take is to **ensure the head of the bed is at 30 degrees** to **reduce intracranial pressure** followed by **administering an osmotic diuretic** to **reduce intracranial pressure**.

Rationales: Elevating the head of the bed would be the first action because elevation will immediately assist in the drainage of fluid from the cranium. In addition, it will only take a moment to perform this action. The nurse would next administer the osmotic diuretic keeping in mind that the goal is to decrease the intracranial pressure. Once these are instituted, the nurse would prepare the client for surgery.

Clinical Judgment Cognitive Skill: Take Action

References: Ignatavicius et al., 2021, Chapter 40

6-F.

Answers:

Two hours later, the nurse re-assesses the client and finds that his airway remains patent. A quarter-sized amount of clear wetness is noted on the head dressing. Oxygen saturation is 94% (on 2 L oxygen via nasal cannula). The client is awake and states his name, but is unsure where he is, what happened to him, and what day it is. Glasgow Coma Scale score = 10. Vital signs: temperature = 99.2°F (37.3°C), apical heart rate = 70 beats/min and regular, respirations = 18 breaths/min, BP = 155/60 mm Hg. The client reports his headache is now 8/10 on a 0 to 10 pain intensity scale. He opens his eyes in response to pain. Pupils equal and react to light slowly.

Rationales: Clear drainage on the head dressing is a possible sign of a cerebrospinal fluid (CSF) leakage and the drainage should be tested for CSF. This is a complication of cranial surgery and would be immediately reported to the neurosurgeon. Altered neurological status is also an indication of a complication. The client should be oriented to time and place. The Glasgow Coma Scale score has worsened decreasing to a 10, and the client's headache has also worsened. The blood pressure is elevated and shows a widened pulse pressure. Oxygen saturation, apical heart rate, and respirations are normal. The client's temperature is only slightly elevated and this is expected following a surgical procedure.

Clinical Judgment Cognitive Skill: Evaluate Outcomes

Reference: Ignatavicius et al., 2021, Chapter 40

NGN Unfolding Case Study #7: ST Elevation Myocardial Infarction (STEMI) (Concept of Perfusion)

7-A.

Answers:

Assessment Finding	Assessment Finding that Requires Immediate Follow-Up
Pain level = 8/10	X
Temperature = 99.2 °F (37.3 °C)	
Apical heart rate = 98 beats/min and irregular	X
Respirations = 20 beats/min	
Blood pressure (BP) = 154/84 mm Hg	
Oxygen saturation = 93% (on 3 L/min)	X
ST elevations on initial ECG	X

Rationales: In an ST elevation myocardial infarction (STEMI), a coronary artery is completely blocked and a large part of the heart muscle is unable to receive blood. The ischemia can lead to necrosis if blood flow is not restored. Manifestations include crushing substernal chest pain. The client's pain level of 8/10 requires immediate follow-up because although the client received nitroglycerin by EMS and received morphine sulfate IV in the ED, the pain intensity has decreased by only 2 points (10/10 to 8/10). Cardiac dysrhythmias is a primary complication following STEMI and an apical heart rate that has changed from a regular rhythm to an irregular one is a concern. A pulse oximetry of 89%, although unchanged, indicates hypoxia. ST elevations on ECG is a concern because is indicates coronary artery blockage in an MI. The temperature reading is elevated from normal but is unchanged. The blood pressure is elevated from normal but has decreased from the previous reading. In addition, pain can affect the blood pressure causing it to increase.

Clinical Judgment Cognitive Skill: Recognize Cues

Reference: Ignatavicius et al., 2021, Chapter 40

7-B.

Answers: C, D, E, G, H

Rationales: Following MI, the nurse needs to monitor the client very closely because of the many complications that can follow. These include dysrhythmias, heart failure, pulmonary edema, cardiogenic shock, thrombophlebitis, pericarditis, mitral valve insufficiency, postinfarction angina, and ventricular rupture. Sepsis, pneumonia, and hypovolemic shock are not likely to occur following MI unless another coexisting health problem that causes these conditions is present.

Clinical Judgment Cognitive Skill: Analyze Cues

Reference: Ignatavicius et al., 2021, Chapter 40

7-C.

Answers:

Based on the nurse's assessment findings, the nurse determines that the client's temperature reading **is an expected finding** and the client's BP reading **is decreased due to medication.** The ST elevation noted on the initial ECG **most likely indicates acute myocardial infarction.**

Rationales: Following an MI, an elevation in temperature may be noted and is a response to the cardiac injury, deprivation of oxygen, and ischemia. An elevation in the white blood cell count may also be noted on the second day following MI. Although a blood pressure reading of 154/84 mm Hg is higher than a normal reading, it has decreased from the initial reading of 178/98 mm Hg. The decrease is likely due to the administration of nitroglycerin and IV morphine sulfate. The ST elevation on the ECG along with the client presentation indicates acute myocardial infarction.

Clinical Judgment Cognitive Skill: Prioritize Hypotheses

Reference: Ignatavicius et al., 2021, Chapter 40

7-D.

Answers:

Nursing Action	Indicated	Contraindicated	Non-Essential
Begin cardiopulmonary resuscitation (CPR).		X	
Check vital signs.	X		
Be sure the client is in a semi-Fowler position.	X		
Obtain a 12-lead ECG.	X		
Stop the reperfusion therapy.		X	
Obtain a chest x-ray.			X
Prepare to administer IV diltiazem.	X		
Prepare to administer IV amiodarone.	X		
Prepare to administer IV digoxin.	X		

Rationales: The cardiac rhythm shows that the client is experiencing atrial fibrillation. In atrial fibrillation, multiple rapid impulses from many foci depolarize in the atria in a totally disorganized manner at a rate of 350 to 600 times per minute. The atria quiver and thrombi formation is a concern. The client is placed in a semi-Fowler position to ease the work of breathing and to assist in providing oxygenation to all body tissues. Vital signs are checked and the pulse oximetry is monitored to ensure adequate perfusion. An ECG is obtained to check the rhythm. Medications are administered with the goal of converting the rhythm back to normal. These medications may include digoxin (cardiac glycoside), diltiazem (calcium channel blocker), and amiodarone (class III antidysrhythmic). Reperfusion therapy is not stopped because the client is at risk for thrombi formation. There is no reason to perform CPR. A chest x-ray may be helpful in assessing heart size but is a nonessential intervention at this time.

Clinical Judgment Cognitive Skill: Generate Solutions

Reference: Ignatavicius et al., 2021, Chapters 31 & 40

7-E.

Answers:

The *immediate* action that the nurse would take is to **place the client in a semi-Fowler position** to **provide oxygen and circulation to all body tissues** followed by **checking vital signs** to **determine a baseline status and specific plan for treatment**.

Rationales: The client would immediately be placed in a semi-Fowler position, if not already in that position, to ease the work of breathing and to assist in providing oxygenation to all body tissues. The nurse would then check vital signs to determine a baseline status and specific plan for treatment. In addition, the nurse would not administer cardiac medications without knowledge of the client's pulse rate and blood pressure. If these measurements are too low, the medications may be contraindicated.

Clinical Judgment Cognitive Skill: Take Action

Reference: Ignatavicius et al., 2021, Chapters 31 & 40

7-F.

Answers:

Client Finding	Effective	Ineffective	Unrelated
Temperature = 99.2°F (37.3°C)			X
Apical heart rate = 80 beats/min and regular	X		
Respirations = 20 breaths/min			X
Oxygen saturation = 90% (on 3 L/min oxygen)		X	
Blood pressure (BP) = 130/72 mm Hg	X		
Cardiac rhythm = Normal sinus rhythm	X		
Dyspnea		X	
Chest pain 5/10 on 0 to 10 pain intensity scale		X	

Rationales: The goal of treatment for atrial fibrillation is to convert the abnormal rhythm to a normal one. Conversion of atrial fibrillation to a normal sinus rhythm, as shown on the cardiac rhythm strip, indicates effectiveness. An apical heart rate that is 80 beats/min and is regular indicates that treatment was effective. The blood pressure, although it is not in the normal range, is lower than the previous measurement, which shows improvement. A pulse oximetry of 89% indicates hypoxia, and dyspnea indicates respiratory distress and require xfollow-up. The temperature is unchanged yet unrelated to the treatment. Respirations are normal and are also an unrelated finding.

Clinical Judgment Cognitive Skill: Evaluate Outcomes

Reference: Ignatavicius et al., 2021, Chapters 31 & 40

NGN Unfolding Case Study #8: Diabetes Mellitus Type 2 (Concepts of Metabolism and Fluid and Electrolyte Balance)

8-A.

Answers:

Vital signs: temperature = 101°F (38.3°C), apical heart rate = 96 beats/min and regular, respirations = 20 breaths/min, oxygen saturation = 92% on room air (RA), blood pressure = 104/68 mm Hg. Skin dry with decreased turgor. Finger stick blood glucose (FSBG) = 450 mg/dL (25 mmol/L). Client reports thirst and tolerating oral fluids without nausea. Weight = 112 lb (50.8 kg) which is a weight loss of 8 lb (3.6 kg) since 2 weeks ago. Fine crackles noted bilaterally in the lungs. Denies shortness of breath. No cyanosis; capillary refill 3 seconds. Pedal pulses 2+ bilaterally; 2+ edema bilaterally in feet and ankles; neck vein distention noted. Abdomen soft, bowel sounds present × 4, states last bowel movement yesterday (soft, brown, moderate amount). Has low abdominal discomfort on palpation; 3/10 on a 0 to 10 pain intensity scale. States she is urinating every 3 to 4 hours with no burning. Moves all extremities but is weak and needs assistance with standing and ambulating. Is alert and oriented. States no numbness or tingling in extremities; PERRLA.

Rationales: Fever is indicative of the presence of a urinary tract infection and warrants immediate follow-up to prevent urosepsis. An apical heart rate of 96 beats/min is not expected in a client with heart failure who is taking cardiac medications. This is an abnormal finding and can be an indication of a complication of the heart failure because an increased heart rate places a burden on the workload of the heart. The remaining vital signs are normal. Skin status and thirst are expected manifestations of HHS and once treatment for HHS is initiated these should resolve. Weight loss is also a manifestation of HHS and needs to be addressed but does not require immediate follow-up. Point-of-care glucose level is extremely elevated. Although it is a manifestation of HHS, it requires immediate follow-up with treatment to stabilize the client. Fine crackles noted bilaterally in the lungs, edema in the feet and ankles, and neck vein distension could be indications of worsening heart failure and require immediate follow-up. The client is weak and needs assistance with standing and ambulation. This is an indication that the client is at risk for injury and safety precautions need to be implemented immediately. It is always a concern if a client has pain and this requires immediate follow-up. The remaining assessment findings are normal or expected and do not require follow-up.

Clinical Judgment Cognitive Skill: Recognize Cues

Reference: Ignatavicius et al., 2021, Chapter 35 & 59

8-B.

Answers:

Assessment Finding	Heart Failure	HHS	UTI
Confusion and lethargy	X	X	X
States she is thirsty		X	
Temperature = 101°F (38.3°C)			X
Fine crackles bilaterally in lung bases	X		
FSBG = 450 mg/dL (25 mmol/L)		X	
2+ edema bilaterally in the feet and ankles	X		
Weight loss		X	
Neck vein distention	X		

Rationales: Heart failure is the inability of the heart to maintain adequate cardiac output to meet the metabolic needs of the body. Therefore, it works harder to pump blood through the body. Because of this workload on the heart, the client has feet and ankle edema, neck vein distention, and fine crackles. The client is probably hypoxic which can cause confusion, particularly in older adults. All of these health problems can cause lethargy. Manifestations of HHS include altered central nervous system function with neurological symptoms such as confusion and lethargy, fever higher than 100.4°F (38°C), and weight loss. Thirst and dry skin with decreased turgor occurs because of the dehydration state that develops. Fever, confusion, and lethargy, particularly in an older person, are characteristics of a UTI.

Clinical Judgment Cognitive Skill: Analyze Cues

Reference: Ignatavicius et al., 2021, Chapter 59

8-C.

Answers: B, C, D, E, F, H

Rationales: Although weight loss is a concern and needs to be addressed, it is not a primary and immediate concern because it may be due to dehydration. Lung sounds reveal fine crackles bilaterally and are a priority because the client has a history of heart failure. Bilateral edema in her feet and ankles and neck vein distention can be an indication of worsening heart failure. Dehydration is a concern and needs to be treated to restore circulating blood volume and protect against cerebral, coronary, and renal hypoperfusion. The urinary tract infection is a primary concern because of the risk of urosepsis so treatment needs to be initiated. Fever may be due to UTI and/or HHS. A concern of treatment for HHS (causing hyperglycemia) is cerebral edema and increased intracranial pressure. If the blood glucose falls too far too fast before the brain has time to equilibrate, water is pulled from the blood to the cerebrospinal fluid and brain, causing cerebral edema and increased intracranial pressure.

Clinical Judgment Cognitive Skill: Prioritize Hypottheses

Reference: Ignatavicius et al., 2021, Chapter 59

8-D.

Answers:

Nursing Action	Indicated	Contraindicated	Non-Essential
Monitor intake and output carefully.	X		
Maintain continuous bedrest.			X
Maintain the client in a flat position.		X	
Place the client on a continuous cardiac monitor.	X		
Monitor vital signs frequently.	X		
Perform frequent FSBGs.	X		
Limit fluids to 240 mL every 8 hours.		X	
Send urine for urinalysis daily.			X
Monitor lung sounds every shift.	X		

Rationales: Intake and output measurements need to be performed for the client with heart failure and HHS to ensure fluid balance and to monitor for impending fluid overload. Continuous bedrest is nonessential although safety precautions need to be implemented because the client is weak and needs assistance with ambulating. A flat position is contraindicated because this will place stress on the heart and make it difficult for the client to breathe. A continuous cardiac monitor should be attached to the client because the client has heart failure and will receive treatment for HHS. Treatment for HHS affects electrolytes, specifically the potassium level, and altered potassium levels can cause cardiac irritability and dysrhythmias. Vital signs need to be monitored because of the treatment instituted for the heart failure and HHS; they also provide an indication of client tolerance to treatment. FSBG measurements are necessary because of HHS and to monitor response to treatment. Limiting fluids is contraindicated and can be harmful. A follow-up urinalysis may be done to check for resolution of the UTI but daily urinalysis is nonessential. Lung sounds need to be monitored because of the heart failure and will provide an indication of fluid overload and worsening of the heart failure.

Clinical Judgment Cognitive Skill: Generate Solutions

Reference: Ignatavicius et al., 2021, Chapter 59

8-E.

Answers:

The *immediate* action that the nurse would take is to **elevate the head of the bed to 30 to 40 degrees** to **decrease intracranial pressure** followed by **checking the blood glucose level** to **determine the change in status**.

Rationales: A concern of treatment for HHS is cerebral edema and increased intracranial pressure. If the blood glucose falls too far too fast before the brain has time to equilibrate, water is pulled from the blood to the cerebrospinal fluid and brain, causing cerebral edema and increased intracranial pressure. Neurological changes such as confusion and lethargy, headache and nausea, a rise in blood pressure with a widened pulse pressure are manifestations of this complication. Therefore, the nurse would first elevate the head of the bed to 30 to 40 degrees to decrease intracranial pressure and then check the blood glucose level to determine the change in status. Following this and additional necessary assessments, the nurse would contact the physician. There is no useful reason to stop the infusion of ciprofloxacin. Increasing the IV flow of normal saline could worsen the condition. An antiemetic may be needed but would not be an immediate action.

Clinical Judgment Cognitive Skill: Take Action

Reference: Ignatavicius et al., 2021, Chapter 59

8-F.

Answers:

Assessment Finding	Effective	Ineffective	Unrelated
BP = 140/70 mm Hg	X		
FSBG = 275 mg/dL (15.3 mmol/L)	X		
Urine output = 20 mL/hr		X	
Sodium = 145 mg/dL (145 mmol/L)	X		
Potassium = 5.5 mEq/L (5.5 mmol/L)		X	
Blood osmolarity = 350 mOsm/kg (0.28 mmol/kg)	X		
Oxygen saturation = 92%			X
Fine crackles noted bilaterally in the lungs			X
2+ edema bilaterally in feet and ankles			X

Rationales: Although not within the normal range, the client's blood pressure has decreased. The blood glucose level 275 mg/dL (15.3 mmol/L) is decreasing. The sodium level is at the high end of normal. The blood osmolarity has returned to an acceptable value. These are all indications that the treatment is effective. A urine output of 20 mL/hr is not a normally acceptable standard and treatment for HHS should lead to a higher urine output. The potassium level of 5.5 mEq/L (5.5 mmol/L) indicates hyperkalemia; with treatment for HHS, the potassium level is expected to decrease. Although the pulse oximetry is normal, it is an unrelated finding. Fine crackles, edema and neck vein distension are abnormal findings but are unrelated to the treatment for HHS.

Clinical Judgment Cognitive Skill: Evaluate Outcomes

Reference: Ignatavicius et al., 2021, Chapter 59

NGN Unfolding Case Study #9: Peptic Ulcer Disease (Concepts of Infection and Fluid and Electrolyte Balance)

9-A.

Answers:

Client Finding	Client Finding that Requires Immediate Follow-Up
Has some difficulty swallowing and feels full after meals	
Abdomen is soft and tender on palpation with no guarding	
Stools are black and tarry	
Skin color is pale	
History of coronary artery disease	X
Drinks alcohol on the weekends	
Has lost weight	
Takes aspirin daily	X
B/P = 98/60 mm Hg	X
Vomited red blood this morning	X

Rationales: A client with coronary artery disease could be more susceptible to the adverse effects of anemia and may need to be have a higher hemoglobin level maintained than a client without this health problem. The use of aspirin or other NSAIDs predispose to peptic ulcer disease; this requires immediate follow-up so that the possible cause of the bleeding can be considered. The presence of abdominal pain, especially if severe and associated with rebound tenderness or involuntary guarding, raises concern for perforation. Although this client has a tender abdomen, there is no guarding. The client's temperature and respiration rate are normal and are not of concern at this time. However, the apical heart rate 96 beats/min, indicating tachycardia, the BP is lower than normal at 98/60 mm Hg, and the oxygen saturation is low at 89%; these findings indicate blood loss. Having some difficulty swallowing and feeling full after meals, constipation and black and tarry stools, and weight loss are expected manifestations of an upper GI bleed. A pale appearance is expected with anemia and although this needs to be addressed, it does not require immediate follow-up. The fact that the client states he drinks alcohol on weekends will also need to be addressed but it is not an immediate concern.

Clinical Judgment Cognitive Skill: Recognize Cues

Reference: Ignatavicius et al., 2021, Chapter 50

9-B.

Answers:

Assessment Finding	Peptic Ulcer Disease	GI Bleeding	Coronary Artery Disease
Heartburn or a gnawing or burning feeling	X		
Abdominal pain = 3/10	X		
Black and tarry stool		X	
Skin color is pale		X	X
Feeling tired		X	X
Apical heart rate = 96 beats/min		X	
Blood pressure (BP) = 98/60 mm Hg		X	
Oxygen saturation = 89%		X	

Rationales: The client with a peptic ulcer will experience epigastric pain after meals and will describe it as heartburn or a gnawing or burning feeling. The client will also report some difficulty swallowing and feeling full after eating. Abdominal tenderness and pain are another manifestation of peptic ulcer. In GI bleeding, manifestations such as vomiting red blood and black and tarry stools are obvious signs. As blood loss progresses, the client will exhibit signs of anemia such as feeling tired and a pale appearance. In addition, vital sign changes will occur and the client will experience tachycardia, hypotension, and a decreased oxygen saturation as blood is lost. In CAD, the client is likely to experience feelings of tiredness and exhibit a pale appearance. This is likely due to the pathophysiological disease process and side effects of the medication.

Clinical Judgment Cognitive Skill: Analyze Cues

Reference: Ignatavicius et al., 2021, Chapter 50

9-C.

Answers: A, D

Rationales: GI bleeding is a major concern because it is an active client problem (the client vomited blood) which is causing hypovolemia as evidenced by hypotension and tachycardia. Anemia is present because of GI bleeding. Epigastric pain is manageable at 3/10 and he is prone to constipation. Neither of these findings is a priority concern for the nurse at this time. Dysphagia and weight loss are problems that will need to be addressed but can be at a later time because they do not present an immediate threat to the client.

Clinical Judgment Cognitive Skill: Prioritize Hypotheses

Reference: Ignatavicius et al., 2021, Ch. 50

9-D.

Answers:

Provider Order	Anticipated	Contraindicated	Non-Essential
Insertion of a nasogastric tube			X
Preparation for endoscopy	X		
Cardiologist consult	X		
Administration of a proton pump inhibitor and prokinetic agent	X		
Administration of a blood transfusion			X
Administration of IV morphine		X	
Administration of IV ondansetron			X

Rationales: Endoscopy is a diagnostic test to determine the cause of the upper GI bleeding. The gastroenterologist will be able to locate and identify the bleeding lesion and once it has been identified, therapeutic endoscopy can be performed to achieve hemostasis and prevent recurrent bleeding. The goal of using a prokinetic agent is to improve gastric visualization at the time of endoscopy by clearing the stomach of blood, clots, and food residue and the proton pump inhibitor will decrease acid production to assist in visualization. A cardiologist consultation is anticipated because the client has coronary disease and cardiac medication changes may be necessary. Insertion of a nasogastric tube with lavage may be done in some client situations but is not an essential prescription since the client is not vomiting blood consistently. Usually the goal is to maintain hemoglobin at a level of ≥9 g/dL (90 g/L) even for clients with CAD, so at this time a blood transfusion in nonessential. Ondansetron is an antiemetic and its administration is not essential since the client is not currently experiencing any further nausea or vomiting. The administration of IV morphine sulfate would be contraindicated because IV sedating medications would be given prior to endoscopy.

Clinical Judgment Cognitive Skill: Generate Solutions

Reference: Ignatavicius et al., 2021, Chapter 50

9-E.

Answers:

The *priority* action that the nurse would take is **check vital signs** to **determine any changes** followed by **administering a proton pump inhibitor and prokinetic agent** to **improve stomach visualization and to suppress acid secretion.**

Rationales: Vital signs are always checked as a priority before a diagnostic procedure to obtain a baseline. These are also checked before administering medications to ensure that the medication is safe to administer. The nurse would next administer a proton pump inhibitor and prokinetic agent to improve stomach visualization for the endoscopy and to suppress acid secretion. A cardiologist consult is needed but since the client's cardiac status is stable the consult is not necessarily needed for approval but rather for adjustments in the cardiac medication regimen. There is no reason to administer ondansetron. Ondansetron is an antiemetic and the client is not currently experiencing any further nausea or vomiting.

Clinical Judgment Cognitive Skill: Take Action

Reference: Ignatavicius et al., 2021, Chapter 50

9-F.

Answers:

Client Statement	Understood	Requires Further Teaching
"I will cut my daily aspirin dose in half."		X
"It may be a good idea to eat some foods with probiotics such as yogurt."	X	
"I can continue to drink alcohol as long as it is only on the weekends."		X
"I should avoid any foods that contain vitamin C."		X
"I may have to take some more medications if my biopsies are positive for infection."	X	
"It is a good thing that I stopped smoking a while back because smoking can increase the acid in my stomach."	X	
"I can't skip any doses of my prescribed medications because they are needed to protect my stomach and help my ulcer heal."	X	
"I may have another black and tarry bowel movement next time I go but if I continue to see these kind of bowel movements or see any blood, I need to notify my doctor."	X	
"If I should feel lightheaded, dizzy, and weak, it is probably from the new medication and I don't need to worry about that."		X

Rationales: Probiotics may be helpful to promote the growth of "good" bacteria in the GI tract. Some helpful foods include yogurt and aged cheese. If the stomach biopsies done during endoscopy show *Helicobacter pylori* infection, the client may need to take a combination of antibiotics to kill the bacteria. Smoking also increases stomach acid and can alter the protective lining of the stomach, making it more susceptible to the development of an ulcer. Medications must be taken as prescribed or the risk of developing an ulcer or reoccurrence of an ulcer exists. Usually a proton pump inhibitor, a histamine (H2) blocker, and a cytoprotective agent are prescribed. The client may have residual stool that may need to be passed and it may be black and tarry, but if the client continues to have these type of bowel movements or sees blood, the physician needs to be notified because this could indicate further GI bleeding. The client should not take aspirin because this is very irritating to the stomach lining and can cause bleeding. Alcohol needs to be limited or avoided and the client needs to consult with the physician on restrictions. There is no healthy reason to avoid vitamin C. Not eating vitamin C will delay healing. If the client feels lightheaded, dizzy, and weak, it could be an indication of bleeding and resultant anemia and this warrants primary health care notification.

Clinical Judgment Cognitive Skill: Evaluate Outcomes

Reference: Ignatavicius et al., 2021, Chapter 50

NGN Unfolding Case Study #10: Bowel Obstruction (Concepts of Elimination and Fluid and Electrolyte Balance)

10-A.

Answers:

Nursing assessment findings include:

- Vital signs: temperature = 99.2°F (37.3°C), apical heart rate = 90 beats/min and irregular with an occasional skipped beat, respirations = 24 beats/min blood pressure (BP) = 168/90 mm Hg, oxygen saturation = 93% (on RA), abdominal pain level = 5/10 on a 0 to 10 pain intensity scale
- Reports loss of appetite, vomiting, constipation with diarrhea containing blood streaks, abdominal distention and tenderness; mass in mid-abdomen palpated, bowel sounds are high-pitched tinkling sounds; last bowel movement was during the night; weight is 145 lb (65.8 kg); reports a loss of 10 lb (4.5 kg) in the last month
- Breath sounds are clear bilaterally and client denies dyspnea or chest pain
- Skin is intact, dry, with poor turgor; sore white patches on mucous membranes in the mouth
- Reports urine output has decreased over the past week; denies burning or difficulty

- Moves all extremities and is able to ambulate independently; reports general fatigue and weakness
- Alert and oriented, coherent and responds appropriately; denies forgetfulness or memory loss; reports numbness and tingling in the ankles and feet bilaterally

Rationales: The client has major GI signs and symptoms, including moderate abdominal pain, vomiting, bloody stool, abdominal distention, and abnormal bowel sounds. He also has a palpable mass in the middle of his abdomen. All of these findings indicate the presence of a major GI problem. In addition, the client has findings consistent with dehydration likely resulting from diarrhea and vomiting. These findings include dry skin with poor turgor, a loss of body weight (likely water weight), rapid pulse, and decreased kidney function.

Clinical Judgment Cognitive Skill: Recognize Cues

Reference: Ignatavicius et al., 2021, Chapter 51

10-B.

Answers:

Assessment Finding	Bowel Obstruction	Chemotherapy
Sore white patches on mucous membranes of the mouth		X
Abdominal pain of 5/10 on a 0 to 10 pain intensity scale	X	
Loss of appetite and weight loss	X	X
Numbness and tingling in the ankles and feet bilaterally		X
High-pitched tinkling bowel sounds	X	
Apical heart rate = 90 beats/min	X	
BP = 168/90 mm Hg	X	

Rationales: The side effects and adverse effects of chemotherapy result from the effects of antineoplastic medication on normal cells. Side and adverse effects include mucositis, anorexia, nausea, vomiting, diarrhea, neutropenia, thrombocytopenia, and neuropathy. Sore white mouth sores can indicate a fungal infection from neutropenia. Abdominal pain and loss of appetite are manifestations of a bowel obstruction. Abdominal pain occurs as a result of blockage and the obstruction compressing the nerves in the area. High-pitched tinkling sounds are characteristic depending on the type and location of the obstruction. Because of the pain, the nurse would expect to note that the apical heart rate would be elevated as well as blood pressure.

<u>Clinical Judgment Cognitive Skill:</u> Analyze Cues

<u>Reference:</u> Ignatavicius et al., 2021, Chapter 51

10-C.

<u>Answers:</u> A, B, H

<u>Rationales:</u> Pain is a priority immediate concern because it causes physical distress in the client and needs to be addressed. It is also indicative of the bowel obstruction. Dehydration and electrolyte imbalances are also a priority and evidenced by physical assessment findings and the levels of BUN, creatinine, sodium, and potassium. BUN, creatinine, and sodium levels are elevated and indicative of fluid volume deficit. The potassium level is low indicating an electrolyte imbalance. Other signs of dehydration that the client exhibits are the elevated heart rate, decreased urine output, and dry skin with poor skin turgor. These manifestations should return to normal once the dehydration and electrolyte imbalances are treated. Normally the BP is low in dehydration; however, pain has an effect on the BP and will increase it. The BP reading is not a primary immediate concern at this time and will likely stabilize once the pain is controlled and once the dehydration and electrolyte imbalances are corrected, kidney function values should return to normal. The ECG finding is not a concern because it shows occasional PVCs which are not harmful. Intestinal perforation is a complication of bowel obstruction. This is not a primary immediate concern at this time because the client is not exhibiting signs of perforation and because diagnostic testing shows that the obstruction is a partial one.

<u>Clinical Judgment Cognitive Skill:</u> Prioritize Hypotheses

<u>Reference:</u> Ignatavicius et al., 2021, Chapter 51

10-D.

<u>Answers:</u>

Nursing Action	Anticipated	Contraindicated	Non-Essential
Sips of clear liquids only		X	
Administration of a laxative		X	
Bowel rest	X		
IV potassium replacement	X		
Vital signs every 30 minutes			X
Prepare for surgery	X		
Antibiotic administration	X		
Insertion of a nasogastric tube	X		
Increase the IV flow rate to 100 mL/hr	X		

<u>Rationales:</u> To treat a bowel obstruction, the client is placed on an NPO status and not allowed any food or fluid. This allows the bowel to rest. A nasogastric tube is inserted to remove excess gas from the stomach. In some cases, a partial bowel obstruction is treated conservatively and surgical intervention is unnecessary because the obstruction may resolve on its own. However, since this client's obstruction is due to tumor, surgery will be necessary. Administration of a laxative is contraindicated because of the NPO status and the obstruction, and could also further alter fluid and electrolyte balance. Fluid and electrolyte replacement are necessary to correct the imbalances. Thus, the IV flow rate would be increased and potassium would be administered by the IV route. Vital sign monitoring is important but it is not essential to measure the vital signs every 30 minutes unless a change warrants doing so.

<u>Clinical Judgment Cognitive Skill:</u> Generate Solutions

<u>Reference:</u> Ignatavicius et al., 2021, Chapter 51

10-E.

Answers:

The nurse is prioritizing actions. The nurse would first **increase the flow rate of the IV to 100 mL/hr and administer IV potassium**, and then would **insert a nasogastric tube** followed by **preparing the client for surgery**.

Rationales: The nurse would first address the fluid deficit and the electrolyte imbalance that the client is experiencing and would increase the flow rate of the IV to 100 mL/hr and administer IV potassium. This is an important first action because a fluid deficit can affect fluid volume in the body and lead to hypovolemia, affecting all body tissues. Likewise, a potassium imbalance affects all body tissues and their function, and can cause cardiac irritability resulting in dysrhythmias. The nurse would next insert the nasogastric tube to remove excess gas from the stomach and possibly provide some pain relief for the client. The nurse would then prepare the client for surgical intervention.

Clinical Judgment Cognitive Skill: Take Action

Reference: Ignatavicius et al., 2021, Chapter 51

10-F.

Answers:

Client Statement	Understood	Requires Further Teaching
"I should eat small amounts of food every day rather than 3 large meals."	X	
"It is okay to take a mild laxative if I don't have a bowel movement in 4 days."		X
"I need to contact my surgeon if I see any oozing of clear yellow drainage coming from my incision or if the incision edges seem to be separating."	X	
"The pain medication that I take may make it difficult to have a bowel movement."	X	
"I would like to plan some walks outside because the weather is so beautiful right now, but I know that I have to limit my activity."		X
"I need to check my temperature every day. If it is ever 101°F (38.3°C) or higher, I need to call my surgeon."	X	

Rationales: The client is instructed to eat small amounts of food several times a day and to avoid eating three large meals. Meals need to be spaced out and the client should add new foods into the diet slowly avoiding foods that may cause gas, loose stools, or diarrhea. It is also important to be sure that protein is consumed daily for healing. The client should not take a laxative without specific advice from the surgeon to do so. A laxative could be harsh on the sensitive intestinal lining and disrupt the suture line. The client needs to contact the surgeon if any oozing of clear yellow drainage is seen coming from the incision or if the incision edges seem to be separating; this is a sign of dehiscence. It is important for the client to know that many pain medications can cause constipation and measures, as approved by the surgeon, should be taken. Some surgeons prescribe the use of stool softeners. Progressive walking is extremely important in the postoperative period to prevent postoperative complications such as thrombus formation. For other activities, the client should consult with the surgeon. Wound infection is a postoperative complication. The client should monitor his or her temperature every day. If the temperature is 101°F (38.3°C) or higher, the client needs to contact the surgeon.

Clinical Judgment Cognitive Skill: Evaluate Outcomes

Reference: Ignatavicius et al., 2021, Chapter 51